124.75

NUTRITION SUPPORT for the CRITICALLY ILL PATIENT

A GUIDE TO PRACTICE

NUTRITION SUPPORT for the CRITICALLY ILL PATIENT

A GUIDE TO PRACTICE

Edited by

GAIL CRESCI

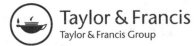

Taylor & Francis
Taylor & Francis Group

Boca Raton   London   New York   Singapore

A CRC title, part of the Taylor & Francis imprint, a member of the
Taylor & Francis Group, the academic division of T&F Informa plc.

Published in 2005 by
CRC Press
Taylor & Francis Group
6000 Broken Sound Parkway NW
Boca Raton, FL 33487-2742

Library of Congress Cataloging-in-Publication Data

Nutrition support for the critically ill patient: a guide to practice / edited by Gail Cresci
    p. cm.
  Includes bibliographical references and index.
  ISBN 0-8493-2153-0 (alk. paper)
  1. Critically ill—Nutrition. 2. Diet therapy.
  [DNLM: 1. Critical Illness—therapy. 2. Nutritional Suppoort. 3. Nutritional Requirements. WB 410 N9751 2005]
I. Cresci, Gail.
RM217.N65 2005
615.8'54—dc22

                                         2004058493

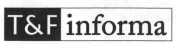

This book is dedicated

*To my parents, who taught me to appreciate
the opportunity to learn.
To my loving husband Tony, who wholeheartedly supports
and encourages my goals and educational endeavors.
To my precious sons, Adrian and Marius, in whom I hope
to instill the value of learning and who I hope
will strive for excellence in all they pursue.
To my teachers and mentors, for all their unconditional
guidance and support.*

*A special dedication to Peter Furst, M.D. (1936–2004).
His commitment to science, education, and nutrition has
greatly influenced the practice of nutrition support as
we know it today.*

Preface

The practice of nutrition support has gone through many changes since its inception in 1968. Because it closely interfaces with medicine, the science of nutrition is very dynamic as it evolves with advances in medical care. This contributes to making nutrition support a very exciting and challenging field in which to practice. In the current medical environment, nutritionists face the many challenges of providing optimal patient care while working within the constraints of managed care. In order to accomplish this, they must not only possess a keen comprehension of nutrition, but also of physiology, pharmacology, research, and health care administration.

No single therapeutic plan is applicable to all patient populations. The critically ill patient is unique from the general hospitalized or long-term care patient receiving nutrition support. Medical intervention, including nutritional therapy, varies significantly among patient acuity levels. There are significant alterations in the physiologic and metabolic pathways in critical illness. These variances, with the potential systemic and organ dysfunctions that may result, affect provision of optimal medical nutritional therapy. The goal of this book is to provide a comprehensive reference on the principles and practice of nutrition support for the critically ill population through evidence-based medicine. The primary target audience for this book is any critical care practitioner, to include physicians, dietitians, pharmacists, nurses, respiratory therapists, and those studying and researching the science of critical care nutrition. This book will also be helpful to those practicing in rehabilitation or long-term care settings, because it will provide insight into the metabolic conditions their patients have undergone while in the acute care setting.

The book has a progressive structure, beginning with an in-depth review of the metabolic alterations that occur during critical illness. Next follows discussion of energy, macronutrient, micronutrient, and fluid and electrolyte requirements, as well as specialized nutrients that can be applied to a general critical care population. This is followed by discussion of the delivery of nutrition support to the critically ill and all the issues and challenges that accompany it. Separate chapters outline the unique nutritional needs and issues that occur throughout the lifecycle. Included are chapters on physiologic and systemic conditions encountered in the intensive care unit, to include trauma, burns, systemic inflammatory response, and sepsis. Next come special considerations for the various disease states and complications that can occur in critically ill patients, including renal, hepatic, and pulmonary disease and pancreatitis. Several professional issues are presented, including ethical considerations, quality improvement, and the economic considerations of nutrition support. Unique features of this book include the extensive list of current references and the inclusion of protocols, tables, figures, and case studies, allowing the reader to apply the science-based information directly to clinical practice.

The chapters have been written by a prominent group of authors, who not only have committed their careers to nutrition support but who also currently practice in the subject area about which they wrote. This allows for insight into the nuances of the practice of nutrition support for the critically ill. It is my goal that this volume be *the* reference book of choice as a practice guide for nutrition support in the critically ill. With the commitment and enthusiasm of the authors and publisher, this vision is a reality.

Gail Cresci, M.S., R.D., C.N.S.D.

Editor

Gail Cresci received her Bachelor of Science degree from the University of Akron in Ohio and her Master of Science degree from Chicago Medical School/Finch University of Health Sciences. Gail completed her dietetic internship at Walter Reed Army Medical Center in Washington, D.C. She then served on active duty in the Army for six years as a registered dietitian, with the final Army rank of Captain. Currently, Gail is an assistant clinical professor and codirector of the Surgical Nutrition Service at the Medical College of Georgia (MCG) in Augusta, Georgia. For more than 11 years, Gail has worked at MCG with the department of surgery, providing nutritional care for the surgical and trauma intensive care unit patients and the surgical subspecialty patients requiring specialized nutrition (gastrointestinal; vascular; oncology; cardiothoracic; ear, nose, and throat; neurosurgery; trauma; orthopedics). Gail plays an integral role in promoting and instituting early enteral nutrition, not only by rounding with the physicians and working closely with the nursing and pharmacy staff, but also by placing small bowel feeding devices at the bedside.

Gail is involved with many nutrition organizations, including the American Society of Parenteral and Enteral Nutrition (ASPEN), where she serves as the membership liaison and reviewer for the publication *Nutrition in Clinical Practice*. She has served on the Dietitians Committee and the Standards Committee. She is also a member of the American Dietetic Association (ADA) and the Dietitians in Nutrition Support (DNS) Practice Group, as well as the Georgia Dietetic Association and Georgia ASPEN.

Gail is involved in clinical research and has presented her research at several national and international conferences. She speaks locally, nationally, and internationally on nutrition support topics. Over the past several years, she has authored more than 12 textbook chapters and numerous peer reviewed journal articles in the area of nutrition support.

Gail enjoys spending time with her husband, twin boys, and two dogs, as well as family and friends. Other personal interests include cooking, running, cycling, reading, and traveling.

Contributors

Christoph Beglinger, M.D.
Professor of Gastroenterology
GI Unit
University Hospital Basel
Basel, Switzerland

Stig Bengmark, M.D., Ph.D.
Senior Professor
Honorary Visiting Professor
University College London (UCL), London
  University
London, United Kingdom

Suzanne Benjamin, R.Ph., B.C.N.S.P.
Clinical Pharmacist
Nutrition Support Service
Indiana University Hospital
Indianapolis, Indiana

Jatinder Bhatia, M.B.B.S. (corresponding author)
Professor and Chief
Section of Neonatology
Vice-Chair for Clinical Research
Department of Pediatrics
Medical College of Georgia
Augusta, Georgia

Patricia J. Bishop, M.S.N., R.N.
Ursuline College
Breen School of Nursing
Cleveland, Ohio

Beverley Borjas, R.D.
The University Hospital, Cincinnati
Cincinnati, Ohio

Rex O. Brown, Pharm.D., F.C.C.P., B.C.N.S.P.
Professor and Executive Vice-Chair
Department of Pharmacy
University of Tennessee Health Science
  Center
Nutrition Support Pharmacist
Regional Medical Center at
  Memphis/University of Tennessee Bowld
  Hospital
Memphis, Tennessee

Alice E. Buchanan, M.S., R.D.
Clinical Dietitian
Vanderbilt Center for Human Nutrition
Nashville, Tennessee

Ayaz J. Chaudhary, M.D., F.A.C.P., F.A.C.G.
Assistant Professor of Medicine
Director of Endoscopy
Division of Gastroenterology and Hepatology
Department of Internal Medicine
Medical College of Georgia
Augusta, Georgia

Srinath Chinnakotla, M.D.
Transplant Surgeon
Baylor Institute of Transplantation Sciences
Waco, Texas

Michael L. Christensen, Pharm.D.
Professor
Pediatric Research Unit
Departments of Pharmacy and Pediatrics
University of Tennessee Health Science Center
  and LeBonheur Children's Medical Center
Memphis, Tennessee

Katherine Connor, R.D.
St. Joseph's Hospital and Medical Center
Phoenix, Arizona

Maria Isabel Toulson Davisson Correia, M.D., Ph.D.
Professor of Surgery
Alfa Institute of Gastroenterology
Federal University of Minas Gerais
Belo Horizonte, Brazil

Gail Cresci, M.S., R.D., C.N.S.D.
Assistant Clinical Professor
Medical College of Georgia
Augusta, Georgia

Jorge I. Cué, M.D., F.A.C.S.
Associate Professor of Surgery
Surgical Director
Surgical Intensive Care Unit
Medical College of Georgia
Augusta, Georgia

Nicole M. Daignault, R.D., L.D., C.N.S.D.
Nutrition and Metabolic Support Service
Emory University Hospital
Atlanta, Georgia

Frank Davis M.D., F.A.C.S.
Associate Professor of Surgery
Memorial Health University Medical Center
Savannah, Georgia

Carolina Trancoso de Almeida
General Surgeon
Trauma Center Hospital João XXIII
ATLS, PHTLS, and ACLS Instructor
Belo Horizonte, Brazil

Letícia De Nardi, R.D.
Dietitian, Food Technician
Laboratory of Metabology and Nutrition in
 Surgery
Gastroenterology Department
University of São Paulo Medical School
São Paulo, Brazil

Concepcion Fernandez Estivariz, M.D.
Emory University School of Medicine
Atlanta, Georgia

David Frankenfield, M.S., R.D., C.N.S.D.
Chief Clinical Dietitian, Nutrition Support
 Specialist
Penn State's Milton S. Hershey Medical Center
Hershey, Pennsylvania

Vanessa Fuchs, M.Sc., R.D.
Mexico's General Hospital
American British Cowdray Medical Center
Mexico City, Mexico

M. Patricia Fuhrman, M.S., R.D., L.D., F.A.D.A., C.N.S.D.
Area Clinical Nutrition Marketing Director
Coram Healthcare
St. Louis, Missouri

Peter Fürst, M.D., Ph.D.
Institute of Nutrition Science
University of Bonn
Bonn, Germany

Michele M. Gottschlich, Ph.D., R.D.
Director
Nutrition Services
Shriners Hospital for Children
Cincinnati, Ohio

Daniel P. Griffith, R.Ph., B.C.N.S.P.
Clinical Coordinator
Nutrition and Metabolic Support Service
Program Director
Nutrition Support Residency
Department of Pharmacy
Emory University Hospital
Atlanta, Georgia

Naren Gupta, M.D.
Resident
Department of Surgery
Medical College of Georgia
Augusta, Georgia

Jeanette Hasse, Ph.D., R.D., L.D., F.A.D.A., C.N.S.D.
Transplant Nutrition Specialist
Baylor Institute of Transplantation Sciences
Waco, Texas

A. Christine Hummell, M.S., R.D., C.N.S.D., L.D.
The Cleveland Clinic Foundation
Critical Care Dietitian
Cleveland, Ohio

Gordon L. Jensen, M.D., Ph.D.
Director and Professor of Medicine
Vanderbilt Center for Human Nutrition
Nashville, Tennessee

L. Lee Jimenez, R.D., C.N.S.D.
Sodexho Food Services
North Potomac, Maryland

Troy F. Kimsey, M.D.
Department of Surgery
Medical College of Georgia
Augusta, Georgia

Lori Kowalski, M.S., R.D., L.D.N., C.N.S.D.
Clinical Dietitian
Children's Hospital of Pittsburgh
Pittsburgh, Pennsylvania

Rosemary A. Kozar, M.D., Ph.D.
Department of Surgery
University of Texas — Houston Medical School
Houston, Texas

Joseph Krenitsky M.S., R.D.
Nutrition Support Specialist
University of Virginia Health System
Digestive Health Center of Excellence
Charlottesville, Virginia

Kenneth A. Kudsk, M.D., F.A.C.S.
Professor of Surgery
Vice-Chairman of Surgical Research
University of Wisconsin — Madison
Madison, Wisconsin

Carolyn Kusenda M.S., R.D., C.N.S.D.
Nutrition Support Specialist
University of Virginia Health System
Charlottesville, Virginia

Jonathan P. Kushner, M.D., F.A.C.P., C.N.S.P.
Assistant Professor of Medicine
Division of Digestive Diseases
The University Hospital, Cincinnati
Cincinnati, Ohio

Joseph Lacy, R.D.
Clinical Dietitian
The University Hospital, Cincinnati
Cincinnati, Ohio

Rebecca Lee, R.N.
Nutrition Support Nurse
The University Hospital, Cincinnati
Cincinnati, Ohio

Jennifer Lefton, R.D., L.D./N., C.N.S.D.
Clinical Dietitian II
Jackson Health System
Miami, Florida

Joanna Lipp, M.S., R.D., C.N.S.D., C.D.E.
Clinical Nutrition Specialist
Nutrition Support Service
University of Rochester
Rochester, New York

Peter P. Lopez, M.D., C.N.S.P.
Assistant Professor of Surgery
DeWitt Daughtry Family Department of
  Surgery
University of Miami School of Medicine
Miami, Florida

Maria R. Lucarelli, M.D.
Fellow
Division of Pulmonary/Critical Care
  Medicine
Department of Internal Medicine
The Ohio State University Medical Center
Columbus, Ohio

Ainsley M. Malone, M.S., R.D.
Mount Carmel West Hospital
Columbus, Ohio

Mary Marian, M.S., R.D.
Clinical Nutrition Research Specialist and
　Clinical Lecturer
University of Arizona, College of Medicine
Tucson, Arizona

Robert G. Martindale, M.D., Ph.D.
Professor of Surgery
Chief, Gastrointestinal Surgery Section
Medical College of Georgia
Augusta, Georgia

Theresa Mayes, R.D.
Clinical Dietitian
Shriners Hospital for Children
Cincinnati, Ohio

John E. Mazuski, M.D., Ph.D., F.C.C.M.
Associate Professor
Department of Surgery
Barnes-Jewish Hospital, Trauma, Surgery,
　Critical Care Division
Washington University Medical School
St. Louis, Missouri

**Mary S. McCarthy, Ph.(C.), R.N.,
C.N.S.N.**
Nursing Research Service
Madigan Army Medical Center
Tacoma, Washington

Tom Stone McNees, M.S., R.D., C.N.S.D.
Nutrition Support Dietitian
Neuroscience — Critical Care Cluster
Clarian Nutrition Support/Methodist
　Hospital
Indianapolis, Indiana

**Margaret M. McQuiggan, M.S., R.D.,
C.S.M.**
Shock Trauma Intensive Care Unit
Memorial Hermann Hospital
Houston, Texas

Rémy Meier, M.D., Ph.D.
Head
GI Department
Kantonsspital Liestal
Liestal, Switzerland

**Jay M. Mirtallo, M.S., R.Ph., B.C.N.S.P.,
F.A.S.H.P.**
Specialty Practice Pharmacist, Nutrition
　Support/Surgery
Department of Pharmacy
The Ohio State University Medical Center
Clinical Associate Professor of Pharmacy
College of Pharmacy
The Ohio State University
Columbus, Ohio

Frederick A. Moore, M.D.
Department of Surgery
University of Texas — Houston Medical School
Houston, Texas

Sandor Nagy, M.D.
Fellow
Neonatal Perinatal Medicine
Department of Pediatrics, Section of
　Neonatology
Medical College of Georgia
Augusta, Georgia

Anita Nucci, Ph.D., R.D., L.D.N.
Manager
Clinical Nutrition/Nutrition Support and
　Intestinal Care Center
Children's Hospital of Pittsburgh
Pittsburgh, Pennsylvania

Mark H. Oltermann, M.D., C.N.S.P.
Assistant Professor
Department of Internal Medicine
Texas Tech Medical Center — Amarillo
Amarillo, Texas

Carol Rees Parrish, R.D., M.S.
Nutrition Support Specialist
University of Virginia Health System
Digestive Health Center of Excellence
Charlottesville, Virginia

Lindsay J. Pell, Pharm.D.
Specialty Practice Pharmacist
Critical Care/Rehabilitation
Department of Pharmacy
The Ohio State University Medical Center
Columbus, Ohio

Marie-Andrée Roy, M.Sc.
Research Assistant
Vanderbilt Center for Human Nutrition
Nashville, Tennessee

Mary Krystofiak Russell, M.S., R.D., L.D.N., C.N.S.D.
Director of Nutrition Services
Duke University Hospital
Durham, North Carolina

Jose L. Sandoval
Mexico's National Institute of Respiratory
   Diseases
Mexico City, Mexico

Harry C. Sax, M.D., F.A.C.S.
Professor of Surgery
Department of Surgery
University of Rochester School of Medicine
   and Dentistry
Rochester, New York

Hank Schmidt, M.D., Ph.D.
Resident
Department of Surgery
Medical College of Georgia
Augusta, Georgia

Teresa R. Schmidt, R.D., L.D.
Pharmaceuticals Sales Specialist — Oncology
AstraZeneca
Victoria, Minnesota

Elizabeth B. Sedlak, M.S.N., R.N.
Coordinator
ALL ABOUT WOMEN
Bedford Medical Center
Bedford, Ohio

Mary Beth Shirk, Pharm.D.
Specialty Practice Pharmacist, Critical Care
Department of Pharmacy
The Ohio State University Medical Center
Columbus, Ohio

Krishnan Sriram, M.D., F.A.C.S., F.R.C.S.(C.)
Director, Surgical Critical Care
Department of Surgery
John H. Stroger Jr. Hospital of Cook County
Chicago, Illinois

Elaina E. Szeszycki, Pharm.D., B.C.N.S.P.
Staff Pharmacist
CVS Pharmacy
Pharmacist
Coram Healthcare
Indianapolis, Indiana

Beth Taylor, M.S., R.D., C.N.S.D., F.C.C.M.
Clinical Dietitian Specialist
Barnes-Jewish Hospital
St. Louis, Missouri

Raquel S. Torrinhas, R.B., M.S.
Biologist Chief
Laboratory of Metabology and Nutrition in
   Surgery
University of São Paulo Medical School
Department of Gastroenterology
São Paulo, Brazil

Dan L. Waitzberg, M.D., Ph.D.
Associate Professor of Gastroenterology
Laboratory of Metabology and Nutrition in
   Surgery
University of São Paulo Medical School
Department of Gastroenterology
São Paulo, Brazil

Adam D. Waller, M.D.
Senior Gastroenterology Fellow
Division of Gastroenterology and Hepatology
Department of Internal Medicine
Medical College of Georgia
Augusta, Georgia

Marion F. Winkler, M.S., R.D., L.D.N., C.N.S.D.
Surgical Nutrition Specialist
Department of Surgery and Nutritional Support
  Service
Rhode Island Hospital
Senior Teaching Associate of Surgery
Brown University School of Medicine
Providence, Rhode Island

Thomas R. Ziegler, M.D.
Associate Professor of Medicine
Director of Emory Center for Clinical and
  Molecular Nutrition
Emory University School of Medicine
Atlanta, Georgia

Table of Contents

Section I

Metabolic Alterations in the
Critically Ill

1 Metabolic Response to Stress

Maria Isabel Toulson Davisson Correia
Federal University of Minas Gerais

Carolina Trancoso de Almeida
Trauma Center Hospital João XXIII

CONTENTS

1.1 INTRODUCTION

The metabolic response to stress was first described in 1942, by Sir David Cuthbertson, who introduced the terms *ebb* and *flow* to describe the phases of hypo- and hypermetabolism that follow traumatic injury. The metabolic response is triggered by multiple stimuli, including arterial and venous pressure and volume, osmolality, pH, arterial oxygen content, pain, anxiety, and toxic mediators from infection and tissue injury (Table 1.1). These stimuli reach the hypothalamus and then stimulate the sympathetic nervous system and the adrenal medulla. Indeed, the metabolic response to stress is a physiological response to an insult that might become pathological, depending on the intensity and duration of injury. Actually, the metabolic response can be seen as the "fight or flight" response to adverse phenomena that can become highly associated with increased morbidity and mortality if perpetuated for long periods. The ultimate goal of the metabolic response is to restore homeostasis. Intermediate goals are to limit further blood loss; to increase blood flow, allowing greater delivery of nutrients and elimination of waste products; to debride necrotic tissue; and to initiate wound healing.

TABLE 1.1
Metabolic Response to Stress — Triggering Factors

Arterial and venous pressure
Volume
Osmolality
pH
Arterial oxygen content
Pain
  Anxiety
  Toxic mediators
  Infection
  Tissue injury

With the development of medical science, the once seemingly simple metabolic response to stress (represented by the ebb and flow phases) has evolved into a complicated and intricate web of responses that enroll several body compartments. Although one cannot fully go against the development of the metabolic response to stress, recognizing its magnitude and knowing its different particularities might help to minimize the risks of perpetuating its duration. Thus, the reduction of morbidity and mortality related to metabolic stress might be ensured. Indeed, mortality from prolonged critical illness is high: almost three out of ten adult patients with an intensive-care stay of more than three weeks do not survive.[1] Despite the fact that modern surgery has become less aggressive with the so-called minimal approach procedures, trauma has greatly increased due to urban violence and wars. Thus, it is extremely important to be acquainted with the complex mechanisms of the stress response (Figure 1.1) in order to act early and perhaps prevent some of its deleterious effects. The magnitude of the response and adequate initial approach are determinant factors that might influence the patient's outcome. The severity of hypermetabolic phenomena thereafter might lead to the systemic inflammatory response syndrome (SIRS), the amplified generalized body response.

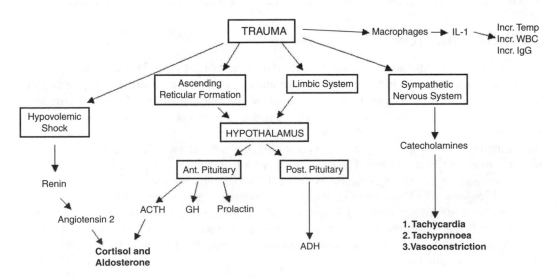

FIGURE 1.1 Metabolic response to stress.

TABLE 1.2
Contributors to Metabolic Stress

The Stress Response Is Related To:

Magnitude (severity)
Duration (the longer the more severe)
Nutritional status of the patient (malnourished patients do worse)
Associated diseases (increase morbidity and mortality)
    Diabetes
    Heart disease
    Pulmonary
    Immunologic
    Others

1.2 STRESS

Stress is a term applied in the fields of physiology and neuroendocrinology to refer to those forces or factors that cause disequilibrium to an organism and therefore threaten homeostasis.[2] The stressors might be a consequence of physical injury, mechanical disruption, chemical changes, or emotional factors. The body's response to these factors will depend on their magnitude, the duration of the events, and the nutritional status of the patient (Table 1.2). Complex sensory systems trigger reflex nervous system responses to the stressors that alert the central nervous system (CNS) of the disturbance. In the CNS, neurons of the paraventricular nucleus of the hypothalamus elaborate corticotropin-releasing hormone (CRH) and activate the hypothalamic–pituitary–adrenal axis (HPA). In addition, other areas of the brain signal the peripheral autonomic nervous system. These last two systems elicit an integrated response, referred to as the *stress response*, which primarily controls bodily functions such as arousal, cardiovascular tone, respiration, and intermediate metabolism.[2] Other functions, such as feeding and sexual behavior, are suppressed, while cognition and emotion are activated. In addition, gastrointestinal activity and immune/inflammatory responses are altered.

1.3 HISTORICAL PERSPECTIVE

Sir David Cuthbertson, a chemical pathologist in Glasgow, was the first physician to study the metabolic response to injury in the early part of the 20th century, by following patients with long bone fractures.[3] Long before Cuthbertson's studies, however, John Hunter, in *Treatise on the Blood, Inflammation and Gunshot Wounds*, was the first to question the paradox of the response to injury: "Impressions are capable of producing or increasing natural actions and are then called *stimuli*, but they are likewise capable of producing too much action, as well as depraved, unnatural, or what we commonly call diseased action."[4] Hunter must have perceived intuitively that nature might have created these responses in order to have some advantages in terms of recovery, but he also noticed that if the responses were exaggerated, then life could be jeopardized.

The concept that illness was associated with an increased excretion of nitrogen leading to negative nitrogen balance was defined in the late 19th century. During the First World War, studies carried out by DuBois showed that an increase in 1°C in temperature was associated with a 13% increase in the metabolic rate.[5]

Cuthbertson's findings were derived from questions asked by orthopedic surgeons who were eager to find out why patients with fractures of the distal third of the tibia were slow to heal. His studies were negative in the sense that he could not offer the exact explanation of the phenomenon, but at the same time he came up with something much more interesting and fundamental. He measured the excretion of calcium, phosphorus, sulfate, and nitrogen in the urine and found that the amount of excreted phosphorous and sulfate in relation to calcium was higher than expected if all these elements had come from the bone.[3] Cuthbertson went on to show that this was a catabolic phenomenon related to breakdown of protein, reflecting an increase in metabolic rate.[3] The association between the systemic metabolic response and hormonal elaboration was soon sought, but this approach was initially hampered by methodological problems. The investigations carried out by Cannon on the autonomic nervous system suggested the increased catecholamine response to illness as one of the explanations of the physiologic responses seen by Cuthbertson.[6] Later, Selye proposed corticosteroids as the main mediators of the protein catabolic response.[7]

But what was the signal that initiated and propagated the immediate elaboration of the adrenal cortical hormones? Hume and Egdahl showed that in injured dogs (operative injury or superficial burn to the limbs) that had intact sciatic nerves or spinal cords, there was an increase of adrenal hormones, contrary to what happened in those animals with transected nerves or spinal cords, in which the response was abated.[8,9] From the investigative setting, it was possible to identify afferent nervous signals as essential components to trigger the HPA stress response.

Allison et al. depicted that the metabolic response was also associated with suppression of insulin release followed by a period of insulin resistance and with high glucagon and growth hormone levels.[10–12] Recently, the metabolic response has been associated not only with neuroendocrine alterations but with the accompaniment of inflammatory responses and mediators plus immunologic dysfunctions.[13,14]

1.4 METABOLIC RESPONSE TO STRESS

1.4.1 THE EBB AND FLOW PHASES

Cuthbertson originally divided the metabolic response into an ebb phase and a flow phase (Figure 1.2 and Table 1.3).[3] The ebb phase begins immediately after injury and typically lasts 12 to 24 hours. However, this phase may last longer, depending on the severity of trauma and the adequacy of resuscitation. The ebb phase we may equate with prolonged and untreated shock, a circumstance that is more often seen in experimental animals than in clinical practice. It is characterized by tissue hypoperfusion and a decrease in overall metabolic activity. In order to compensate for this, catecholamines are discharged, with norepinephrine being the primary mediator of the ebb phase. Norepinephrine is released from peripheral nerves and binds to beta$_1$ receptors in the heart and to alpha and beta$_2$ receptors in peripheral and, to a lesser degree, splanchnic vascular beds. The most important effects are cardiovascular, because norepinephrine is a potent cardiac stimulant, causing increased contractility and heart rate and vasoconstriction. These phenomena attempt to restore blood pressure, increase cardiac performance, and maximize venous return.

Hyperglycemia may be seen during the ebb phase. In patients with trauma, the degree of hyperglycemia parallels the severity of injury. Hyperglycemia is promoted by hepatic glycogenolysis secondary to catecholamine release and by direct sympathetic stimulation of glycogen breakdown.

Some authors have investigated the ebb phase in experimental animals and human beings and have noticed important aspects,. For example, after sustained long fractures with concomitant great loss of blood, there is an impairment of vasoconstriction that is not seen in bleeding events alone, such as that seen in duodenal ulcer bleeding.[15] In another study, Childs showed an effect of injury on impairing thermoregulation in injured subjects and showed reduced vasoconstriction in response to cold stimulus.[16]

The onset of the flow phase, which encompasses the catabolic and anabolic phases, is signaled by high cardiac output with the restoration of oxygen delivery and metabolic substrate. The duration of this phase depends on the severity of injury or the presence of infection and development of complications. It typically peaks at around three to five days, subsides by seven to ten days, and merges into an anabolic phase over the next few weeks. During this hypermetabolic phase, insulin

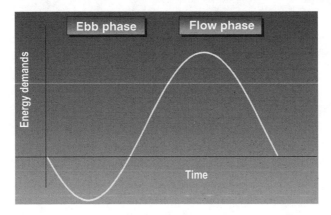

FIGURE 1.2 Metabolic response to stress. (From Cuthbertson et al., *Adv. Clin. Chem.*, 1969. With permission.)

TABLE 1.3
Metabolic Response to Stress

The ebb and flow phases
Glucose and protein metabolism
Fluid and electrolyte response
Endocrine response
    Hypothalamic–pituitary–adrenal axis (HPA)
    Thyrotropic axis
    Somatotropic axis
    Lactotropic axis
    Luteinizing hormone–testosterone axis
Inflammatory response
Immunologic response

---

release is high, but elevated levels of catecholamines, glucagon, and cortisol counteract most of its metabolic effects.

Increased mobilization of amino acids and free fatty acids from peripheral muscles and adipose tissue stores is a result of this hormonal imbalance. Some of these released substrates are used for energy production – either directly as glucose or through the liver as triglyceride. Other substrates contribute to the synthesis of proteins in the liver, where humoral mediators increase production of acute phase reactants. Similar protein synthesis occurs in the immune system for the healing of damaged tissues. Although this hypermetabolic phase involves both catabolic and anabolic processes, the net result is a significant loss of protein, characterized by negative nitrogen balance and decreased fat stores. This leads to an overall modification of body composition, characterized by losses of protein, carbohydrate, and fat stores, accompanied by enlarged extracellular (and, to a lesser extent, intracellular) water compartments.

1.4.2 GLUCOSE AND PROTEIN METABOLISM

During starvation, glucose infusion inhibits hepatic gluconeogenesis, but after injury, despite the high concentration of circulating glucose, gluconeogenesis prevails. The amino acids released from protein catabolism in muscle are largely taken up by the liver for new glucose production, rather than being used as fuel to meet energy demands. The latter are provided by the fat reserve (about 80 to 90%).[17] Why injured patients need such a high rate of endogenous glucose production may

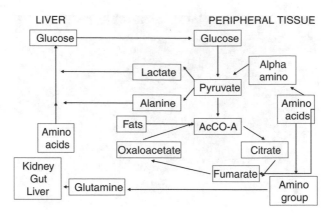

FIGURE 1.3 Aerobic glycolysis and Cori cycles.

be explained by the high demand of injured tissues for glucose. Wilmore et al. showed that patients with severe burns in one leg with minor injury to the other had a fourfold increase of glucose uptake by the burned limb.[18] At the same time, the burned leg produced higher amounts of lactate, suggesting that it respires anaerobically. The lactate is then returned to the liver for gluconeogenesis, in the so-called Cori cycle, which is metabolically expensive. One mol of glucose yields 2 ATP through glycolysis but via gluconeogenesis costs 3 ATP. This may contribute to the underlying increase in the metabolic rate (Figure 1.3).

Insulin has an anabolic or storage effect by synthesizing large molecules from small molecules and inhibiting catabolism. It also promotes glucose oxidation and glycogen synthesis, whereas it inhibits glycogenolysis and gluconeogenesis. On the other hand, the catabolic hormones, such as catecholamines, cortisol, and glucagons, enhance glycogenolysis and gluconeogenesis.

1.4.3 Fluid and Electrolyte Response

Hypovolemia prevails in the ebb phase and is entirely reversible with appropriate fluid administration. However, in the absence of volume resuscitation, within 24 hours, mortality is nearly uniform.[19] The patient's initial response to hypovolemia is targeted to keep adequate perfusion to the brain and the heart in detriment of the skin, fat tissue, muscles, and intraabdominal structures. The oliguria, which follows injury, is a consequence of the release of antidiuretic hormone (ADH) and aldosterone. Secretion of ADH from the supraoptic nuclei in the anterior hypothalamus is stimulated by volume reduction and increased osmolality. The latter is mainly due to an increased sodium content of the extracellular fluid. Francis Moore coined the terms *sodium retention phase* and *sodium diuresis phase* of injury to describe the antidiuresis of both salt and water in the flow phase.[20] Volume receptors are located in the atria and pulmonary arteries, and osmoreceptors are located near ADH neurones in the hypothalamus. ADH acts mainly on the connecting tubules of the kidney but also on the distal tubules to promote reabsorption of water. Aldosterone acts mainly on the distal renal tubules to promote reabsorption of sodium and bicarbonate and increased excretion of potassium and hydrogen ions. Aldosterone also modifies the effects of catecholamines on cells, thus affecting the exchange of sodium and potassium across all cell membranes. The release of large quantities of intracellular potassium into the extracellular fluid is a consequence of protein catabolism and may cause a rise in serum potassium, especially if renal function is impaired. Retention of sodium and bicarbonate may produce metabolic alkalosis with impairment of oxygen delivery the tissues. After injury, urinary sodium excretion may fall to 10 to 25 mmol/24 h and potassium excretion may rise to 100 to 200 mmol/24 h. Intracellular fluid and exogenously administered fluid accumulate preferentially in the extracellular third space because of increased vascular permeability and a relative increase in interstitial oncotic pressure; this is why most patients become so edematous after the first days following injury and resuscitation.

1.4.4 ENDOCRINE RESPONSE

1.4.4.1 Hypothalamic–Pituitary–Adrenal Axis

The hypothalamus secretes corticotropin-releasing hormone (CRH) in response to the stress stimuli. CRH stimulates the production, by the pituitary, of adrenocorticotropic hormone (ACTH), also known as corticotropin, which, as its name implies, stimulates the adrenal cortex. More specifically, it triggers the secretion of glucocorticoids, such as cortisol, and has little control over the secretion of aldosterone, the other major steroid hormone from the adrenal cortex. Corticotropin-releasing hormone itself is inhibited by glucocorticoids, making it part of a classical negative feedback loop (Figure 1.1 and Figure 1.4). It seems that the secretion of aldosterone is most likely under the control of an activated rening-angiotensin system.[21]

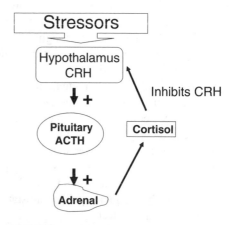

FIGURE 1.4 The hypothalamic–pituitary–adrenal axis (HPA).

Hypercortisolism acutely shifts carbohydrate, fat, and protein metabolism, so that energy is instantly and selectively available to vital organs such as the brain, and anabolism is thus delayed. Intravascular fluid retention and the enhanced inotropic and vasopressor response to catecholamines and angiotensin II offer hemodynamic advantages in the "fight or flight" response. This hypercortisolism can be interpreted as an attempt of the organism to mute its own inflammatory cascade, thus protecting itself against overresponses.[21]

Serum ACTH was found to be low in chronic critical illness while cortisol concentrations remained elevated, suggesting that cortisol release may be driven through alternative pathways, possibly involving endothelin.[22]

1.4.4.2 Thyrotropic Axis

Within two hours after surgery or trauma, serum levels of T3 decrease, whereas T4 and TSH briefly increase. Apparently, low levels of T3 are due to a decreased peripheral conversion of T4. Subsequently, circulating levels of TSH and T4 often return to "normal" levels, whereas T3 levels remain low. It is important to mention that the magnitude of T3 decrease has been found to reflect the severity of illness. Several cytokine mediators, mainly tumor necrosis factor (TNF), interleukin-1 (IL-1), and interleukin-6 (IL-6), have been investigated as putative mediators of the acute low T3 levels. Teleologically, the acute changes in the thyroid axis may reflect an attempt to reduce energy expenditure, as in starvation.[21]

A somewhat different behavior is seen in patients remaining in intensive care units for longer periods. It has been seen that there are low-normal TSH values and low T4 and T3 serum concentrations. This seems to be due to reduced hypothalamic stimulation of the thyrotropes, in turn leading to reduced stimulation of the thyroid gland. Endogenous dopamine and prolonged hypercortisolism may play a role in this phenomenon. When exogenous dopamine and glucocorticoids are given, hypothyroidism is provoked or aggravated in critical illness.[23]

1.4.4.3 Somatotropic Axis

Throughout the first hours or days of an insult — be it surgery, trauma, or infection — circulating levels of growth hormone become elevated and the normal GH profile, consisting of peaks alternating with virtually undetectable troughs, is altered (peak GH and interpulse concentrations are high and the GH pulse frequency is elevated). In physiological situations, GH is released from the pituitary somatotropes in a pulsatile fashion, under the interactive control of the hypothalamic GH-releasing hormone (GHRH), which is stimulatory, and somatostatin, which exerts an inhibitory effect.[21] After stress, it seems that withdrawal of the inhibitory effect of somatostatin and increased availability of stimulatory GH-releasing factors (hypothalamic or peripheral) could hypothetically be involved. It has also been suggested that there seems to be acquired peripheral resistance to GH and that these changes are brought about by the effects of cytokines, such as TNF, IL-1, and IL-6.[21] Growth hormone exerts direct lipolytic, insulin-antagonizing, and immune-stimulating actions; such changes would prioritize essential substrates such as glucose, free fatty acids, and amino acids toward survival rather than anabolism.

In chronic illness, the changes in the somatotropic axis are different. GH secretion is chaotic and reduced, compared with the acute phase. Although the nonpulsatile fraction is still elevated and the number of pulses is high, mean nocturnal GH serum concentrations are scarcely elevated and are substantially lower than in the acute phase of stress. One possibility that explains this situation is that the pituitary is taking part in the "multiple organ failure syndrome," becoming unable to synthesize and secrete GH.[21] Another explanation could be that the lack of pulsatile GH secretion is due to increased somatostatin tone or a reduced stimulation by endogenous releasing factors, such as GHRH.

1.4.4.4 Lactotropic Axis

Prolactin was among the first hormones known to have increased serum concentrations after acute physical or psychological stress.[21] This increase might be mediated by oxytocin, dopaminergic pathways, or vasoactive intestinal peptide (VIP). Cytokines may be the triggering factor. Changes in prolactin secretion in response to stress might contribute to altered immune function during the course of critical illness. In mice, inhibition of prolactin release results in impaired lymphocyte function, depressed lymphokine-dependent macrophage activation, and death from normally non-lethal exposure to bacteria.[24,25] It remains unclear whether hyperprolactinemia contributes to the vital activation of the immune cascade after the onset of critical illness.

In the chronic setting of critical illness, serum prolactin levels are no longer as high as in the acute phase.

1.4.4.5 Luteinizing Hormone–Testosterone Axis

Testosterone is the most important endogenous anabolic steroid hormone. Therefore, changes within the luteinizing hormone–testosterone axis in the male may be relevant for the catabolic state in critical illness, in which there are low testosterone levels. The exact cause is unclear, but cytokines may once again be enrolled in this phenomenon.[23,26] A hypothesis about the low testosterone levels is that it may be important to switch off anabolic androgen secretion in acute stress, in order to conserve energy and metabolic substrates for vital functions.[21]

In chronic states, circulating testosterone levels become extremely low, in fact almost unde-tectable.[21,23] Endogenous dopamine, estrogens, and opiates might be the cause of the low levels.

1.4.5 Inflammatory Response

The inflammatory response is part of the body's phenomena following injury in the attempt to restore homeostasis. In most situations after injury, healing is successful. However, sometimes this is not the case and deviations occur, leading to a perpetuated response that may jeopardize survival. In systemic inflammatory response syndrome (SIRS), inflammation is triggered at sites remote from the site of initial injury. In some cases, SIRS progresses to multiple organ dysfunction syndrome (MODS), which is associated with high mortality rates.

The physiologic response to trauma is a complex cellular and molecular event, in which inflammatory cells, such as polymorphonuclear cells (PMNs), macrophages, and lymphocytes, are

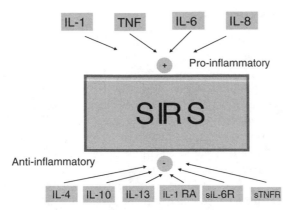

FIGURE 1.5 The inflammatory response.

recruited to the site of injury and secrete inflammatory mediators. The endothelium at the site of injury also participates. PMNs are the first cells to arrive at the site of injury and release potent oxidizing molecules, including hydrogen peroxide, hypochlorous acid, oxygen free radicals, proteolytic enzymes, and vasoactive substances, such as leukotrienes, eicosanoids, and platelet activating factor (PAF). There is evidence that PAF is partially responsible for the increased permeability in sepsis and shock.[27] Oxygen free radicals are proinflammatory molecules causing lipid peroxidation, inactivation of enzymes, and consumption of antioxidants. PMNs release proteolytic enzymes that activate the kinin/kallikrein system, which, in turn, stimulates the release of angiotensin II, bradykinin, and activated plasminogen. Bradykinin causes vasodilation and mediates increased vascular permeability.

Macrophages are activated by cytokines and engulf invading organisms. They also debride necrotic host tissue and elaborate additional cytokines. Tumor necrosis factor alpha (synthesized by macrophages) and IL-1 beta (synthesized by macrophages and endothelial cells) are the proximal proinflammatory mediators (Figure 1.5). These cytokines initiate elaboration and release of other cytokines, such as IL-6. They also stimulate the hepatic acute phase response. IL-6 is secreted by monocytes and macrophages, neutrophils, T and B cells, endothelial cells, smooth muscle cells, fibroblasts, and mast cells. This cytokine is probably the most potent inductor of acute phase response, although its exact role in the inflammatory response remains unclear.[28] On the other hand, it is considered to be the most reliable prognostic indication of outcome, particularly in sepsis, because it reflects the severity of injury.[19]

IL-8 belongs to a group of mediators known as *chemokines* because of their ability to recruit inflammatory cells to the sites of injury. It is synthesized by monocytes, macrophages, neutrophils, and endothelial cells. IL-8 is also used as an index of magnitude of systemic inflammation, and it seems to be able to identify those patients who will develop multiple organ dysfunction syndrome (MODS). Muehlstedt et al. observed high levels of IL-6 and IL-8 in alveolar washouts two hours after injury, suggesting that the alveoli might be the first structures suffering the metabolic response to stress.[29] These high levels might be used in the future as prognostic factors to the development of MODS.

IL-4 and IL-10 are anti-inflammatory cytokines, synthesized by lymphocytes and monocytes and exerting similar effects. They inhibit the synthesis of TNF-α, IL-1, IL-6, and IL-8.

Nitric oxide (NO) is elaborated by various cell types, including endothelial cells, neurons, macrophages, smooth muscle cells, and fibroblasts. NO mediates vasodilation and regulates vascular tone. NO is probably a key mediator in the pathophysiology of stress and shock.

Acute-phase reactants are produced in the liver in response to injury in order to maintain homeostasis; their production is induced by cytokines. These proteins function as opsonins (C-reactive protein), protease inhibitors (alpha$_1$-proteinase), hemostatic agents (fibrinogen), and transporters (transferrin). Albumin is a negative acute-phase protein, and its synthesis is curtailed by inflammation.

1.4.6 IMMUNOLOGIC RESPONSE

As an integral part of the body's response to infection and injury, the inflammatory mediators (TNF-α, IL-1, and IL-6) release substrate from host tissues to support T and B lymphocyte activity, thereby creating a hostile environment for invading pathogens.[30] These inflammatory mediators raise body temperature and produce oxidant substrates that initiate downregulation of the process once invasion has been defeated. Nonetheless, this mechanism poses considerable cost to the host and, according to its magnitude and duration, might lead to SIRS. The latter might cause MODS in some patients. The majority of patients survive SIRS without developing early MODS and, after a period of relative clinical stability, manifest a compensatory anti-inflammatory response syndrome (CARS) with suppressed immunity and diminished resistance to infection.[14] The interaction between the innate and the adaptive immune systems seems to be an important inductor of both SIRS and CARS. It seems that T cells from the adaptive immune system play a role in the early SIRS response to injury and in CARS. Other possible mediators of CARS include prostaglandins of the E series. Also, products of complement activation seem to induce TNF-α production.[14] In summary, SIRS, which regularly occurs after serious injury and in some cases proves fatal to the injured individual, has been partially characterized by both clinical and animal research. However, the triggering mechanisms and signaling systems involved in inducing and maintaining SIRS are incompletely understood and defined.

1.5 CONCLUSIONS

The stress response aims to provide higher organisms with homeostatic adjustments to any kind of injury, such as cold exposure, volume loss, hypoglycemia, and inflammation. Therefore, the stress response is a physiological phenomenon that tries to protect the body against any aggression. However, when the stress response is too intense and lasts for long periods, it is associated with higher morbidity and mortality. In order to avoid such situations, it is of utmost importance to be aware of the different facets of the stress response and to comply with several attitudes that might be able to decrease its magnitude. Pharmacological and nutritional interventions, which will be discussed in other chapters of this book, can be used to attenuate the metabolic response to stress, thus decreasing morbidity and mortality. Nonetheless, these interventions, especially new treatments, should be viewed with caution and under protocol control, because attenuating or abolishing the metabolic response is not without risk. Care providers must be fully aware of the possible side effects.

Future research, especially in the area of genetics and molecular biology, will no doubt help us to understand several aspects of stress not yet known.

REFERENCES

1. Van den Berghe, G., Baxter, R.C., Weekers, F., et al. A paradoxical gender dissociation within the growth hormone insulin-like growth factor I axis during protracted critical illness. *J. Clin. Endocrinol. Metab.*, 85, 183, 2000.
2. Wilmore, D.W. From Cuthbertson to fast-track surgery: 70 years of progress reducing stress in surgical patients. *Ann. Surg.*, 236, 643, 2002.
3. Cuthbertson, D. Effect of injury on metabolism. *Biochem. J.*, 2, 1244, 1930.
4. Hunter, J. *A Treatise on the Blood, Inflammation and Gunshot wounds.* G. Nichol, 1794 .
5. DuBois, E.F. *Basal Metabolism in Health and Disease.* Lea and Febiger, Philadelphia, 1924.
6. Cannon, W.B. *The Wisdom of the Body,* 2nd ed. Norton, New York, 1932.
7. Selye, H. The general adaptation syndrome and the diseases of adaptation. *J. Clin. Encocrinol.*, 6, 117, 1946.

8. Hume D.M. The neuro-endocrine response to injury: present status of the problem. *Ann. Surg.,* 46, 548, 1953.

9. Egdahl R.H. Pituitary-adrenal response following trauma to the isolated leg. *Surgery,* 46, 9, 1959.

10. Allison, S.P., Hinton, P., Chamberlain, M.J. Intravenous glucose tolerance, insulin and free fatty acid levels in burned patients. *Lancet,* 2, 1113, 1968.

11. Wilmore, D.W., Moylan, J.A., Pruitt, B.A., et al. Hyperglucagonaemia after burns. *Lancet,* 1, 73, 1974.

12. Ross, H., Johnstone, I.D.A., Welborn, T.A., et al. Effect of abdominal operations on glucose tolerance and serum levels of insulin, growth hormone and hydrocortisone. *Lancet,* 2, 563, 1966.

13. Epstein, J., Breslow, M.J. The stress response to critical illness. *Crit. Care Clin.,* 15, 17, 1999.

14. Mannick, J.A., Rodrick, M.L., Lederer, J.A. The immunologic response to injury. *J. Am. Coll. Surg.,* 193, 237, 2001.

15. Little, R.A., Stoner, H.B. Effect of injury on the reflex control of pulse rate in man. *Circ. Shock,* 10, 161, 1983.

16. Childs, C., Stoner, H.B., Little, R.A. A comparison of some thermoregulatory responses in healthy children and in children with burn injury. *Din. Sci.,* 77, 425, 1989.

17. Kinney, J.M., Duke, J.H., Long, C.L., et al. Tissue fuel and weight loss after injury. *J. Clin. Path.,* 23, 65, 1970.

18. Wilmore, D.W., Taylor, J.W., Hander, E.W., et al. Influence of burn wound on local and systemic responses to injury. *Ann. Surg.,* 186, 444, 1977.

19. Kim, P.K., Deutschman, C.S. Inflammatory responses and mediators. *Surg. Clin. N. Am.,* 80, 885, 2000.

20. Moore, F.D. *The Metabolic Care of the Surgical Patient.* Saunders, Philadelphia, 1959.

21. Van den Berghe, G. Endocrine evaluation of patients with critical illness. *End. Met. Clin.,* 32, 385, 2003.

22. Vermes, I., Bieshuizen, A., Hampsink, R.M., et al. Dissociation of plama adrenocorticotropin and cortisol levels in critically ill patients: possible role of endothelin and atrial natriuretic hormone. *J. Clin. Endocrinol. Metab.,* 80, 1238, 1995.

23. Van den Berghe, G., de Zegher, F., Vlasselaers, D., et al. Thyrotropin releasing hormone in critical illness: from dopamine-dependent test to a strategy for increasing low serum triiodothyronine, prolactin and growth hormone concentrations. *Crit. Care. Med.,* 24, 590, 1996.

24. Russell, D.H. New aspects of prolactin and immunity: a lymphocyte-derived prolactin-like product and nuclear protein kinase C activation. *Trends Pharmacol. Sci.,* 10, 40, 1989.

25. Weinmann, M. Endocrine and metabolic dysfunction syndromes in the critically ill. *Crit. Care Clin.,* 17, 1, 2001.

26. Guo, H., Calckins, J.H., Sigel, M.M., et al. Interleukin-2 is a potent inhibitor of Leydig cell steroidogenesis. *Endocrinology,* 127, 1234, 1990.

27. Dinarello, C.A. Proinflammatory and anti-inflammatory cytokines as mediators in the pathogenesis of septic shock. *Chest,* 112 (S), 321, 1997.

28. Hack, C.E., deGroot, E.R., Felt-Bersma, R.J.F., et al. Increased plasma levels of interleukin-6 in sepsis. *Blood,* 74, 1704, 1989.

29. Muehlstedt, S.G., Richardson, C.J., Lyte, M., Rodriguez, J.L. Systemic and pulmonary effector cell function after injury. *Crit. Care Med.,* 30, 1322, 2002.

30. Grimble, R.F. Nutritional therapy for cancer cachexia. *Gut,* 52, 1391, 2003.

2 Carbohydrate Metabolism

Mary Marian
University of Arizona

Katherine Connor
St. Joseph's Hospital and Medical Center

CONTENTS

2.1 INTRODUCTION

The primary function of carbohydrates (CHOs) is to yield energy (4 kcal/g substrate) for human metabolism. Glucose, the preferred source of energy for cells, is an essential fuel for the brain and other nervous tissue. CHOs are also vital to the composition of RNA and DNA, coenzymes, glycoproteins, and glycolipids.[1] Defined chemically as an aldehyde or ketone derivative of polyhydric alcohol, or compounds that yield such molecules on hydrolysis, CHOs exist in several forms, including monosaccharides, di- and oligosaccharides, and polysaccharides, such as starch and fibers.[1]

Glucose concentration in the blood is maintained within a narrow range (70 to 100 g/dl) and is probably the most regulated of all of the body's substances.[1] This tight regulation ensures a steady source of glucose, which the brain requires as a continuous source of energy. Blood glucose levels are regulated by both metabolic and hormonal mechanisms. The major hormones controlling blood glucose levels are insulin, glucagon, and epinephrine, but glucocorticoids, thyroid hormone, and growth hormone can also play a role.[1]

2.2 FED STATE

Carbohydrate metabolism during the fed state is characterized by an increase in blood glucose levels, fats, amino acids, and their metabolites. After a meal containing carbohydrates is ingested, carbohydrates are digested and absorbed. The monosaccharide glucose is the primary form of CHO found in the blood. Glucose is either oxidized by the tissues for energy, stored in the liver and

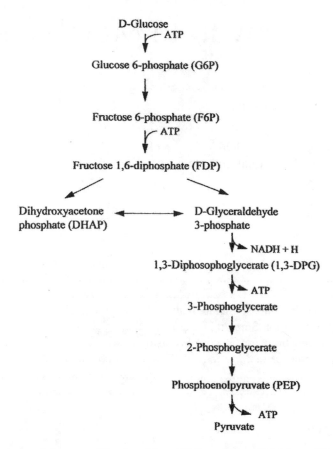

FIGURE 2.1 Two stages of glycogen. (Reprinted from Welborn MB and Moldawer LL, in *Clinical Nutrition Enteral and Tube Feeding,* WB Saunders, Philadelphia, 1997, 61–80. With permission.)

muscles as glycogen, or stored in the adipocytes as an available energy source when needed, as triacylglycerols.

Excess glucose in the blood is stored in the liver and muscles as the branched polymer glycogen.[1] Glycogen plays a principal role in metabolism, serving as a ready source of glucose to maintain blood glucose levels. Although glycogen stores account for as much as 6% of liver mass and only 1% of muscle mass, overall muscle stores represent 3 to 4 times the glycogen stores available in the liver.[1] Muscle glycogen is used primarily by the muscles for energy, whereas hepatic glycogen can either be stored or released into the systemic circulation.

Glucose is metabolized through glycolysis. During glycolysis, glucose is converted to pyruvate, resulting in the production of adenosine triphosphate (ATP) (see Figure 2.1).[2] Pyruvate can be metabolized under anaerobic conditions to form lactate. During anaerobic metabolism, six molecules of ATP are formed. Additionally, pyruvate can be transaminated to the amino acid alanine, carboxylated to oxaloacetate, or decarboxylated to acetyl CoA (see Figure 2.2).[3]

The Krebs cycle, as illustrated in Figure 2.3, serves as the final common pathway for the oxidation of many fuel molecules. Carbohydrates, amino acids, and lipids can enter the Krebs cycle after being converted to acetyl CoA.[3]

Following increases in blood glucose levels, the pancreas secretes the anabolic hormone insulin. Insulin secretion is prompted by the absorption of carbohydrates and amino acids, resulting in the disposal of glucose within the tissues as glycogen in the liver, glucose transport and glycogen synthesis in the muscle, triglyceride synthesis, and amino acid transport and synthesis into proteins in the insulin-sensitive peripheral tissues, primarily the skeletal musculature. Typically, following

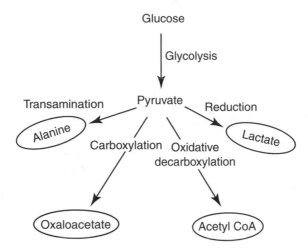

FIGURE 2.2 Possible fates of pyruvate. (Reprinted from DeLegge MH and Ridley C, in *The Science and Practice of Nutrition Support: A Case-Based Core Curriculum*, Kendall/Hunt, Dubuque, IA, 2001, 1–16. With permission.)

cellular glucose update, glucose is subsequently metabolized to pyruvate via glycolysis, with glucose possibly stored as glycogen (see Figure 2.1).[2]

Increases in blood glucose levels suppress pancreatic secretion of glucagon. Glucagon, the major counterregulatory hormone of insulin, is primarily responsible for signaling the production of glucose from endogenous sources through the activation of hepatic glycogenolysis and gluconeogenesis and through mobilization of fatty acids from the adipose tissue.[1] The glucocorticoids such as cortisol, secreted by the adrenal cortex, also stimulate the secretion of glucagon and secretion of gluconeogenic precursors from the peripheral tissues. Glucocorticoids also inhibit glucose utilization by extrahepatic tissues.

Gluconeogenesis, when noncarbohydrate substrates are converted to glucose or glycogen, serves as a mechanism to ensure that a steady source of glucose is always available. Gluconeogenesis occurs during stress and when inadequate glucose substrate is available. The hormones glucagon, cortisol, and epinephrine stimulate the process, whereas insulin suppresses it. Gluconeogenesis can also be inhibited by hyperglycemia, independent of hormonal levels.[4] During times of stress, enhanced gluconeogenesis persists despite elevated serum glucose and insulin levels.

During the postabsorptive state, the body relies on endogenous fuel production to meet metabolic requirements. This state is characterized by the release, interorgan transfer, and oxidation of endogenous fatty acids and by the continued release of glucose from liver glycogen stores and skeletal release of amino acids. Glycogen stores within the musculature serve as a ready source of glucose within the muscle. Circulating insulin levels remain low.

Additionally during this phase, tissue glucose uptake occurs at a rate of approximately 8 to 10 g/h, with the free body glucose pool (about 16 g) requiring replacement every two hours.[5] When blood glucose levels fall below a critical level, headache, slurred speech, confusion, seizures, unconsciousness, coma, and death can result if the energy substrate for brain activity is reduced.[5] To avoid these circumstances, in healthy individuals glucose levels are generally tightly regulated by a variety of physiological controls.

Blood glucose and insulin levels start declining, with blood glucagon levels increasing, approximately an hour after meal consumption.[5] During the fasted state, both blood glucose and serum insulin levels continually decline. As a result, glucose transport into the muscle and fat stores also declines. Due to changes in the plasma glucose-to-glucagon ratio, glycogenolysis ensues, resulting in inhibition of hepatic glycogen synthesis. Figure 2.4 summarizes the substrate fluxes associated with both the fasted and fed states.[6]

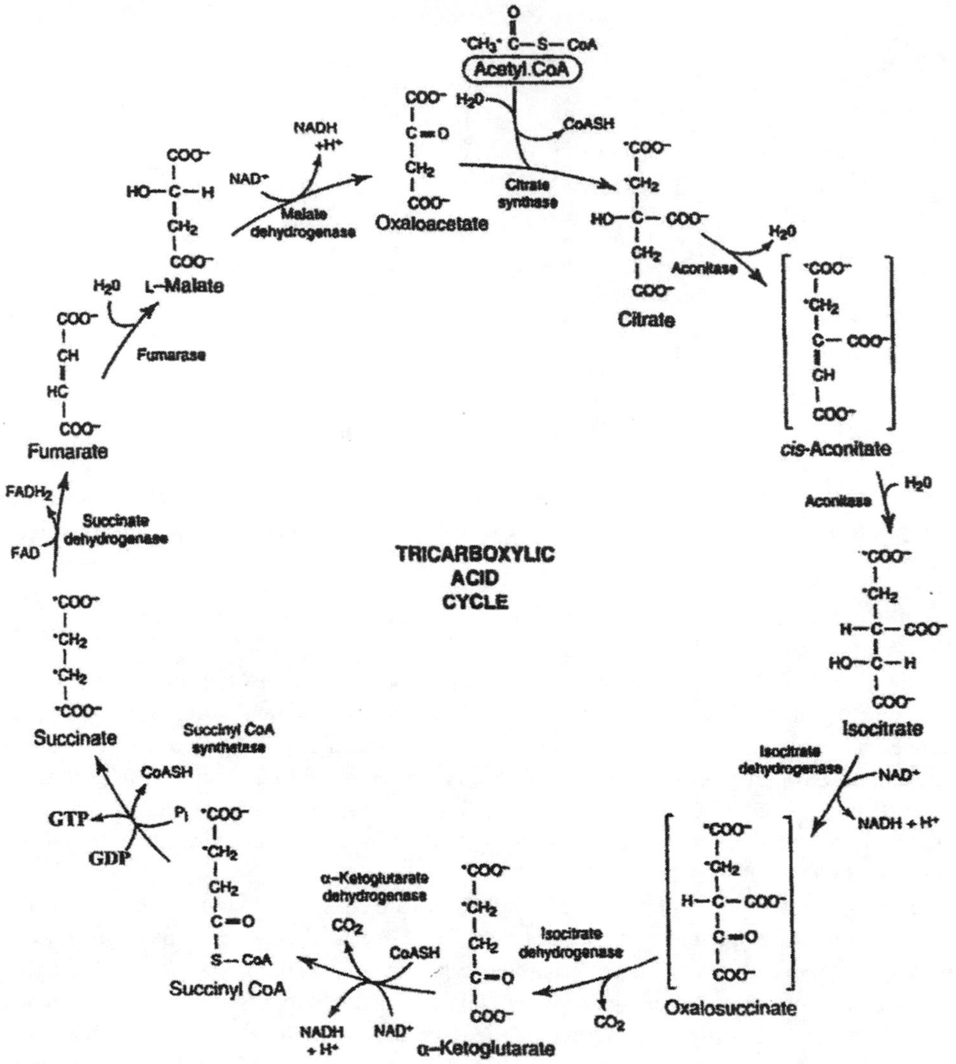

FIGURE 2.3 Krebs cycle. (Reprinted from DeLegge MH and Ridley C, in *The Science and Practice of Nutrition Support: A Case-Based Core Curriculum,* Kendall/Hunt, Dubuque, IA, 2001, 1–16. With permission.)

2.3 STARVATION

To meet the body's energy needs during starvation or fasting, the liver and skeletal muscle glycogen stores are gradually exhausted when a fast continues longer than two to three days.[5] Once glycogen depletion has occurred, deamination of the gluconeogenic amino acids, such as alanine and glutamine, accounts for an increasingly greater percent of the total glucose production to meet the preferential needs for glucose by the brain and central nervous system. Although glucose levels are elevated, the total rate of gluconeogenesis does not increase during this time because the total amount of glucose released into the circulation decreases by 40 to 50%, with the overall glucose use declining.[5] Glucose production thereafter results due to the utilization of endogenous noncarbohydrate sources such as glycerol (as well as lactate and pyruvate) because body proteins cannot serve as a long-term source of fuel because of their structural and functional importance. Protein depletion in excess of 20% is not compatible with life. However, some tissues continue to require glucose as fuel, so gluconeogenesis continues at low levels to meet these needs.

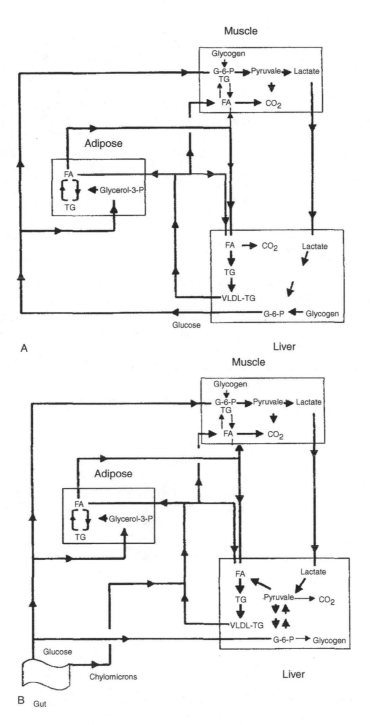

FIGURE 2.4 Substrate fluxes in fasted (A) and fed (B) critically ill patients. (Reprinted from Wolfe RR and Martini WZ, *World J. Surg.*, 24, 639–647, 2000. With permission.)

Fat mobilization during starvation, which likely results from decreasing insulin levels, inhibits lipase and allows for intracellular hydrolysis of triglycerides. Because the liver only partially oxidizes most of the fatty acids it receives, serum levels of acetoacetate, β-hydroxybutyrate, and acetone (collectively known as *ketone bodies*) increase.[5] Ketone bodies, released by the liver, can be oxidized to CO_2 and H_2O by tissues such as the kidneys and muscles. To compensate for this reduction in glucose availability, the brain also converts to using ketoacids as an energy source. This was corroborated by Hasselbalch and colleagues, who investigated glucose metabolism by the brain in fasted subjects.[7] The investigators reported that brain metabolism decreased by 25% during a 3.5 day fast, and ketone body utilization increased from 16 to 160 kcal/d.

The body requires approximately 100 g of CHO daily to prevent the formation of ketone bodies. As the body gradually converts to utilizing ketone bodies as an energy source, the demand for glucose diminishes and hepatic gluconeogenesis decreases, sparing muscle protein. Within approximately two weeks, the body fully adapts to starvation and protein oxidation is minimal.[5] Although the brain and the central nervous system can convert to utilizing ketoacids for fuel in the face of starvation, these by-products of incomplete fatty acid metabolism eventually become toxic.

In summary, during the fasted or starvation state, energy expenditure is reduced, protein stores are conserved, and alternative fuel sources are utilized for energy.

2.4 STRESS RESPONSE

The stress response to injury or acute infection is characterized by a syndrome exhibiting a predictable physiologic response (see Table 2.1). This syndrome was first noted in the 1860s, but the details were not fully described until studied by Cuthbertson in the 1930s.[8] Cuthbertson found increased urinary losses of nitrogen, potassium, and phosphorus that were not reduced with aggressive oral nutrition following injury.[8] A gradual increase in oxygen consumption, paralleled by increases in body temperature, was also noted. The predictable physiological changes were also observed to occur in two distinct phases, subsequently named the *ebb* and *flow* phases. Occurring shortly after injury, the ebb phase is generally of short duration, lasting from 12 to 24 hours. The ebb phase is also associated with a reduction in oxygen consumption, body temperature, and cardiac output, as well as hypoperfusion and lactic acidosis.[8]

Following resuscitation, the ebb phase gradually gives way to the flow phase, which is characterized by hypermetabolism; alterations in glucose, protein, and fat metabolism; and a hyperdynamic cardiovascular response (see Table 2.1). Elevated ADH and aldosterone levels also result in sodium and fluid retention, leading to increases in body weight. Generally, the stress response peaks several days following insult and slowly diminishes as recovery ensues. Excess fluid and sodium accumulations are also excreted, and reductions in body weight occur.

The duration of the flow phase depends on the severity of injury, presence of infection, and development of complications, but typically peaks around three to five days, subsides by seven to

---

TABLE 2.1
Clinical Manifestations of the Stress Response

Ebb Phase	Flow Phase
Reduced oxygen consumption	Increased oxygen consumption
Reduced body temperature	Body temperature increases
Reduced cardiac output	Increased cardiac output
Elevated blood glucose levels	Normal or slightly increased glucose
Glucose production normal	Glucose production increased
Increased free fatty acids	Release of free fatty acids increased
Low insulin levels	Insulin levels increase
Increased catecholamine levels	Elevated catecholamine levels
Increased glucagon levels	Elevated glucagon levels
Increased blood lactate levels	Normal blood lactate levels

---

ten days, and abates with transition into the anabolic phase.[8] Although this stress response, a fundamental physiologic response to preserve organ function and repair damaged tissue, occurs following uncomplicated procedures such as elective surgery, with trauma and severe infections the response can be especially prolonged, having a deleterious impact on health as protein and fat stores are depleted, resulting in malnutrition, especially in unfed patients. If the stress response is allowed to continue unabated, multiorgan failure and death follow. The intensity of the stress response generally parallels the severity of illness and injury.

2.4.1 ALTERATIONS IN GLUCOSE METABOLISM

As discussed, alterations in CHO metabolism are commonly associated with trauma, sepsis, burns, and surgery. Although the precise mechanisms resulting in the hypermetabolic response are not completely understood, a predictable milieu, mediated by a variety of hormones and cytokines, generally results in hypercatabolism (see Figure 2.5).[9]

This stress response results in major metabolic alterations as the body shifts from an anabolic state of storing glucose as glycogen to a catabolic state and significant increases in energy expenditure. To meet the increased demands in energy, body nutrient stores are mobilized to provide substrates to meet the increased energy demands. The body's glycogen stores are quickly depleted in the first 24 hours.[9] Fat and protein stores serve as energy sources thereafter. Although triglyceride stores are also mobilized and oxidized for energy, they do not inhibit the catabolism of protein. In a way similar to starvation, hypercatabolism leads to the loss of lean body mass.

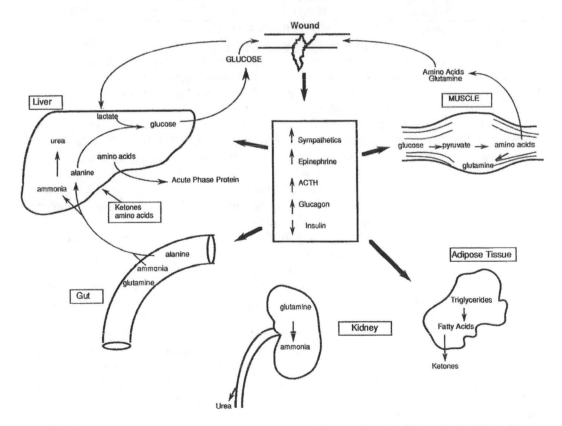

FIGURE 2.5 Neuroendocrine and metabolic consequences of injury. (Reprinted from Smith MK and Lowry SF, in *Modern Nutrition in Health and Disease*, Williams & Wilkins, Baltimore, 1999, 1555–1568. With permission.)

The alterations in carbohydrate metabolism commonly associated with the hypermetabolic response include:

- Hyperglycemia
- Enhanced peripheral glucose uptake and utilization
- Hyperlactatemia
- Increased glucose production via glyconeolysis and gluconeogenesis
- Suppressed glycogenesis
- Glucose intolerance
- Insulin resistance, as reflected by persistent hyperglycemia in spite of elevated insulin levels

Initially during the ebb phase, glucose production is slightly increased, with low insulin levels.[9] Although insulin levels increase during the flow phase, glucose levels continue elevated, as characterized by hyperglycemia, suggesting an alteration in the relationship between insulin sensitivity and glucose disposal. Studies involving trauma patients reflect that hepatic glucose production results from utilization of 3-carbon precursors, including glycerol, pyruvate, lactate, and amino acids, primarily glutamine and alanine.[10] Lactate, produced as a result of anaerobic metabolism and released from the skeletal muscle and other tissues, is recycled to glucose via the Cori cycle, whereas glucose is reconstituted from alanine in the glucose–alanine cycle.[4] The utilization of lactate for gluconeogenesis via the Cori cycle is metabolically expensive: 1 mol of glucose yields 2 ATP through glycolysis but costs 3 ATP via gluconeogenesis.[5] This may also contribute to the increased energy requirements associated with the flow phase.

In spite of this built-in protective mechanism, it appears that during times of sepsis, hypoglycemia can result. Wilmore et al. observed that in burn patients who developed septic complications, glucose production decreased, whereas production was maintained in patients with burns not developing sepsis.[11] It thus appears that a factor inhibiting glucose production is present during sepsis that is not apparent during nonseptic stress.

Elevated glucose levels typically parallel the severity of the illness or injury. Although glucose utilization by the central nervous system appears normal in the injured patient, the kidneys and the wound appear to be the primary consumers of glucose.[12] Wilmore et al. reported that patients with severe burns to one leg compared with minor injuries sustained by the other leg experienced a fourfold uptake of glucose by the burned limb.[13] Furthermore, the wound released large amounts of lactate, due to the significant amounts of glucose consumed. Although, as discussed previously, lactate is converted back to glucose, this again results in greater utilization of energy.

A marked rise in the counterregulatory hormones glucagon, glucocorticoids, and catecholamines accompanies all phases of injury. With the onset of the flow phase and hypermetabolism, these hormones exert a constellation of metabolic effects, as exhibited in Figure 2.5.

Glucagon, epinephrine, and norepinephrine are the catabolic hormones primarily responsible for stimulating endogenous glucose production. In clinical studies, administration of any of a number of combinations utilizing these hormones results in mimicking the metabolic alterations associated with critical illness.[13] Glucagon has been shown as the primary hormone responsible for producing hepatic gluconeogenesis and glycogenolysis, whereas epinephrine appears to be the primary culprit in stimulating glycogenolysis.[14,15] Cortisol mobilizes amino acid efflux from the skeletal muscle, thereby providing substrate for hepatic gluconeogenesis. The catecholamines stimulate hepatic gluconeogenesis and glycolysis, increase lactate production from the peripheral tissues, and increase metabolic rate and lipolysis.[12]

Many of the hormonal changes manifested with injury or infection appear to be mediated by a variety of cytokines. Tumor necrosis factor (TNF); interleukins (IL)-1, 2, and 6; and interferon-γ are the cytokines most studied, with TNF thought to be the primary initiator of many of the responses that occur following injury and infection.[12]

2.5 IMPLICATIONS FOR NUTRITION SUPPORT

When starvation is superimposed on injury or critical illness, the metabolic alterations commonly associated with starvation that allow for a reduction in energy expenditure and protein sparing do not occur. Conversely, lean body mass is catabolized as an energy source to meet the increased energy needs. Additionally, hyperglycemia and glucosuria are seen in critically ill patients. Hence, alterations in glucose metabolism can have a significant impact on the administration of exogenous glucose provided via parenteral or enteral nutrition and other glucose-containing solutions. Typically, in healthy subjects the exogenous provision of glucose or insulin results in suppression of glucose production. In contrast, studies have found that exogenous provision of glucose or insulin failed to suppress hepatic glucose production in trauma patients with gluconeogenesis prevailing.[17,18] In burn patients, Wolfe and colleagues reported that endogenous glucose (2.6 mg/kg/min) was only able to suppress glucose production by 73%; in healthy volunteers, this glucose provision resulted in total suppression.[19] Exogenous glucose administration also does not appear to suppress lipolysis in trauma patients.[3, 12]

Although the precise etiology underlying insulin resistance and altered glucose disposal is unclear, peripheral insulin resistance is thought to occur as a result of physiological alterations at the cellular level associated with the stress response, including an impairment in insulin receptor binding, a postreceptor defect in glucose utilizations, or both.[3] Koruda and colleagues noted that the counterregulatory hormones catecholamines and glucagon reduced glucose uptake by the adipocytes by decreasing glucose transporter activity in the rat.[21] Additionally, a variety of post-transport defects in cellular metabolism have been described in insulin-resistant diabetes, including alterations in glucose oxidation and musculature enzymatic activities.[4] Depressed glycogenesis and excess cortisol, catecholamine, and cytokine secretion, commonly seen in stressed conditions, are also thought to be contributory factors.[4]

2.5.1 RECOMMENDATIONS FOR GLUCOSE PROVISION

An understanding the alterations in glucose metabolism associated with critical illness is important when determining the macronutrient contributions provided during nutritional support. The optimal amount of CHO needed is the amount adequate to spare the use of protein for energy while also avoiding hyperglycemia. The minimum requirements have been estimated to be 1 mg/kg/min, with the maximal amount of CHO generally tolerated to be approximately 4 to 7 mg/kg/min, or 50% to 60% of total energy needs in critically ill patients.[23] Fat synthesis occurs when glucose oxidation rates are exceeded. This may also result in excess CO_2 production. Measurement of the respiratory quotient through indirect calorimetry can also provide feedback on CHO utilization, because an R.Q. > 1 reflects lipogenesis and excessive CHO administration.

Hyperglycemia is the most common complication associated with nutrition support, particularly parenteral support. A variety of factors have been cited, such as a reduction in glucose utilization with diabetes, stress, sepsis, liver disease, aging, and some medications. Reportedly, hyperglycemia or insulin deficiency during critical illness may be linked to complications such as severe infections, multiple organ failure, polyneuropathy, and mortality.[22] Van den Berghe and colleagues also found that the use of intensive insulin therapy to maintain blood glucose values at levels 110 mg/dl substantially reduced morbidity and mortality in intensive care patients, regardless of whether they had a history of diabetes.[22] Intensive insulin management also prevented other comorbidities, such as acute renal failure.

Rosmarin and colleagues retrospectively evaluated 102 patients receiving total parenteral nutrition (TPN).[24] When patients (N = 19) received a dextrose provision of 4 mg/kg/min, none experienced hyperglycemia; five patients experienced hyperglycemia with glucose provisions of 4.1 to 5.0 mg/kg/min; and 18 to 19 patients receiving dextrose 5 mg/kg/min experienced hyperglycemia.

This was statistically significant. To promote optimal glucose tolerance, the dextrose provision for critically ill patients should not exceed 4 mg/kg/min, which can be calculated as follows:

$$\text{mg/kg/minute dextrose load} = \frac{\text{Dextrose (mg)}}{\text{Body weight (Kg)} \times 1440 \text{ minutes}}$$

Note that 24 hours = 1440 minutes.

To minimize the potential for hyperglycemia associated with parenteral nutrition, others recommend initiating support with approximately half of the carbohydrate needs, approximately 150 to 200 g, for the first 24 hours.[25]

Hyperglycemia may also result due to factors other than glucose intolerance, such as chromium deficiency in some patients. Because hyperglycemia is multifactorial, all factors should be considered when determining the appropriate treatment.

2.6 REFEEDING SYNDROME

Refeeding syndrome may result in malnourished patients with the initiation of aggressive specialized nutrition support. A potentially lethal condition, refeeding syndrome can be defined as "the metabolic and physiologic consequences of depletion, repletion, compartmental shifts, and interrelationships of phosphorus, potassium, magnesium, glucose metabolism, vitamin deficiency, and fluid resuscitation" in malnourished patients undergoing refeeding orally, enterally, or parenterally.[27] The common conditions associated with refeeding are illustrated in Table 2.2.

Refeeding syndrome is thought to occur as a result of the body's shifting from utilizing stored body fat for energy to carbohydrates, when energy is provided following starvation.[27] As blood glucose levels rise, serum insulin levels also increase, causing the intracellular movement of electrolytes from the systemic circulation. Circulating levels of potassium, phosphorus, and magnesium subsequently are reduced. The stimulation of insulin secretion also alters the action of glucagon in the liver, with inhibition of fatty acid mobilization and reductions in gluconeogenesis and glycogenolysis.

Refeeding syndrome symptoms generally manifest as generalized malaise, edema, muscle weakness, hyperglycemia, and cardiac arrhythmia.[27] Refeeding is associated with sodium retention and expansion of the extracellular space, resulting in weight gain and thereby leading to an increase in cardiovascular demands. Fluid shifts can result in cardiac failure, dehydration or fluid overload, hypotension, prerenal failure, and sudden death.[28,29] Furthermore, reductions in available circulating potassium, phosphorus, and magnesium, coupled with an expansion of the intravascular volume, lead to a significant risk of developing cardiopulmonary decompensation.

Patients at risk for developing refeeding syndrome include malnourished individuals, especially patients with a weight loss of greater than 10% over a few months, and critically ill patients who have not been fed for 7 to 10 days.[27] Additionally, refeeding syndrome is also common following prolonged fasting, significant weight loss in obese individuals following certain types of gastric bypass surgery, prolonged intravenous fluid repletion, alcohol abuse, and anorexia nervosa.

Because refeeding syndrome can be dangerous, resulting in increased morbidity and mortality, overzealous feeding with specialized nutrition support should be avoided.[29] Prior to the initiation of specialized nutrition support, electrolyte and mineral abnormalities should be corrected and fluid status adequately resuscitated. Specialized nutrition support should also be advanced slowly, with patients monitored closely for signs of heart failure.[25] Malnourished patients with cardiac or pulmonary difficulties are at high risk for developing congestive heart failure with refeeding. Serum electrolyte, mineral, and glucose levels, in addition to fluid status, should be monitored closely for several days to allow for repletion of suboptimal levels, control of blood glucose should hyperglycemia occur, and restoration of fluid balance as needed. Identification of patients at high risk and anticipation of potential development are keys to prevention.

TABLE 2.2
Conditions Commonly Associated
with Refeeding Syndrome

Hypokalemia
Provision of insulin
Steroids and diuretics
Amphotericin B
Hypomagnesemia
Prolonged nasogastric tube suctioning
Prolonged vomiting
Severe diarrhea

Hypophosphatemia
Diabetic ketoacidosis
Chronic alcoholism
Respiratory alkalosis
Provision of insulin
Nasogastric tube suctioning
Malnutrition
Severe diarrhea

Hypomagnesemia
Malnutrition
Chronic alcoholism
Cisplatin
Prolonged nasogastric tube suctioning
Severe diarrhea
Gastrointestinal fistulas
Pancreatitis
Hypoparathyroidism

2.7 CONCLUSION

Carbohydrates are usually the primary energy substrates in human diets. A thorough understanding of the differences between carbohydrate metabolism in starvation and fed states vs. a stress state is critical when designing nutrition support regimens for critically ill patients. This will minimize the potential complications associated with glucose administration and promote positive clinical outcomes.

REFERENCES

1. Owen OE. Regulation of energy and metabolism. In *Nutrition and Metabolism in Patient Care.* WB Saunders Co., Philadelphia, 1988, 35–59.
2. Welborn MB and Moldawer LL. Glucose metabolism. In *Clinical Nutrition Enteral and Tube Feeding*, 3rd ed. Rombeau JL and Rolandelli RH (eds). WB Saunders Co., Philadelphia, 1997, 61–80.
3. DeLegge MH and Ridley C. Nutrient digestion, absorption, and excretion. In *The Science and Practice of Nutrition Support: A Case-Based Core Curriculum.* Gottschlich MM, Fuhrman MP, Hammond KA, Holcombe BJ, and Seidner DL (eds). Kendall/Hunt Publishing Co., Dubuque, IA, 2001, 1–16.
4. Mizock BA. Alterations in carbohydrate metabolism during stress: a review of the literature. *Am. J. Med.*, 98:75–84, 1995.

5. Wolfe, R, Allsop, J, and Burke, J. Glucose metabolism in man: responses to intravenous glucose infusion. *Metabolism*, 28:210–220, 1979.
6. Wolfe RR and Martini WZ. Changes in intermediary metabolism in severe surgical illness. *World J. Surg.*, 24:639–647, 2000.
7. Hasselbalch SG, Knudsen GM, Jakobsen J, et al. Brain metabolism during short-term starvation in humans. *J. Cereb. Blood Flow Metab.*, 14:125–131, 1994.
8. Cuthbertson DP. Observations on disturbance of metabolism produced by injury to the limbs. *Q. J. Med.*, 25:233–246, 1932.
9. Smith MK and Lowry SF. The hypercatabolic state. In *Modern Nutrition in Health and Disease*, 9th ed. Shils ME, Olson JA, Shike M, and Ross AC (eds). Williams & Wilkins, Baltimore, 1999, 1555–1568.
10. Zhang XF, Kunkel KR, Jahoor F, and Wolfe RR. Role of basal insulin the regulation of protein kinetics and energy metabolism in septic patients. *J. Parenter. Enteral Nutr.*, 15:394, 1991.
11. Okabe N and Hashizume N. Drug binding properties of glycosylated human serum albumin as measured by fluorescence and circular dichroism. *Biol. Pharm. Bull.*, 17:16–21, 1994.
12. Wilmore DW, Goodwin CW, Aulick LH, et al. Effect of injury and infection on visceral metabolism and circulation. *Ann. Surg.*, 192:491–504, 1980.
13. Souba W and Wilmore D. Diet and nutrition in the care of the patient with surgery, trauma, and sepsis. In *Modern Nutrition in Health and Disease*, 9th ed. Shils ME, Olson JA, Shike M, and Ross AC (eds). Williams & Wilkins, Baltimore, 1999, 1589–1641.
14. Wilmore D. Nutrition and metabolism following thermal injury. *Clin. Plast. Surg.*, 1:603–619, 1974.
15. Webber J. Abnormalities in glucose metabolism and their relevance to nutrition support in the critically ill. *Curr. Opin. Clin. Nutr. Metab. Care*, 1:191–194, 1998.
16. McGuiness OP, Shau V, Benson EM, et al. Role of epinephrine and norepinephrine in the metabolic response to stress hormone infusion in the conscious dog. *Am. J. Physiol.*, 273:674–681, 1997.
17. Chu CA, Sindelar DK, Neal DW, et al. Comparison of the direct and indirect effects of epinephrine on hepatic glucose production. *J. Clin. Invest.*, 99:1044–1056, 1997.
18. Black PR, Brooks DC, Bessey PQ, et al. Mechanisms of insulin resistance following injury. *Ann. Surg.*, 196:420–433, 1982.
19. Wilmore DW and Aulick LH. Systemic responses to injury and the healing wound. *J. Parenter. Enteral Nutr.*, 4:147–151, 1980.
20. Wolfe RR, Durkot MJ, Allsop JR, et al. Glucose metabolism in severely burned patients. *Metabolism*, 28:1031–1039, 1979.
21. Koruda M, Honnor RC, Cushman SW, et al. Regulation of insulin-stimulated glucose transport in the isolated rat adipocyte. *J. Biol. Chem.*, 262:245–253, 1987.
22. American Society for Parenteral and Enteral Nutrition Board of Directors. Guidelines for the use of parenteral and enteral nutrition in adult and pediatric patients. *J. Parenter. Enteral Nutr.*, 26(S):1S–110S, 2002.
23. Van den Berghe G, Wouters P, Weekers F, et al. Intensive insulin therapy in critically ill patients. *N. Engl. J. Med.*, 345:1359–1367, 2001.
24. Rosmarin DK, Wardlaw GM, Mirtallo J. Hyperglycemia associated with high, continuous infusion rates of total parenteral nutrition dextrose. *Nutr. Clin. Pract.*, 11:151–156, 1996.
25. Matarese LE. Metabolic complications of parenteral nutrition therapy. In *The Science and Practice of Nutrition Support A Case-Based Core Curriculum*, Gottschlich MM, Fuhrman MP, Hammond KA, Holcombe BJ, and Seidner DL (eds). Kendall/Hunt Publishing Co., Dubuque, IA, 2001, 269–286.
26. Solomon SM and Kirby DF. The refeeding syndrome: a review. *J. Parenter. Enteral Nutr.*, 14:90–97, 1990.
27. Peters AI and Davidson MB. Effects of various enteral feeding products on postprandial glucose response in patients with type 1 diabetes. *J. Parenter. Enteral Nutr.*, 16:69–74, 1992.
28. Ladage E. Refeeding syndrome. *ORL Head Neck Nurs.*, 21:18–20, 2003.
29. Crook MA, Path FRC, Hally V, and Panteli JV. The importance of the refeeding syndrome. *Nutrition*, 17:632–637, 2001.
30. Weinsier RL and Krumdieck CL. Death resulting from overzealous total parenteral nutrition: the refeeding syndrome. *Am. J. Clin. Nutr.*, 34:393, 1980.

3 Protein and Amino Acid Metabolism: Comparison of Stressed and Nonstressed States

Peter Fürst
University of Bonn

CONTENTS

... there is a circumstance attending accidental injury which does not belong to a disease, namely that the injury done has in all cases a tendency to produce both, the disposition and means of cure.

John Hunter, *Blood, Inflammation and Gunshot Wounds*, 1794

3.1 INTRODUCTION

Critical illness due to trauma, injury, or infection is a major health problem in industrialized society: some 8% of the population dies each year as the result of injuries (1,2). Because trauma affects young people disproportionately, it claims as many years of productive life as cardiovascular diseases and cancer combined (3).

The care of injured patients has improved over the past decade. Some of the responsible factors include effective management of shock and of fluid and electrolyte balance, as well as new nutritional means. As both common and specific mechanisms for alterations in substrate metabolism are being covered, unique opportunities arise to intervene in the disease process (4). Undoubtedly, the efficacy of providing substrate to the injured, immunocompromised, or malnourished host has caused a renaissance in the clinical application of dietary intervention in the treatment and prevention of disease (5,6). Presently, it has become feasible to employ specialized nutritional support and to modify the metabolic response to stress by using pharmacologic doses of specific nutrients, especially those related to protein metabolism. Pharmacological nutrition is a novel concept that has introduced a new dimension into the fascinating field of modern clinical nutrition. The explosion of new information related to this exciting approach is certainly only a prelude to its use in routine clinical settings (7).

Indeed, aggressive nutritional support plays a major role in the comprehensive care of injured or critically ill patients (8,9). The purpose of this chapter is to present a general approach to protein (amino acid) metabolism of severely injured and critically ill patients. The approach is based on our current understanding of biochemical and physiological alterations that occur in such patients and that are known as the metabolic response to trauma, injury, and infection.

3.2 THE NEUROENDOCRINE AND METABOLIC RESPONSES TO STRESS AND THEIR EFFECT ON PROTEIN METABOLISM

Trauma, injury, and infection are insults to a living body caused by certain external forces and may range from minor elective surgery to massive damage, such as severe burns or multiple-system injury. The pathophysiological and biochemical responses from moderate to severe trauma exhibit a very complex picture, influenced by the local effect and the systemic response.

In the majority of cases, the local effects are more easily resolved with adequate treatment. In contrast, the systemic effects are highly dependent on the nature and magnitude of the local injury and thus represent a stereotyped response, which is difficult to treat and stands for the factor that frequently may jeopardize survival (10). After a variety of insults (e.g., shock, trauma, burns, sepsis, or pancreatitis), patients develop a systematic inflammatory response that is presumably beneficial and resolves as the patient recovers. However, if the systematic inflammatory response is exaggerated or perpetuated, severe disturbances in protein metabolism may arise. The resulting hypermetabolism and catabolism can cause acute protein malnutrition, with impairment in immune function and subclinical multiple organ dysfunction, including acute renal failure (11).

The florid protein wasting response seen early after injury or burns (12), which appears to require adrenaline as well as cortisol and growth hormone, is obviously a catabolic response. Nevertheless, catecholamines also possess general anabolic effects, which appear to be mediated through β-receptors of an unusual kind (13–15). The anabolic effects of catecholamines are not well understood, and there is substantial confusion in the literature concerning the exact mechanisms of these effects. Consequently, at present it is difficult to come to a satisfactory, integrated view of the role of catecholamines in the regulation of protein metabolism and lean body mass.

The hypermetabolism of the stressed patient, whether from injury or infection, is associated with increases in muscle proteolysis, hepatic ureagenesis associated with enhanced glucose production, and increased mobilization of fat. Both injured and septic patients reveal an increased rate of whole-body protein catabolism, with a more modest increase in protein synthesis, leaving a negative nitrogen (N) balance. Infusion with an adequate amount of amino acids partially improved the synthesis rate, but the extent of protein catabolism was insensitive to intravenous nutrition (16,17). Metabolic rate and nitrogen excretion are related to the extent of injury. The two responses generally parallel each other, as shown in Figure 3.1.

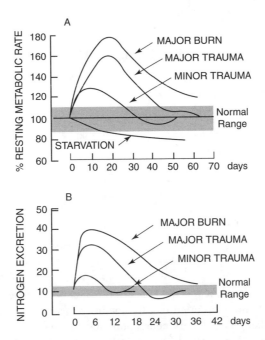

FIGURE 3.1 Metabolic rate (**a**) and nitrogen excretion (**b**) are related to the extent of injury. The two responses generally parallel each other (patients received 12 g nitrogen daily). (From Wilmore D.W., *The Metabolic Management of the Critically Ill*, Plenum Medical Books, New York, 1977. With permission.)

It has been demonstrated that the infusion of a combination of cortisol, epinephrine, and glucagon could produce the hyperglycemia seen in stress, as well as the increased thermogenesis and N loss, a catabolic picture not shown with the administration of any single hormone (18). However, some important inflammatory features of the metabolic response could not be reproduced by the hormone infusion (19). Frayn questioned the importance of the counterregulatory hormones in stress, emphasizing that the high levels of these hormones occurred early after injury and returned to essentially normal values before the peak of the catabolic response (20).

The cascade of alterations in neuroendocrine control mechanisms resulting from critical illness profoundly influences protein and amino acid metabolism and thus body protein components.

3.3 THE EFFECT OF CRITICAL ILLNESS ON BODY PROTEIN MASS — THE NEGATIVE NITROGEN BALANCE

Following an acute injury without a low flow state, lean body mass is first mobilized and then lost. The major reservoir is skeletal muscle. Superimposed on this are the effects of diseases of the kidney, liver, or intestinal tract, which have been considered more specifically in other chapters. Loss of lean body mass (LBM) or, more specifically, body cell mass (BCM) can result in impaired host defense and increased morbidity and mortality with critical illness (17,21). The clinical impressions of muscle loss after injury were placed on a quantitative basis by the early work of Cuthbertson, who reported the increase in resting metabolism and the excretion of nitrogen, sulfur, phosphorous, and creatine following leg-bone fracture in man (22). These observations were extended by subsequent metabolic balance studies, which emphasized a negative nitrogen balance as the hallmark of the response to injury and infection (23).

In severe traumatic conditions like acute renal failure, urinary excretion of nitrogen may reach 35 to 40 g N per day, the equivalent of more than 1 kg lean body mass (24). Efforts made by various investigators to improve the nutrition of acute surgical patients have produced conflicting

TABLE 3.1
Nitrogen Balance (Mean ± SD) During 5% Dextrose Infusion

Pathophysiological State	Nitrogen Balance	
	$mg \cdot kg^{-1} \cdot day^{-1}$	$g \cdot 70\ kg^{-1} \cdot day^{-1}$
Severe burns	−380 ± 70	−27.0 ± 5.0
Severe injury	−260 ± 90	−18.0 ± 6.0
Post–radical bladder cystectomy	−172 ± 47	−12.0 ± 1.3
Sepsis	−162 ± 84	−11.4 ± 5.9
Post–total hip replacement	−96 ± 25	−6.7 ± 1.8
Malnourished	−90 ± 20	−3.2 ± 0.2
Normal subjects	−45 ± 3	−3.2 ± 0.2
Normal subjects after a 10 to 14 day fast	−30 ± 1	−2.1 ± 0.1

Source: From (28–31).

results. According to one opinion, it was not conceivable to expect nitrogen utilization at the height of the catabolic response; others reported that the majority of the postoperative nitrogen loss was due to starvation, rather than to obligatory neuroendocrine responses (25). Later, it was established that an improved nitrogen balance could be approached in severe catabolic states with increasing nitrogen provision, though the augmented nitrogen loss is not reduced by the nitrogen intake (26). The patient whose problem is primarily partial starvation can be put into positive N balance with good nutrition support, whereas the strongly catabolic patient cannot achieve a positive N balance by nutritional means until the peak of the catabolic drive has passed. Kinetic studies indicate that the provision of a protein intake of up to 1.5 $g \cdot kg^{-1} \cdot day^{-1}$ can improve the N balance, but going above that level of intake merely increases the rate of protein synthesis and breakdown without improving the nitrogen balance (27).

In standardized conditions (28), negative nitrogen balance is eight times higher in patients with severe burns and six times higher in those with severe injury than in normal subjects (Table 3.1). Nitrogen balance in postoperative patients is between the normal value and that of accidental injury and depends on the severity of the operation, being more negative after cystectomy than after total hip replacement. The nitrogen balance of septic patients is comparable to that of patients after radical cystectomy. Normal subjects, who are fasted prior to infusion of a 5% dextrose solution, had about 50% reduction in N excretion (Table 3.1). Malnourished patients who were not septic and were remote from injury or surgery, nevertheless revealed rates of N excretion twice those of normal subjects and about three times those of normal subjects with prior fasting (28–31).

Indeed, the development of clinical nutrition reveals a remarkable picture. Increased nitrogen loss associated with hypermetabolism attracted scientific attention because of the new interest in adrenocortical hormones and the possibility that injury induces cortisol secretion, which then causes muscle breakdown and negative nitrogen balance (32). This argument has been used repeatedly to emphasize the futility of providing extra nutrition when the metabolic response had been shown to be obligatory. When protein hydrolysates were given to surgical patients, however, the N loss seemed to remain high, although the N balance was somewhat improved depending on the severity of the stress. Later, Wretlind produced an improved protein hydrolysate for intravenous use but felt that the utilization of such a material would always be limited until more calories could be administered than could be given by glucose solutions in a peripheral vein. The majority of presently available preparations lack glutamine, tyrosine, and cysteine. This might seriously limit optimum protein synthesis. Short-chain synthetic dipeptides containing these amino acids are available, enabling optimum composition and proportion of amino acids for support of critically ill, catabolic patients.

3.4 CHANGES IN PROTEIN TURNOVER

The manner in which net protein catabolism takes place is a subject of great debate. Although the classic text by Waterlow and coworkers contains a detailed account of the underlying theory (33), more recent reviews discuss the difficulties identified as a result of modern work (16,34,35). Unidirectional rates of protein synthesis and degradation might be measured by the following methods:

- Whole-body turnover studies in which isotopic amino acids are given by bolus or constant infusion and the specific activities of precursor and degradation products (CO_2, urea, ammonia) are determined as a function of time in blood, urine, and breath
- Measurement of synthesis rates in muscle and blood by sampling protein from these tissues in studies similar to whole-body studies
- Measurement of 3-methylhistidine excretion in urine, or arteriovenous difference of 3-methylhistidine, as a measure of the unidirectional rate of muscle protein breakdown

Previous data indicate that changes in both protein synthesis and catabolism depend on the severity of injury. Severe burn (36), skeletal trauma, and sepsis (37) appear to cause increases in both synthesis and catabolism. Mild burns (36) and elective operation (38–40) result in only minimal changes. Unfortunately, these early studies have not been corrected for nutrient intake, which is a major factor influencing protein synthesis (7).

More recent patterns are summarized in Figure 3.2. Critical illness or endocrine diseases, which result in lean tissue wasting over a long period of time, also depress muscle protein turnover through reduced protein synthesis and protein breakdown. Whole-body protein turnover is, therefore, also depressed, although in some circumstances visceral protein turnover may be elevated (e.g., liver and kidney disease). Under these circumstances, it makes sense that any attempts to replenish depleted cell mass should aim to increase muscle protein synthesis rather than to decrease muscle protein breakdown (16). In circumstances in which there is excessive muscle wasting associated with increased whole-body energy expenditure — as in severe injury, after burns of more than about 10% of body surface area (41–44), in polymyositis (45), during infection (46), and with some kinds of cancer (45,47) — whole-body nitrogen balance is markedly negative, probably because of changes that include an increase of protein breakdown in different tissues. Whether muscle protein synthesis also falls, as might be expected, or rises (possibly as an adaptive response to the rise in protein breakdown) is not known. The major change is a marked acceleration of lean tissue proteolysis (48), probably including muscle proteolysis.

Excretion of 3-methylhistidine has been measured during burn injury and sepsis, and both indicate marked increase in muscle catabolism (49–51). Patients after minor operative procedures and with hyperketonuria after trauma had slightly increased or normal rates of 3-methylhistidine excretion (51,52). In traumatized patients, the response of nitrogen balance and 3-methylhistidine excretion to exogenously administered amino acids is of interest. Parenteral nutrition with adequate levels of amino acids and energy markedly improves nitrogen balance, compared to administration of energy substrate alone. Measurement of 3-methylhistidine excretion under each of these conditions, however, indicates no difference in skeletal muscle catabolic rates (52). These data suggest that exogenous nutritional support is effective in increasing protein synthesis in the presence of increased protein catabolism, and that increased protein synthesis results in improved nitrogen balance (52). Urinary 3-methylhistidine excretion must be interpreted with caution, because under some conditions the gut may be a major contributor. It is also now realized that myofibrillar and sarcoplasmic proteins are regulated separately (16,53,54). Nevertheless, these considerations do not restrict the usefulness of the method for specific measurement of myofibrillar protein breakdown. It is to be remembered that all the implicated methods rely on many assumptions that have not yet been verified, and the problem of precursors and their measurements is still a vexed question.

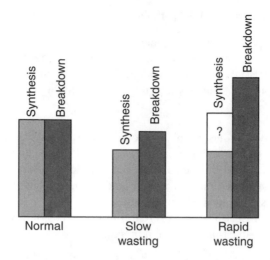

FIGURE 3.2 Extent of protein synthesis and protein breakdown. The slow wasting condition is found in mild injury, malnutrition, cancer, immobilization, etc. Rapid wasting occurs after severe injury, burns, and infection. The responses are, for the most part, well grounded in patient observations. It is not certain to what extent protein synthesis can rise in injury associated with inflammatory disease. (Reproduced from Rennie, M.J. and Cuthbertson, D.J.R., in *Artificial Nutrition Support in Clinical Practice*, Greenwich Medical Media Limited, London, 2002, 25–50. With permission.)

Recently, the implication of mass isotopomer analysis has been advocated (55,56). The use of this novel theoretical approach to the analysis of tracer appearance in polymeric molecules (such as proteins) may, in the future, render redundant the need to measure precursor labeling (16).

3.5 PLASMA AND MUSCLE AMINO ACID CHANGES IN RESPONSE TO INJURY AND INFECTION

3.5.1 PLASMA AMINO ACIDS

Although circulating plasma amino acids constitute a small fraction of the free amino acid pool in the body, they are important because of their role in transport of nitrogen to body organs and because their concentration pattern reflects the net amino acid metabolism. In the 1940s, Man and coworkers monitored plasma α-amino acid nitrogen in patients undergoing operative procedures. They observed decline following the operation, and the values slowly returned to normal during convalescence (57). Interestingly, malnourished patients exhibited lower preoperative α-amino nitrogen concentrations, the values remaining depressed for a longer period of time following the operation. At this early time, little attention was paid to nutritional factors. However, in recent, carefully conducted studies, the preceding postoperative decline of most plasma free amino acids has been confirmed, although certain essential amino acids showed an increase with time (58,59). In patients who had suffered a severe injury, amino acid concentrations have been reported to rise, fall, or remain within normal limits (60). In reports in which the measurements were obtained during the flow phase and under defined conditions, a more consistent response emerged (61). In burn patients receiving rigorous nutritional support during their hospitalization, most plasma free amino acid levels were found to be decreased, although phenylalanine was elevated (62).

It is notable that the branched-chain amino acid concentrations were not distinguishable from control values. Other investigators noted similar results but, apart from the elevation of phenylalanine, enhanced concentrations of glutamic acid, methionine, aspartic acid, and hydroxyproline were occasionally noted. Profound hyperaminoacidemia has been noted during the radiation period in patients who have undergone bone marrow transplantation (63). Thermal injury induces time-dependent variations in plasma amino acids that is, an initial hyperaminoacidemia reflecting proteolysis in the wounded areas, a decrease in gluconeogenic amino acids as a consequence of excessive usage in the liver, and a progressive return to normal (64,65). There is also a durable hyperphenylalaninemia, reflecting increased protein turnover and specific alterations of sulfur amino acids. The finding of high levels of aromatic (phenylalanine and tyrosine) and sulfur-containing (methionine and cysteine) amino acids in sepsis and severe trauma certainly suggest impaired liver function (66,67).

3.5.2 INTRACELLULAR MUSCLE-FREE AMINO ACIDS

It is obvious that the maintenance of the plasma amino acid steady state depends on the net balance of the released amino acids from endogenous protein stores and is also contingent on their subsequent utilization in the peripheral tissues. It is further to be expected that the extent of proteolysis in various tissues will be influenced by the catabolic stimuli and thereby contribute to the characteristic changes of circulating amino acids and their turnover during the catabolic state.

In carefully conducted flux studies, it was demonstrated that amino acid release by the skeletal muscle in severely ill patients highly exceeded that observed in a healthy control group (68). This augmented influx of amino acids into the extracellular compartment is accompanied by a corresponding influx of amino acids from plasma to the visceral tissues. This means that amino acids released from peripheral tissue (skeletal muscle) compare favorably with the uptake in splanchnicus and confirms the marked translocation of amino acid nitrogen from carcass to viscera. In other words, changes in the extracellular compartment depend on amino acids derived from the free intracellular pool, the concentration of this pool being determined by muscle protein breakdown, intracellular intermediary metabolic pathways, and the efflux to the plasma compartments. Consequently, changes in plasma compartment must be evaluated on the basis of the magnitude of intracellular oxidation, the rate of gluconeogenesis, and the extent of intracellular reutilization. It is conceivable that the study of the intracellular compartment will promote the understanding of amino acid metabolism in catabolic states. Skeletal muscle contains the largest pool of intracellular free amino acids. In normal humans, most amino acids have a much higher concentration in intracellular water than in plasma (69).

The pattern of changes in amino acid concentration in muscle shows many similarities during catabolism (70). In all cases, there is an increase in branched-chain amino acids (BCAA), aromatic amino acids, and methionine, and a decrease in glutamine and basic amino acids (lysine and arginine). Regarding the changes observed in neutral amino acids, there is a graduation of response, with minimal changes seen in muscle with bed rest and maximal changes in sepsis (71).

A uniform reduction of approximately 50% of free muscular glutamine associated with negative nitrogen balance seems to be one of the most typical features of the response to trauma and infection (Figure 3.3). The marked intracellular glutamine depression has been demonstrated after elective operation (72), major injury (61,73), burns (60,61), infections (73–75), and pancreatitis (76), irrespective of nutritional attempts at repletion. Reduction of the muscle free glutamine pool thus appears to be a hallmark of the response to injury, and its extent and duration is proportional to the severity of the illness. Recent studies have underlined that the tissue glutamine depletion is caused mainly by stress-induced alterations in the interorgan glutamine flow (77). Muscles, and probably lung glutamine effluxes, are accelerated to provide substrate for the gut, immune cells, and kidneys (78,79), explaining at least in part the profound decline in muscle free glutamine concentration.

Most of the liver free amino acid concentrations are lower in critically ill patients than in control groups, the BCAA levels being decreased by 35% (80). In nonsurviving patients, the hepatic concentrations of total amino acids, BCAA, gluconeogenic amino acids, and basic amino acids are lower than in surviving patients. The liver amino acid pattern reflects the plasma rather than the

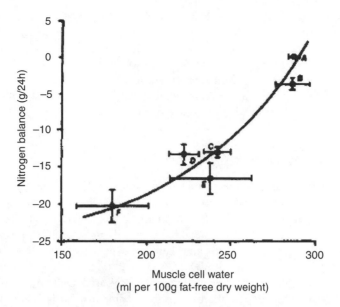

FIGURE 3.3 Trauma-induced intracellular glutamine depletion in human muscle tissue (mean ± SEM). (Combined data from Fürst, P., *Proc. Nutr. Soc.*, 42, 451–462, 1983, and Fürst, P. and Stehle, P., in *Metabolic and Therapeutic Aspects of Amino Acids in Clinical Nutrition*, CRC Press, Boca Raton, FL, 2004, 613–631. With permission.)

muscle amino acid patterns (80). The elevated hepatic phenylalanine levels are in agreement with muscle and plasma data and may indicate that during critical illness, the liver cannot metabolize the amount of phenylalanine released by muscle tissue. In experimental studies, a remarkably uniform response of decreased levels in all intestinal amino acids was elicited by trauma. Glutamine, which is one of the major amino acid components of the muscle (27%) and liver (22%), reveals relatively low contents in the intestine (3.3%). This low level in the intestine may be due to high GDH activity of the mucosa. The BCAA contents in rat liver and intestine are 2.6 and 6.4 times, respectively, the BCAA present in the muscle. Trauma elicits a minor reduction (6%) in muscle BCAA but a marked increase (22%) in liver BCAA and a decrease (27%) in intestinal BCAA (80,81).

Human adipose tissue *in vivo* is a consistent net exporter of both alanine and glutamine, and a consumer of glutamate (82). After an overnight fast, adipose tissue seems to contribute about one-third as much as muscle to whole-body alanine and glutamine production, and more than one-half as much as muscle to glutamate uptake. No data are available for the influence of injury on the adipose tissue amino acid content and release, which may play a substantial role in whole-body production during episodes of stress.

Similarly, little is known about the altered amino acid concentrations due to injury of the actively metabolizing leukocyte cells (83) and cerebrospinal fluid (CSF) (84). Trauma, remote from the brain, enhances the total amino acid levels in CSF, in contrast to the well known decline in plasma. Glutamine and glutamate account for 73% of this increase in CSF. The systemic trauma enhances the levels of excitatory neurotransmitters — glutamate and aspartate in CSF (84).

3.6 CELLULAR HYDRATION

A fascinating recent hypothesis emphasizes the essential importance of the cellular hydration state as a determinant of protein catabolism in health and disease (85). It is postulated that an increase in cellular hydration (swelling) acts as an anabolic proliferate signal, whereas cell shrinkage is

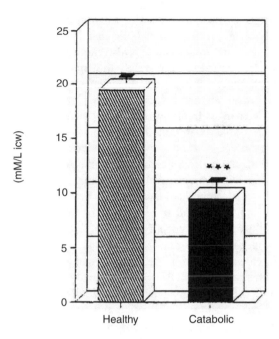

FIGURE 3.4 Whole-body nitrogen balance and cellular hydration of skeletal muscle. Healthy subjects (n = 17). Catabolic patients include those with liver tumors, polytrauma, burns, necrotizing pancreatitis (n = 26). Skeletal muscle cell water was measured in a needle biopsy sample from quadriceps femoris by the chloride distribution method. Extra- and intracellular distributions were calculated by the chloride method, assuming normal membrane potential of 87.2 mV. (Reproduced from Häussinger, D. et al., *Lancet*, 341, 1330–1332, 1993. With permission.)

catabolic and antiproliferate. The authors put forward the hypothesis that changes in cellular hydration state might be the variable linking muscle glutamine content with protein turnover and, because of the large muscle mass, the whole-body nitrogen balance. Data from previous studies of the relation between intracellular glutamine content and catabolism in patients with various underlying disorders enabled the evaluation of the relation between muscle–cell water content and whole-body nitrogen balance, showing an inverse relation (Figure 3.4). The concentrative uptake of glutamine into muscle and liver cells would be expected to increase cellular hydration, thereby triggering a protein anabolic signal. Indeed, glutamine (dipeptides) supplementation may facilitate aggressive therapeutic interventions, in order to improve cellular hydration state and subsequently modify or reverse catabolic changes (86).

3.7 THE CONCEPT OF CONDITIONALLY ESSENTIAL AMINO ACIDS IN CRITICAL ILLNESS — REQUIREMENTS

During episodes of various acute and chronic wasting diseases, the classical definition of the essentiality of amino acids is seriously challenged. In 1962, Mitchell pointed out in the first volume of his treatise *Comparative Nutrition of Man and Domestic Animals* that an "amino acid may be a dietary essential even if an animal is capable of synthesizing it, provided that the demand for it exceeds the capacity for synthesis" (87). Thus, the strict nutritional classification of the common amino acids formulated by Rose, and later by Jackson, Chipponi, and others, is not acceptable as we attempt to understand how dietary protein serves to meet our nutritional needs in disease (86,88).

Grimble proposes that, regardless of the definition used, final judgment about the usefulness of an essential amino acid will be on the grounds of clinical and nutritional efficacy (89). A more general proposition is that "a possible and useful direction might put more emphasis on metabolic control and its regulation of tissue and organ function and nutritional status" (86–88). This definition offers suggestions about how certain shared metabolic characteristics might be used to differentiate the various nutritionally important amino acids. It also implies that the dietary "essentiality" of a given amino acid is dependent on the ratio of supply to demand; the distinction between *essential* and *nonessential* largely disappears because it depends on conditions (86,88). In this context, chronic and acute wasting diseases are associated with particular amino acid deficiencies and imbalances causing specific changes in amino acid requirements. Thus, the new approach categorizes amino acids as indispensable, conditionally indispensable, or dispensable, according to their functional and physiological properties and considering the ratio of supply to demand under various pathological conditions (86). Indeed, administration of the required conditionally indispensable amino acid might greatly facilitate an anabolic response to life-threatening disease (90).

The major question is which amino acids are to be considered conditionally essential (indispensable) during diseased conditions and in what amounts they should be administered. Amino acid requirements are carefully investigated and defined for healthy individuals (91). Critical illness, however, considerably influences amino acid requirements. Remarkably, there are no conclusive data available relative to changes of amino acid requirements induced by episodes of infection, injury, trauma, multiple organ failure (MOF), or acute renal or liver failure. Consequently, future research evaluating amino acid requirements in these conditions using modern methods must receive high priority. Indeed, the requirements of glutamine and cysteine (and perhaps those of arginine and taurine) are apparently very different in critically ill patients (7). Higher requirements of branched-chain amino acids have been repeatedly claimed in controversial debates, yet their benefits could not be confirmed in well controlled studies (92).

In the following section, the potentially indispensable amino acids (glutamine, cysteine, arginine, and taurine) will be discussed and their function scrutinized. Their possible clinical application and tentative requirements will be suggested.

3.7.1 GLUTAMINE

Glutamine is the most prevalent free amino acid in the human body, constituting more than 60% of the total free amino acid pool in skeletal muscle (69). As described previously, there is much evidence that hypercatabolic and hypermetabolic situations are accompanied by marked depression of muscle intracellular glutamine (70,93). Furthermore, during catabolic stress or when tumors are proliferating, peripheral glutamine stores are rapidly diminished and the amino acid is preferentially shunted as a fuel source toward visceral organs or tumor tissue. This creates a glutamine-depleted environment, the consequences of which include enterocyte and immunocyte starvation (94). Consequently, glutamine is considered conditionally indispensable and should be endogenously administered during episodes of catabolic stress and undernutrition.

Two unfavorable chemical properties of free glutamine hamper its use as a nutritional substrate in routine clinical settings:

- Instability, especially during heat sterilization and prolonged storage
- Limited solubility (~ 3 g/100 ml at 20°C)

The rate of breakdown of free glutamine depends on temperature, pH, and anion concentration. The decomposition of free glutamine yields the cyclic product pyroglutamic acid and ammonia. All these drawbacks can be overcome by use of synthetic glutamine-containing dipeptides (93,95).

Leaving aside such considerations, several studies show that free glutamine may be provided by adding the crystalline amino acid to a commercially available amino acid solution before administration. However, appropriate preparation of such a solution requires a daily procedure at 4°C, under strictly aseptic conditions in a local pharmacy, followed by laborious sterilization

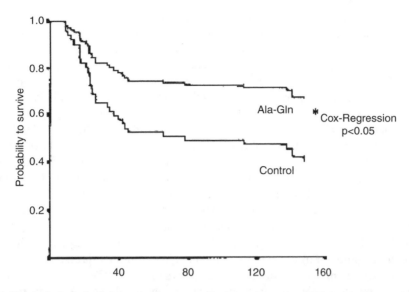

FIGURE 3.5 Survival plot of a subgroup of parenterally fed patients treated for nine days and longer under standardized conditions. Ala-Gln: 1.2 g of standard amino acid solution per kilogram of body weight plus 0.3 g of alanyl-glutamine per kilogram of body weight per day. Control: 1.5 g of standard amino acid solution per kilogram of body weight. (Reproduced from Goeters, C. et al., *Crit. Care Med.*, 30, 2032, 2002. With permission.)

through membrane filtration (96). In addition, to diminish the risk of precipitation, glutamine concentrations in such solutions should not exceed 1 to 2%.

Many clinical investigations showed improved nitrogen economy and maintained intracellular glutamine concentration with glutamine or glutamine-containing dipeptide supplementation. More importantly, numerous well controlled clinical studies, directed to investigate primary endpoints such as morbidity, mortality, and length of hospital stay, have demonstrated obvious improvements in clinical outcome in both surgical and critically ill patients (for references see 7,93).

In a recent comprehensive meta-analysis, Novak and coworkers examined the relationship between glutamine supplementation and length of hospital stay, morbidity, and mortality in patients undergoing surgery and experiencing critical illness (97). They reviewed 550 titles, abstracts, and papers. There were 14 randomized trials showing lower risk ratio with glutamine supplementation; the rate of infectious complications was also lower, and hospital stays shorter, with glutamine nutrition. With respect to mortality, the treatment benefit was observed in studies of parenteral glutamine and high-dose glutamine, compared to studies of enteral glutamine and low-dose glutamine, respectively. With respect to length of hospital stay, all of the treatment benefit was observed in surgical patients compared to critically ill patients (-3.5 days vs. 0.9 day). That a longer period on the control and treatment and parenteral feeds is required to affect survival has been emphasized by a study involving 144 ICU patients (98). Consistent with previous results, there was no difference in clinical outcomes in those patients fed for a shorter period, but for those fed for more than 9 days, the survival measured at 6 months was significantly better: 22 out of 33 vs. 13 out of 35 (Figure 3.5).

The lack of any effect on mortality with enteral glutamine supplementation is a consistent observation (99–101) and may reflect the limited systemic availability of glutamine (102). Another reason in the critically ill might be the presence of bacterial overgrowth: the bacteria preferentially consume glutamine (99). Because glutamine is absorbed in the upper part of the small intestine and subsequently metabolized in the liver, glutamine thus might not be available for the target mucosal tissue in the lower sites of the intestine (99).

A further recent meta-analysis reports results in studies with bone marrow transplantation patients receiving parenteral nutrition supplemented with glutamine vs. standard parenteral nutrition (103). The findings indicated that glutamine supplementation can significantly reduce length of hospital stay and decrease incidence of positive blood cultures. Indeed, it is difficult to extrapolate this result with confidence to the critically ill patient. However, many of these patients have a significant degree of immunosuppression or susceptibility to infection, particularly late in the course of illness.

In a new analysis of clinical and microbiological data of the Griffiths study (104), the authors report that the nature and overall rates of intensive care–acquired infections (ICAIs) related mostly to reduced mortality for the MOF in the ICU (105). Glutamine-treated patients developed fewer Candida infections after longer stays and, importantly, none of those infected died, whereas many control patients on standard TPN not only became infected sooner but also had more infections and died from MOF. Overall, only 38% of ICAIs who died were in glutamine groups, compared with 74% in controls. These new data show that glutamine is significantly associated with improved survival (105,106). Indeed, preventing nosocomial infections is a valuable goal resulting in reduced ICU stays, reduced duration of mechanical ventilation and antibiotic pressure, fewer side effects, lower costs, and fewer emergences of resistant microorganisms (107).

Recently the question was raised: "Glutamine save lives! What does it mean?" (108). The underlying mechanisms of supplemental glutamine (dipeptide) in causing reversal of severe illness might be due to support of the mucosa, the immune system, and the hepatic biosynthesis of glutathione (109–111). According to another proposal, glutamine plays a more global regulatory role by modifying the endogenous inflammatory responses. These mechanisms might be due to attenuation of the elaboration of proinflammatory mediators and up-regulation of anti-inflammatory factors (108,112). The contribution of glutamine to protein anabolism and through acid–base homeostasis may elicit a further defense mechanism of the host, but the specific role of these functions to the host defense has not been quantified.

According to the current *Canadian Clinical Practice Guidelines for Nutrition Support in Mechanically Ventilated Critically Ill Patients*, parenteral supplementation with glutamine is recommended (113). As a consequence of the available evidence, Wilmore, in a current editorial, defines glutamine "as a highly unique and important nutrient, one that serves as both an important metabolite and a metabolic switch or regulator, essential to human health and survival" (114).

3.7.2 CYSTEINE

In healthy adults, the sulfur-containing amino acid cysteine can be synthesized from methionine using the liver-specific transsulfuration pathway. In liver tissue of fetuses and of preterm and term infants, the activity of cystathionase, the key enzyme in the transsulfuration pathway, is low or undetectable (115,116). In liver disease, the body's cysteine requirements cannot be met due to the diminished transsulfurating capacity (117). Consequently, cysteine should be considered an essential amino acid in immature infants and a conditionally essential amino acid in liver disease. In both cases, it should be provided exogenously. The tentative requirements are estimated to be 20 mg/kg (91).

Cyst(e)ine is a potent antioxidant *per se* and a precursor for glutathione (118,119). Glutathione and cysteine inhibit the expression of the nuclear transcription factor in stimulated T-cell lines (118,119). This might provide an interesting approach to the treatment of AIDS, because the transcription factor enhances HIV mRNA expression. In fact, *in vitro* studies show that the stimulatory effects of TNF, induced by free radicals, on HIV replication in monocytes can be inhibited by sulfur-containing antioxidants (120). These basic studies indicate that treatment of inflammatory diseases and AIDS with sulfhydryl antioxidants may be beneficial, and powerful arguments have been advanced in favor of such treatment (121,122). Clinical studies using this strategy are not yet available.

Route of administration seems to influence the rate of hepatic cysteine synthesis by altering the delivery of cysteine precursors to the liver. Steginck and Den Besten (123) demonstrated in healthy men that intravenous infusion of solutions containing methionine but not cyst(e)ine resulted in depressed concentrations of all three forms of circulating cysteine (free cysteine, free cystine, and protein-bound cysteine). This result suggests that parenteral solutions should contain not only methionine but additional amounts of cyst(e)ine. Supplementation with cyst(e)ine may also improve taurine concentrations during long-term TPN. However, addition of cyst(e)ine to TPN solutions is problematic. At neutral or slightly alkaline pH, cysteine is rapidly oxidized during heat sterilization, and storage of cysteine yields the dimer cystine, which itself is very poorly soluble and which precipitates in the solution. Acidic conditions may lead to a reduction of the sulfhydryl group and the formation of hydrogen sulfide.

N-acetyl-cysteine has been proposed as a cysteine replacement in the ICU, especially in the treatment of sepsis. Nevertheless, the results are strikingly poor (102). The reason is that humans lack tissue acylases, except in the kidney (7,93). Consequently, following long-term infusion, the compound will accumulate in body fluids and be excreted in the urine (7,93). A recent study confirmed that N-acetyl-cysteine metabolism is disturbed in sepsis, resulting in impaired cardiac performance (124).

Future use of synthetic cysteine containing dipeptides will be the solution. Studies with highly soluble cysteine peptides (L-cysteine-L-alanine and L-cysteine-glycine) have provided evidence that these cysteine peptides are well utilized in experimental animals (125,126). Their synthesis in industrial-scale and subsequent human studies is still warranted (112).

3.7.3 ARGININE

Arginine is a precursor of polyamine and nucleic acid synthesis, a promoter of thymic growth, and an endocrinologic secretagogue stimulating release of growth hormone, prolactin, insulin, and glucagons (127). It is metabolized within the enterocyte by the arginase pathway to ornithine and urea and by the arginine deaminase pathway to citrulline (128). Arginine metabolism in enterocytes may participate in the support of gut morphology and function by acting as a substrate for nitric oxide synthesis (129). Inhibition of nitric oxide synthesis increases intestinal mucosal permeability in experimental models of ischemia and reperfusion intestinal injury (130) and acute necrotizing enterocolitis (131). In addition, administration of arginine reverses the effect of nitric oxide synthase inhibition (130). These results suggest that basal nitric oxide production is important in minimizing the mucosal barrier dysfunction in these models.

During major catabolic insults such as trauma or surgery, an increase in urinary nitrogen — excreted largely as urea — represents the end product of increased lean body tissue catabolism and reprioritized protein synthesis. During these stress situations, arginine is claimed to become conditionally essential in that demand is greater than endogenous supply (132). Arginine may be of significance in the critically ill because of its potential role in immunomodulation (133,134), and it is hypothesized that high-dose arginine enhances the depressed immune response of individuals suffering from injury, surgical trauma, malnutrition, or sepsis. On the basis of animal and *in vitro* experiments, however, the results derived from critically ill patients are controversial. Clinical studies on enteral arginine administration have shown moderate net nitrogen retention and protein synthesis, compared with isonitrogenous diets in critically ill and injured patients. After surgery for certain malignancies in elderly postoperative patients, supplemental arginine (25 g/day) enhanced T-lymphocyte responses to phytohemagglutinin and concavalin A and increased the CD4 phenotype number (135). Interestingly, insulin-like growth factor 1 levels were increased by about 50%, reflecting the growth hormone secretion induced by arginine supplementation. A large oral arginine intake (30 g/day) improved wound healing (136) and enhanced the blastogenic response to several mitogens (137). Overall, however, there was no improvement in patient outcome or length of hospital stay (138).

Studies involving immunomodulating diets enriched with ample amounts of arginine but also n-3 fatty acids, nucleotides, and sometimes glutamine are available, yet the specific effects of the different compounds in the diets are difficult to distinguish (132,139,140). One potential complication of arginine administration is its known competition with the essential amino acid lysine for tubular reabsorption (141). Thus, large doses of arginine induce lysine deficiency by increasing its renal excretion. There is also the concern that arginine supplementation in critically ill patients increases the systemic inflammatory response syndrome (SIRS) due to enhanced NO release, additionally generated during SIRS, sepsis, or burn injury (4). High concentration of NO formed increases epithelial permeability. The endothelial damage is due to the reaction with NO and superoxide, resulting in peroxinitrite, which nitrosylates the aromatic amino acids in the endothelial membrane, thereby causing an impairment of the endothelial barrier function, and finally may result in septic shock (142). This, presumably, is one reason that even a suggestion of an increased mortality risk has been reported in recent analyses (143). Consequently, universal use of immune nutrients is not currently recommended for critically ill patients and should be confined to the surgical and trauma populations (113,143,144).

3.7.4 TAURINE

Taurine (2-aminoethane sulfonic acid) is the most abundant free amine in the intracellular compartment (69). Taurine has a functional role in stabilizing the membrane potential and in bile salt formation, growth modulation, osmoregulation, antioxidation, promotion of calcium transport, and calcium binding to membranes. It exerts positive ionotropic effects on the heart and has antiarrhythmic and antihypertensive effects. It is involved in many metabolic responses in the central nervous system, has an anticonvulsant action, may have an insulinogenic action, and is required for eye function (145). Taurine is capable of influencing programmed cell death in various cell types, depending on the initiating apoptotic stimulus (146), and can affect Fas (CD95/APO-1)-mediated neutrophil apoptosis through the maintenance of calcium homeostasis (147).

There is some evidence that taurine might be indispensable during episodes of catabolic stress. We and others found low extracellular and intracellular taurine concentrations after trauma and infection (70). Low taurine concentrations in plasma, platelets, and urine have been described in infants and children and also in adult trauma patients undergoing taurine-free long-term parenteral nutrition (148–150). Plasma taurine deficiency after intensive chemotherapy or radiotherapy is more severe in patients receiving taurine-free parenteral nutrition than in orally fed patients (151). Low intracellular taurine concentrations in muscle are a typical feature in patients with chronic and acute renal failure, probably because of impaired metabolic conversion of cysteine sulfinic acid to taurine (152,153). Intracellular taurine depletion may be associated with the well known muscle fatigue and arrhythmic episodes that occur in uremia.

3.7.4.1 Taurine Supplementation

Taurine has been characterized as a conditionally essential amide in preterm infants and neonates and is currently incorporated in most neonatal dietary regimens (154). Our understanding of the role of taurine in various pathological functions is based largely on animal studies. More recently, however, there have been a few human studies that provide some insight into possible therapeutic applications. Taurine is obviously important in several medical conditions, such as sepsis, ischemia-reperfusion states, postoperative states, pulmonary fibrosis, cardiac failure, and other conditions (154).

The question arises as to whether taurine supplementation could be beneficial in acute and chronic renal failure, during episodes of catabolic stress, and in other conditions in which it might have a beneficial effect on morbidity or outcome. Free crystalline taurine is available for inclusion in intravenous or enteral preparations. However, we hypothesize that the extremely high intracellular to extracellular transmembrane gradient (250:1) might limit the cellular uptake of taurine. We have proposed a novel binding of taurine to a suitable amino acid carrier in the form of a synthetic taurine conjugate (155). Experimental data strongly suggest improvement in transmembrane transport and intracellular utilization with this conjugate (156).

Taurine might possess biological properties that enable it to act as a potent molecule in the regulation of inflammatory and immunological processes; it also serves as a powerful antioxidant. Taurine is worth considering as a future important member in the growing family of pharmacological nutrients.

3.8 CONCLUSION

More than 300 years ago, John Hunter summarized the paradox of the response to injury: "Impressions are capable of producing or increasing natural actions and are then called *stimuli*, but they are likewise capable of producing too much action, as well as depraved, unnatural, or what we commonly call diseased action" (*Treatise on the Blood Inflammation and Gunshot Wounds*, John Hunter, 1794). Presumably, Hunter perceived that nature must have designed these responses to promote healing and recovery but realized that when responses exceed normal limits, they threaten and jeopardize the life of the host. Therefore, a major goal of modern clinical nutrition is indeed to modify stress response below the extreme and thereby positively influence recovery.

Optimum nutrition support with proteins (amino acids) should be adjusted to the undergoing metabolic state of the patient. The metabolic state is the result of some blend of the response to starvation and the response to injury (insult), infection, or a specific disease. In all cases, adequate energy and protein (nitrogen substrates) are provided to meet the increased requirements of hypercatabolic, hypermetabolic, malnourished (depleted) patients. With current techniques, appropriate nutritional support may be provided with a low incidence of complication. Improved understanding of regulatory mechanisms may lead to novel therapies that could modify the intensity or nature of the injury response, thus altering the consequent metabolic demands. Specific modifications of the composition of amino acid intake might have clinical benefit in certain disease states; such modification is known as disease-specific therapy.

The main focus of this chapter has been the evaluation of the clinical use of protein and amino acids, as well as new nitrogen-containing substrates (dipeptides, conjugates), exerting specific actions on the immune system, maintaining gut integrity, and modifying the metabolic response to trauma, thereby reducing morbidity and mortality. From the experimental and clinical studies to date, the strongest candidate would appear to be glutamine containing dipeptide. Cysteine and taurine are highly interesting substrates with several new functional properties. The growing body of evidence seen in experimental studies should be critically evaluated in future clinical investigations, using highly soluble cysteine containing dipeptides and taurine conjugates.

This compilation may well illustrate how far we have advanced in our knowledge of the importance of changed composition and new nitrogen-containing substrates in modern artificial nutrition. An attempt was also made to highlight directions that hold promise for advancing conditionally essential amino acids in future patient care. There is little question that efforts made to modify the response to disease by nutritional means will be rewarded with improved patient outcome. Surprising and exciting medical progress of yesterday belongs to the medical exercise.

REFERENCES

1. Trunkey, D.D., On the nature of things that go bang in the night, *Surgery*, 92, 123–132, 1982.
2. Trunkey, D.D., In search of solutions, *J. Trauma*, 53, 1189–1191, 2002.
3. Centers for Disease Control, Annual summary I 98: Reported morbidity and mortality in the United States, *Morbidity Mortality WKLY Rep.*, 111, 1983.

4. Suchner, U., Kuhn, K.S., and Fürst P., The scientific basis of immunonutrition, *Proc. Nutr. Soc.*, 59, 553–563, 2000.
5. Abbott, W.C. et al., Nutritional care of the trauma patient, *Surg. Gynecol. Obstet.*, I 57, 1–13, 1983.
6. Biffl, W.L., Moore, E.E., and Haenel, J.B., Nutrition support of the trauma patient, *Nutrition*, 18, 960–965, 2002.
7. Fürst, P. and Stehle, P., Parenteral nutrition substrates, in *Artificial Nutrition Support in Clinical Practice*, Payne-James, J., Grimble, G., and Silk, D., Eds., Greenwich Medical Media Limited, London, 2001, 401–434.
8. Bessey, P.Q., What's new in critical care and metabolism, *J. Am. Coll. Surg.*, 184, 115–125, 1997.
9. Bessey, P.Q., Parenteral nutrition and trauma, in *Parenteral Nutrition*, Rombeau, J.L. and Caldwell, M.D., Eds., W.B. Sanders, Philadelphia, 1986, 471–488.
10. Hasselgren, P.O., Catabolic response to stress and injury: implications for regulation, *World J. Surg.*, 24, 1452–1459, 2000.
11. Trujillo, E.B., Robinson, M.K., and Jacobs, D.O., Feeding critically ill patients: current concepts, *Crit. Care Nurse*, 21, 60–69, 2001.
12. Wernerman, J. and Vinnars, E., The effect of trauma and surgery on interorgan fluxes of amino acids in man, *Clin. Sci.* 73, 129–133, 1987.
13. Martinez, J.A., Portillo, N.I.P., and Larralde, J., Anabolic actions of a mixed beta-adrenergic agonist on nitrogen retention and protein turnover, *Horm. Metab. Res.*, 23, 590–593, 1991.
14. Mantle, D., Delday, M.I., and Maltin, C.A., Effect of clembuterol on protease activities and protein levels in rat muscle, *Muscle Nerve*, 15, 471–478, 1992.
15. Mantle, D. and Reedy, V.R., Adverse and beneficial functions at proteologic enzymes in skeletal muscle: an overview, *Adverse Drug React. Toxicol. Rev.*, 21, 31–49, 2002.
16. Rennie, M.J. and Cuthbertson, D.J.R., Protein and amino acid metabolism in the whole body and in the tissue, in *Artificial Nutrition Support in Clinical Practice*, Payne-James, J.J., Grimble, G., and Silk, D.B.A., Eds., Greenwich Medical Media Limited, London, 2002, 25–50.
17. Douglas, R.G. and Shaw, J.H., Metabolic response to sepsis and trauma, *Br. J. Surg.*, 7, 281–289, 1989.
18. Bessey, P.Q. et al., Combined hormonal infusion simulates the metabolic response to injury, *Ann. Surg.*, 200, 264–281, 1984.
19. Watters, J.M. et al., Introduction of interleukin-l in humans and its metabolic effects, *Surgery*, 98, 298–306, 1985.
20. Frayn, K.N., Hormonal control of metabolism in trauma and sepsis, *Clin. Endocrinol.*, 24, 577–599, 1986.
21. Elwyn, D.H., Nutritional requirements of stressed patients, in *Textbook of Critical Care*, The Society of Critical Care Medicine, Eds., W.B. Saunders, Philadelphia, 1988.
22. Cuthbertson, D.P., The distribution of nitrogen and sulfur in the urine during conditions of increased catabolism, *Biochem. J.*, 25, 236–244, 1931.
23. Cuthbertson, D.P., Observation on the disturbances of metabolism produced by injury to the limbs, *Q. J. Med.*, 1, 223–230, 1932.
24. Duke, J.H. et al., Contribution of protein to caloric expenditure following injury. *Surgery*, 68, 168–174, 1970.
25. Moore, F.D. and Brennan, M.R., Intravenous amino acids, *N. Engl. J. Med.*, 293, 194–195, 1975.
26. Shenkin, A. et al., Biochemical changes associated with severe trauma. *Am. J. Clin. Nutr.*, 33, 2119–2127, 1980.
27. Shaw, J.H.F., Wildbore, M., and Wolfe, R.R., Whole body protein kinetics in severely septic patients, *Ann. Surg.*, 205, 288–294, 1987.
28. Takala, J. and Klossner, J., Branched chain enriched parenteral nutrition in surgical patients, *Clin. Nutr.*, 5, 167–170, 1986.
29. Kinney, J.M. et al., The intensive care patient, in *Nutrition and Metabolism in Patient Care*, Kinney, J.M. et al., Eds., W.B. Saunders, Philadelphia, 1988, 656–671.
30. Rodriguez, D.J. et al., Obligatory negative nitrogen balance following spinal cord injury, *JPEN*, 15, 319–322, 1991.
31. Takala, J., Suojaranta-Ilinen, R., and Pitkänen, O., Nutrition support in trauma and sepsis, in *Artificial Nutrition Support in Clinical Practice*, Payne-James, J., Grimble, G. and Silk, D., Eds., Greenwich Medical Media Limited, London, 2001, 511–522.

32. Kinney, J.M. and Elwyn, D.H., Protein metabolism and injury, *Annu. Rev. Nutr.*, 3, 433–466, 1983.
33. Waterlow, J.C., Garlick, P.J., and Millward, D.J., *Protein Turnover in Mammalian Tissues and in the Whole Body*, Elsvier-North Holland, Amsterdam, 1978.
34. Bier, D.M., Intrinsically difficult problems, the kinetics of body proteins and amino acid in man, *Diab. Metab.*, 5, 111–132, 1989.
35. Pacy, P.J. et al., Stable isotopes as tracers in clinical research, *Ann. Nutr. Metab.*, 33, 65–78, 1989.
36. Kien, C.L. et al., Increased rates of whole body protein synthesis and breakdown in children recovering from burns, *Ann. Surg.*, 187, 383–391, 1978.
37. Long, C.L. et al., Whole body protein synthesis and catabolism in septic man, *Am. J. Clin. Nutr.*, 30, 1340–1344, 1977.
38. Crane, C.W. et al., Protein turnover in patients before and after elective orthopaedic operations, *Br. J. Surg.*, 64, 129–133, 1977.
39. Tashiro, T. et al., Whole body turnover, synthesis and breakdown in patients receiving parenteral nutrition before and after recovery from surgical stress, *JPEN*, 9, 452–455, 1985.
40. O'Keefe, S.J.D., Sender, P.M., and James, W.P.T., Catabolic loss of body nitrogen in response to surgery, *Lancet*, 2, 1035–1037, 1974.
41. Golden, M., Waterlow, J.C., and Picou D., The relationship between dietary intake, weight change, nitrogen balance and protein turnover in man, *Am. J. Clin. Nutr.*, 30, 1345–1350, 1977.
42. Biolo, G. et al., Mechanisms of altered protein turnover in chronic diseases: a review of human kinetic studies, *Curr. Opin. Clin. Nutr. Metabol. Care*, 6, 55–63, 2003.
43. Donati, L. et al., Nutritional and clinical efficacy of ornithine-α-ketoglutarate in severe burn patients, *Clin. Nutr.*, 18, 307–311, 1999.
44. Wolfe, R.R., Relation of metabolic studies to clinical nutrition: the example of burn injury, *ASCN*, 64, 800–808, 1996.
45. Rennie, M.J., Muscle protein turnover and the wasting due to injury and disease, *Br. Med. Bull.*, 41, 257–264, 1985.
46. Tomkins, A.M. et al., The combined effects of infection and malnutrition on protein metabolism in children, *Clin. Sci.*, 65, 313–324, 1983.
47. Mitchell, L.A. and Norton, L.W., Effect of cancer plasma on skeletal muscle metabolism, *J. Surg. Res.*, 47, 423–426, 1989.
48. Arnold, J. et al., Increased whole-body protein breakdown predominates over increased whole-body protein synthesis in multiple organ failure, *Clin. Sci.*, 84, 655–661, 1993.
49. Blazes, C. et al., Quantitative contribution by skeletal muscle on elevated rates of whole-body protein breakdown in burned children as measured by 3-methylhistidine output, *Metabolism*, 27, 671–676, 1978.
50. Long, C.L. et al., Urinary excretion of 3-methylhistidine: an assessment of muscle protein catabolism in adult normal subjects and during malnutrition, sepsis and skeletal trauma, *Metabolism*, 30, 765–776, 1981.
51. Williamson, D.H. et al., Muscle-protein catabolism after injury in man, as measured by urinary excretion of 3-methylhistidine, *Clin. Sci. Mol. Med.*, 52, 527–533, 1977.
52. Neuhäuser, M. et al., Urinary excretion of 3-methylhistidine as an index of muscle protein catabolism in postoperative trauma: the effect of parenteral nutrition, *Metabolism*, 29, 1206–1213, 1980.
53. Kettelhut, I.C., Wing, S.S., and Goldberg, A.L., Endocrine regulation of protein breakdown in skeletal muscle, *Diab. Metab. Rev.*, 4, 751–772, 1988.
54. Hasselgren, P.O., Muscle protein metabolism during sepsis, *Biocehm. Soc. Trans.*, 23, 1019–1025, 1995.
55. Hellerstein, M.K. and Neese, R.A., Mass isotopomer distribution analysis: a technique for measuring biosynthesis and turnover of polymers, *Am. J. Physiol.*, 263, E988–E1001, 1992.
56. Hellerstein, M.K. and Neese, R.A., Mass isotopomer distribution analysis at eight years: theoretical analytic and experimental considerations, *Am. J. Physiol.*, 276, E1146–E1170, 1999.
57. Man, E.B. et al., Plasma α-amino acid nitrogen and serum lipids of surgical patients, *J. Clin. Invest.*, 25, 701–708, 1946.
58. Askanazi, J. et al., Muscle and plasma amino acids after injury: hypocaloric glucose vs. amino acid infusion, *Ann. Surg.*, 191, 465–472, 1980.

59. Dale, G. et al., The effect of surgical operation on venous plasma free amino acids, *Surgery,* 81, 295–301, 1977.
60. Stinnett, J.D. et al., Plasma and skeletal muscle amino acids following severe burn injury in patients and experimental animals, *Ann. Surg.*, 195, 75–89, 1982.
61. Fürst, P. et al., Influence of amino acid supply on nitrogen and amino acid metabolism in severe trauma, *Acta Chir. Scand.*, 494, 136–138, 1979.
62. Aulick, L.H. and Wilmore, D.W., Increased peripheral amino acid release following burn injury, *Surgery,* 85, 560–565, 1979.
63. Hutchinson, M.L., Clemans, G.W., and Detter, F., Abnormal plasma amino acid profiles in patients undergoing bone marrow transplant, *Clin. Nutr.*, 3, 133, 1984.
64. Cynober, L., Amino acid metabolism in thermal burns, *JPEN*, 13, 196–205, 1989.
65. Cynober, L. et al., Plasma and urinary amino acid pattern in severe burn patients: evolution throughout the healing period, *Am. J. Clin. Nutr.*, 36, 416–425, 1982.
66. Woolf, L.I. et al. Arterial plasma amino acids in patients with serious postoperative infection and in patients with major fractures, *Surgery,* 79, 283–292, 1976.
67. Jeevanandam, M., Trauma and sepsis, in *Amino Acid Metabolism and Therapy in Health and Nutritional Disease*, Cynober, L., Ed., CRC Press, Boca Raton, FL, 1995, 245–255.
68. Wilmore, D.W. et al., Effect of injury and infection on visceral metabolism and circulation, *Ann. Surg.*, 192, 491–504, 1980.
69. Bergström, J. et al., Intracellular free amino acid concentration in human muscle tissue, *J. Appl. Physiol.*, 36, 693–697, 1974.
70. Fürst, P., Intracellular muscle free amino acids: their measurement and function, *Proc. Nutr. Soc.*, 42, 451–462, 1983.
71. Fürst, P., Alvestrand, A. and Bergström, J., Branched-chain amino acids and branched-chain keto acids in uremia, in *Branched Chain Amino Acids: Biochemistry, Physiopathology and Clinical Science,* Schauder, P. et al., Eds., Raven Press Ltd., New York, 1992, 173–186.
72. Askanazi, J. et al., Muscle and plasma amino acids after injury: the role of inactivity, *Ann. Surg.*, 188, 797–803, 1978.
73. Askanazi, J. et al., Muscle and plasma amino acids following injury: influence of intercurrent infection, *Ann. Surg.*, 192, 78–85, 1980.
74. Milewski, P.J. et al., Intracellular free amino acids in undernourished patients with and without sepsis, *Clin. Sci.*, 62, 83–91, 1982.
75. Roth, E. et al., Metabolic disorders in severe abdominal sepsis: glutamine deficiency in skeletal muscle, *Clin. Nutr.*, 1, 5–41, 1982.
76. Roth, E. et al., Amino acid concentrations in plasma and skeletal muscle of patients with acute hemorrhagic necrotizing pancreatitis, *Clin. Chem.*, 31, 1305–1309, 1985.
77. Souba, W.W., Glutamine: a key substrate for the splanchnic bed, *Annu. Rev. Nutr.*, 11, 285–308, 1991.
78. Rennie, M.J. et al., Skeletal muscle glutamine transport, intramuscular glutamine concentration, and muscle protein turnover, *Metabolism*, 38, 47–51, 1989.
79. Plumley, D.A., Souba, W.W., and Hautamaki, R.D., Accelerated lung amino acid release in hyperdynamic septic surgical patients, *Arch. Surg.*, 125, 1761, 1990.
80. Roth, E. et al., Liver amino acids in sepsis, *Surgery,* 97, 436–442, 1985.
81. Jeevanandam, M. and Ali, M.R., Altered tissue amino acid levels in traumatized, growing rats due to ornithine-alpha-ketoglutarate supplemented oral diet, *J. Clin. Ntr. Gastroenterol.*, 6, 23–28, 1991.
82. Caballero, B., Gleason, R.E., and Wurtman, R.T., Plasma amino acid concentrations in healthy elderly men and women, *Am. J. Clin. Nutr.*, 53, 1249–1252, 1991.
83. Wells, F.E. and Smits, B., Leucocyte amino acid concentrations and their relationships to changes in plasma amino acids, *JPEN*, 4, 264–268, 1980.
84. Ali, R. et al., Altered amino acid (AA) levels due to remote trauma in cerebrospinal fluid (CSF), *FASEB J.*, 7, A646, 1993.
85. Häussinger, D. et al., Cellular hydration state: an important determinant of protein catabolism in health and disease, *Lancet*, 341, 1330–1332, 1993.
86. Fürst, P., Old and new substrates in clinical nutrition, *J. Nutr.*, 128, 789–796, 1998.
87. Mitchell, H.H., *Comparative Nutrition of Man and Domestic Animals*, vol. 1, Academic Press, New York, 1962.

88. Young, V.E. and Tharakan, J.F., Nutritional essentiality of amino acids and amino acid requirements in healthy adults, in *Metabolic and Therapeutic Aspects of Amino Acids in Clinical Nutrition*, Cynober, L., Ed., CRC Press, Boca Raton, FL, 2004, 439–464.

89. Grimble, G.K, The significance of peptides in clinical nutrition, *Annu. Rev. Nutr.,* 14, 419–447, 1994.

90. Wilmore, D.W., The practice of clinical nutrition: how to prepare for the future, *JPEN*, 13, 337–343, 1989.

91. Fürst P. and Stehle, P., What are the essential elements needed for the determination of amino acid requirements in humans?, *J. Nutr.*, 2004, 134, 1558S–1565S.

92. Brennan, M.F. et al., Report of a research workshop: branched chain amino acids in stress and injury, *JPEN*, 10, 446–452, 1986.

93. Fürst, P. and Stehle, P., Glutamine and glutamine-containing dipeptides, in *Metabolic and Therapeutic Aspects of Amino Acids in Clinical Nutrition*, Cynober, L., Ed., CRC Press, Boca Raton, FL, 2004, 613–631.

94. Bode, B.P. and Souba, W.W., Modulation of cellular proliferation alters glutamine transport and metabolism in human heptoma cells, *Ann. Surg.*, 220: 411–424, 1994.

95. Fürst P., New developments in glutamine delivery, *J. Nutr.*, 131, 2562S–2568S, 2001.

96. Khan, K. et al., The stability of L-glutamine in total parenteral nutrition, *Clin. Nutr.*, 10, 193, 1991.

97. Novak, F. et al., Glutamine supplementation in serious illness: a systematic review of the evidence, *Crit. Care Med.*, 30, 2022–2029, 2002.

98. Goeters, C. et al., Parenteral L-alanyl-L-glutamine improves 6-month outcome in critically ill patients, *Crit. Care Med.*, 30, 2032, 2002.

99. Fürst, P., Conditionally indispensable amino acids in enteral feeding and the dipeptide concept, in *Proteins Peptides and Amino Acids in Enteral Nutrition*, Fürst, P. and Young, V., Eds., Karger, Basel, 2000, 199–219.

100. Hondijk, A.P. et al., Randomized trial of glutamine-enriched enteral nutrition on infections morbidity in patients with multiple trauma, *Lancet*, 352, 772–776, 1998.

101. Conejero, R. et al., Effect of a glutamine-enriched enteral diet on intestinal permeability and infectious morbidity at 28 days in critically ill patients with systemic inflammatory response syndrome: a randomized single-blind, prospective, multicenter study, *Nutrition*, 18, 716–721, 2002.

102. Griffiths, R.D., Nutrition support in critically ill septic patients, *Curr. Opin. Clin. Nutr. Metabol. Care*, 6, 203–210, 2003.

103. Murray, S.M. and Pindoria, S., Nutrition support for bone marrow transplant patients, *Cochrane Database Syst. Rev.*, CD002920, 2002.

104. Griffiths, R.D., Jones, C., and Palmer, T.E., Six-month outcome of critically ill patients given glutamine-supplemented parenteral nutrition, *Nutrition*, 13, 295–302, 1997.

105. Griffiths, R.D. et al., Infection, multiple organ failure, and survival in the intensive care unit: influence of glutamine-supplemented parenteral nutrition on acquired infection, *Nutrition*, 18, 546–552, 2002.

106. Hardy, G., Does glutamine enable severely ill intensive care patients to cope better with infection and increase their chance of survival?, *Nutrition*, 18, 712–713, 2002.

107. Vincent, J., Nosocomial infection and outcome, *Nutrition*, 18, 713–714, 2002.

108. Wilmore, D.W., Glutamine saves lives! What does it mean?, *Nutrition*, 13, 375, 1997.

109. Harward, T.R. et al., Glutamine preserves gut glutathione levels during intestinal ischemia/reperfusion, *J. Surg. Res.*, 56, 351, 1994.

110. Yun, J.C. et al., Alanyl-glutamine preserves hepatic glutathione stores after 5-FU treatment, *Clin. Nutr.*, 15, 261, 1996.

111. Fläring, U.B. et al., Glutamine attenuates post-traumatic glutathione depletion in human muscle, *Clin. Sci.* (Lond.), 104, 275–282, 2003.

112. Fürst, P., A thirty-year odyssey in nitrogen metabolism: from ammonium to dipeptides, *JPEN*, 24, 197–209, 2000.

113. Heyland, D.K. et al., Canadian clinical practice guidelines for nutrition support in mechanically ventilated, critically ill patients, *JPEN*, 27, 355–373, 2003.

114. Wilmore, D.W., Why should a single nutrient reduce mortality? *Crit. Care Med.*, 30, 2153–2154, 2002.

115. Gaull, G., Sturman, J.A., and Räihä, N.C.R., Development of mammalian sulfur metabolism: absence of cystathionase in human fetal tissues, *Pediatr. Res.*, 6, 538–547, 1972.

116. Di Buono, M. et al., Dietary cysteine reduces methionine requirement in men, *Am. J. Clin. Nutr.,* 74, 761–766, 2001.

117. Chawla, R.K. et al., Plasma cysteine, cystine and glutathione in cirrhosis, *Gastroenterology,* 87, 770–776, 1984.

118. Mihm, S. and Dröge, W., Intracellular glutathione level controls DNA binding activity of NFB-like proteins, *Immunobiology,* 181, 245–247, 1990.

119. Mihm, S., Ennen, J., and Pessagra, U., Inhibition of HIV-1 replication and NFB activity by cysteine and cysteine derivatives, *AIDS,* 5, 497–503, 1991.

120. Grimble, R.F. and Grimble, G.K., Immunonutrition: role of sulfur amino acids, related amino acids, and polyamines, *Nutrition,* 14, 605–610, 1998.

121. Roederer, M. et al., N-acetylcysteine: potential for AIDS therapy, *Pharmacology,* 46, 121–129, 1992.

122. Dröge, W., Cysteine and glutathione deficiency in AIDS patients: a rationale for the treatment with N-acetyl-cysteine, *Pharmacology,* 46, 612–615, 1993.

123. Steginik, L.D. and Den Besten, L., Synthesis of cysteine from methionine in normal adult subjects: effect of route of alimentation, *Science,* 178, 514–516, 1972.

124. Spapen, H.D. et al., N-acetylcysteine and cardiac dysfunction in human septic shock, *Clin. Intens. Care,* 13, 27–32, 2002.

125. Fürst, P. et al., Design of parenteral synthetic dipeptides for clinical nutrition: *in vitro* and *in vivo* utilization, *Ann. Nutr. & Metab.,* 41, 10–21, 1997.

126. Stehle P. et al., Intravenous dipeptide metabolism and the design of synthetic dipeptides for clinical nutrition, in *Peptides in Mammalian Protein Metabolism,* Grimble, G.K. and Backwell, F.R.C., Eds., Portland Press Ltd., London, 1998, 103–118.

127. Barbul, A., Arginine: biochemistry, physiology and therapeutic implications, *J. Parenter. Enter. Nutr.,* 10, 227–238, 1986.

128. Blachier, F. et al., Arginine metabolism in rat enterocytes, *Biochem. Biophys. Acta,* 1092, 304–310, 1991.

129. Cynober, L., Can arginine and ornithine support gut functions?, *Gut,* 35, S42–S45, 1994.

130. Kubes, P., Ischemia-reperfusion in feline small intestine: a role for nitric oxide, *Am. J. Physiol.,* 264, G143–G149, 1993.

131. Miller, M.J. et al., Nitric oxide release in response to gut injury, *Scand. J. Gastroenterol.,* 28, 149–154, 1993.

132. Schmidt, M. and Martindale, R., Nutraceuticals in critical care nutrition, in *Nutrition and Critical Care,* Cynober, L. and Moore, F.A., Eds., Karger, Basel, 2003, 245–265.

133. Kirk, S.S. and Barbul, A., Role of arginine in trauma, sepsis and immunity, *JPEN,* 14, 226–229, 1990.

134. Evoy, D., Lieberman, M., Fahey III, T., and Daley, J., Immunonutrition: the role of arginine, *Nutrition,* 14, 611–617, 1998.

135. Daly, J.M., Reynolds, J., and Thom, A., Immune and metabolic effects of arginine in the surgical patient, *Ann. Surg.,* 298, 512–523, 1988.

136. Barbul, A. et al., Arginine enhances wound healing and lymphocyte response in humans, *Surgery,* 108, 331–337, 1990.

137. Sodeyama, M. et al., Sepsis impairs gut amino acid absorption, *Am. J. Surg.,* 165, 150–154, 1993.

138. Lin, E., Goncalves, J.A., and Lowry, S.F., Efficacy of nutritional pharmacology in surgical patients, *Curr. Opin. Clin. Nutr. Metab. Care,* 1, 41–50, 1998.

139. Atkinson, S., Seiffert, E., and Bihari, D., A prospective randomized double-blind clinical trial of enteral immunonutrition in the critically ill, *Crit. Care Med.,* 26, 1164–1172, 1998.

140. Kudsk, K.A. et al., A randomized trial of isonitrogenous enteral diets after severe trauma: an immune-enhancing diet reduces septic complications, *Ann. Surg,* 224, 531–540, 1996.

141. Vinnars, E., Fürst, P., and Hallgren, B., The nutritive effect in man of non-essential amino-acids infused intravenously (together with the essential ones). I. Individual non-essential amino acids, *Acta Anaesthesiol. Scand.,* 14, 147–172, 1972.

142. Frank, J., Pompella, A., and Biesalski, K.H., Histochemical visualisation of oxidant stress, *Free Radic. Biol. Med.,* 29, 1096–1105, 2000.

143. Heyland, D.K. and Samis, A., Does immune nutrition in septic patients do more harm than good?, *Int. Care Med.,* 29, 669–671, 2003.

144. Heyland, D.K. et al., Should immunonutrition become routine in critically ill patients? A systematic review of the evidence, *JAMA*, 286, 944–953, 2001.
145. Huxtable, R.I., Physiological actions of taurine, *Physiol. Rev.*, 72, 101–163, 1992.
146. Wang, J.H. et al., The beneficial effect of taurine on the prevention of human endothelial cell death, *Shock*, 6, 331–338, 1996.
147. Condron, C., Taurine attenuates calcium-dependent, Fas-mediated neutrophil apoptosis, *Shock*, 19, 564–569, 2003.
148. Geggel, H.S. et al., Nutritional requirement for taurine in patients receiving long-term parenteral nutrition, *N. Engl. J. Med.*, 312, 142–146, 1985.
149. Heird, W.C. et al., Pediatric parenteral amino acid mixture in low birth weight infants, *Pediatrics*, 81, 41–50, 1988.
150. Kopple, J.D. et al., Effect of intravenous taurine supplementation on plasma, blood cell and urine taurine concentrations in adults undergoing long-term parenteral nutrition, *Am. J. Clin. Nutr.*, 52, 846–853, 1990.
151. Desai, T.I.C. et al., Taurine deficiency after intensive chemotherapy and/or radiation, *Am. J. Clin. Nutr.*, 55, 708–711, 1992.
152. Bergström, J. et al., Sulfur amino acids in plasma and muscle in patients with chronic renal failure: evidence for taurine depletion, *J. Intern. Med.*, 226, 189–194, 1989.
153. Suliman, M.E., Anderstam, B., and Bergström, J., Evidence of taurine depletion and accumulation of cysteinesulfinic acid in chronic dialysis patients, *Kidney Int.*, 50, 1713–1717, 1996.
154. Redmond, H.P. et al., Immunonutrition: the role of taurine, *Nutrition*, 14, 599–604, 1998.
155. Fürst et al., Reappraisal of indispensable amino acids. Design of parenteral synthetic dipeptides: synthetic and characterization, *Ann. Nutr. & Metab.*, 41, 1–9, 1997.
156. Hummel, M. et al., Intestinal taurine availability from synthetic amino acid-taurine conjugates: an *in vitro* perfusion study in rats, *Clin. Nutr.*, 16, 137–139, 1997.

4 Lipid Metabolism: Comparison of Stress and Nonstressed States

Dan L. Waitzberg, Raquel S. Torrinhas, and Letícia De Nardi
University of São Paulo Medical School

CONTENTS

4.1 BASIC CONCEPTS

4.1.1 DEFINITION

The word *lipid* is derived from the Greek *lipos*, meaning fat. The lipids are products of biological origin, consisting of groups of fatty acids (FAs): carboxylic acids with long, unbranched chains, formed by an even number of carbon atoms connected by simple or double bonds. They can be found in various forms, as described in Table 4.1.

TABLE 4.1
Various Forms of Fats

Form	Examples
Oils	Esters formed from fatty acids (FAs) that present in liquid form
Fats	Esters formed from FAs that present in solid form
Waxes	The principal components are esters formed from FA and long-chain alcohols
Steroids	Cholesterol and sex hormones
Others	Soaps, detergents, and biliary salts

4.1.2 NOMENCLATURE/CLASSIFICATION

The following list shows how fatty acids are characterized:

- By the number of atoms in the carbon chain:
  - Long chain — 14 to 20 carbon atoms
  - Medium chain — 6 to 12 carbon atoms
  - Short chain — Up to 6 carbon atoms
- By the number of double bonds:
  - Saturated fats — No double bonds
  - Monounsaturated fats — One double bond
  - Polyunsaturated fats — More than one double bond
- In the case of unsaturated fatty acids, by the position of the first double bond counting from the methyl radical (represented by the Greek letter omega: ω) or starting from its functional group (represented by the letter delta: Δ).[2] See the example in Figure 4.1.

The various types of fatty acids and their principal sources are described briefly in Table 4.2.[3]
The lipids can be further classified into simple, composite, or variable, according to their composition:[4]

- Simple — FAs, neutral fats (steroids of FAs with glycerol, such as triglycerides), waxes (steroids of FAs with alcohols, such as cholesterol esters)
- Composite — Phospholipids (composed of phosphoric acid, FA, and a nitrogenated base), glycolipids (composed of FA, monosaccharide, and a nitrogenated base), lipoprotein (lipid particles and protein)
- Variable — Steroids (such as cholesterol, vitamin D, biliary salts), vitamins A, E, K.

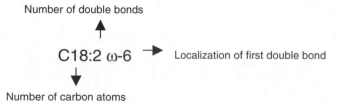

FIGURE 4.1 Linoleic acid: 18 carbons in the chain (long-chain fatty acid) and with two double bonds (polyunsaturated), of which the first is located in the sixth carbon.

TABLE 4.2
Types of Fatty Acids and their Principal Sources

Saturated			Monounsaturated	Polyunsaturated	
Short Chain	Medium Chain	Long Chain	ω-9	ω-6	ω-3
Acetic	Capric	Myristic	Oleic	Linoleic 18:2	α-Linolenic
Propionic	Caprylic	Palmitic	Palmitoleic		
Butyric	Capric	Stearic		γ-Linolenic 18:3	EPA 20:5
	Lauric	Arachidic		DHA 22:6	
				Arachidonic 20:4	
		Sources			
Butter	Coconut	Animal fat	Olive oil	Safflower oil	Fish oil
Fibers	Palms	Cocoa	Rapeseed oil	Soybean oil	Nut oil
				Corn oil	Rapeseed oil
				Cotton oil	Soybean oil
				Sunflower oil	

TABLE 4.3
Main Functions of Lipids

Energy supply through foods (9.3 Kcal/g), essential fatty acids, and liposoluble vitamins (A, D, E, K)
Stored combustible energy (where 95% is in the form of triglycerides), principally for periods of fasting
Mechanical protection (bones and organs) and maintenance of body temperature
Synthesis of cellular structures, such as phospholipid membrane
Synthesis of hormones
Transport of liposoluble vitamins
Intra- and extracellular mediators of immune response
Participation in inflammatory process and in oxidative stress

4.1.3 FUNCTION

In basic terms, the lipids are a source of energy with a high caloric density (9.3 Kcal/g). They also have a role in the synthesis of hormones and cellular structures, the transportation of liposoluble vitamins, intracellular and extracellular signaling, and the supply of essential fatty acids.[3] The main functions of the lipids are outlined in Table 4.3.

4.2 BASIC HUMAN PHYSIOLOGY AND LIPID BIOCHEMISTRY

4.2.1 INGESTION

The daily energy requirement of humans is generally provided by FAs ingested in the diet. However, when necessary, FAs (saturated or monounsaturated) can be synthesized from glucose and amino acids through enzymatic elongation reactions (by adding units of two carbons) and desaturation (creation of new double bonds).[3] The desaturation mechanism is stimulated by insulin and inhibited by glucose, adrenaline, and glucagon.[3]

However, we do not produce specific desaturating enzymes (-12 and -15 desaturase) responsible for adding a double bond before the ninth carbon at the end of the methyl (distal) extremity.

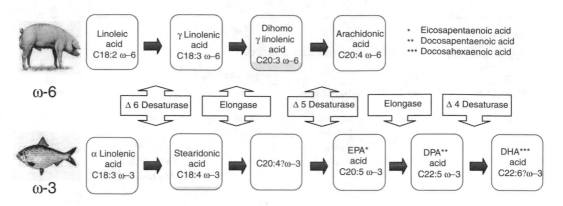

FIGURE 4.2 Formation of new long chain ω-6 and ω-3 polyunsaturated fatty acids from α-linoleic and α-linolenic essential fatty acids.

Consequently, the long-chain polyunsaturated fatty acids (PUFAs), namely ω-6 (α-linoleic acid) and ω-3 (α-linolenic acid), cannot be produced endogenously. These are obtained exclusively from diet and are therefore denominated essential.[3]

The daily requirements of ω-6 and ω-3 essential fatty acids are 3% and 5%, respectively, of the total caloric ingestion. However, the diet typical of Western nations and other industrialized countries is rich in ω-6 PUFA (7 to 10%) and contains little ω-3 PUFA, which explains the great predominance of the former in cellular membrane structures.

By sequential enzymatic processes of elongation and desaturation, linoleic acid forms γ-linolenic acid, which is in turn converted into arachidonic acid. By the same metabolic pathway and in a competitive manner, α-linolenic acid is converted into eicosapentaenoic acid (EPA) and docosahexaenoic acid (DHA), as shown in Figure 4.2. These FAs participate in the composition of cellular membranes and are precursors of eicosanoids, which regulate the immune and inflammatory functions.[5]

Certain derivatives of essential FAs, such as dihomogammalinolenic and arachidonic acid (both ω-6) and eicosapentaenoic acid (ω-3) are especially important because they are precursors of lipid mediators involved in many physiological functions.[5]

Insufficient ingestion of essential FAs can cause immunological dysfunction, dermatitis, alopecia, thrombocytopenia, and poor cicatrization. The main symptoms and clinical signs of ω-6 and ω-3 deficiency are given in Table 4.4.

4.2.2 DIGESTION

Fats are frequently consumed in the form of triglycerides (three molecules of fatty acids and one of glycerol). Due to their molecular complexity and hydrophobic nature, triglycerides require the action of various enzymes and mechanical movement in order to be broken down and absorbed by the digestive system.

The process of digesting lipids begins in the stomach, with emulsification by physical movements (propulsion, retropropulsion, and mixing) and by enzymatic action (through the lingual and gastric lipases). The lingual and gastric lipases are efficient in the emulsification and breaking down of medium-chain fatty acids.[6]

The digestion of food and nutrients principally takes place in the small bowel, where the secretion of cholecystokinin (CCK) occurs in response to the presence of fats and proteins. CCK stimulates the secretion and release of bile by the liver and gall bladder. The bile (rich in biliary salts and phospholipids) intensifies the emulsification process, thereby increasing the surface area and favoring the enzymatic action on the fats.[7]

TABLE 4.4
Clinical Symptoms of the Deficiency of Essential Fatty Acids

Deficiency	Clinical Symptoms
Omega-6 fatty acids	Skin lesions
	Anemia
	Augmented platelet aggregation
	Thrombocytopenia
	Hepatic steatosis
	Delayed cicatrization
	Increased susceptibility to infections
	In children: growth retardation and diarrhea
Omega-3 fatty acids	Neurological symptoms
	Reduction in visual acuity
	Skin lesions
	Growth retardation
	Impaired learning capacity
	Abnormal electroretinogram

The principal enzymes involved in the duodenal digestion of lipids are pancreatic lipase, phospholipase-A$_2$, and cholesterol esterase.[7]

4.2.3 ABSORPTION

The absorptive process of FAs varies in relation to the length of their carbon chains. The long-chain fatty acids (LCFAs) are absorbed in the brush border of the enterocytes and migrate to the smooth endoplasmic reticulum, where the resynthesis of the triglycerides (TGs) occurs. The TGs are incorporated into the apolipoproteins, resynthesized phospholipids, and cholesterol, forming the lipoproteins that reach the circulation through the lymphatic system.

After passing through the enterocytes, the medium-chain fatty acids (MCFAs) bind to albumin. Most of the MCFAs are conducted to the liver by the blood stream and not by lymphatic transport, which is used mainly for the LCFAs.[3] The short-chain fatty acids (SCFAs) can be produced via the bacterial fermentation of fibers, especially the soluble ones; they are absorbed directly in the large intestine and used as a source of energy. The SCFAs produced in the intestine are acetic, butyric, and propionic acid.[8] SCFAs absorbed in the intestinal lumen do not necessarily reach the circulation, because in general they are used in the metabolism of the colonocytes. The absorption of the liposoluble vitamins A, D, E, K, all the fats, and cholesterol occurs in the ileum.

4.2.4 TRANSPORT

After their intestinal absorption, the FAs are transported in the blood stream to be used by the liver and peripheral tissues, or for storage in the adipose tissue.

The FAs are conducted in various forms: free fatty acids (bonded to albumin), chylomicrons, and lipoproteins (composed of cholesterol esters, phospholipids, and triglycerides). The transportation pathway can be either exogenous (transport of the dietary lipids from the intestine to the liver) or endogenous (transport of the lipoproteins synthesized in the hepatocytes to the peripheral tissues).[9,10]

The LCFAs have a strong affinity for binding with albumin, unlike MCFAs and SCFAs, which do not need to bind with this protein in order to be transported.

The FAs can be transported through the blood stream by lipoproteins of various densities, depending on the locality of production:[11]

- When originating from intestinal absorption, they are transported in the form of chylo-microns (lipoprotein rich in dietary triglycerides with a density of 0.92 to 0.96 g/l).
- When produced by the liver, they are transported through VLDL (very low-density lipoprotein with a density of 0.95 to 1.0 g/l), LDL (low-density lipoprotein with a density of 1.0 to 1.06 g/l), and HDL (high-density lipoprotein with a density of 1.06 to 1.21 g/l).

The VLDLs are formed in the liver and transported to the adipocytes, where hydrolysis, reesterification, and storage of TG occur. Hepatic lipase action transforms VLDL into LDL by removal of TG.

The LDLs are a part of the metabolic pathway of cholesterol-rich lipoproteins. They remain longer in the vascular compartment and are responsible for the distribution of cholesterol to the extrahepatic tissues.

Cholesterol released by LDL is incorporated into the cellular membranes and stored in the form of cholesterol ester or used for synthesis of steroid hormones. In hypercholesterolemia, elevated levels of LDL favor the generation of an oxidized form (LDL-ox), which is extremely atherogenic.

HDLs play a fundamental role in the reverse transport of cholesterol, by removing excess from the peripheral tissues and transporting it to the liver, where it is metabolized and eliminated in the form of acid and biliary salts.[12]

The principal function of the chylomicrons is to supply energy to the peripheral tissues through the release of free FAs. Contact with the capillary endothelium stimulates the lipoprotein lipase (LPL) enzyme, which releases TGs and generates free FAs that are used as energy substrate or stored.[13]

Recently, a family of proteins known as *fatty acid–binding proteins* (FABPs) has been identified that seems to have an important role in the transfer of these acids through the membrane, besides making them available for metabolizing. When managing the distribution of FAs through the organelles, FABPs modulate their utilization as metabolites of energy and storage.[14] Furthermore, they have an effect on cellular differentiation and functionality, besides the proliferation and regulation of genetic transcription.[15,16]

4.2.5 CELLULAR UTILIZATION OF LIPIDS

Lipids can be used as an energy source through a β-oxidation reaction within the mitochondria. Upon reaching the cells to be oxidized, the FAs pass through the cellular membrane to the cytosol. However, before oxidation can effectively take place in the matrix, they must also cross the barrier represented by the mitochondrial membrane. For this, LCFAs need the aid of carnitine, which is activated by specific enzymes (Figure 4.3). MCFAs are more soluble in water than LCFAs and can get into the mitochondria with partial independence from the aid of carnitine (only 10 to 20%). Nevertheless, in muscle tissue MCFAs are totally dependent on the activity of carnitine as a carrier. Once inside the mitochondria, FAs serve as substrate for beta oxidation and energy synthesis.[3]

FAs can also be useful, in a selective manner, in the synthesis of the phospholipids of cellular and organelle membranes. In humans, the predominant FAs incorporated in the membranes are EPAs and DHAs (ω-3), arachidonic acid (ω-6), and oleic acid (ω-9).[17] The lipids' cellular distribution is generally specific, but it can be altered by the availability of fats in the diet, especially PUFAs.[18]

The essential FAs can cause structural and functional alterations in the phospholipidic membrane (including immune system cells), modifying their stability, their permeability, the activity of receptors and enzymes, their transport, regulatory functions, and cellular metabolism.[19,20] In addition, they can activate intracellular routing of signals by the formation of biologically active molecules that act as secondary messengers and inflammatory mediators called *eicosanoids*.[17,21]

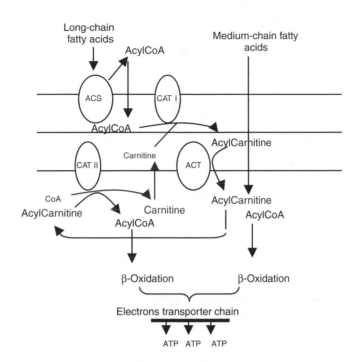

FIGURE 4.3 The long-chain fatty acids cross the mitochondrial membrane with the help of carnitine, after activation of the CoA-fatty acids by acetyl-CoA synthesis (ACS), where CoA is exchanged for carnitine by the action of carnitine acetyltransferase I (CATI). The carnitine fatty acid is then transported into the intramitochondrial space, where the inverse effect occurs through the action of carnitine acetyltransferase II (CATII). The carnitine group returns to the intermembrane space through the action of carnitine acylcarnitine translocase (ACT). Once inside the mitochondria, the fatty acids become substrate for the machinery of beta oxidation to provide energy.

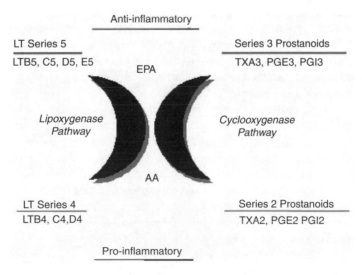

FIGURE 4.4 LT = leukotriene; TX = thromboxane; PG = prostaglandin; EPA = elcosapentaenoic acid; AA = arachidonic acid.

There are two pathways for the synthesis of eicosanoids: cyclooxygenase and lipoxygenase, which, respectively, produce prostanoids (thromboxane, prostaglandin) and leukotriene and lipoxin (Figure 4.4).

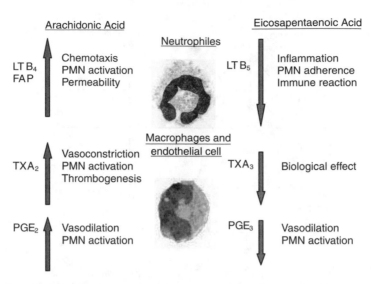

FIGURE 4.5 The role of eicosanoids, resulting from the metabolism of arachidonic acid and eicosapentaenoic acid, on the functions of phagocytic cells.[27] PMN = polymorphonuclear, LTB = leukotriene B, TXA = thromboxane, PGE = prostaglandin, FAP = platelet aggregation factor.

The eicosanoids participate in various cellular and physiological events, modulating processes such as platelet aggregation, smooth muscle contraction, leukocyte chemotaxis, inflammatory cytokine production, and immune functions.[22] In an inflammatory picture, there is an increase in the even number series eicosanoids, produced by the metabolism of ω-6 FAs. High levels of some of these eicosanoids are also found in patients with inflammatory conditions or sepsis and in critically ill patients.

The eicosanoids modulate the inflammatory response in different ways. Eicosanoids originating from the metabolism of PUFA-type ω-6 are potent inflammatory mediators, but those of the odd number series, originating from the metabolism of ω-3 PUFA, result in an attenuated inflammatory response.[23] This indicates that ω-3 FAs have the capacity to inhibit an acute inflammatory response induced or aggravated by eicosanoids derived from the metabolism of ω-6 FAs. The role of eicosanoids, resulting from the metabolism of arachidonic acid and eicosapentaenoic acid, on phagocytic cells is depicted in Figure 4.5.

The eicosanoids regulate the production of several cytokines involved in inflammation. Prostaglandin 2, originating from ω-6 FAs, produces several proinflammatory effects that include fever, increased vascular permeability, and vasodilation, but inhibits the production of IL-1, IL-2, IL-6, and TNF-α.[24] On the other hand, leukotrienes of series 4 increase the production of IL-1, IL-2, and IL-6 and augment lymphocyte proliferation.[24] With the increased offer of ω-3 PUFAs in relation to ω-6 PUFAs, the synthesis of prostaglandins and leukotrienes of the even number series is reduced, thereby modulating the inflammatory cytokines, particularly in humans.[25–27]

The capacity of ω-3 FAs in antagonizing the production of eicosanoids derived from the metabolism of ω-6 FAs constitutes a key point in the anti-inflammatory effect attributed to ω-3 FAs, but these fatty acids also exert other effects that seem to be independent of the modulation of eicosanoid production. Preliminary scientific evidence indicates that, in cellular culture models, ω-3 FAs can influence the production of cytokines, thus directly inhibiting the production of TNF-α and interleukins IL-1β and IL-6 by immunocompetent cells.[28]

Inhibition of the liberation of proinflammatory cytokines by ω-3 FAs appears to be associated with their participation in the activation of perixome proliferator-activated receptors (PPARs), nuclear receptors that can antagonize the signaling pathways of nuclear transcription factor NFkB.[29]

NFkB is responsible for the transcription of genes involved in the inflammatory response, including cytokines, adhesion molecules, and other mediators of proinflammatory signals. PPARs also control the duration and intensity of the inflammatory response, because they induce the expression of genes that codify proteins involved in the catabolism of lipid proinflammatory mediators.[30–32] Additionally, multiple genes that modulate lipid metabolism are regulated by PPARs and their ligand activators through adjustment of the expression of gene encoding for proteins.[33]

4.2.6 Storage

Lipids are stored in the form of triglycerides, which are molecules comprising three esters of FA (saturated, monounsaturated, or polyunsaturated) and an alcohol (glycerol). The deposit of triglycerides occurs mainly in the adipose tissue, a specialized type of connective tissue that acts primarily as a major fat deposit. In humans, adipose tissue accounts for approximately 15% of the body weight of a normal adult male and is equivalent to about two months of energy reserve.

There are two types of adipose tissue: white and brown. Brown, tan, or multilocular adipose tissue has a special function in the regulation of the body temperature in newborns, whereas deposits of this tissue are practically nonexistent in adults.[34] White, yellow, or unilocular adipose tissue is widely distributed in the subcutaneous tissues. The blood flow for this tissue varies depending on the body weight and nutritional state, because it increases during fasting. It also possesses nerve fibers, comprising part of the sympathetic nervous system.[35] TGs ingested in food are the main components of the fat deposits, but excess carbohydrate and dietary proteins can also be converted into fatty acids in the liver through lipogenesis.

Under certain metabolic circumstances, a breaking down of triglycerides (lipolysis) can occur, with the release of FAs from the adipose tissue for cellular use in the synthesis of energy. This process prevails over lipogenesis when there is a greater demand for energy. Lipolysis in the adipose tissue can occur through the action of the lipoprotein lipase enzyme or of a lipase sensitive to a hormone, through the stimulation of lipolytic hormones: adrenocorticotropic hormone (ACTH), catecholamines (adrenaline and noradrenaline), growth hormone (GH), glucagon, cortisol, and leptin.

Lipolytic hormones bind to receptors present in the cellular membrane of the adipocytes, triggering a cascade of activation, through cyclic adenosine monophosphate (cAMP), which transports them to the activation of the enzyme hormone-sensitive lipase and consequent hydrolysis of the fatty acids (see schematic representation in Figure 4.6). The concentrations of the lipolytic hormones are directly related to the degree of activation of the sympathetic nervous system (SNS). The antilipolytic hormone is insulin.

In this way, hormones released by nerve stimulation can stimulate lipolysis, through the activation of the hormone-sensitive lipase in the adipocytes, and thereby influence the regulation of the lipid metabolism.

4.3 ALTERATIONS IN METABOLISM DURING FASTING WITHOUT COMPLICATIONS

The response to chronically inadequate alimentary ingestion (fasting) aims to preserve fat-free body mass. It is characterized by a decrease in the expenditure of energy, the use of alternative sources of fuel, and a reduced expenditure of protein. Low seric glucose levels (between 60 and 80 mg/dl) trigger a signal to the brain, notifying it of a hypoglycemia state. In response, counterregulating hormones are released (i.e., cortisol, glucagon, GH, and adrenaline).[13]

A reduction of the plasma insulin concentration, in conjunction with an increase in counterregulating hormones, activates the hormone-sensitive lipase present in the cytoplasm of the adipocytes and of the muscle tissue. In the adipose tissue, the action of this enzyme releases FAs and glycerol from the deposit of triacylglycerol.[13,36]

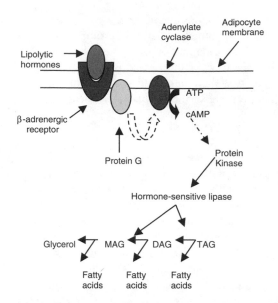

FIGURE 4.6 Action of the lipolytic hormones on the lipolysis of triglycerides. Lipolytic hormones (epinephrine, glucagon, and glucocorticoids) bind to the specific receptor, triggering the activation of the adenylate cyclase enzyme, with consequent increases in the cAMP. The increased cAMP leads to the activation of protein kinase A, which phosphorylates and activates hormone-sensitive lipase. This, in turn, hydrolyzes fatty acids from triacylglycerols (TAGs), diacylglycerols (DAGs), and monoacylglycerols (MAGs). The fatty acids are then released from the MAGs through the action of monoacylglycerol lipase.

The reserves of glycogen last approximately 24 hours; therefore, the glucose must be synthesized again, using protein as a substratum. The protein in the muscles and other sources is broken down, and amino acids (alanine and glutamine) are released and transported to the liver, where glyconeogenesis takes place. After 24 hours of fasting, the oxidation of FAs becomes, progressively, the main source in the production of energy for the tissues; however, the nervous system and red blood cells continue to use glucose partially as an energetic fuel.

The oxidation of FAs produces an accumulation of it acetyl-CoA, which is then converted to ketone bodies (KBs) through the ketogenic pathway. The production of KBs during fasting is regulated by the high ratio of plasma glucagon–insulin and also by the reduced concentration of malonyl-CoA of the hepatocyte. (This metabolite has the function of inhibiting the activity of carnitine palmitoyl transferase [CPT], which is the key enzyme in the β-oxidation.)[36]

The KBs present in the circulation, together with free FAs, are used for production of ATP by the peripheral and principally muscular tissues.

During the first week of fasting, intense muscular catabolism occurs for glucose production by the liver. Following this, there is an adaptation response to the prolonged fasting, such that after about four weeks of fasting, the consumption of body protein is considerably reduced, mainly due to the adaptation of using KBs as an alternative fuel in response to prolonged fasting.[13,36]

The use of KBs during prolonged fasting and the consequent inhibition of the utilization of glucose occurs not only in the central nervous system, but also in the muscles, renal cortex, mammary glands, and small intestine, thus enabling a normal adult to survive for up to two months of fasting.[13,36]

4.4 LIPID METABOLISM IN A STRESSED STATE

The term *stress* is frequently employed in scientific literature in the area of nutrition to describe certain clinical situations. *Physiological stress* is characterized by neurological and endocrinological alterations that affect the normal physiological function of the organism. *Pathological stress* may be defined as that which emerges from prolonged physiological stress or an additional stress due to disease or trauma. Pathological stress is also called severe stress. In this section, we will consider stress as a pathological response to an illness or injury.

4.4.1 Alterations in the Metabolism of Lipids during Stress

In critically ill patients, the ingestion of fats and other nutrients may be reduced, or even completely absent, in relation to the increased energy needs of the organism. This is because individuals in a condition of stress frequently suffer a significant loss of appetite, a syndrome known as *anorexia*. Although the causes of anorexia are complex, there are indications that factors such as leptin and proinflammatory cytokines are involved.[37,38]

Leptin is a hormone that is synthesized and secreted by adipocytes and bound to receptors in the hypothalamus and other tissues. Leptin may act as a regulator of the mass of body fat. A decrease in the fat deposits reduces the production of leptin. In the hypothalamus, a low concentration of leptin leads to a greater expression of neuropeptide Y, which increases alimentary ingestion.[39] However, under stress there is an increase of leptin release, despite the reduction in fat reserves, with a consequent decrease in appetite.[37,38]

In fasting situations, the organism resorts to compensatory mechanisms that protect it from the possible damage caused by the lack of nutrients. These mechanisms include a breaking down of protein and fat and a reduction in the use of energy. However, in the presence of stress, these mechanisms of adaptation to prolonged fasting do not occur. The presence of tissue damage leads to the installation of a catabolic picture in a desperate attempt to recover homeostasis in the organism. The magnitude of the catabolic reaction seems to be related more to the intensity of the tissular injury than to the type of stress.

During stress, the liberation of catabolic hormones leads to an increase in lipolytic activity. Paralleling this is a preferential oxidation of fat by various tissues, such as the muscles, where a resistance to insulin is developed.[40,41] However, nervous and immune cells continue to need glucose as an energy source, but this is supplied by neoglycogenesis.

Despite the intense lipolysis observed during the metabolic response to stress, there is not always an increase in the plasma concentrations of free FAs, suggesting that the clearance rate of free FAs in the plasma is increased.[42] On the other hand, under certain conditions, the activity of lipoprotein lipase is inhibited by the production of proinflammatory cytokines (such as INF-γ and IL-1), impairing the clearance of TGs from the circulation and installing a picture of hypertriglyceridemia.[43]

The increased rates of lipolysis previously described are so intense that they frequently exceed the energy requirements of the organism. The fatty acids that are not oxidized can be reesterified into TGs in the liver and inserted into the VLDLs. The hepatic production of TGs may be increased in stress situations, propitiating the development of hepatic steatosis. VLDLs, in turn, seem to have protective effects against endotoxemia through their capacity to bind with endotoxins and enable their degradation in hepatic parenchymal cells.[44,45]

In relation to the metabolic alterations of lipids in stress conditions, there is a decrease in the concentrations of plasma cholesterol, in spite of the increase in its hepatic production. Likewise, probably due to the increased catabolism, there is a decrease in the concentration of plasma LDL together with HDL. The decrease in HDL seems to be related to the increase of its subendothelial uptake and retention.[44,45]

In addition, cytokines liberated during stress can modify the composition of HDL and LDL, influencing functional properties of these lipoproteins. In this way, alterations of proteins associated with HDL, for instance, can lead to a reduced capacity for actuating in the reverse transport of cholesterol.[44,45]

TABLE 4.5
Main Functions of Insulin on Fat

Activity	Effect
Anticatabolic (to prevent degradation)	Inhibit lipolysis, prevent excessive ketone and ketoacidosis production
Anabolic (to promote storage)	Facilitate pyruvate reduction into free FAs by stimulating lipogenesis
Transport	Activate the lipoprotein lipase, facilitating the transport of TGs to adipose tissue

4.4.2 MODULATION OF THE METABOLISM OF LIPIDS INDUCED BY STRESS

4.4.2.1 Hormonal Response to Stress and the Metabolism of Lipids

The neural–endocrine alterations released in a stress situation are characterized by the high presence of neural stimuli, as much from the central nervous system as from autonomous nerves that activate the endocrine system to liberate glucagon, cortisol, and catecholamines, thereby significantly increasing the plasmatic levels of these hormones. Consequently, there is an alteration of the balance between insulin, the principal anabolic hormone (the functions of which are outlined in Table 4.5), and these important catabolic hormones, favoring catabolism. In burn patients, the amount of glucagon may double, cortisol may increase fourfold, and catecholamines may increase by eight to ten times, compared with normal controls. These changes are related to the metabolic effects of the disease, which include a significant increase in lipolysis.[46]

There are indications that adipocytes may have direct contact with nerve endings that, when stimulated, provoke an increase in lipolysis. Therefore, it is possible that the stimulation of these nerves does not alter metabolism by the modulation of endocrine functions alone, but also by direct effects on peripheral tissues.[47]

4.4.2.1.1 Cortisol

Cortisol produces important effects in energy metabolism during sepsis and trauma. Its effects on lipid metabolism, however, are not well understood. Hypercortisolemia increases the arterial concentration of nonesterified ("free") fatty acids (NEFAs) and their organic turnover. However, arterial–venous studies have shown that hypercortisolemia reduces the efflux of NEFAs from some deposits of fatty tissue. This inhibition of lipid mobilization seems to be associated with a reduction in the rate of activity of the hormone-sensitive lipase in these deposits.[48] The increase in the arterial concentration of NEFA may be explained by the higher rate of lipoprotein lipase activity, because the plasma concentrations of triglycerides are reduced. Another possible effect on metabolism might be through specific sites of cortisol activity.

4.4.2.1.2 Catecholamines

The infusion of adrenaline in humans leads to an increase in the efflux of NEFA from adipose tissue, due to the increase of its transcapillary efflux resulting from the increase of lipolysis in the adipose tissue.[49] Adrenaline also causes an important elevation in the blood flow in adipose tissues, which results in an increased presentation of the triacylglycerol lipoprotein as a substratum for lipoprotein lipase, to be hydrolyzed in the vascular component.

The effect of noradrenaline on lipid metabolism in adipose tissue is similar to that of adrenaline. The infusion of noradrenaline leads to an increased blood flow in the adipose tissue that, in turn, results in an increase in the efflux of NEFAs and glycerol from the adipose tissue, indicating intense activity of hormone-sensitive lipase.[50] Apparently, the blood flow in the adipose tissue, together with its catecholamines, is an important regulator of the metabolism.[50]

In the presence of severe injury, perfusion of the adipose tissue may be impaired; this can lead to a lower concentration of NEFAs and their reduced turnover. One of the major differences between sepsis and trauma seems to be the hypertriglyceridemia induced by sepsis. This effect during sepsis

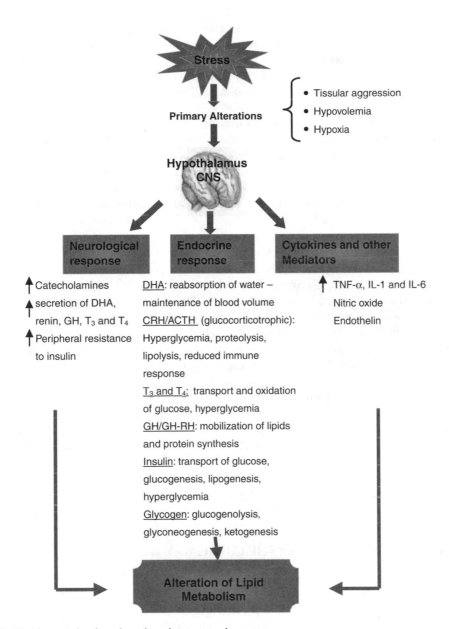

FIGURE 4.7 Neuroendocrine alterations in a stressed state.

seems to be mediated partially through the liver by the selective cleavage of NEFAs into TGs and an increased *de novo* synthesis of TGs. Additionally, the clearance of TGs from peripheral areas is reduced through a decrease in the levels of lipoprotein lipase.[51]

A schematic of the neuroendocrine response to stress is shown in Figure 4.7.

4.4.2.2 The Cytokine Response to Stress and Lipid Metabolism

Injury to tissues interferes with metabolism through the neural–endocrine nervous system and also by the induction of proinflammatory mediators. In sepsis and in trauma, the levels of plasmatic cytokines, which include TNF-α and interleukin 1β and 6, can increase rapidly.[52,53]

TNF-α seems to have an important effect in the induction of anorexia and the loss of adipose tissue. The administration of TNF-α in laboratory animals induces cachexia with anorexia and a depletion of adipose tissue.[54] This cytokine is also involved in the genesis of a resistance to insulin by inhibiting the phosphorylase of receptors.[55] IL-1 presents the same effects as TNF-α by suppressing the activity of lipoprotein lipase and increasing intracellular lipolysis. IL-6 appears to have an important effect in the development of cachexia.[56] This cytokine is an important modulator in human metabolism, which is capable of stimulating lipolysis and fat oxidation without causing hypertriglyceridemia.

The cytokine response to trauma or sepsis may vary according to the nature of the insult. These cytokines can directly affect the metabolism of the adipose tissue, and they can even influence lipid metabolism indirectly through alterations of the counterregulatory hormone plasma concentrations. IL-6 and TNF-α, for example, induce important neuroendocrine alterations by stimulating the secretion of corticotrophin, cortisol, noradrenaline, adrenaline, and glucagon.[57,58] In the last decade, it has been demonstrated that cytokines — such as TNF-α, leptin, and plasminogen activator inhibitor-1, which are produced by adipose tissue — act like endocrines and paracrines, thus allowing the adipose tissue to regulate the metabolism of its lipid content.[59]

In patients with cancer, there is activity of yet another protein, known as lipid mobilization factor (LMF).[60] LMF is produced by tumoral cells and initiates lipolysis through stimulation of the adenylate cyclase enzyme, in a process dependent on guanosine triphosphate and in a manner homologous to the action of the lipolytic hormones.[61] The stimulation of lipolysis by LMF seems to be associated with the selective modulation of the expression of protein G (Figure 4.6), with an increase in protein G of type Gs (a deficiency of which leads to obesity) and with a decrease in Gi (with increased expression in pictures of hyperthyroidism and associated with a reduced fat mobilization). Thus, besides directly stimulating lipolysis, LMF also sensitizes adipose tissue to lipolytic stimulation.[62]

Alterations in the metabolism of lipids induced by the presence of disease are the result of complex interactions involving the central nervous system, hormones, stimulus of autonomous nerves, inflammatory mediators, and peripheral hormones. It has been recognized only recently that receptors beta-2 of the adipose tissue seem to have an important role in the intense lipolysis observed in the metabolic response to stress.[63] The stimulation of these receptors increases the concentrations of cAMP, which in turn stimulates the activity of hormone-sensitive lipase.

Due to the reduced ingestion of fats and alterations in the lipid metabolism frequently found in stress situations, it is necessary to supply these nutrients through appropriate nutritional therapy.

4.5 PROVISION OF LIPIDS TO THE CRITICALLY ILL

There are several distinct advantages to be gained from providing lipids to patients in critical condition. Offering lipids avoids the deficiency of essential fatty acids and its harmful consequences. The high energy density of lipid permits a reduction in the volume of fluids administered without a loss of energy content. Greater provision of lipids allows the administration of less glucose, thus reducing the negative effects of excess glucose contribution, such as hepatic dysfunction, greater production of CO_2, and O_2 consumption of oxygen.[64] In situations of hyperglycemia, the use of lipids offers a safe alternative for better control of the glycemic rate.

4.5.1 FORMULAS FOR ENTERAL NUTRITION

Enteral diets contain a wide variety of triglycerides, originating from several dietary sources. Generally, in these diets, n-6 long-chain triglycerides (LCTs) are provided by soybean, safflower, corn, or sunflower oil. The n-3 LCT are provided by fish oil, sardines, or borage oil. Saturated medium-chain triglycerides (MCTs) come in the form of industrialized MCT, from coconut oil or babassu palm oil, and the monounsaturated fatty acids are usually derived from olive oil and rapeseed.[65]

Normally, the emulsifier used is soybean lecithin. Lecithin consists almost entirely of phosphatidylcholine and phosphatidylethanolamine.[65]

It is worth noting that enteral diets have distinct concentrations of lipids, which may vary from 1.5 g/l, in certain elementary diets, to 93.7 g/240 ml, in specialized formulas for seriously ill patients in the ICU with adult respiratory distress syndrome.

Regarding critically ill patients, randomized studies, both prospective and controlled, have indicated that the provision of an enteral diet enriched with ω-3 fatty acid, arginine, and derivatives of RNA was accompanied by a decrease in the rate of infection and a shorter hospital stay.[66–68] However, these effects cannot be attributed exclusively to the dietary content of ω-3 fatty acids, because these diets also provide other nutrients with immunomodulating properties. In these patients, it is important to determine the amount and the type of available fat in each product of the enteral diet offered.

4.5.2 Parenteral Formulas: Lipid Emulsions

Lipid emulsions (LEs) have been an integral part of parenteral nutritional therapy for more than 30 years and are composed of triglycerides, which constitute the central part of exogenous chylomicrons, emulsified and covered by a layer of phospholipids, which helps to maintain the fats in an aqueous phase in the emulsion. Antioxidants such as liposoluble vitamins (vitamin E) and vegetable esters are also present. The chylomicrons' diameter present in the LE generally ranges from 200 to 350 nm.[65]

In recent decades, the clinical use of parenteral lipid emulsions gained momentum with the development of a safe and effective lipid emulsion for clinical practice, consisting of a soybean oil derivative combined with egg phosphatide.[69]

The LEs offer advantages in having a high energy density and a neutral pH and in being isosmotic with the plasma. For optimal use, some days of adaptation are necessary. Occasionally, patients may present episodes of fever. Anaphylactic reactions are very rare. It is advisable to measure the plasma triglycerides to verify that they are clearing adequately, especially in conditions in which the metabolism of fats might be impaired.[65]

The lipid emulsions available for clinical use are differentiated by the content of FAs, which should be determined and taken into consideration before indicating them to patients in critical condition.[65] Recently, soybean LE has been contraindicated for critical patients because this LE is rich in ω-6 PUFAs and this type of FA can impair immune functions.[65]

Lipid emulsions may be composed of LCT present in soybean, sunflower, or cottonseed oils, together with phospholipids of egg yolk or of soybeans as emulsifying agents. The composition of these emulsions may contain only LCT (10% and 20%) or may be a physical mixture in equal parts of MCT and LCT, or even a chemical mixture of MCT and LCT, known as *structured lipids*.[70]

In any parenteral nutritional strategy, the lipid emulsions should supply 15 to 40% of the total caloric intake. In clinical practice, the use of LCT is recommended at between 25 and 35% of the total consumption of nonproteins (30 to 60 g/day).[71] Levels greater than 50% of the total nonprotein calories can impair phagocyte cell function.[72,73]

A weekly measurement of triglycerides is recommended in order to monitor the supply of parenteral LE.

4.5.3 ω-3 and ω-9 Lipid Emulsions (LEs)

Despite the controversy in the literature, it is now recognized that an excess of ω-6 PUFAs can contribute to aggravating the condition of critically ill patients, compromising their clinical course, probably due to the synthesis of proinflammatory eicosanoids, intense lipid peroxidation, and slow plasmatic clearance (because it is an LCFA). In an attempt to reduce the supply of ω-6 fatty acids to patients in critical condition, new alternatives are being developed for nutritional therapies, which include the supply of various fatty acids.

Most lipid emulsions for parenteral use are based on soybean oil, rich in LCT. A lipid emulsion containing 50% of MCT and 50% LCT has been used as an alternative for parenteral nutrition in critical patients. Its biochemical profile can offer some advantages for immunodeficient patients because it contains a smaller amount of ω-6 LCT.[74,75]

Recently, a lipid emulsion with an olive oil base, which is rich in monounsaturated ω-9 FA, has been developed for clinical use in order to reduce the supply of ω-6 in parenteral therapy. The new emulsion consists of a mixture of soybean oil (20%) and olive oil (80%) with only 18% of ω-6 PUFA, an amount sufficient to prevent or to correct essential FA deficiency.[76,77]

The provision of a parenteral lipid emulsion with an olive oil base is an attempt to reduce the undesirable effects of the excessive availability of PUFAs. Those effects include an increase in lipid peroxidation, inhibition of the synthesis of homologs of essential FAs, alterations in the cellular membrane structures, and alterations in the immune system.[78–80]

A fish oil–based LE (rich in ω-3 FA) is already available in Europe and in Latin America for clinical use. This appears to preserve immune functions better than total parenteral nutrition, by partially preventing some aspects of the inflammatory response. Due to its high cytotoxicity, LE with a 10% fish oil base should not be administered in isolation, but always as 10 to 20% of the total lipids offered per day.

The parenteral use of fish oil–enriched LEs in surgical patients inhibits the inflammatory picture and preserves or improves the immunological alterations normally induced by surgical stress.[81,82]

Thus, modern nutritional planning should consider the provision of lipids as a source of energy and of essential FAs and also as a modulator of the immuno-inflammatory response.

4.6   PERSPECTIVES

Much has been learned in the last few decades about the biochemistry of lipids and their metabolism during stress. The administration of approximately 1 g of lipids per kilogram of body weight is safe, provided it is done slowly and continually.

New LEs containing mixtures of soybean oil, olive oil, fish oil, and MCT are being tested by specialized laboratories and services.[83] It is probable that new, stimulating lipid emulsions will soon be available for use in critically ill patients.

REFERENCES

1. Holum, J.R., Lipids, in *Fundamentals of General, Organic and Biological Chemistry*, Holum, J.R., ed., John Wiley & Sons, New York, 1994, 566–582.
2. Gunstone, F., Fatty acids: nomenclature, structure, isolation and structure determination, biosynthesis and chemical synthesis, in *Fatty Acid and Lipid Chemistry*, Black Academic & Professional, Glasgow, 1996, 1–33.
3. Borges, V. and Waitzberg, D.L., Gorduras, in *Nutrição enteral e parenteral na prática clínica*, Waitzberg D.L., ed., Atheneu, São Paulo, 1995, 21–32.
4. Gunstone, F., Fatty acids: nomenclature, structure, isolation and structure determination, biosynthesis and chemical synthesis, in *Fatty Acid and Lipid Chemistry*, Black Academic & Professional, Glasgow, 1996, 35–59.
5. Calder, P.C., Long-chain n-3 fatty acids and inflammation: potential application in surgical and trauma patients, *Braz. J. Med. Biol. Res.*, 36, 433, 2003.
6. Liao, T.H., Hamosh, P., and Hamosh, M., Fat digestion by lingual lipase: mechanism of lipolysis in the stomach and upper small intestine, *Pediatr. Res.*, 18, 402, 1984.
7. Corey, M.C., Small, D.M., and Bliss, C.M., Lipid digestion and absorption, *Ann. Ver. Physiol.*, 45, 651, 1983.

8. Livesey, G. and Elia, M., Short-chain fatty acids as an energy source in the colon: metabolism and clinical applications, in *Physiological and Clinical Aspects of Short-Chain Fatty Acid,* Cumings, J.H., Rombeau, J.L., and Sakata, T., eds., Cambridge University Press, Cambridge, 1995, 427–481.

9. Havel, R.J. and Kane, J.P., Introduction: structure and metabolism of plasma proteins, in *The Metabolic and Molecular Bases of Inherited Disease,* 7th ed., vol. II, Scriver, C.R., Beaudet, A.L., Sly, W.S., and Valle, D., eds., McGraw-Hill, New York, 1995, 1841–1851.

10. Dominiczak, M.H., Apolipoproteins and lipoproteins, in *Handbook of Lipoprotein Testing*, Rifai, N., Russel Warnick, G., and Dominiczak, M.H., eds., AACC Press, Washington, DC, 1997, 123–134.

11. Chylomicron's density. http://www.afh.bio.br/digest/digest2.asp.

12. Barter, P.J. and Rye, K.A., High-density lipoproteins and coronary artery disease, *Atherosclerosis*, 121, 1, 1996.

13. Ettinger, S., Macronutrients: carboidratos, proteinas e lipideos, in Kraus: *Alimentos, Nutricao e Dietoterapia*, Mahan, L.K. and Escott-Stump, S., Eds., Editora Roca, São Paulo, 2002, 3, 30–64.

14. Glatz, J.F.C. and Van der Vusse, G.J., Cellular fatty acid binding protein: their function and physiological significance, *Pro. Lipid Res.,* 35, 243, 1996.

15. Graber, R., Sumida, C., and Nunez, E.A., Fatty acids and cell signal transduction, *J. Lipid Mediators Cell Signal*, 9, 91, 1994.

16. Sumida, C., Graber, R., and Nunez, E.A., Role of fatty acids in signal transduction: modulators and messengers, *Prostaglandins Leukot. Essent. Fatty Acids*, 48, 117, 1993.

17. Alexander, J.W., Immunonutrition: the role of omega-3 fatty acids, *Nutrition*, 14, 627, 1998.

18. Sprecher, H., An update on the pathways of polyunsaturated fatty acid metabolism, *Curr. Opin. Clin. Nutr. Met. Care,* 2, 135, 1999.

19. Calder, P.C. and Deckelbaum, R.J., Dietary lipids: more than just a source of calories, *Curr. Opin. Clin. Nutr. Metab. Care.,* 2, 105, 1999.

20. Kinsella, J.E., Lipids, membrane receptors, and enzymes: effects of dietary fatty acids, *JPEN*, 14 (suppl.), 200S, 1990.

21. Calder, P.C. and Grimble, R.F., Polyunsaturated fatty acids, inflammation and immunity, *Eur. J. Clin. Nutr.*, 56 (suppl.), S14, 2002.

22. Calder, P.C., Lipid metabolism in critically ill, in *Nutrition and Critical Care*, Nestlé Nutrition Workshop Series Clinical & Performance Program, 8, 75, 2003.

23. James, M.J., Gibson, R.A., and Cleland, L.G., Dietary polyunsaturated fatty acids and inflammatory mediator production, *Am. J. Clin. Nutr.*, 71 (suppl.), S343, 2000.

24. Calder, P.C., N-3 polyunsaturated fatty acids and cytokine production in health and disease, *Ann. Nutr. Metab.*, 41, 203, 1997.

25. Endres, S. et al., The effect of dietary supplementation with n-3 polyunsaturated fatty acids on the synthesis of interleukin-1 and tumor necrosis factor by mononuclear cells, *N. Engl. J. Med.*, 320, 265, 1989.

26. Meydani, S.N., Oral (n-3) fatty acid supplementation suppresses cytokine production and lymphocyte proliferation: comparison between young and older women, *J. Nutr.*, 121, 547, 1991.

27. Meydani, S.N., Modulation of cytokine production by dietary polyunsaturated fatty acids, *Proc. Soc. Exp. Biol. Med.*, 200, 189, 1992.

28. Calder, P.C., Long chain n-3 fatty acids and inflammation: potential application in surgical and trauma patients, *Braz. J. Med. Biol. Res.*, 36, 433, 2003.

29. Poynter, M.E. and Daynes, R.A., Peroxissome proliferator-activated receptor alpha activation modulates cellular redox status, represses nuclear factor-kappa B signaling, and reduces inflammatory cytokine production in aging, *J. Biol. Chem.* 273, 32833, 1998.

30. Mascaro, C. et al., Control of human muscle-type carnitine palmitoyltransferase I gene transcription by peroxisome proliferator-activated receptor, *J. Biol. Chem.* 273, 8560, 1998.

31. Rodriguez, J.C. et al., Peroxisome proliferator-activated receptor mediates induction of the mitochondrial 3-hydroxy-3-methylglutaryl-CoA synthase gene by fatty acids, *J. Biol. Chem.,* 269, 18767, 1994.

32. Baillie, R.A. et al., Coordinate induction of peroxisomal acyl-CoA oxidase and UCP-3 by dietary fish oil: a mechanism for decreased body fat deposition, *Prostaglandins Leukot. Essent. Fatty Acids*, 60, 351, 1999.

33. Desvergne, B. and Wahli, W., Peroxissome proliferator-activated receptors: nuclear control of metabolism, *Endocrinol Rev.*, 20, 249, 1999.

34. Nichols, D.G. and Locke, L., Thermogenic mechanism in brown adipose tissue, *Physiol. Rev.*, 64, 1, 1984.

35. Pénicaud, L. et al., The autonomic nervous system, adipose tissue plasticity, and energy balance, *Nutrition,*16, 903, 2000.

36. Otton, R. and Curi, R., Metabolismo dos acidos graxos no jejum e diabetes, in *Entendendo a Gordura,* Cupri, R., Pompeia, C., Miyasaka, C.K., and Procópio, J., Eds., Manole, São Paulo, 2002, 15, 187–197.

37. Grunfeld, C. and Feingold, K.R., Regulation of lipid metabolism by cytokines during host defense, *Nutrition,* 12 (suppl.), S24, 1996.

38. Gaillard, R.C. et al., Cytokines, leptin, and the hypothalamo-pituitary-adrenal axis, *Ann. N. Y. Acad. Sci.*, 917, 647, 2000.

39. Inui, A., Cancer anorexia-cachexia syndrome: current issues in research and management, *CA Cancer J. Clin.*, 52, 72, 2002.

40. Shaw, J.H.F. and Wolfe, R.R., Fatty acid and glycerol kinetics in septic patients and in patients with gastrointestinal cancer, *Ann. Surg.,* 205, 368, 1987.

41. Stoner, H.B. et al., The relationships between plasma substrates and hormones and the severity of injury in 277 recently injured patients, *Clin. Sci.*, 56, 563, 1979.

42. Martinez, A. et al., Assessment of adipose tissue metabolism by means of subcutaneous microdialysis in patients with sepsis or circulatory failure, *Clin. Physiol. Funct. Imaging*, 23, 286, 2003.

43. Hardardottir, I., Grunfeld, C., and Feingold, K.R., Effects of endotoxin and cytokines on lipid metabolism, *Curr. Opin. Lipidol.,* 5, 207, 1994.

44. Khovidhunkit, W. et al., Infection and inflammation-induced proatherogenic changes lipoproteins, *J. Infect. Dis.*, 181 (suppl.), S462, 2000.

45. Carpentier, Y.A. and Scruel, O., Changes in concentration and composition of plasma lipoproteins during the acute phase response, *Curr. Opin. Clin. Nutr. Metab. Care*, 5, 153, 2002.

46. Wolfe, R.R. et al., Regulation of lipolysis in severely burned children, *Ann. Surg.*, 206, 214, 1987.

47. Youngstrom, T.G. and Bartness, T.J., Catecholaminergic innervation of white adipose tissue in Siberian hamsters, *Am. J. Physiol.*, 268, 744, 1995.

48. Samra, J.S. et al., Effects of physiological hypercortisolemia on the regulation of lipolysis in subcutaneous adipose tissue, *J. Clin. Endocrinol. Metab.*, 83, 626, 1998.

49. Samra, J.S. et al., Effects of adrenaline infusion on the interstitial environment of subcutaneous adipose tissue as studied by microdialysis, *Clin. Sci.,* 91, 425, 1996.

50. Kurpad, A. et al., Effect of noradrenaline on glycerol turnover and lipolysis in the whole body and subcutaneous adipose tissue in humans *in vivo, Clin. Sci.,* 86, 177, 1994.

51. Feingold, K.R. et al., Endotoxin rapidly induces changes in lipid metabolism that produce hypertriglyceridemia: low doses stimulate hepatic triglyceride production while high doses inhibit clearance, *J. Lipid. Res.*, 33, 1765, 1992.

52. Michie, H.R. et al., Detection of circulating tumor necrosis factor after endotoxin administration, *N. Engl. J. Med.*, 318, 1481, 1988.

53. Maass, D.L., White, J., and Horton, J.W., IL-1beta and IL-6 act synergistically with TNF-alpha to alter cardiac contractile function after burn trauma, *Shock*, 18, 360, 2002.

54. Tisdale, M.J., Biology of cachexia, *J. Natl. Cancer. Inst.*, 89, 1763, 1997.

55. Uysal, K.T. et al., Protection from obesity-induced insulin resistance in mice lacking TNF alpha function, *Nature*, 389, 610, 1997.

56. Barton, B.E. and Murphy, T.F., Cancer cachexia is mediated in part by the induction of IL-6-like cytokines from the spleen, *Cytokine*, 16, 251, 2001.

57. Van der Poll, T. et al., Tumor necrosis factor mimics the metabolic response to acute infection in healthy humans, *Am. J. Physiol.*, 261, 457, 1991.

58. Stouthard, J.M. et al., Endocrinologic and metabolic effects of interleukin-6 in humans, *Am. J. Physiol.*, 268, 813, 1995.

59. Diamond, F., The endocrine function of adipose tissue, *Growth Genetics & Hormones*, 18, 2, 17–22, 2002, http://www.gghjournal.com/pdf/volume_18/18-2/18-2pdfcolor.pdf.

60. Todorov, P.T. et al., Purification and characterization of a tumor lipid-mobilizing factor, *Cancer Res.*, 58, 2353, 1998.

61. Tisdale, M.J., Biochemical mechanisms of cellular catabolism, *Curr. Opin. Clin. Nutr. Metab. Care*, 5, 401, 2002.

62. Islam-Ali, B. et al., Modulation of adipocyte G-protein expression in cancer cachexia by a lipid-mobilizing factor (LMF), *Br. J. Cancer*, 85, 758, 2001.

63. Herndon, D.N. et al., Lipolysis in burned patients is stimulated by the beta 2-receptor for catecholamines, *Arch. Surg.*, 129, 1301, 1994.

64. Ribeiro, P.C., Terapia nutricional na sepse, http://www.einstein.br/sepse/pdf/4_4.pdf.

65. Carpentier, Y.A. et al., Recent developments in lipid emulsions: relevance to intensive care, *Nutrition*, 13, 9 (suppl.), S73, 1997.

66. Heyland, D.K. et al., Should immunonutrition become routine in critically ill patients? A systematic review of the evidence, *JAMA*, 286, 944, 2001.

67. Gianotti, L. and Braga, M., Perioperative nutrition in cancer patients, *Nutr. Clin. Metabol.*, 15, 298, 2001.

68. Gianotti, L. et al., A randomized controlled trial of preoperative oral supplementation with a specialized diet in patients with gastrointestinal cancer, *Gastroenterol.*, 122, 1763, 2002.

69. Wretlind, A., Development of fat emulsions. *J. Parenter. Enteral. Nutr.*, 5, 230, 1981.

70. Mascioli, E.A. et al., Medium chain triglycerides and structured lipids as unique nonglucose energy sources in hyperalimentation, *Lipids*; 22, 421, 1987.

71. Silva, M.L.T. and Waitzberg, D.L., NPT sistema lipídico. Mistura 3 em 1. in *Nutrição Enteral e Parenteral na Prática Clínica*, Waitzberg D.L., ed, São Paulo, Atheneu, 1995, 257–260.

72. Waitzberg, D.L. et al., Influence of medium chain triglyceride-based lipid emulsion on rat polymorphonuclear cell functions, *Nutrition*, 12, 93, 1996.

73. Waitzberg, D.L. et al., Parenteral lipid emulsions and phagocytic systems. *Br. J. Nutr.*, 87 (suppl.), S49, 2002.

74. Bach, A.C. and Babayan, V.K., Medium-chain triglycerides: an update, *Am. J. Clin. Nutr.*, 36, 950, 1982.

75. Ulrich, H. et al., Parenteral use of medium-chain triglycerides: a reappraisal, *Nutr.*, 12, 231, 1996.

76. Goulet, O. et al., Long-term efficacy and safety of a new olive oil-based intravenous fat emulsion in pediatric patients: a double-blind randomized study, *Am. J. Clin. Nutr.*, 70, 338, 1999.

77. Granato, D., Effects of parenteral lipid emulsion with different fatty acid composition on immune cell functions *in vitro*, *J. Parenter. Enteral. Nutr.*, 24, 113, 2000.

78. Martinez, M. and Ballabriga, A., Effects of parenteral nutrition with high doses of linoleate on the developing human liver and brain, *Lipids*, 22, 133, 1987.

79. Pitkanen, O. Hallman, M., and Andersson, S., Generation of free radicals in lipid emulsion used in parenteral nutrition, *Pediatr. Res.*, 29, 56, 1991.

80. Halliwell, B. and Chirico, S., Lipid peroxidation: its mechanism, measurement and significance, *Am. J. Clin. Nutr.*, 57 (suppl.), 715, 1993.

81. Schauder, P. et al., Impact of fish oil enriched total parenteral nutrition on DNA synthesis, cytokine release and receptor expression by lymphocytes in the postoperative period, *Br. J. Nutr.*, 87 (suppl.), S103, 2002.

82. Weiss, G. et al., Immunomodulation by perioperative administration of n-3 fatty acids. *Br. J. Nutr.*, 87 (suppl.), S89, 2002.

83. Torrinhas, R.S. et al., Effect of multiple fatty acids parenteral lipid emulsion on the expression of functional immunological surface molecules on human monocytes/macrophages, 26th Clinical Congress — ASPEN. San Diego, February 23–27, 2002, poster session.

Section II

Nutrients for the Critically Ill

5 Nutrition Assessment and Monitoring

Marion F. Winkler
Rhode Island Hospital, Brown University

CONTENTS

5.1 OVERVIEW

Nutrition assessment of the critically ill patient presents a unique challenge to the practitioner. Traditional methods of assessing nutritional status are of limited value in the intensive care unit (ICU) setting. No simple recommendation can be given regarding the best test for nutrition assessment; therefore, the use of any method can be appropriate provided the limitations are clearly understood.[1] Severely ill patients, no matter what assessment tool is used, will likely be identified as malnourished or at nutritional risk.[2] These patients will almost always exhibit decreased nutrient intake, increased energy and nutrient requirements, altered nutrient utilization, or all of these. The diagnosis of a malnourished state must be interpreted cautiously. It is important to judge whether the assessment indicates a state induced by nutrient deficiency that will improve with nutrition support or whether it reflects the severity of the metabolic derangement caused by the underlying illness or injury.[2] Both conditions often coexist for the majority of critically ill patients. The purpose of nutrition assessment in the ICU is to identify evidence of preexisting nutritional deficiency, evaluate the risk of nutrition-related complications that may affect outcome, and establish the need for specialized nutrition support. Reassessment should be completed periodically due to the prolonged course of ICU patients and must incorporate monitoring adequacy of intake and response to therapy.

5.2 THE CRITICALLY ILL PATIENT

Critical illness comprises a wide spectrum of life-threatening medical or surgical conditions usually requiring ICU-level care.[2] Most critically ill patients exhibit at least severe single organ failure and require active therapeutic support. Patients admitted to an ICU typically have one or more of the following conditions:

- Acute hemodynamic instability
- Acute respiratory distress
- Severe acid–base disorders
- Acute change in level of consciousness
- Life-threatening fluid and electrolyte imbalance
- The need for invasive procedures to assess physiologic function
- Postoperative state with major comorbidity, such as cardiac or pulmonary failure
- Intraoperative bleeding, thrombolysis, or risk of immediate bleeding
- Severe burns, multiple trauma, or head injury

In a substantial number of critically ill patients, systemic inflammatory response syndrome (SIRS) or sepsis is present. The American College of Chest Physicians and the Society of Critical Care Medicine describes SIRS as "a systemic response to non-specific insults which may include infection, pancreatitis, trauma, and burns."[3] Assigning a point for each of the following variables present makes the diagnosis of SIRS:

- Fever ($> 38°C$) or hypothermia ($< 36°C$)
- Tachycardia (heart rate > 90)
- Tachypnea (respiratory rate > 20)
- $PaCO_2 < 32$ mm HG
- Abnormal white blood cell count ($> 12,000$ mm^3 or $< 4,000$ mm^3 or 10% bands)

In sepsis, the site of infection is known. Severe sepsis is associated with signs of at least one acute organ dysfunction, hypoperfusion, or hypotension. Multiple organ dysfunction syndrome (MODS) is a frequent complication of SIRS. The syndrome is present when there is altered function of two or more organs in an acutely ill patient requiring intervention. MODS can be primary, resulting from direct injury to an organ from trauma, or it may be secondary, occurring in the presence of inflammation or infection in organs remote from the initial injury. In a study of 7602 trauma patients, a SIRS score greater than 2 on admission was a significant independent predictor of outcome and need for ICU admission in trauma.[4] A number of tools are available to assess severity of illness, including the Acute Physiology and Chronic Health Evaluation (APACHE) II score and the Therapeutic Intervention Scoring System (TISS-28).[5,6] The Glasgow Coma Score (GCS) is a frequently used tool for quantifying a patient's state of consciousness.[7] Severity of illness scores can be incorporated into nutrition risk screening and assessment.

A thorough understanding of the metabolic response to injury and critical illness is essential for the practitioner who conducts nutrition assessment. These principles are described in detail in other chapters of this book. There is a well defined endocrine and metabolic response to stress characterized by increased resting energy expenditure (REE), whole-body proteolysis, and lipolysis. Clinical manifestations of this state may include fever, high cardiac output, increased oxygen consumption, hyperglycemia, decreased peripheral vascular resistance, and increased ureagenesis with high urinary nitrogen excretion. A strongly positive fluid balance with edema is often present. The combined impact of the metabolic alterations that occur in stress, coupled with bed rest and lack of adequate nutritional intake, can lead to rapid and severe depletion of lean body mass. Specialized nutrition support cannot fully prevent or reverse the metabolic alterations and disruption in body composition associated with critical illness, but it may ameliorate the rate of net protein catabolism.

5.3 DETERMINING NUTRITIONAL RISK

In the ICU, optimization of the patient's metabolic state is the initial objective of clinical management. During this time, the nutrition support practitioner should assess the patient's preexisting nutritional status. ICU patients are a heterogeneous group of patients. Many patients will be able to resume full oral feeding after a short ICU stay; others, suffering from major trauma, operative complications, or severe infection, may require enteral or parenteral nutrition.[8] Identifying the patient who will be able to eat and the one who may require early and prolonged nutrition support helps to establish nutritional risk. Patients at increased nutritional risk in the ICU tend to be those who have:[9]

- Clinical evidence of malnutrition
- Chronic disease
- Acute conditions accompanied by sepsis, trauma, or emergent surgery
- Advanced age
- Length of ICU stay exceeding five days due to the increased risk of death and morbidity

A prospective cohort study of ICU patients aged 70 and older, screened upon admission and six months after discharge, demonstrated that impaired nutritional status upon admission, in addition to severity of illness, was related to six-month mortality.[10] Results such as these emphasize the need for systematic nutrition assessment in the ICU.

5.4 NUTRITION ASSESSMENT

All of the traditional nutrition assessment parameters lose their specificity in the critically ill patient. Although they are not sensitive or specific indicators of nutritional status *per se*, many parameters do provide useful prognostic information.

5.4.1 ANTHROPOMETRICS AND BODY COMPOSITION

Anthropometric measurements are not sensitive to acute changes and are of limited value following fluid resuscitation or when a patient has pleural effusions, generalized edema, or anasarca. In a study of 10 critically injured and 12 severely septic patients over a 3 to 4 week period, Hill documented a net accumulation of 4.73 and 12.5 liters of total body water in trauma and septic patients, respectively.[11] Most of the changes in body weight could be accounted for by changes in extracellular water. Of interest, elderly patients took more than three weeks to correct this overexpansion of extracellular water, compared to younger patients in whom diuresis occurred in half the time. Hill also determined that trauma patients lost 16% and septic patients lost 13% of their total body protein during the first 21 days following injury or insult.[11] In the first 10 days, two-thirds of this protein loss came from skeletal muscle, but beyond 10 days the loss was primarily viscera. Changes in body fat mass reflected energy balance. Hill found that body fat was oxidized with insufficient energy intake, but body fat mass was preserved when energy intake was equal to total energy expenditure.[11]

Preinjury weight and weight history often are the most useful assessment data, but because the patient may be sedated and intubated, this information is best obtained from a family member. If fluid resuscitation or edema obscure weight loss, family members may be questioned regarding change in clothing size as well as weight history.[12] A driver's license may also provide self-reported height and weight. Nutritional status can be classified by body mass index (BMI). A BMI less than

16 is associated with severe undernutrition and may define preexisting malnutrition.[1,13] Serial weights do provide useful monitoring information over the course of the patient's hospitalization and recovery, provided scales are accessible and calibrated and patients are actually weighed. Despite protocols requiring weight measurement two times per week in one hospital, only 60% of patients had recorded weights.[14] Some clinicians advocate the use of arm circumference measurement (provided it is correctly interpreted), because this measurement is simple to teach and perform and utilizes an inexpensive nonstretchable flexible tape. Ravasco et al. found that midarm circumference less than the fifth percentile was the only anthropometric parameter associated with a high mortality rate in critically ill patients.[15] Bed rest alone may cause loss or atrophy of muscle, regardless of nutritional status or intake. Clinicians should inspect fat and muscle stores, body habitus, edema, and overall muscle tone and palpate skinfold thickness.

Bioelectrical impedance (BIA) has been used to determine fluid status and changes in lean body mass. BIA is portable, easy to perform, inexpensive, and noninvasive. This technique measures the electrical resistance or opposition of flow to a small current. Because relationships between changes in lean body mass and total body water are unpredictable in critically ill patients, results must be carefully interpreted.[16] Interestingly, the measurement of bioelectrical impedance vector analysis has been investigated for bedside monitoring of fluid status in the ICU.[17] Central venous pressure correlated with direct impedance measurements more than with total body water prediction. This may offer a less invasive approach for guiding fluid management in critically ill patients.

In summary, anthropometry reflects chronic changes in body composition and functions best as a measure of the amount of change in total body energy stores and lean body mass over extended periods of time.[18] It does not perform well as an index of the functional capacity or metabolic health of acutely ill patients.

5.4.2 SERUM PROTEINS

Laboratory tests, primarily serum proteins, are influenced by hepatic dysfunction, protein-losing states, acute infection, and inflammation (see Table 5.1). Interpretation of laboratory measurements is affected by intercompartmental fluid shifts, the acute-phase response, and provision of exogenous blood products. Hepatic acute-phase response is an orchestrated cascade of events initiated by proinflammatory cytokines that result in an increase in acute-phase protein production by the liver with a concomitant decrease in serum protein levels.[19]

Serum albumin is likely to be abnormal in the critical care setting because of the "intermingled effects of both undernutrition and the severity of illness or underlying disease."[2] Prolonged hypoalbuminemia in critically ill patients is associated with poor outcome, and serum albumin levels correlate with increased morbidity and mortality. Serum albumin levels less than 2.8 gm/dl were associated with a higher mortality in 44 nontrauma ICU patients requiring mechanical ventilation.[15] Survivors following a prolonged ICU stay (> 7 days) had a significantly higher overall mean serum albumin concentration than nonsurvivors and were able to recover to a higher mean serum albumin level.[20] In a similar study, ICU nonsurvivors had lower albumin concentrations on admission to the ICU, which decreased more rapidly within the first 48 hours; the value of serum albumin at 24 to 48 hours was as accurate as APACHE II in predicting mortality in this patient population.[21] Albumin levels consistently increased in burn survivors with less than 50% total body surface area, whereas patients who ultimately died had further decline of protein levels.[22] Preoperative serum albumin concentration was a strong predictor of systemic sepsis, pneumonia, and deep wound infection in a study of 54,000 patients.[23] When measured daily, trends in serum albumin concentration have been used to predict outcome (mechanical ventilation dependency) in ICU patients.[24]

Septic ICU patients have been shown to have significantly lower levels of retinol-binding protein and prealbumin than nonseptic patients.[2] These more rapid turnover proteins are best used as measures of efficacy of nutrition therapy or adequacy of intake in critically ill patients. In a study of 120 ICU patients, Bauer et al. demonstrated that prealbumin was sensitive to adequacy of caloric

TABLE 5.1
Selected Proteins, Characteristics, and Evaluation of Results

Protein	Function	Half-Life	Normal Range[a]	Interpreting Results
Albumin	Binds and transports small molecules; Maintains oncotic pressure	20 days	3.5 to 5.0 mg/dl	Synthesized in liver; altered by liver disease; Alterations occur in kidney disease with glomerular damage; Elevated in dehydration; Levels fall with protein-losing enteropathy; may be low in chronic, long-term, unstressed malnutrition; Negative acute-phase reactant; levels drop in inflammation, shock
C-reactive protein	General marker of infection and inflammation	5 hours	0.2 to 8 mg/l	Synthesized by the liver; Present during episodes of acute inflammation; Levels increase in acute inflammation, infection; Levels decrease as inflammation subsides
Prealbumin (transthyretin)	Thyroxine-binding protein	2 days	18 to 38 mg/dl	Highly sensitive to dietary deprivation and refeeding; used to monitor response to nutrition therapy; Elevated in renal failure; Negative acute-phase reactant
Retinol-binding protein	Vitamin A transport; bound to prealbumin	12 hours	2 to 6 mg/dl	Used to monitor response to nutrition therapy; Elevated in renal failure; Negative acute-phase reactant; Decreased in vitamin A deficiency
Transferrin	Iron-binding protein	8 days	202 to 336 mg/dl	Levels fall when diet is deficient in protein; Synthesized in liver; altered by liver disease; Elevated in iron deficiency; chronic blood loss; pregnancy; Levels low in chronic diseases, cirrhosis, nephrotic syndrome, protein-losing enteropathy; Negative acute-phase reactant

[a] Normal ranges based on lifespan, pathology and laboratory medicine, Rhode Island Hospital, Providence, RI.

Sources: Lab Tests Online. http://www.labtestsonline.org, accessed 5/11/04; Pi-Sunyer, F.X. and Woo, R., Laboratory assessment of nutritional status, in *Nutrition Assessment,* Simko, M.D., Cowell, C., and Gilbride, J.A. (Eds.), Aspen Publishers, Rockville, MD, 1984; Ross Products Division, Abbott Laboratories, *Laboratory Utilization for Nutritional Support: Current Practice, Requirements, Expectations,* 14th Annual Ross Roundtable on Medical Issues, 1994; Winkler, M.F., Nutrition assessment in critical care, in *Nutrition Assessment,* Simko, M.D., Cowell, C., and Gilbride, J.A. (Eds.), Aspen Publishers, Gaithersburg, MD, 1995.

intake.[25] Prealbumin levels increased 4 mg/l within a week of initiating adequate nutrition support (25 kcal/kg), compared to 2 mg/l increases in patients receiving half the calories (11 kcal/kg). A consensus panel report noted that prealbumin less than 5 mg/dl or failure to increase more than 4 mg/dl per week is associated with poor prognosis.[26] An upward trend in prealbumin and retinol-binding protein may suggest reversing catabolism toward anabolism.[27] The magnitude of prealbumin response to nutrition support could be used to assess adequacy of the intervention.

Other acute-phase reactants are markers of the injury response and its intensity. C-reactive protein (CRP) is associated with infection and inflammation. CRP characteristically rises within hours after an acute stimulus and returns to near normal levels with resolution of infection.[28] Reny et al. found that CRP, in combination with SIRS, is a useful way to diagnose infection in ICU patients.[29] A decrease in CRP of ≥ 50 mg/l between admission and day 4 has been shown to be a good predictor of recovery.[29] The determination of CRP in conjunction with prealbumin may help distinguish an acute-phase response from malnutrition.[18]

5.4.3 OTHER PARAMETERS

Skin testing or delayed cutaneous hypersensitivity has limited value in the ICU patient because of underlying disease, immunocompromise, selected medications, and technical application and interpretation. Respiratory muscle strength assessed by airway pressures, endurance, and vital capacity may be reduced in malnourished patients. This technique is also of limited value in the ICU because it requires a patient who is awake and alert. Hypercapnia, hypoxia, medications, and intrinsic muscle disease may impact interpretation of these data.[30] An increased understanding of cellular abnormalities associated with disease and the impact of nutritional therapies on stress states has vast implications for metabolic assessment.[18] Magnetic resonance spectroscopy allows detection and monitoring of changes in muscle energy metabolism associated with both starvation and refeeding. Changes in skeletal muscle energetics may improve understanding of skeletal muscle catabolism and the resultant loss of both structural and functional proteins, impaired muscle function, and body composition alteration.[18] Microdialysis, a minimally invasive tool that allows sampling and determination of solutes of low molecular weight in the interstitial space, may provide new insight for regulation of lipolysis and glucose metabolism at the tissue level.[31]

5.4.4 NITROGEN BALANCE

Nitrogen balance reflects net protein synthesis, the difference between whole-body protein synthesis and breakdown. Nitrogen balance studies are best used not to determine nutritional status *per se* but to determine whether nutrition support has been sufficient to prevent net catabolism or to promote anabolism. Ideally, total urinary nitrogen measurements should be made; however, estimations of nitrogen loss can be obtained from urine urea nitrogen (UUN) and approximation of nonurinary nitrogen losses. In the critically ill patient, abnormal nitrogen losses may occur through burn wound exudate, fistula drainage, gastrointestinal fluid loss, diarrhea, or dialysis. Measurement of 24-hour UUN excretion has been used to evaluate the degree of hypermetabolism. When used to determine degree of stress, the most sensitive and specific measure of nitrogen excretion is obtained in the fasting state. The efficacy of nutritional parameters is often tested against nitrogen balance.[32] Table 5.2 describes factors to consider when interpreting nitrogen balance in the clinical setting.

5.5 INDIRECT CALORIMETRY

Indirect calorimetry is the preferred standard for measurement of oxygen consumption in severely injured patients.[33,34] Many investigators have documented substantial increases in REE and the inaccuracy of predictive equations in the assessment of energy expenditure in critical illness. The

TABLE 5.2
Interpretation of Nitrogen Balance

Balance	Interpretation	Factors to Consider
Intake = output	Nitrogen equilibrium (steady state)	Caloric intake = caloric requirement Usual goal for maintaining a well nourished individual
Intake > output	Positive nitrogen balance (nitrogen retention)	Indicates growth, anabolic state Typical finding for growing child, pregnancy, intensively training athletes Evaluate renal function if nitrogen excretion is unexpectedly low
Intake < output	Negative nitrogen balance (catabolic state)	If intake is zero or negligible, nitrogen balance will be negative (even in a well nourished, nonstressed individual). Goal = improve intake. If intake is reasonable and nitrogen balance is negative in a nonstressed individual, evaluate adequacy of caloric intake. Evaluate renal function if nitrogen excretion is unexpectedly high (may reflect resolving renal insufficiency). In hypermetabolic states, urinary nitrogen excretion will be very high. Provide adequate calories and protein. Goal = less negative over time. If calorie and protein intakes are adequate, the best way to minimize nitrogen excretion is to reduce the source of stress (e.g., treat infection, stabilize fractures, cover open wounds, drain pus, control environmental temperature).

Fick equation can also be used to measure oxygen consumption in severely injured patients; however, it may underestimate whole-body oxygen consumption and may be episodic, not always reflecting fluctuations post injury.[33] In the ICU setting, indirect calorimetry may be inaccurate when FIO_2 exceeds 60% or in spontaneous breathers requiring supplemental oxygen. Metabolic measurements provide beneficial information when the critically ill patient fails to respond adequately to estimated nutritional needs, has organ dysfunction, is in need of long-term nutrition support, or is being weaned from mechanical ventilation.[35] It is particularly useful in determining energy requirements in the obese critically ill patient. Indirect calorimetry can be an important aspect of nutrition assessment. Its role is to identify individual caloric requirements, minimize consequences of overfeeding, and serve as a benchmark for adequate intake and achievement of goal calories. Serial monitoring of caloric delivery as a percent of requirements should be a routine component of nutrition assessment and reassessment.[36]

5.6 SUBJECTIVE GLOBAL ASSESSMENT

Subjective global assessment (SGA), which encompasses the patient history and physical examination, is a validated and reproducible clinical method to evaluate nutrition status.[2] There are clinical studies demonstrating SGA as a good predictor of complications for patients undergoing gastrointestinal surgery, liver transplantation, and dialysis.[2,37,38] SGA was been found to be more specific than sensitive and may miss mild degrees of malnutrition. Although it has not been formally evaluated in critical care, it may help to assess the impact of disease or treatment on nutrition status or risk. The use of SGA in the ICU is illustrated in Table 5.3.

SGA begins with a thorough review of food intake and how it differs from normal. This information is typically obtained from family members, because ICU patients may be intubated and sedated. A significant number of patients may enter the ICU after a prolonged admission in the hospital. In this situation, a review of calorie counts or adequacy of specialized nutrition support intake is necessary. A thorough evaluation of the underlying reason that a patient is not eating may

TABLE 5.3
Use of Subjective Global Assessment in the Intensive Care Unit

Patient History: Mr. H. is a 50-year-old male who presents with abdominal pain, hypotension, tachycardia, and shortness of breath. Findings on CT scan reveal free air and stool in the abdomen. He is actively resuscitated. He undergoes exploratory laparotomy, small bowel resection, and ileostomy revision with findings of perforated ileum, gangrenous small bowel, and fecal peritonitis. The patient has a past medical history of pneumatosis intestinalis resulting in ischemic bowel. He is status post previous small bowel resection (1 1/2 feet terminal ileum) and creation of end ileostomy. His medical history is significant for heart disease with previous angioplasty, emphysema, steroid-dependent chronic obstructive pulmonary disease, and cirrhosis. His social history is positive for tobacco and alcohol abuse. He has no known allergies. His medications at home include aspirin, plavix, cardizem, prednisone, prevacid, lexapro, advair, and albuterol. He is admitted to the intensive care unit. On postoperative day 1, the patient is intubated, sedated, and requiring pressors to maintain blood pressure.

Food intake compared to usual: The patient is NPO. He was eating well up until the day prior to admission, when he had onset of acute abdominal pain.

Gastrointestinal symptoms (frequency, duration, intensity): Nasogastric tube output is approximately 1000 ml/day; there is a small amount of green effluent from ileostomy. By history, the patient had usual ileostomy output of 1600 ml/day with report of increasing output depending on food intake.

Weight history: On admission, the patient weighed 90.9 kg. His weight six months prior was 81.8 kg. He had no reports of edema prior to admission. His height is 167.64 cm. Body mass index is 32.3, consistent with obesity. Weight in the intensive care unit, postoperative day 2 is 98 kg, consistent with fluid resuscitation.

Performance status: Prior to admission, patient was ambulatory and independent in activities of daily living. He is now intubated, sedated, and bedridden.

Nutrition-focused physical exam:

HEENT	Anicteric, no cervical adenopathy
Chest	Coarse, crackles
COR	RRR
Abdomen	Obese, soft, nondistended, incision intact, ostomy dusky; nasogastric tube draining 1 liter
Extremities	Warm, 2+ edema, decreased muscle tone

Clinical (impact of disease, metabolic demands, treatment): The patient has ischemic bowel disease and has undergone multiple small bowel resection, including 1 1/2 feet of terminal ileum, resulting in an end ileostomy. He has significant cardiac disease, pulmonary disease, and alcoholic cirrhosis. He is currently critically ill, requiring mechanical ventilation and pressors. He was found to have fecal peritonitis. His measured energy expenditure is consistent with hypermetabolism (approximately 30% above predicted). He is edematous with 8 kg weight gain. He has history of alcoholic abuse.

Overall assessment: The patient is classified as previously well nourished (obese) with increased nutritional risk due to clinical impact of disease, metabolic demands of critical illness, and history of substance abuse. The patient will not likely be extubated within 48 to 72 hours. The patient has a "dusky"-appearing ostomy site. He has an unpredictable return of gastrointestinal function and advancement to oral diet. He will likely require specialized nutrition support.

be more informative than quantifying the actual intake. Byers et al. found that the initial clinical decision to admit a patient to the ICU had the highest impact on time taken to initiate normal oral feeding, taking 17 days in ICU vs. 3 days on a regular floor.[39] Other risk factors associated with patients unable to take a regular oral diet for 5 days were the need for neurosurgery, endotracheal intubation, pelvic fracture, laparotomy, and emergency surgery. This component of SGA should also focus on adequacy of enteral intake if the patient is being fed by tube. It is well documented that enteral nutrition delivery is frequently low in the ICU because of inappropriate prescription rate, inadequate delivery, mechanical problems with the feeding tube, interruptions for airway management and diagnostic procedures, and GI dysfunction.[36,40] Factors significantly associated with low enteral nutrition prescription rate in one study were use of vasoactive drugs, insertion of central venous catheters, and need for extrarenal replacement.[40]

The second component of SGA is evaluation of frequency, intensity, and duration of gastrointestinal symptoms. This history can and should be obtained in conjunction with the abdominal exam. The presence of diarrhea should prompt a thorough review of the medication list, in addition to the patient's history and clinical course. The presence of gastric and intestinal drainage tubes and volume of output may impact the ability to feed enterally, and the quantity and content of drainage may help guide fluid and electrolyte replacement and design of the feeding formulation.

The third component of SGA is the weight history. As previously discussed, weight is often difficult to assess accurately in the ICU due to fluid balance; however, history of weight loss and the underlying mechanism of how the weight loss occurred provides useful assessment data. Patients with pulmonary disease often have severe weight loss due to decreased intake, early satiety, shortness of breath, fatigue, and increased energy expenditure due to the work of breathing. Performance status and function is the fourth component of SGA. Although many critical care patients are bedridden, preillness or preinjury performance status is a useful indicator of health and functioning and can serve as a benchmark to monitor recovery and response to nutritional intervention.

The nutrition-focused physical examination is an essential component of SGA, not only to identify signs and symptoms of nutrient deficiency or excess but also to help determine how patients can be fed. In the ICU patient, the review of systems provides significant information to help guide nutritional care. Focus on general overall appearance, cognition, oral cavity, abdominal exam, and organ system function.

The impact of disease, metabolic demands, and treatment — the final component of SGA in the ICU patient — is often the factor that places the patient at nutritional risk. ICU medical admissions are typically because of a cardiopulmonary event, diabetic ketoacidosis, GI bleeding, drug overdose, or sepsis with multiple organ system failure. Assessment and monitoring of this population should include the following:[41]

- Preadmission nutritional status
- Diagnosis
- Presence of SIRS
- Organ function
- Use of vasopressors
- Inotropic medications and paralytic agents
- Aspiration risk
- The clinician's ability to predict the clinical course and the need for specialized nutrition support

The admission to a surgical ICU is frequently due to risk of bleeding, postoperative or intraoperative complication, major surgery, or surgery with major comorbidity. Assessment and monitoring of this population should include preoperative nutritional status, diagnosis, type of surgery and effect on absorption and digestion, ability to predict return of GI function, and nutrition support access options.[41] The preinjury nutritional status of a trauma patient is often well nourished, as many of these individuals are young adults in some type of accident. Patients in whom preinjury nutritional status is likely poor are those with history of alcohol or substance abuse, or elderly patients with chronic disease. Factors to consider in the assessment include type of trauma, severity of injury, extent of surgery, comorbidities, complications including SIRS, MODS, GI function, enteral access options, and whether the patient will be able to meet increased nutritional requirements spontaneously.[41]

5.7 SUMMARY

Nutrition assessment should be performed in all critically ill patients. Because most of the traditional markers used in nutrition assessment lose their specificity in illness, injury, infection, and inflammation, they must be interpreted cautiously. The clinical history and nutrition-focused physical examination, coupled with clinical judgment and the ability to predict when a patient will eat, are useful assessment tools in the ICU. Establishing screening and assessment guidelines, as well as nutrition support protocols, is an integral step in ensuring the timeliness of patient evaluation and initiation of therapy.[42] The goals of nutrition support should be stated clearly following interpretation of the nutrition assessment. In addition to establishing energy and nutrient goals, clinicians should focus on minimizing the deleterious effects of bed rest and reduced physical activity on muscle catabolism.

REFERENCES

1. Cerra, F.B. et al., ACCP consensus statement: applied nutrition in ICU patients, *Chest,* 111, 769, 1997.
2. ASPEN Board of Directors and Clinical Guidelines Task Force, Guidelines for the use of parenteral and enteral nutrition in adult and pediatric patients, *JPEN*, 26(1), 15A–65A, 95A–125A, 2002.
3. Bone, R.C. et al., Definitions for sepsis and organ failure and guidelines for the use of innovative therapies in sepsis: the ACCP/SCCM Consensus Conference Committee, *Crit. Care Med.*, 20, 864, 1992.
4. Malone, D.L. et al., Back to basics: validation of the admission systemic inflammatory response syndrome score in predicting outcome in trauma, *J. Trauma,* 51, 458, 2001.
5. Knaus, W.A. et al., APACHE II: a severity of disease classification, *Crit. Care Med.*, 13, 818, 1985.
6. Culles, D.J., Civetta, J.M., and Briggs, B., Therapeutic intervention scoring system: a method for quantitative comparison of patient care, *Crit. Care Med.*, 2, 57, 1974.
7. Jennett, B. et al., Predicting outcome in individual patients after severe head injury, *Lancet,* 1(7968), 1031, 1976.
8. Chiolero, R.L. and Fink, M.P., Nutritional and metabolic care in the intensive care unit: a feeling of some uncertainty? *Curr. Opin. Clin. Nutr. Metab. Care,* 5, 159, 2002.
9. Boles, J.-M. et al., Nutritional status in intensive care unit patients: evaluation in 84 unselected patients, *Crit. Care Med.*, 11, 87, 1983.
10. Dardaine, V. et al., Outcome of older patients requiring ventilatory support in intensive care: impact of nutritional status, *J. Am. Geriatr. Soc.*, 49, 564, 2001.
11. Hill, G.L., Implications of critical illness, injury, and sepsis on lean body mass and nutritional needs, *Nutrition*, 14, 557, 1998.
12. Berry, J.K. and Braunschweig, C.A., Nutritional assessment of the critically ill patient, *Crit. Care Nurs. Q.*, 21, 33, 1998.
13. McWhirter, J.P. and Pennington, C.R., Incidence and recognition of malnutrition in the hospital, *Br. Med. J.*, 308, 945, 1994.
14. Kondrup, J. et al., Incidence of nutritional risk and causes of inadequate nutritional care in hospitals, *Clin. Nutr.*, 21, 461, 2002.
15. Ravasco, P. et al., A critical approach to nutritional assessment in critically ill patients, *Clin. Nutr.*, 21, 73, 2002.
16. Roos, A.N. et al., Weight changes in critically ill patients evaluated by fluid balances and impedance measurements, *Crit. Care Med.*, 21, 871, 1993.
17. Piccoli, A. et al., Relationship between central venous pressure and bioimpedance vector analysis in critically ill patients, *Crit. Care Med.*, 28, 132, 2000.
18. Jacobs, D.O. and Wong, M., Metabolic assessment, *World J. Surg.*, 24, 1460, 2000.
19. Cioffi, W.G., What's new in burns and metabolism, *J. Am. Coll. Surg.*, 192, 241, 2001.
20. Blunt, M.C., Nicholson, J.P., and Park, G.R., Serum albumin and colloid osmotic pressure in survivors and non-survivors of prolonged critical illness, *Anaesth.*, 53, 755, 1998.

21. McCluskey, A. et al., The prognostic value of serial measurements of serum albumin in patients admitted to an intensive care unit, *Anaesth.*, 51, 724, 1996.
22. Manelli, J.C. et al., A reference standard for plasma proteins is required for nutritional assessment of adult burn patients, *Burns*, 24, 337, 1998.
23. Gibbs, J. et al., Preoperative serum albumin level as a predictor of operative mortality and morbidity, *Arch. Surg.*, 134, 36, 1999.
24. Sapijaszco, M.J.A. et al., Non respiratory predictor of mechanical ventilation dependency in intensive care unit patients, *Crit. Care Med.*, 24, 601, 1996.
25. Bauer, P. et al., Parenteral with enteral nutrition in the critically ill, *Intens. Care Med.*, 26, 893, 2002.
26. Bernstein, L., Measurement of visceral protein status in assessing protein and energy malnutrition: standard of care, *Prealbumin in Nutritional Care Consensus Group*, 11, 169, 1995.
27. Raguso, C.A., Dupertuis, Y.M., and Pichard, C., The role of visceral proteins in the nutritional assessment of intensive care unit patients, *Curr. Opin. Clin. Nutr. Metab. Care*, 6, 211, 2003.
28. Young, B., Gleeson, M., and Cripps, A.W., C-reactive protein: a critical review, *Pathology*, 23, 118, 1991.
29. Reny, J-L. et al., Diagnosis and follow-up of infections in intensive care patients: value of C-reactive protein compared with other clinical and biological variables, *Crit. Care Med.*, 30, 529, 2002.
30. Chan, S., McCowen, M.B., and Blackburn, G.L., Nutrition management in the ICU, *Chest*, 115, 145S, 1999.
31. Binnert, C. and Tappy, L., Microdialysis in the intensive care unit: a novel tool for clinical investigation or monitoring? *Curr. Opin. Clin. Nutr. Metab. Care*, 5, 185, 2002.
32. Lopez-Hellin, J. et al., Usefulness of short-lived proteins as nutritional indicators in surgical patients, *Clin. Nutr.*, 21,119, 2002.
33. Epstein, C.D. et al., Comparison of methods of measurements of oxygen consumption in mechanically ventilated patients with multiple trauma: the Fick method versus indirect calorimetry, *Crit. Care Med.*, 28, 1363, 2000.
34. Headley, J.M., Indirect calorimetry: a trend toward continuous metabolic assessment, *AACN Clin. Issues,* 14, 155, 2003.
35. Brandi, L.S., Bertolini, R., and Calafa, M., Indirect calorimetry in critically ill patients: clinical applications and practical advice, *Nutrition,*13, 349, 1997.
36. McClave, S.A., McClain, C.J., and Snider, H.L., Should indirect calorimetry be used as part of nutritional assessment? *J. Clin. Gastroenterol.*, 33, 14, 2001.
37. Detsky, A.S. et al., What is subjective global assessment of nutritional status? *JPEN*, 11, 8, 1987.
38. Hasse, J. et al., Subjective global assessment: alternative nutrition-assessment technique for liver-transplant candidates, *Nutrition*, 9, 339, 1993.
39. Byers, P.M. et al., The need for aggressive intervention in the injured patient: the development of a predictive model, *J. Trauma*, 39, 1103, 1995.
40. DeJonge, B. et al., A prospective survey of nutritional support practices in intensive care unit patients. What is prescribed? What is delivered? *Crit. Care Med.*, 29, 8, 2001.
41. Winkler, M.F. and Malone, A.M., Medical nutrition therapy for metabolic stress: sepsis, trauma, burns, and surgery, in *Krause's Food, Nutrition, and Diet Therapy,* 11th ed., Mahan, L.K. and Escott-Stump, S., Eds., W.B. Saunders, Philadelphia, 1058–1078, 2003.
42. Aihara, R. et al., Guidelines for improving nutritional delivery in the intensive care unit, *J. Healthcare Qual.*, 24, 22, 2002.

6 Energy Requirements in the Critically Ill Patient

David Frankenfield
Penn State's Milton S. Hershey Medical Center

CONTENTS

6.1 INTRODUCTION

Accurate determination of energy needs is an important part of the nutritional assessment of critically ill patients. Provision of calories equal to energy expenditure is usually the goal, but under some circumstances hypocaloric feeding is acceptable or maybe even desirable [1]. Under no circumstances is overfeeding a critically ill person a good thing. The goal of this chapter is to describe the energy requirements of the critically ill patient, to examine the methods for determining energy requirements, and to discuss situations in which hypocaloric feeding might be appropriate and which therefore do not require an accurate reckoning of metabolic rate.

6.2 THE INFLAMMATORY RESPONSE IN CRITICALLY ILL PATIENTS

As a result of traumatic or surgical injury, infection, cancer, and other illness, the human body produces an inflammatory response [2]. At the mediation level, several interacting systems are involved. The central nervous system, hormones, cytokines, eicosanoids, growth factors, and catabolic factors all play a role [3]. Clinically apparent hallmarks of the response include fever, tachycardia, tachypnea, and leukocytosis [2]. These patients tend to be hyperdynamic. Blood chemistry hallmarks of the inflammatory response include fasting hyperglycemia, hypertriglyceridemia (but hypocholesterolemia), and hypoalbuminemia (but increased acute-phase proteins) [4]. Metabolically, the patient undergoing an inflammatory response has an increase in resting metabolic rate, an increase in muscle catabolism and nitrogen loss, enhanced gluconeogenesis that is resistant to feeding, a blunting of ketone production if the patient is starved, and an increase in peripheral glutamine production — but an even greater increase in glutamine consumption centrally. This chapter will emphasize the changes in resting metabolic rate brought about by the inflammatory response in critically ill patients.

6.3 SOME HISTORY

Many of the pioneers in human energy metabolism pursued not only studies of metabolic rate in healthy people but also in people with fevers due to infections or other causes. (Francis Benedict even reported on the effect of fever on resting metabolic rate in healthy subjects made acutely ill by mercury poisoning caused accidentally by contamination of the air in the respiration calorimeter he was using to study metabolic rate in healthy volunteers) [5,6]. These and other early works consistently showed that fever, no matter the origin, increases resting metabolic rate (Figure 6.1) [7]. In fact, the rule of thumb still in use today, which states that resting metabolic rate increases by 13% per degree centigrade, can be traced back to the work of DuBois in the 1910s and 1920s [7]. The concept of hypermetabolism and hypercatabolism after injury was crystallized in the seminal work of Cuthbertson in the 1930s [8].

In the 1960s and 1970s, John Kinney and many researchers who trained under him made major contributions to our understanding of the hypermetabolic response after illness and injury [9,10]. Common recommendations at this time were to provide calorie support at $1\,^1\!/_2$ times measured resting metabolic rate [11]. It was under such conditions that the concept of carbohydrate-driven carbon dioxide production as a cause for respiratory distress came about and was studied [11,12] and how the relative influence of carbohydrate load vs. overfeeding became confused.

In 1979, Calvin Long (one of Kinney's protégés) published stress factors for illness and injury that are still widely used today [13]. These factors were intended as multipliers for the Harris–Benedict equation for healthy resting metabolic rate [14]. For the impact the Long study had on the way metabolic rate is calculated in intensive care units, it was remarkably small. Thirty-nine nonventilated patients were studied and categorized into five groups, and a separate group of burn patients was abstracted from an earlier publication (1970) to fill the Long study's burn group. Table 6.1 gives the stress factors as originally published.

Soon after the publication of Long's study, commercially available, portable, indirect calorimeters came onto the market, resulting in many, often conflicting, publications on metabolic rate in critical illness [15–22]. Some investigators found that resting metabolic rate was more than 150% of expected healthy resting metabolism; others found almost no elevation in resting metabolic rate at all. The conflicting nature of these works may be an indication of the extent to which care practices at individual hospitals affect resting metabolic rate of the patients being cared for there, or they might represent the heterogeneity of published study groups sorted by disease type without considering underlying variability in the degree of inflammation.

6.4 IS HYPERMETABOLISM LINKED TO ILLNESS PER SE OR TO THE INFLAMMATORY RESPONSE TO ILLNESS?

Most research on resting metabolic rate in critically ill patients categorizes those patients based on their reason for being critically ill (trauma vs. surgery vs. pancreatitis, etc.). Long's seminal paper [13] is a good example of this, with division of subjects into elective surgery, blunt and

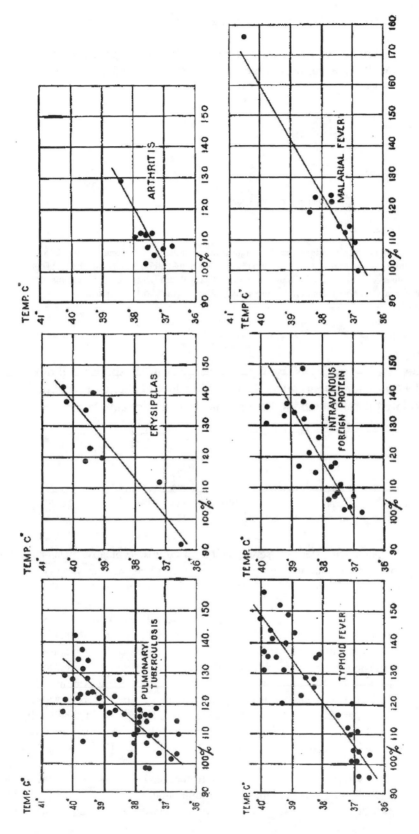

FIGURE 6.1 The metabolic rate response to fever from various causes, as reported by Eugene DuBois in 1915 to 1921 [7]. Data points enhanced for this reproduction. Erysipelas is a hemolytic streptococcal skin infection that causes fever. (From DuBois, E.F., JAMA, 77, 352, 1921. With permission.)

TABLE 6.1
Stress and Activity Multipliers for Injury and Illness Suggested by Long in 1979 (Multiply Basal Metabolic Rate by Harris–Benedict Equation by Activity Factor and by Injury Factor)

Activity Factor	
Confined to bed	1.2
Out of bed	1.3
Injury factor	
Minor operation	1.2
Skeletal trauma[a]	1.35
Major sepsis (fever, hypotension, tachypnea, tachycardia, [i.e., SIRS])	1.6
Severe thermal burn	2.10

[a] This appears to be an average of skeletal trauma (auto crashes without brain injury) at ×1.32, blunt trauma (gunshot wounds) at ×1.37, and trauma with steroids (brain injury) at ×1.61. It should also be pointed out that the major sepsis and severe thermal burn stress factors do not match the percent increase over basal measured in the study (1.32 for burns and 1.79 for sepsis).

TABLE 6.2
Influence of Injury or Disease Type vs. Inflammatory Response to Illness as the Cause for Hypermetabolism in Critically Ill Patients (Percent of Calculated Basal Metabolic Rate by Harris–Benedict Equation)

Injury Group	Maximum Body Temperature > 38°C		All
	Yes	No	
Trauma	145 ± 22	123 ± 14	134 ± 23
Major surgery	138 ± 22	125 ± 14	132 ± 22
Medical	139 ± 20	125 ± 20	132 ± 20
All	141 ± 24	124 ± 17	

penetrating trauma, trauma with steroids, sepsis, and burn groups. Typically, burns and sepsis are found to be the most hypermetabolic condition, followed by blunt trauma, surgery, and medical conditions. However, categorization by illness type alone does not explain all of the variability in resting metabolic rate in critically ill patients.

Frankenfield et al. [23] examined inflammatory response relative to injury type in a diverse group of nonburn trauma, surgery, and medical intensive care unit patients. Presence of fever was used as a marker of inflammatory response. It was found that cause of illness made relatively little difference in resting metabolic rate once the effect of fever was controlled for. In afebrile subjects, hypermetabolism was less pronounced than in febrile subjects and there was almost no difference by injury type (Table 6.2). There was more separation by illness type in febrile subjects (trauma being somewhat more hypermetabolic than either surgery or medicine), but when subjects' body temperature was controlled by covariate analysis, resting metabolic rates among the febrile subjects were $137 \pm 21\%$ of healthy resting metabolic rate for trauma, $135 \pm 20\%$ for surgery, and $135 \pm 21\%$ for medicine.

In heavily sedated, severely brain-injured patients, Bruder et al. found that the percent elevation in measured total metabolic rate was determined by body temperature [24]. In fact, metabolic rate increased by an average of 10% per degree centigrade of temperature elevation (similar to DuBois's observation more than 80 years earlier that metabolic rate increased by 13% per degree centigrade). On the other hand, Bruder also found that total metabolic rate as a percentage of healthy resting rate was higher in septic brain-injury patients than in nonseptic brain-injury patients (142 ± 28% vs. 123 ± 19% of healthy resting metabolic rate) and that controlling for differences in body temperature blunted but did not eliminate this difference (128 ± 22 vs. 119 ± 16% healthy resting metabolic rate).

Another way of examining the relation of resting metabolic rate and fever is to examine the change in resting metabolic rate as febrile patients are cooled. Metabolic rate has been found to drop in sedated febrile patients being cooled by external cooling. A 10% decrease in resting metabolic rate occurred as body temperature was lowered from 39.2 to 37.2 degrees centigrade [25]. The fact that the patients were sedated during cooling is critical, because if they were not sedated, shivering would have occurred, resulting in increased metabolic rate.

Thus, it seems that the presence of an inflammatory response is a major factor in determining the degree of hypermetabolism in critically ill patients. Within any disease category, fever denotes an increase in resting metabolic rate. This points out the importance of body temperature as a feature of clinical nutrition assessment and practice in the ICU.

6.5 WHAT IS THE IMPACT OF PHYSICAL ACTIVITY AND SEDATION ON METABOLIC RATE?

Intuitively, sedation and medical paralysis should be associated with a decrease in resting metabolic rate. Indeed, in a randomized trial on the effect of propofol vs. midazolam on time to sedation and time to awakening, Kress et al. [26] used 33 medical ICU patients as their own controls to determine the change in oxygen consumption as subjects went from the awake to the sedated state. Oxygen consumption dropped from 4.58 ml/min/kg body weight to 3.89 ml/min/kg body weight (equivalent to an 18% drop in metabolic rate from 32 kcal/kg to 27 kcal/kg body weight), with no difference noted between the propofol and the midazolam.

Similarly, Marik and Kaufman [27] used eight medical ICU patients as their own controls as medical paralysis was induced. In these subjects, oxygen consumption fell 34% from 200 ± 77 ml/min/m² body surface area to 149 ± 35 ml, with no change in body temperature. Paradoxically, septic trauma patients in whom a clinical decision had been made to medically paralyze have been observed to have higher resting metabolic rates than septic trauma patients in whom medical paralysis was not clinically indicated (48 ± 16 vs. 42 ± 6 kcal/kg body weight) [22]. The most likely explanation of this observation is that the medically paralyzed patients were more seriously ill and therefore had more inflammatory injury and higher resting metabolic rate. Thus, it is safe to say that sedation and medical paralysis will decrease resting metabolic rate in an individual as he or she goes from a conscious to a drugged state, but it is not true to state that subjects requiring heavy sedation or paralysis are less hypermetabolic than those not requiring such drug therapy, because those requiring therapy are probably sicker.

Physical activity also contributes to the total metabolic rate of critically ill patients. Activities such as bathing, chest physiotherapy, and dressing changes may increase metabolic rate by 20 to 35% [28,29]. However, because these activities are usually short lived, the overall impact on daily metabolic rate is more on the order of about 5% [22].

6.6 WHAT IS THE LINK BETWEEN HYPERMETABOLISM AND HYPERCATABOLISM?

Increased muscle catabolism and nitrogen loss are hallmarks of critical illness [4]. Hypermetabolism is thought to go hand in hand with this catabolic state, because both are consequences of the inflammatory response. In Frankenfield's series of trauma patients [30], there was in fact a linear

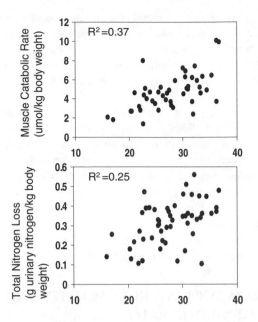

FIGURE 6.2 Relationship between muscle catabolic rate and resting metabolic rate, and between urinary nitrogen loss and resting metabolic rate in critically ill trauma patients (from data in reference 43).

association between resting metabolic rate and muscle catabolic rate and between resting metabolic rate and total urinary nitrogen loss in patients receiving nutrition support (Figure 6.2). The mean ratio of energy expenditure per gram of nitrogen lost was about 100:1, but the correlation between the two was quite low, so the range in this ratio was wide (49:1 to 319:1), making such a ratio useless in estimating nitrogen loss from metabolic rate. Thus, one can safely say that as resting metabolic rate rises, catabolic rate and nitrogen loss tend to rise, but quantification cannot be made without measurement.

6.7 HOW IS RESTING METABOLIC RATE PREDICTED?

Although measurement of resting metabolic rate in the ICU is possible, it is seldom done, leaving the clinician with little choice but to determine metabolic needs by estimation. It is not possible to list or comment on all of the estimation methods, so this chapter discusses only a few pertinent methods.

Common practice for predicting resting metabolic rate in critically ill patients is to calculate healthy resting metabolic rate (often using the Harris–Benedict equations) [14] and then to multiply this rate by a stress factor. Calvin Long's stress factors from 1979 are still used for this purpose today. In the 1990s a different approach emerged, which deemphasized patient categorization into stress factors and instead used dynamic physiologic variables in regression equations to predict resting metabolic rate. Swinamer [31] was one of the first to report such an equation, developed from 112 mechanically ventilated critical care patients (47% trauma):

$$RMR = BSA(941) - age(6.3) + Temp(104) + RR(24) + V_T(804) - 4243 \qquad (6.1)$$

in which BSA is body surface area (m^2), age is in years, Temp is body temperature (degrees centigrade), RR is respiratory rate in breaths/minute, and V_T is tidal volume in liters/breath.

This is the prototypical form of resting metabolic rate equations in critical care in that the body surface area and age terms reflect the classic determinants of healthy resting metabolic rate (i.e., metabolic body size), and the Temp, RR, and V_T terms reflect the effect of inflammatory response on metabolic rate. Of note is the absence of a factor for type of injury, even though a heterogeneous patient population was used to develop the equation.

Soon after the release of the Swinamer equation, Ireton-Jones [32] published an equation in regression form that also accounted for the typical predictors of healthy resting metabolism (body weight, age, sex) and added categories of illness (trauma, burn injury) but did not utilize clinical variables such as body temperature, respiratory rate, or tidal volume to account for degree of inflammation:

$$RMR = wt(5) - age(10) - sex(281) + trauma(292) + burn(851) + 1925 \qquad (6.2)$$

This equation was developed from a group of 65 ventilator-dependent ICU patients. Fifty-two percent were burn victims. In 1997, an amended equation was published from the same data, but with corrections to the statistics [33]:

$$RMR = wt(5) - age(11) - sex(244) + trauma(239) + burn(804) + 1784 \qquad (6.3)$$

In 1994, Frankenfield et al. [34] published an equation developed from 423 measurements in 56 mechanically ventilated trauma and septic trauma patients that again relied on a marker of healthy resting metabolic rate (RMR[healthy], in this case the Harris–Benedict equation), physiologic variables (V_E, minute ventilation in L/min), and disease category (SMOF, septic multiple organ failure):

$$RMR = RMR(healthy)(1.3) + V_E(100) + SMOF(300) - 1000 \qquad (6.4)$$

A more recent equation published by Frankenfield was constructed retrospectively from the data in [24] and referred to as the Penn State equation. This equation was developed based on a broad mix of trauma, surgical, and medical ICU patients [35]:

$$RMR = RMR(healthy)(1.1) + V_E(32) + Tmax(140) - 5340 \qquad (6.5)$$

The RMR(healthy) term is the Harris–Benedict equation using actual weight for nonobese and adjusted weight for obese patients, V_E is minute ventilation in L/min, and Tmax is maximum body temperature in the previous 24 hours (degrees centigrade). The investigators later found that use of adjusted body weight in the Harris–Benedict equation caused significant underestimation of healthy resting metabolic rate [36], so the Penn State ICU equation was recomputed from the original data using actual body weight for obese and nonobese people both [37]:

$$RMR = RMR(healthy)(0.85) + V_E(33) + Tmax(175) - 6433 \qquad (6.6)$$

6.7.1 VALIDATION

The number of calculation equations published over the years is legion. The number of validation studies of published equations is not (probably numbering fewer than ten). One of the first validation studies of any of the preceding equations was conducted by Flancbaum [38], in which the 1992 Ireton-Jones and Frankenfield equations (Equation 6.2 and Equation 6.4) were examined. Neither equation performed particularly well. Correlation coefficients between measured and predicted resting metabolic rate were low ($R^2 = 0.15$ for Frankenfield and 0.07 for Ireton-Jones). The Ireton-Jones equation was prone to underestimation (doing so in 89% of cases vs. 37% for

Frankenfield). On the other hand, the Frankenfield equation could markedly overestimate true resting metabolic rate (by 1617 kilocalories in one case).

Similarly, MacDonald [39], using continuous gas exchange technology (thus probably measuring total metabolic rate, which is greater than resting metabolic rate) in 76 critically ill patients with body mass index < 30 kg/m², tested the validity of the Swinamer, 1992 Ireton-Jones, Frankenfield, and Penn State equations (Equations 6.1, 6.2, 6.4, and 6.5). The 1992 Ireton-Jones equation underestimated measured metabolic rate (on average 85 ± 16% of total metabolic rate) with low correlation ($R^2 = 0.23$), whereas the Frankenfield equation correlated with total metabolic rate ($R^2 = 0.52$) and on average was 90 ± 20% of measured. In both the Ireton-Jones and Frankenfield equations, only 63% of subjects were predicted to within 20% of measured metabolic rate. The Penn State equation correlated with measured total metabolic rate ($R^2 = 0.66$) and on average calculated at 87 ± 11% of measured total metabolic rate. Seventy-two percent of subjects were estimated to within 20% of measured total metabolic rate. The Swinamer equation predicted total metabolic rate to within 20% of measured in 88% of subjects, and on average metabolic rate was predicted at 93 ± 12% of measured.

In another validation study, the Ireton-Jones and Penn State equations (Equations 6.2, 6.3, 6.5, and 6.6) were tested against measured resting metabolic rate in 47 critically ill patients (trauma, surgical, and medical ICU, with no restriction on body mass index) [37]. Defining an accurate prediction of resting metabolic rate as one lying within 10% of measured and defining a clinically important error as a prediction that was more than 15% above or below measured resting metabolic rate, the modified Penn State equation (Equation 6.6) was accurate 72% of the time vs. 60% of the time for the Ireton-Jones equation, and made a clinically important error 11% of the time vs. 28% of the time for the Ireton-Jones equation. Table 6.3 summarizes the validation work performed on these equations, categorizing each by the percentage of times an accurate estimate is made and the percentage of times that a large error is made.

TABLE 6.3
Summary of Validation Studies of Equations for Resting Metabolic Rate in Critical Care Patients (Subjects with Body Mass Index < 30 kg/m², Except where Indicated)

Equation	Validation Paper	Measured Parameter	% of Subjects Predicted to within 10% of Measured	% of Subjects Predicted within 11 to 15% of Measured	% of Subjects Predicted Greater than 15% of Measured
Ireton-Jones [32]	MacDonald [39]	Total metabolic rate	28	15	57
Ireton-Jones [32]	Frankenfield [37]	Resting metabolic rate	52 (72)*	14 (0)*	34 (28)*
Frankenfield [34]	MacDonald [39]	Total metabolic rate	43	9	48
Swinamer [31]	MacDonald [39]	Total metabolic rate	55	9	36
Penn State [35]	MacDonald [39]	Total metabolic rate	39	18	43
Penn State [35]	Frankenfield [37]	Resting metabolic rate	69 (67)*	17 (16)*	14 (17)*
Penn State (revised) [37]	Frankenfield [37]	Resting metabolic rate	79 (61)*	21 (11)*	0 (28)*

Note: The data presentation in the validation study by Flancbaum [38] did not lend itself to the format of this table.

* Percentages in parentheses are for subjects with body mass index > 30 kg/m².

6.8 HOW DOES OBESITY AFFECT THE PREDICTION OF RESTING METABOLIC RATE?

Fifty percent of Americans are obese [40]. Obesity predisposes to various illnesses and increases operative and anesthesia risk. It is therefore quite common to encounter obese patients in the ICU. As with other aspects of critical care in the obese person, nutrition assessment in obesity is often extrapolated from data from normal-weight patients or is based on conjecture and assumption.

Just as it is with their normal-weight compatriots, total metabolic rate in obese people is often calculated from predicted resting metabolic rate (often Harris–Benedict) multiplied by stress factors. Unlike for normal-weight people, resting metabolism calculations are usually modified by using an obesity-adjusted body weight rather than the actual weight of the patient [41]. Obesity-adjusted body weight is most often calculated as a percentage of the excess body weight added to the ideal body weight. The percentage of excess body weight added to ideal can range from 25 to 45% and seems to be based on empiricism rather than on data.

Jeevanandam et al. [42], in a small but detailed study of intermediary metabolism in obese trauma patients (n = 7 with 10 control subjects), included information on resting metabolic rate and body composition. These investigators found that total resting metabolic rate between obese (mean body mass index 36 kg/m^2) and nonobese subjects (mean body mass index 25 kg/m^2) was similar (2550 ± 172 vs. 2538 ± 162 kcal/day) and that the caloric expenditure per kg lean body mass was also not different between the groups (43.6 ± 2.9 kcal/kg vs. 39.0 ± 2.5 kcal/kg). On a per-kilogram body weight basis, however, the obese subjects' metabolic rate was only 25 kcal/kg to the nonobese's 33 kcal/kg.

In a larger group of trauma victims (11 obese, 41 nonobese), Frankenfield [43] found a measured resting metabolic rate of 1999 ± 120 vs. 2114 ± 66 kcal/day (N.S.) in obese vs. nonobese subjects. Indexing to lean body mass revealed a similar resting metabolic rate between the groups (32 ± 3 kcal/kg vs. 35 ± 1 kcal/kg, not significant) but a significant difference when indexed to total body weight (22 ± 1 vs. 29 ± 1 kcal/kg).

The similarity in resting metabolic rate per kilogram of lean body mass in obese vs. nonobese people belies the fact that resting metabolic rate is more difficult to predict in the obese than in the nonobese person. First, lean body mass and body cell mass are very difficult to measure clinically. Second, as shown in Table 6.3, the rate of accurate prediction using the Penn State equation dropped from 79% in nonobese subjects to 61% in obese subjects, and the rate of large errors increased from 0 to 28% [37], even though the database used to develop the Penn State equations included obese people.

6.9 DOES AGE AFFECT RESTING METABOLIC RATE IN THE CRITICALLY ILL?

Just as the general population is getting heavier, it is also growing older [44]. The elderly make up a substantial percentage of the population in a critical care unit. Typical aging is associated with a drop in fat-free mass (although those who maintain physical activity can minimize this change) [44]. Because fat-free mass is the "engine" of the body, which burns all the fuel and performs all the work [45], it follows that resting metabolic rate decreases with typical aging. Indeed, most predictive equations for resting metabolic rate include a negative age multiplier to account for the attenuation in resting metabolic rate.

Changes in the metabolic response to critical illness in the elderly have not been extensively studied. In one investigation [43], elderly trauma patients were found to have a lower incidence of fever on days 5 to 7 post injury. In young trauma patients, more than 80% were febrile, whereas in the elderly, fewer than 50% were. This was true despite higher infection rates in the elderly group. Resting metabolic rate was 12% lower in the elderly than in the young. Controlling for body compositional differences in the elderly only partly reduced the difference (an 8% difference remained).

In the validation study of predictive equations for resting metabolic rate in the ICU [37], the Penn State equation accurately predicted resting metabolic rate in 85% of elderly subjects, whereas the Ireton-Jones equation accurately predicted resting metabolic rate in only 45% of elderly subjects.

6.10 IS IT NECESSARY TO ACHIEVE ENERGY BALANCE IN CRITICALLY ILL PATIENTS?

In simple starvation, nitrogen balance is a function of both nitrogen (protein) intake and energy intake [46]. At constant but inadequate protein intake, nitrogen balance will improve linearly with increasing energy intake, plateauing in the negative range when energy balance is achieved. When adequate energy is consumed, nitrogen balance will improve linearly with increasing protein intake and will plateau in the positive range. Thus, achievement of energy balance is an important goal in the nutrition support of non-ICU patients.

In critically ill patients, however, nitrogen balance and energy balance appear to be uncoupled. Starvation is associated with increased muscle catabolism and nitrogen loss, whereas aggressive calorie support has been shown to promote weight gain as fat and water but not muscle [47]. Hypocaloric feeding in critical care spares nitrogen and reduces net catabolic rate compared to starvation [48], but at least three studies have shown that feeding calories equal to or in excess of metabolic rate does not improve nitrogen balance or decrease catabolic rate compared to hypocaloric feeding [30,49,50]. There is no linear relationship between calorie intake and nitrogen balance in critically ill patients, as there is in simple starvation. Two of these studies were performed on obese subjects, and the third was performed on a mix of obese and nonobese subjects. All of the studies used parenteral nutrition as the feeding route. Most subjects had postoperative complications or were trauma patients, though in only one of the studies is it mentioned specifically that subjects were cared for in an intensive care unit. Table 6.4 shows a comparison of the parameters of the three studies of hypocaloric feeding. Hypocaloric feeding has not been studied in critically ill, underweight patients, and it would be imprudent to assume that the data for normal-weight and obese people are generalizable to the underweight patient. Hypocaloric feeding may be desirable in the obese patient, with the goal of avoiding large overestimations of true metabolic rate and thus markedly overfeeding the patient.

6.11 IS IT BETTER TO MEASURE OR TO ESTIMATE METABOLIC RATE IN CRITICALLY ILL PATIENTS?

As reviewed previously, estimation of resting metabolic rate in critically ill patients has important limitations. Measurement of metabolic rate is possible clinically by use of indirect calorimetry. However, the equipment is expensive, the technique can be time consuming, and there are some patients who cannot be measured accurately. Furthermore, precise knowledge of resting metabolic rate has not been shown to improve clinical outcome. Measurement of metabolic rate may have a role in the clinical care of patients in whom a reasonable estimate of metabolic rate cannot be expected. Examples of this are significant change in body shape or composition (amputation, severe obesity, spinal cord injury with quadriplegia, scoliosis, very small adults as occurs with some forms of retardation, prolonged bed rest with its attendant loss of muscle mass). Another instance in which measurement of metabolic rate may be desirable is when the patient is not progressing as expected (unexplained high minute ventilation, unexplained failure to wean from ventilator) or when hypometabolism is expected (high S_vO_2, shock, hypothermia, spinal cord injury with quadriplegia).

TABLE 6.4
Energy and Nitrogen Balance and Muscle Catabolic Rate Data for Hypocaloric vs. Full Feeding in Critically Ill Patients

	Study					
	Burge [49]		Frankenfield [30]			Dickerson [48]
Parameter	Hypocaloric	Normocaloric	Hypocaloric	Normocaloric	Overfed	Hypocaloric
Resting metabolic rate (kcal/d)	1767	2199	2095	2175	2257	2205
Total calorie intake (kcal/d)	1285	2429	1600	2280	2815	1397
Intake/RMR	0.73	1.13	0.75	1.05	1.24	0.63
Protein intake (g/d)	111	130	120	120	124	129
Nitrogen intake (g/d)	17.8	20.8	19.2	19.2	19.8	20.6
Urea nitrogen output (g/d)	8.1*	10.7*	26.8	24.9	26.6	15.0
Nitrogen balance (g/d)	+1.3	+2.8	−7.9	−7.5	−8.3	+2.4
3-methylhistidine excretion (μmol/d)	255	335	357	422	375	–

* Urine urea nitrogen value is a fasting value.

6.11.1 INDIRECT CALORIMETRY

Indirect calorimetry is the measurement of respiratory gas exchange in order to make inference about cellular gas exchange (which equates to metabolic rate and substrate utilization). The measured parameters of indirect calorimetry are oxygen consumption (VO_2) and carbon dioxide production (VCO_2). From these measurements, respiratory quotient (RQ) and metabolic rate can be calculated. Indirect calorimetry is valid only when the respiratory gas exchange and the cellular gas exchange are equivalent (Figure 6.3). Equivalence is fairly easy to attain for oxygen consumption, because oxygen is not stored in the body and is not used for purposes other than metabolism. Thus, a change in cellular oxygen consumption is quickly detected as a change in respiratory VO_2. Carbon dioxide, on the other hand, is stored extensively in the body and participates in acid–base homeostasis. Therefore, a change in carbon dioxide production in the cells can take time to manifest as a change in respiratory VCO_2 [51], and a need to convert back and forth to bicarbonate or to ventilate carbon dioxide from the blood in order to normalize pH will result in an uncoupling of cellular and respiratory carbon dioxide.

6.11.1.1 Equipment

Most indirect calorimeters in use today are portable, open-circuit devices. Open-circuit refers to the fact that whereas the entire expired air is captured and measured for gas concentration and volume by the calorimeter, the inspired air is only sampled. Total inspired volume is instead calculated from inspired and expired gas concentrations and expired volume. This puts an upper limit on the FIO_2 at which measurements can be conducted, but it makes the calorimetry device much easier to use.

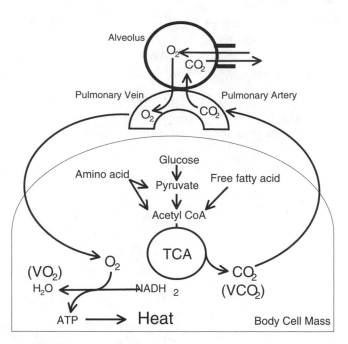

FIGURE 6.3 Diagram illustrating the relationship between pulmonary gas exchange and cellular metabolism. This relationship makes indirect calorimetry possible.

Calorimeters have four basic components. Two of the components relate to analysis of gas concentrations: separate sensors for analyzing carbon dioxide and oxygen consumption in the inspired and expired air. The calorimeter must also have a device for measuring expired air volume. Finally, a computer is used to calculate inspired volume, RQ, and metabolic rate; to run test algorithms; and to manage data output.

6.11.1.2 Measurement Protocols

In order for indirect calorimetry measurements to have meaning, they must be performed under known conditions. Ideally, all clinical indirect calorimetry measurements would be performed continuously, resulting in a value for total daily metabolic rate. Such a measurement would include the effect of physical activity, feeding state, and change clinical condition on the patient's metabolic rate and would average out respiratory artifact (the times when the respiratory and cellular gas exchanges are not equivalent). Systems exist for continuous gas exchange monitoring, some single unit [52] and some multi-unit [53]. However, the most common indirect calorimetry measurement is one in which metabolic rate is measured over a short time period (less than 1 h). In such cases, more attention must be paid to the clinical state of the patient at the time of the measurement, so that the result can be properly interpreted and acted upon.

The most desired measurement condition for a short indirect calorimetry test is that of steady-state rest. Steady-state rest is desirable because it is reproducible, can be accomplished quickly (if due diligence is applied), minimizes the chance of respiratory artifact, and in critical care represents more than 90% of the total metabolic rate unless the patient is agitated or otherwise physically active [22]. The resting state is one in which the patient has been left undisturbed and is lying nearly motionless in bed. This condition should be maintained for at least 30 minutes prior to measurement (less if deeply sedated or medically paralyzed) and continue through the duration of the measurement. In healthy people undergoing indirect calorimetry, resting conditions require a fast, but in the ICU, with patients typically receiving continuous feeding, the fasting state is not supposed to occur, so feeding should not be stopped for indirect calorimeter measurements.

Steady-state refers to a condition in which the subject's gas exchange measurements are varying from minute to minute within a tight range and is another way of assuring that respiratory and metabolic gas exchanges are the same. If a change in respiratory rate, tidal volume (the components of minute ventilation), or FIO_2 has been made recently, the patient will be in a state of change, so indirect calorimetry should not be performed.

When resting conditions are known to exist and it is also known that no ventilator changes have recently been made, an indirect calorimetry measurement can commence. The remaining criterion for steady state (tight variation in VO_2, VCO_2, and minute ventilation) can only be determined after the measurement commences. Typical allowable coefficient of variation to define steady state is 5% in a 10-minute test or 10% coefficient of variation in a 30-minute test (discarding the first five minutes of data automatically). Either protocol has been shown to reflect 24-hour resting metabolic rate [54,55].

If a resting steady state cannot be achieved, the indirect calorimetry measurement can be prolonged over several hours, while typical nursing activities are allowed to occur as usual. The resulting data do not require a minimum coefficient of variation on the gas exchange parameters.

6.11.1.3 Interpretation

There are two aspects to the interpretation of indirect calorimetry studies:

- Assessment of whether the results are technically acceptable
- Integration of the results with clinical conditions at the time of the measurement

The points to note regarding technical acceptability are whether the minute ventilation measured by the calorimeter agrees reasonably with the minute ventilation measured by the mechanical ventilator. (These numbers will not agree 100%, but they should be close to one another.) Other technical aspects are whether steady-state conditions were met and whether the RQ is within the physiologic range (approximately 0.68 to 1.2).

Integration of the measurement with clinical condition entails assessing whether the measurement was performed in a resting state or whether it was prolonged to capture physical activity, whether the patient was sedated or medically paralyzed during the measurement, and whether the patient was febrile or afebrile. The RQ should be at least broadly consistent with the feeding state of the patient. If the patient was measured in the resting state, a factor of 5 to 10% can be added to account for physical activity.

6.12 CONCLUSION

The inflammatory response to critical illness touches off many metabolic changes, one of which is hypermetabolism. The degree of hypermetabolism is largely determined by the degree of inflammatory response to injury rather than by the injury *per se*. Indirect calorimetry is the most accurate way to determine metabolic rate but is not widely available, so predictive methods are usually relied on. Prediction of metabolic rate is most accurate when the influence of body composition and inflammation is taken into account. Obesity makes accurate prediction of metabolic rate more difficult. Therefore, the obese patient may be considered for high-protein, hypocaloric feeding in order to avoid the consequences of overfeeding.

REFERENCES

1. Dickerson R.N., Boschert K.J., Kudsk K.A., et al., Hypocaloric enteral tube feeding in critically ill obese patients, *Nutr.,* 18, 241, 2002.

2. American College of Chest Physicians, Society of Critical Care Medicine Consensus Conference Committee: American College of Chest Physicians, Society of Critical Care Medicine Consensus Conference, Definitions for sepsis and organ failure and guidelines for the use of innovative therapies in sepsis, *Crit. Care Med.*, 20, 864, 1992.

3. Chrousos G.P., The hypothalamic-pituitary-adrenal axis and immune-mediated inflammation, *N. Eng. J. Med.*, 332, 1351, 1995.

4. Chiolero R., Revelly J.P., and Tappy L., Energy metabolism in sepsis and injury, *Nutrition,* 13, 45S, 1997.

5. Carpenter T.M. and Benedict F.G., Mercurial poisoning of men in a respiration chamber, *Am. J. Physiol.,* 24, 187, 1909.

6. Carpenter T.M. and Benedict F.G., Preliminary observations on metabolism during fever, *Am. J. Physiol.,* 24, 203, 1909.

7. DuBois E.F., The basal metabolism of fever, *JAMA,* 77, 352, 1921.

8. Cuthbertson D.P., The disturbance of metabolism produced by bony and non-bony injury, with notes on certain abnormal conditions of bones, *Biochem. J.,* 24, 1244, 1930.

9. Kinney J.M. and Roe F., Caloric equivalent of fever, *Ann. Surg.,* 156, 610, 1962.

10. Kinney J.M., Duke J.H., Long C.L., et al., Tissue fuel and weight loss after injury, *J. Clin. Pathol.,* 23, 65, 1968.

11. Askanazi J., Carpentier Y.A., and Elwyn D.H., Influence of total parenteral nutrition on fuel utilization in injury and sepsis, *Ann. Surg.,* 191, 40, 1980.

12. Askanazi J., Rosenbaum S.H., and Hyman A.I., Respiratory changes induced by the large glucose loads of total parenteral nutrition, *JAMA,* 243, 1444, 1980.

13. Long C.L., Schaffel N., Geiger J.W., et al., Metabolic response to injury and illness: estimation of energy and protein needs from indirect calorimetry and nitrogen balance, *J. Parenter. Enteral. Nutr.,* 3, 452, 1979.

14. Harris J.A. and Benedict F.G., *A Biometric Study of Basal Metabolism in Man*, Publication No. 279, Carnegie Institute, Washington, DC, 1919.

15. Quebbeman E.J., Ausman R.K., and Schneider T.C., A re-evaluation of energy expenditure during parenteral nutrition, *Ann. Surg.,* 195, 282, 1982.

16. Robertson C.L., Clifton G.L., and Grossman R.G., Oxygen utilization and cardiovascular function in head-injured patients, *Neurosurg.,* 15, 307, 1984.

17. Mann S., Westenskow D.R., and Houtchens B.A., Measured and predicted caloric expenditure in the acutely ill, *Crit. Care. Med.,* 13, 173, 1985.

18. Vermeij C.G., Feenstra B.W., and vanLanschot J., Day-to-day variability of energy expenditure in critically ill surgical patients, *Crit. Care. Med.,* 17, 623, 1989.

19. Boulanger B.R., Nayman R., McClean R.F. et al., What are the clinical determinants of early energy expenditure in critically injured patients? *J. Trauma,* 37, 969, 1994.

20. Liggett S.B. and Renfro A.D., Energy expenditures of mechanically ventilated nonsurgical patients, *Chest*, 98, 682, 1990.

21. Roubenoff R.A., Borel C.O., and Hanley D.F., Hypermetabolism and hypercatabolism in Guillain–Barre syndrome, *J. Parenter. Enteral. Nutr.,* 16, 464, 1992.

22. Frankenfield D.C, Wiles C.E., Bagley S., et al., Relationship between resting and total energy expenditure in injured and septic patients, *Crit. Care Med.,* 22, 1796, 1994.

23. Frankenfield D.C., Smith J.S., Cooney R.N., et al., Relative association of fever and injury with hypermetabolism in critically ill patients, *Injury,* 28, 617, 1997.

24. Bruder N., Raynal M., Pellissier D., et al., Influence of body temperature, with or without sedation, on energy expenditure in severe head-injured patients, *Crit. Care Med.,* 26, 568, 1998.

25. Problete B., Romand J.A., Pichard C., et al., Metabolic effects of i.v. propacetamol, metamizol or external cooling in critically ill febrile sedated patients, *Brit. J. Anaesth.,* 78, 123, 1997.

26. Kress J.P., O'Connor M.F., Pohlman A.E., et al., Sedation of critically ill patients during mechanical ventilation, *Am. J. Respir. Crit. Care Med.,* 153, 1012, 1996.

27. Marik P. and Kaufman D., The effects of neuromuscular paralysis on systemin and splanchnic oxygen utilization in mechanically ventilated patients, *Chest*, 109, 1038, 1996.

28. Weissman C., Kemper M., Damask M.C., et al., Effect of routine intensive care interactions on metabolic rate, *Chest*, 86, 815, 1984.

29. Swinamer D.L., Phang P.T., Jones R.L., et al., Twenty-four hour energy expenditure in critically ill patients, *Crit. Care Med.*, 15, 637, 1987.

30. Frankenfield D.C., Smith J.S., and Cooney R.N., Accelerated nitrogen loss after traumatic injury is not attenuated by achievement of nitrogen balance, *J. Parenter. Enteral. Nutr.*, 21, 324, 1997.

31. Swinamer D.L., Grace M.G., Hamilton S.M., et al., Predictive equation for assessing energy expenditure in mechanically ventilated critically ill patients, *Crit. Care Med.*, 18, 657, 1990.

32. Ireton-Jones C.S., Turner W.W., Liepa G.U., et al., Equations for estimation of energy expenditures of patients with burns with special reference to ventilatory status, *J. Burn Care Rehab.*, 13, 330, 1992.

33. Ireton-Jones C.S. and Jones J.D., Why use predictive equations for energy expenditure assessment? *J. Amer. Diet. Assoc.*, 97, A-44, 1997.

34. Frankenfield D.C., Omert L.A., Badellino M.M., et al., Correlation between measured energy expenditure and clinically obtained variables in trauma and sepsis patients, *J. Parenter. Enteral. Nutr.*, 18, 393, 1994.

35. Frankenfield D.C., Energy dynamics, in *Contemporary Nutrition Support Practice: A Clinical Guide,* 2nd ed., Matarese L.E. and Gottschlich M.M., eds., W.B. Saunders, Philadelphia, 2003, p. 89.

36. Frankenfield D.C., Rowe W.A., Smith J.S., et al., Validation of several established equations for resting metabolic rate in obese and nonobese people, *J. Am. Diet. Assoc.*, 103, 1152, 2003.

37. Frankenfield D.C., Smith J.S., and Cooney R.N., Validation of two approaches to predicting resting metabolic rate in critically ill patients, *J. Parenter. Enteral Nutr.,* 28, 259, 2004.

38. Flancbaum L., Choban P.S., Sambucco S., et al., Comparison of indirect calorimetry, the Fick method, and prediction equations in estimating the energy requirements of critically ill patients, *Am. J. Clin. Nutr.,* 69, 461, 1999.

39. MacDonald A. and Hildebrandt L., Comparison of formulaic equations to determine energy expenditure in the critically ill patient, *Nutrition*, 19, 233, 2003.

40. Mokdad A.H., Serdula M.K., Dietz W., et al., The spread of the obesity epidemic in the United States, *JAMA*, 282, 1519, 1999.

41. Cutts M.E., Dowdy R.P., Ellersieck M.R., et al., Predicting energy needs in ventilator-dependent critically ill patients: effect of adjusting weight for edema or adiposity, *Am. J. Clin. Nutr.*, 66, 1250, 1997.

42. Jeevanandam M., Young D.H., and Schiller W.R., Obesity and the metabolic response to severe multiple trauma in man, *J. Clin. Invest.*, 87, 262, 1991.

43. Frankenfield D.C., Cooney R.N., Smith J.S., et al., Age-related differences in the metabolic response to injury, *J. Trauma*, 48, 49, 2000.

44. Johnson R.E. and Chernoff R., Geriatrics, in *Contemporary Nutrition Support Practice: A Clinical Guide*, 2nd ed., Matarese L.E. and Gottschlich M.M., eds., W.B. Saunders, Philadelphia, 376, 2002.

45. Ravussin E., Lillioja S., Anderson T.E., et al., Determinants of 24-hour energy expenditure in man, *J. Clin. Invest.,* 78, 1568, 1986.

46. Calloway D.H. and Spector N., Nitrogen balance as related to caloric and protein intake in young men, *Am. J. Clin. Nutr.*, 2, 405, 1959.

47. Streat S.J., Beddoe A.H., and Hill G.L., Aggressive nutritional support does not prevent protein loss despite fat gain in septic intensive care patients, *J. Trauma*, 27, 262, 1987.

48. Long C.L., Birkhahn R.H., Geiger J.W., et al., Urinary excretion of 3-methyl histidine: An assessment of muscle protein catabolism and nitrogen balance in adult normal subjects during malnutrition, sepsis, and skeletal trauma, *Metabolism*, 30, 765, 1981.

49. Dickerson R.N., Rosato E.F., and Mullen J.L., Net protein anabolism with hypocaloric parenteral nutrition in obese stressed patients, *Am. J. Clin. Nutr.*, 44, 747, 1986.

50. Burge J.C., Goon A., Choban P.S., et al., Efficacy of hypocaloric total parenteral nutrition in hospitalized obese patients: a prospective, double-blind randomized trial, *J. Parenter. Enter. Nutr.*, 18, 203, 1994.

51. Barstow T.J., Cooper D.M., Sobel E., et al., Influence of increased metabolic rate on ^{13}C bicarbonate washout kinetics, *Am. J. Physiol.*, 259, R163, 1990.

52. Headley J.M., Indirect calorimetry: a trend toward continuous metabolic assessment, *AACN J*, 14, 155, 2003.

53. Turney S.Z., McCaslan T.C., and Cowley R.A., The continuous measurement of pulmonary gas exchange and mechanics, *Ann. Thorac. Surg.*, 13, 229, 1972.

54. Frankenfield D.C., Sarson G.Y., Blosser S.A., et al., Validation of a 5-minute steady state indirect calorimetry protocol for resting energy expenditure in critically ill patients, *J. Am. Coll. Nutr.*, 15, 397, 1996.

55. Petros S. and Engelmann L., Validity of an abbreviated indirect colorimetry protocol for measurement of resting energy expenditure in mechanically ventilated and spontaneously breathing critically ill patients, *Inten. Care Med.*, 27, 1164, 2001.

7 Macronutrient Requirements: Carbohydrate, Protein, and Lipid

Jennifer Lefton
Jackson Health System

Peter P. Lopez
University of Miami School of Medicine

CONTENTS

7.1 INTRODUCTION

The metabolic response to critical illness is characterized by hypermetabolism, hyperglycemia, increased lipolysis, and net protein catabolism (1). Skeletal muscle protein is broken down and the amino acids are used for gluconeogenesis and protein synthesis. Synthesis of positive acute-phase proteins (e.g., C-reactive protein) is increased (2). These metabolic changes, along with bed rest and suboptimal nutrient intake, result in depletion of lean body mass. Nutritional support in the critically ill should provide nutrition consistent with the patient's medical condition, nutritional status, and available route of administration; prevent or treat macro- or micronutrient deficiencies; provide doses of nutrients compatible with current metabolism; avoid complications associated with the route of delivery; and improve patient outcomes related to their disease morbidity (body composition, tissue repair, organ function) (3). The patient's response to nutritional support should be monitored so that adjustments can be made to avoid complications and ensure that the goals of nutritional support are met. This chapter reviews the suggested macronutrient (carbohydrate, protein, and lipid) composition of nutritional support provided to critically ill patients.

7.2 CARBOHYDRATES

Carbohydrates are compounds of carbon, hydrogen, and oxygen. They are the chief source of calories in most diets. They are also the main energy source for the body in health and disease states, yielding 4 kcal /g. Carbohydrates play critical roles as constituents of DNA and RNA, coenzymes, glycoproteins, and glycolipids (4). Glucose is the most important carbohydrate, serving as an oxidative fuel for the brain, renal medulla, leukocytes, and erythrocytes (4).

7.2.1 CARBOHYDRATE REQUIREMENTS

The minimum amount of exogenous glucose needed per day is thought to be between 100 and 150 grams (5,6). Optimal carbohydrate delivery should be at a level to allow maximal protein sparing while minimizing hyperglycemia (7). The amount of carbohydrate that can be safely provided to a critically ill patient is a function of the patient's ability to oxidize these carbohydrates. The rate of infusion has been suggested to be no more than 4 to 5 mg/kg/min (8–11). For patients who are diabetic or receiving steroid therapy, or who have stress-induced hyperglycemia, the carbohydrate infusion should be limited to 2.5 to 4.0 mg/kg/min initially until blood sugars are well controlled (Table 7.1) (8). Patients requiring total parental nutrition (TPN) who are at risk for developing refeeding syndrome should be initiated with no more than 100 to 150 g dextrose/d (9,12). Carbohydrate requirements have also been suggested as 30 to 70% of the total calories needed per day (3).

When patients are underfed total energy or carbohydrate needs, adipose and muscle tissue are mobilized for fuel sources and enter into the gluconeogenic pathway to fulfill the body's need for glucose. Unlike adipose tissue, muscle tissue is not considered a stored body fuel, so protein catabolism leads not only to a decrease in skeletal muscle mass, but also to decreased visceral body proteins, the body's structural and metabolically active proteins (4). This can contribute to poor wound healing, impaired immune response, and physiologic exhaustion, leading to total body failure.

Overfeeding of carbohydrates can result in hypercapnia, hyperglycemia, and fatty infiltration of the liver (8). Hyperglycemia as a result of overfeeding carbohydrates may further result in electrolyte imbalances (potassium and phosphorus) due to hyperinsulinemia, which leads to a shift of these electrolytes intracellularly. Respiratory distress (13), hypercapnia during weaning (14), and respiratory failure (15) have been reported in patients receiving excessive carbohydrate loads with TPN. Even death has been reported in malnourished patients given 75 kcal/kg/d as carbohydrates, although this was not in critically ill patients (16). Patients at risk for overfeeding of carbohydrates

---

TABLE 7.1
Calculating Dextrose Infusion Rates

To Calculate the Suggested Daily Maximum Dextrose:
  4 to 5 mg/kg/minute × weight (kg) × 1440 (minutes/24 h) ÷ 1000

  For example:
    How many grams of dextrose should be infused over 24 hours at a rate of 4 mg/kg/min for a 72 kg patient?
        4 mg/kg/minute × 72 kg × 1440 minutes ÷ 1000 = 414 g dextrose/d

To Calculate the Dextrose Infusion Rate:
  g dextrose ÷ weight (kg) ÷ 1440 (minutes/24 hours) × 1000 = dextrose mg/kg/min

  For example:
    What is the dextrose infusion rate for a 72 kg patient receiving 400 grams dextrose daily?
        400 g dextrose ÷ 72 kg ÷ 1440 minutes × 1000 = 3.85 mg/kg/min

include the elderly, those with unusual body sizes or severely malnourished, and those on dialysis containing dextrose (8).

Carbon dioxide (CO_2) retention, increased minute ventilation, difficulty weaning from the ventilator, acute respiratory acidosis or metabolic alkalosis, and a respiratory quotient (RQ) greater than 1 may indicate overfeeding of total calories or carbohydrate (8). The reported low sensitivity and specificity of RQ may limit its use as an indicator of over- and underfeeding (17). A thorough review of the patient's condition, nutritional regimen, and response to therapy must be done frequently in order to avoid over- or underfeeding. When overfeeding is suspected, a reduction in carbohydrate or total caloric intake may prevent elevated CO_2 production and respiratory compromise (18). Strategies to prevent and treat complications associated with overfeeding macronutrients are shown in Table 7.2.

Hyperglycemia may also indicate overfeeding (8); however, critically ill patients may experience hyperglycemia as a result of factors other than nutrition. Blood sugars should be monitored closely and controlled with exogenous insulin if needed. The presence of hyperglycemia may be an independent risk factor for the development of infection (19), and the use of intensive insulin therapy has been shown to reduce morbidity and mortality in surgical patients (20). Therefore, maintaining tight glucose control is an important outcome goal when providing nutritional support in the critically ill.

7.3 PROTEINS

Proteins are essential components of all living cells and are involved in almost every bodily function. Proteins function in tissue, cell, and organelle structure, as enzymes and hormones, and in molecules involved with cell-to-cell communication and in genetic material. The carbon in amino acids can be oxidized, yielding 4 kcal/g (4).

7.3.1 PROTEIN REQUIREMENTS

Protein requirements in the critically ill have not been clearly defined but they generally range between 1.0 and 2.0 g/kg body weight/d. In comparison to the dietary reference intake (DRI) for protein in healthy adults (0.8 g/kg body weight/d) (21), most critically ill patients require almost twice as much protein. Some have suggested protein requirements in the critically ill to be as much as 1.5 to 2.0 g/kg body weight/d (22,23). However, there is little evidence that giving more than 1.0 to 1.5 g/kg body weight/d has any further benefit (24–26). Ishibashi et al. (24) suggest that 1 to 1.2 g/kg body weight/d would provide for optimal protein provision in the first two weeks of critical illness. Larsson et al. (27) also found that provision of 0.2 g nitrogen/kg body weight/d (approximately 1.25 g protein/kg body weight/d) was optimal in the first week post trauma. Providing an exogenous source of protein will reduce nitrogen loss, but protein sparing may not be further improved by providing greater than 1.5 g protein/kg of body weight/d (24–27).

However, this may not apply to patients with substantial protein losses from open wounds, major burns, or GI losses (ostomies and fistulas) (28). High-protein regimens in stable burn patients have shown achievement of nitrogen balance (29,30), increased rates of restored body weight and muscle function (31), and better immune function (fewer bacteremic and antibiotic days) and increased survival (32). High-protein regimens (> 1.5 g protein/kg body weight) are recommended for burn patients until significant wound healing is achieved (1). Critically ill patients will experience substantial losses of body protein regardless of aggressive nutritional support (1,33). One of the goals of nutritional support in critically ill patients is to minimize the loss of and protect lean tissue mass and function.

Initiation of therapy should be started between 1.2 and 1.5 g/kg/d of protein and adjusted as needed (3). Protein requirements have also been suggested as 15 to 20% of total calories coming from protein (3,28). Serum negative acute-phase proteins (e.g., albumin, prealbumin) can be difficult to interpret in the critically ill and may not reflect the adequacy of nutritional support (2,34). Studies

TABLE 7.2

Indicators of Overfeeding, Characteristics and Patients at Risk, and Considerations for Monitoring and Intervention

Complication with Indicator	Patients at Risk	Monitoring and Intervention
Azotemia		
Progressively increasing blood urea nitrogen (BUN) level (30 mg/dl)	Patients ≥ 65 years old Patients given > 2 g protein/kg	Check creatinine clearance; serum creatinine may be less than 2 mg/dl despite renal impairment. Ratio of BUN to creatinine greater than 15 suggests abnormal renal function and/or excessive protein intake, muscle catabolism, or dehydration. Provide adequate energy intake and monitor hydration. Readjust protein as needed.
Fat-Overload Syndrome		
Respiratory distress Sudden hypertriglyceridemia Prolonged prothrombin and partial thromboplastin times Bleeding from orifices Elevated bilirubin level	Patients receiving more than 3 g lipid/kg body weight/d Account for lipid in medications Patients with elevated C-reactive protein (acute-phase response and heightened cytokine production)	Symptoms may arise within a few days of initiating IVLE or after months of tolerance. Monitor triglyceride level; hold lipids when triglyceride is > 300 to 400 mg/dl. Monitor respiratory, hematologic, and hepatic systems. Symptoms abate as lipemia resolves.
Hepatic Steatosis		
Hepatomegaly with or without right-upper quadrant pain or tenderness Abnormal, high-fat liver biopsy	Patients receiving high-carbohydrate, very low fat parenteral nutrition	Liver function tests do not correlate well with hepatic steatosis. Monitor glucose and triglyceride levels and actual feeding. Adjust energy or carbohydrate intake as needed; use mixed fuel feedings that include fat daily. Hepatic steatosis is rarely confirmed.
Hypercapnia		
Elevated $PaCO_2$ Increased minute ventilation; difficulty in weaning from ventilator Acute respiratory acidosis: $PaCO_2$ > 40 mm Hg and pH < 7.40 Acute metabolic alkalosis: $PaCO_2$ 50 to 60 mm Hg, serum bicarbonate > 24 mmol/l, and pH > 7.40	Patients with poor ventilatory status Indirect calorimetry is preferred to estimating energy needs, especially for patients with unusual body sizes and for the elderly	The respiratory quotient is an insensitive indicator of overfeeding, remaining less than 1.0 even with excessive respiratory workload and distress. Adjustments in ventilation may mask elevated carbon dioxide production. Decrease energy intake, particularly from dextrose; add lipid daily. Monitor the patient's response (Paco2, blood pH) to changes in feeding.
Hyperglycemia		
Glucose > 200 mg/dl Insulin administration	Patients with systemic inflammatory response syndrome or pancreatitis, patients on steroids or peritoneal dialysis containing dextrose Infusing more than 4 mg/kg/min	Monitor hydration, blood glucose level, insulin administration, and actual dextrose feeding. Replace some energy from dextrose with energy from lipid.

(continued)

TABLE 7.2 (CONTINUED)
Indicators of Overfeeding, Characteristics and Patients at Risk, and Considerations for Monitoring and Intervention

Complication with Indicator	Patients at Risk	Monitoring and Intervention
Hyperglycemic Hyperosmolar Nonketotic Syndrome		
Glucose level > 600 mg/dl Intravascular dehydration (i.e., plasma level > 350 mOsm/l) Fever Tachycardia, hypotension	Patients receiving high carbohydrate loads followed by prolonged osmotic diuresis Patients with severe burns, reduced renal function, or pancreatitis Patients who underwent cardiopulmonary bypass or are elderly with type 2 diabetes	Monitor central venous pressure or pulmonary capillary wedge pressure. Restore intravascular volume using 0.9% sodium chloride until vital signs stabilize, then 0.45% sodium chloride. Bolus of 10 to 15 U insulin, then 0.1 U per kilogram per hour. When glucose level is < 300 mg/dl, use 5% dextrose in water, 0.45% sodium chloride, and decrease insulin. Manage potassium and other electrolytes.
Hypertonic Dehydration		
Hypernatremia Elevated hematocrit Azotemia	Tube feeding a high-protein formula Loss of large amounts of fluid Elderly	Reduce sodium and protein intake; use isotonic feeding. Provide rehydration over 24 to 48 h or longer. Treatment may require intravenous solutions. Avoid water intoxication. Replenish minerals as needed, especially after the extracellular space has expanded.
Hypertriglyceridemia		
Triglyceride > 300 mg/dl	Patients receiving lipid-based drugs (propofol > 6 mg/kg/h) Lipid loads > 2 g/kg/d Patients with infections, particularly gram-negative sepsis	If triglyceride level rises over 300 to 400 mg/dl, then restrict lipids (e.g., provide 500 ml 10% emulsion at ≤ 21 ml/h once or twice per week). If triglyceride level rises over 500 mg/dl, then hold infusions and monitor essential fatty acid status. Avoid overfeeding energy, fat, and dextrose.
Metabolic Acidosis		
Blood pH < 7.35 Bicarbonate < 21 mEq/l	Patients receiving formulas with low ratios of energy to nitrogen (90:1) Ability to deal with acid loads is diminished in the elderly	Monitor hydration, renal function, pH, bicarbonate, potassium, and BUN. Reduce protein intake and follow the patient's response.
Refeeding Syndrome		
Hypophosphatemia Acute respiratory failure Arterial hypotension Tachycardia	Patients with chronic malnutrition or extended nil per os without nutritional support	Monitor cardiac function. Decrease total energy and dextrose; adjust fluids for appropriate hydration. Monitor minerals in blood and urine. Replenish phosphorus, magnesium, and potassium as needed.

Source: Adapted from: Klein CJ, Stanek GS, Wiles CE. *J. Am. Diet Assoc.* 1998, 98: 795–806.

of these proteins have found them to be good indicators of the severity of illness but not necessarily a good measure of nutrition support outcomes (34). Nitrogen balance can be used to determine protein requirements or to assess the adequacy of current nutrient intake. A nitrogen balance that is +2 to +4 would indicate anabolism. Serial trends in serum hepatic proteins and nitrogen balance studies are more useful than a single measurement, and the trends should reflect improvement as the patient recovers from his or her illness.

Potential adverse effects may occur from underfeeding or overfeeding protein. Providing insufficient amounts of protein will lead to consumption of body protein (4) and greater nitrogen losses. Excess protein is deaminated and the ammonia is excreted as urea (4). Dehydration can result because water is needed for the excretion of urea (35). A protein intake of greater than 1.5 g/kg body weight/d is more likely to result in azotemia for older adults than for younger adults (36,37). Protein intake should be reduced if there is an increase in blood urea nitrogen (BUN) that is greater than 100 mg/dl and a rising ammonia level with worsening encephalopathy (3).

7.4 LIPIDS

Fatty acids perform a wide variety of functions in the body. Fat serves as a source of calories (9 kcal/g) and is a major fuel source after carbohydrate stores are depleted (4). Fat serves to insulate the body and cushion organs. Fats play an important role in cell membrane structure; as a lubricant for body surfaces, joints, and mucus membranes; and in cell signaling components (38). Fat is also needed for fat-soluble vitamin digestion and absorption (4).

7.4.1 FAT REQUIREMENTS

The minimum amount of fat needed is only 2 to 4% of total calories. The only essential fatty acids are the long-chain fatty acids alpha-linolenic acid and linoleic acid (3). When fat is used as a source of calories, generally 15 to 30% of total calories can be provided as fat (3,28). The absolute maximum amount of fat is suggested to be no more than 2.5 g/kg/d (1), or less than 60% of total calories. Some literature suggests that fat be further limited to 1 g/kg/d or less in critically ill patients (1,4,39). The infusion rate for intravenous lipid emulsions (IVLE) is also important to consider and should not exceed 0.11 g/kg/h to avoid metabolic complications (28). Contraindications to the use of IVLE include egg allergy and hypertriglyceridemia. Provision of IVLE is generally considered safe as long as triglyceride concentrations are less than 400 mg/dl (1,12). There is no strong evidence to suggest a benefit in restricting IVLE for patients with thrombocytopenia.

Providing insufficient amounts of lipids over time can result in an essential fatty acid deficiency (EFAD). Three weeks of fat-free TPN has resulted in EFAD (40). Physical signs and symptoms of an essential fatty acid deficiency include diffuse scaly dermatitis, alopecia, thrombocytopenia, anemia, and impaired wound healing. A suspected EFAD can be confirmed by obtaining a triene-to-tetraene ratio that is greater than 0.4. For prevention of essential EFAD, 2 to 4% total daily calorie needs should come from fat (1 to 2% from linoleic acid and 0.5% from alpha-linolenic acid) (1).

Provision of excessive amounts of fat can lead to hypertriglyceridemia and fat overload. Manifestations of fat overload include respiratory distress, coagulopathies, abnormal liver function tests, and impaired reticuloendothelial system (RES) function (8). Overfeeding of IVLE may also be associated with immunosuppression as a result of the breakdown of linoleic acid (an omega-6 polyunsaturated fatty acid) to proinflammatory eicosanoids (41). Battistella et al. (39) found that IVLE provided in the early postinjury period resulted in greater susceptibility to infection, prolonged pulmonary failure, and delayed recovery. However, patients receiving the lipid-free TPN regimen did not have the calories replaced with dextrose. Therefore, it was unclear whether these results were related to the absence of IVLE or the hypocaloric regimen (39). Limiting total fat calories to 15 to 30% should reduce complications related to overfeeding of fat while providing a concentrated source of energy. Monitoring triglyceride clearance is recommended. See Table 7.3 and Table 7.4 for sample calculations for macronutrient needs and a TPN solution.

Further complicating nutrition regimens, is the use of propofol (Diprivan) for sedation in the critically ill population. Propofol is provided in a 10% lipid emulsion and is a calorie source providing 1.1 calories/ml. Calories delivered from propofol should be included in calculations of total nutrient and fat intake and adjustments should be made to the nutrition regimen if needed. Adjustments may include a reduction in the rate of total calories for tube-fed patients or a reduction in the amount IVLE provided with TPN. In some cases, the high amounts of propofol given may negate the need for additional IVLE (Table 7.5) (42).

7.5 SUMMARY

Nutritional support in the critically ill is aimed at supporting the patient through recovery, providing macronutrient substrates appropriate for metabolic alterations, and reducing potential complications associated with nutritional support. Various sources of carbohydrate, protein, and lipid are available (see Chapter 16 and Chapter 17). Provision of macronutrients in the amounts suggested (Table 7.6) will help to achieve outcome goals and avoid complications of under- or overfeeding in critically ill patients.

TABLE 7.3
Calculating TPN Macronutrient Composition

Example
  80 ml/h TPN containing 15% dextrose, 6% amino acids (final concentration) with 250 ml 20% IVLE[a]

To Calculate Dextrose Grams and Carbohydrate Calories:
  80 ml/h × 24 hours = 2000 ml
  2000 ml × 0.15 = 300 g dextrose
  300 g dextrose × 3.4 calories/g = 1020 dextrose calories

To Calculate Amino Acid Grams and Protein Calories:
  2000 ml × 0.06 = 120 g amino acid
  120 g amino acid × 4 calories/g = 480 amino acid calories

To Calculate Lipid Calories:
  250 ml lipid × 2 calories/ml = 500 calories

To Calculate Total Caloric Intake:
  Total calories = 1020 dextrose cals + 480 amino acid cals + 500 lipid calories = 2000 total calories

[a] 20% IVLE provides 2 calories/ml.

TABLE 7.4
Calculating a TPN Solution

Example

A 55-year-old male is status post motor vehicle crash, rendering the GI tract unfit for use.

His height is 5'8" and his weight is 160 lbs (72 kg). The surgical team plans to initiate parenteral nutrition and asks the nutrition support clinician to calculate a formula to meet the patient's needs, providing 1800 ml fluid daily (not including the IV lipids).

The patients' nutritional needs were estimated as:

   25 calories/kg = 1800 calories/d

   1.5 g protein/kg = 108 g protein/d

The following steps can be used to calculate a TPN formulation to meet the patient's macronutrient needs:

1. Calculate the percentage of calories to be delivered as fat and determine the amount of IVLE needed.

   To provide 20% calories as fat:

      1800 calories × 0.20 fat = 360 calories as fat

      360 fat calories = 180 ml 20% IVLE

    2 calories/ml or 360 fat calories ÷ 2 calories ml = 180 ml 20% IVLE

2. Calculate final concentration of amino acids

      108 g protein = 0.06 or 6% amino acids

      1800 ml or 180 g protein ÷ 1800 ml = 0.06 or 6% amino acids

      1800 ml × 0.06 = 108 g protein × 4 calories/g = 432 protein calories

3. Calculate calories left to provide as dextrose

      360 fat calories + 432 protein calories = 792 calories

      1800 total calories – 792 calories = 1008 calories

4. Calculate final concentration of dextrose needed to meet calorie needs

      1008 dextrose calories ÷ 3.4 calories per gram = 296 g dextrose

      296 g dextrose = 0.164 or 16.4% dextrose

      1800 ml or 269 g dextrose ÷ 1800 ml = 0.164 or 16.4% dextrose

The final TPN solution would be for 16.4% dextrose, 6% amino acids, with 180 ml 20% IVLE. This would be started at one-half the goal rate and advanced in increments toward the goal of 75 ml/h if serum glucose and electrolytes remain well controlled.

TABLE 7.5
Calculating TPN Solutions while Patient Is on Propofol

The patient described in Table 7.4 is requiring 20 ml/h propofol for sedation. The nutrition support clinician is consulted to reformulate a TPN solution to avoid overfeeding fat and total calories.

The following steps can be used to calculate a TPN formulation to meet the patient's calorie and macronutrient needs.

1. Calculate fat calories from propofol

      20 ml/h propofol × 24 hours/d = 480 ml propofol/d

      480 ml propofol × 1.1 calorie/ml = 528 fat calories

2. Calculate final concentration of amino acids

      108 g protein = 0.06 or 6% amino acids

      1800 ml or 108 g protein ÷ 1800 ml = 0.06 or 6% amino acids

3. Calculate calories left to provide as dextrose

      528 fat calories + 432 protein calories = 960 calories

      1800 calories – 960 calories = 840 calories as dextrose

4. Calculate final concentration of dextrose needed to meet calorie needs

      840 dextrose calories ÷ 3.4 calories/gram = 247 grams dextrose

      247 g dextrose = 0.137 or 13.7% dextrose

      1800 ml or 247 g dextrose ÷ 1800 ml = 0.137 or 13.7% dextrose

The TPN solution could then be changed to 75 ml/h 13.7% dextrose, 6% amino acids. The IVLE would be held while propofol was given to avoid providing excess fat and total calories.

TABLE 7.6
Macronutrient Requirements in the Critically Ill

Macronutrient	Minimum Requirement	Maximum Requirement	% of Total Calories
Carbohydrate	100–150 g/d	< 4 mg/kg/min	30–70%
Protein	1 g/kg body weight	2 g/kg body weight	15–20%
Fat	2–4% total calories	< 1 g fat/kg/d	15–30%

REFERENCES

1. ASPEN Board of Directors and The Clinical Guidelines Task Force. Guidelines for the Use of Parenteral and Enteral Nutrition in Adult and Pediatric Patients. *J. Parent. Enter. Nutr.* 2002, 26(suppl.): 1SA–138SA.
2. Gabay C, Kushner I. Acute-phase proteins and other systemic responses to inflammation. *N. Engl. J. Med.* 1999, 340: 448–454.
3. Cerra FB, Benitez, MR, Blackburn GL, Irwin RS, Jeejeebhoy K, Katz DP, Pingleton SK, Pomposelli J, Rombeau JL, Shronts E, Wolfe RR, Zaloga GP. Applied nutrition in ICU patients: a consensus statement of the American College of Chest Physicians. *Chest* 1997, 111: 769–778.
4. Frakenfield D. Energy and macrosubstrate requirements. In *The Science and Practice of Nutrition Support: A Case-Based Core Curriculum*. Gottschlich MM (ed.). Kendall/Hunt, Dubuque, IA, 2001, 31–52.
5. Fredstrom S. Carbohydrate. In *Contemporary Nutrition Support Practice: A Clinical Guide*. Matarese LM, Gottschlich MM (eds.). W.B. Saunders, Philadelphia, PA, 1998, 110–116.
6. Skipper A. Principles of parenteral nutrition. In *Contemporary Nutrition Support Practice: A Clinical Guide*. Matarese LM, Gottschlich MM (eds.). W.B. Saunders, Philadelphia, PA, 1998, 227–242.
7. Wilmore DW. Postoperative protein sparing. *World J. Surg.* 1999, 23: 545–552.
8. Klein CJ, Stanek GS, Wiles CE. Overfeeding macronutrients to critically ill adults: metabolic complications. *J. Am. Diet. Assoc.* 1998, 98: 795–806.
9. Skipper A, Millikan KW. Parenteral nutrition implementation and management. In *The ASPEN Nutrition Support Practice Manual*. Merritt RJ (ed.). ASPEN, Silver Spring, MD, 1998, 9.1–9.9.
10. Burke JF, Wolfe RR, Maullny CJ, Mathews DE, Bier DM. Glucose requirements following burn injury. *Ann. Surg.* 1979, 190: 274–285.
11. Guenst JM, Nelson LD. Predictors of total parenteral nutrition-induced lipogenesis. *Chest* 1994, 105: 553–559.
12. Chan S, McCowen KC, Blackburn GL. Nutrition management in the ICU. *Chest* 1999, 115: 145S–148S.
13. Askanazi J, Elwyn DH, Silverberg PA, Rosenbaum SH, Kinney JM. Respiratory distress secondary to a high carbohydrate load: a case report. *Surgery* 1980, 87: 596–598.
14. Dark DS, Pingleton SK, Kerby GR. Hypercapnia during weaning: a complication of nutritional support. *Chest* 1985, 88: 141–143.
15. Covelli HD, Black JW, Olsen MS, Beekman JF. Respiratory failure precipitated by high carbohydrate loads. *Ann. Intern. Med.* 1981, 95: 579–581.
16. Weinsier RL, Krumdieck CL. Death resulting from overzealous total parenteral nutrition: the refeeding syndrome revisited. *Am. J. Clin. Nutr.* 1981, 34: 393–399.
17. McClave SA, Lowen CC, Kleber MJ, McConnell JW, Jung LY, Goldsmith LJ. Clinical use of the respiratory quotient obtained from indirect calorimetry. *J. Parenter. Enter. Nutr.* 2003, 27: 21–26.
18. Talpers SS, Romberger DJ, Bunce SB, et al. Nutritionally associated increased carbon dioxide production: excess total calories vs. high proportion of carbohydrate calories. *Chest* 1992, 102: 551–555.
19. Pomposelli JJ, Baxter JK, Babineau TJ, Pomfret EA, Driscoll DF, Forse RA, Bistrian BR. Early postoperative glucose control predicts nosocomial infection rate in diabetic patients. *J. Parent. Enter. Nutr.* 1998, 22: 77–81.

20. Van den Berghe G, Wouters P, et al. Intensive insulin therapy in critically ill patients. *N. Engl. J. Med.* 2001, 345: 1359–1367.

21. Institute of Medicine, Food and Nutrition Board. *Dietary Reference Intakes for Energy, Carbohydrate, Fiber, Fat, Fatty Acids, Cholesterol, Protein, and Amino Acids (Macronutrients).* National Academy Press, Washington, DC, 2002.

22. Keating KP. Nutritional support in the critically ill. In *Current Surgical Therapy,* 7th ed., Cameron JL (ed). Mosby, St. Louis, MO, 2001.

23. Rombeau JL, et al. Nutritional support. In *Scientific American Surgery,* Wilmore DW, et al. (eds). Scientific American, New York, 1998–2000.

24. Ishibashi N, Plank LD, Sando K, Hill GL. Optimal protein requirements during the first 2 weeks after the onset of critical illness. *Crit. Care Med.* 1998, 26: 1529–1535.

25. Shaw JHF, Wildbore M, Wolfe RR. Whole body protein kinetics in severely septic patients. *Ann. Surg.* 1987, 205: 288–294.

26. Hoffer LJ. Protein and energy provision in critical illness. *Am. J. Clin. Nutr.* 2003, 78: 906–911.

27. Larsson J, Lennmarken C, Martensson J, Sandsedt S, Vinnars E. Nitrogen requirements in severely injured patients. *Br. J. Surg.* 1990, 77: 413–416.

28. Driscoll DF, Bistrian BR. Parenteral nutrition (macronutrient fuels). In *Nutritional Considerations in the Intensive Care Unit: Science, Rationale, and Practice,* Shikora SA, Martindale RG, Schwaitzberg SD (eds). Kendall/Hunt, Dubuque, IA, 2002, 39–49.

29. Matsuda T, Kagan RJ, Hanumadass M, Jonasson O. The importance of burn wound size in determining the optimal calorie–nitrogen ration. *Surgery* 1983, 94: 562–568.

30. Kagan RJ, Matsuda T, Hanumadass M, Castillo B, Jonasson O. The effect of burn wound size on ureagenesis and nitrogen balance. *Ann. Surg.* 1982, 195: 70–74.

31. Demling RH, DeSanti L. Increased protein intake during the recovery phase after severe burns increases body weight gain and muscle function. *J. Burn Care Rehabil.* 1998, 19: 161–168.

32. Alexander JW, MacMillan BG, Stinnett JD, Ogle CK, Bosian RC, Fischer JE, Oakes JB, Morris MJ, Krummel R. Beneficial effects of aggressive protein feeding in severely burned children. *Ann. Surg.* 1980, 192: 505–517.

33. Streat SJ, Beddore SH, Hill GL. Aggressive nutritional support does not prevent protein loss despite fat gain in septic intensive care patients. *J. Trauma* 1987, 27: 262–266.

34. Mueller C. True or false: serum hepatic protein concentrations measure nutritional status. *Support Line* 2004, 26(1): 8–16.

35. Gault MH, Dixon ME, Doyle M, Cohen WM. Hypernatremia, azotemia, and dehydration due to high-protein tube feeding. *Ann. Intern. Med.* 1968, 68: 778–791.

36. Frankenfield D, Cooney RN, Mith JS, Rowe WA. Age-related differences in the metabolic response to injury. *J Trauma* 2000, 48:49–57.

37. Clevenger FW, Rodriguez DJ, Demarest GB, Osler TM, Olson SE, Fry DE. Protein and energy tolerance by stressed geriatric patients. *J. Surg. Res.* 1992, 52: 135–139.

38. Small DM. Structure and properties of lipids. In *Biochemical and Physiologic Aspects of Human Nutrition.* Stipanuk MH (ed.) W.B. Saunders, Philadelphia, 2000, 43–62.

39. Battistella FD, Widegreen JT, Anderson JT, Siepler JK, Weber JC, MacCall K. A prospective, randomized trial of intravenous fat emulsion administration in trauma victims requiring total parenteral nutrition. *J. Trauma* 1997, 43: 52–60.

40. Richardson TJ, Sgoutas D. Essential fatty acid deficiency in four adult patients during total parenteral nutrition. *Am. J. Clin. Nutr.* 1975, 28: 258–263.

41. Alexander JW. Immunonutrition: the role of omega-3 fatty acids. *Nutrition* 1998, 14: 627–633.

42. Eddleston JM, Shelly MP. The effect on serum lipid concentrations of a prolonged infusion of propofol: hypertriglyceridemia associated with propofol administration. *Intensive Care Med.* 1991, 17: 424–426.

8 Micronutrient and Antioxidant Therapy in Critically Ill Patients

Krishnan Sriram
John H. Stroger Jr. Hospital of Cook County

Jorge I. Cué
Medical College of Georgia

CONTENTS

8.1 INTRODUCTION

The term *micronutrient* includes vitamins and trace elements. Vitamins are substances not generally synthesized by the body and are cofactors for various enzymes. Trace elements are metals present in minute quantities that act as cofactors or as part of the structure of specific enzymes. Trace metals (including selenium, zinc, manganese, iron, and copper) and 13 essential vitamins (4 fat soluble and 9 water soluble) are essential in stabilizing or catalyzing homeostatic reactions in the human organism.[2–4] This chapter will discuss the role of micronutrients in critically ill patients and the principles behind their utilization in antioxidant therapy for critical illness. Not every vitamin or trace element deficiency will be addressed individually, except in the tables listed. Otherwise, only the most crucial deficiency states dealing with critical illness will be discussed. The second portion of the chapter will be dedicated to past and current studies highlighting the increasingly important role antioxidant therapy plays in critically ill patients during the acute inflammatory state and oxidative stress state.

Micronutrient deficiencies in critically ill patients may occur as preexisting conditions in patients with poor nutritional status prior to hospitalization, as a result of severe illness with depletion of some of the micronutrients, or iatrogenically, when the physician fails to recognize the nutrient-wasting illness or when there is a failure to institute replacement therapy early in the care of intensive care unit (ICU) patients.[1,2] These deficient states can affect various biochemical processes and enzymatic functions, resulting in organ dysfunction, poor wound healing, and altered immune status — all with deleterious patient outcomes.

Although the American Medical Association has established guidelines for the daily recommended intake of vitamins and trace elements, these have been formulated for a healthy population. The exact formulation of micronutrient replacement required for health maintenance or replacement is not well known in critically ill patients.[5] The FDA has recognized that parenteral vitamin requirements are increased in disease states, and manufacturers have been instructed to modify their products accordingly,[7] but a similar recommendation for trace elements has not been initiated. The American Society for Parenteral and Enteral Nutrition (ASPEN) has taken the lead in establishing guidelines on the administration of parenteral trace element additives.[8] Table 8.1 summarizes the various actions of the essential vitamins and trace elements, the clinical sequelae of the deficient states for each, and the recommendations available for replacement. Table 8.2 gives the suggested composition of parenteral micronutrients for adults.

8.2 ABSORPTION AND INTERACTIONS

8.2.1 VITAMINS

Most water-soluble vitamins are absorbed easily from the proximal gastrointestinal (GI) tract (see Figure 8.1). Fat-soluble vitamins are thought to be absorbed in the mid- and distal ileum, due to the added necessity for fat digestion facilitated by bile and pancreatic lipase. Absorption of fat-soluble vitamins is affected by all conditions with fat malabsorption (pancreatic insufficiency, bile loss), vitamin B_{12} is absorbed in the terminal ileum. Deficiencies can occur with excessive GI losses, such as occur with high-output fistulas and prolonged and excessive diarrhea. Reinstillation of upper GI secretions into the jejunum, either via a nasojejunal tube or jejunostomy,[10] will facilitate absorption of fat-soluble vitamins that require bile and pancreatic secretions for optimal absorption. Additionally, one can avoid the loss of micronutrients that occurs if the aspirated fluid is discarded. Differences between intragastric and intrajejunal administration have not been studied in depth. In the case of vitamin B_{12}, intrajejunal administration actually results in better absorption, even though the stomach (the source of intrinsic factor) is bypassed.[11] This may be due to the increased binding of cobalamin to intrinsic factor at alkaline pH levels seen in the ileum.[12]

Interactions between various vitamins are very complex and not well understood.[13] For example, vitamins E and C are synergistic. Vitamin C recycles vitamin E; thus, vitamin C deficiency decreases the function of the latter. Excess of vitamin E antagonizes vitamin A function. Pyridoxine (vitamin B_6) and riboflavin (vitamin B_2) deficiency increase requirements for niacin. Therefore, single vitamin supplementation can counteract the action of other vitamins. See Table 8.2 for suggested composition of parenteral multivitamin and trace element products for adults.

8.2.2 TRACE ELEMENTS

There is a paucity of information about the exact location in the GI tract where a specific trace element is absorbed. Certain generalizations can be made. Zinc and selenium are absorbed mainly in the duodenum and also in the ileum. The latter location is important, especially when food needs digestion before the Zn is bioavailable. Fe is also absorbed in the duodenum (see Figure 8.1).

Numerous interactions exist between trace elements affecting absorption via the GI tract. Factors affecting bioavailability of trace elements are various:

- Dietary factors include chemical form of nutrient (e.g., the organic form of Cr is better absorbed than the ionic form).
- Antagonistic ligands (e.g., phytate decreases Zn absorption, fiber decreases Zn and Fe absorption, vitamin C decreases Cu absorption but increases Fe absorption).
- Facilitatory ligands (e.g., picolinic acid and citric acid aid absorption of Zn).
- Competitive interactions (e.g., Fe depresses the absorption of Cu and Zn; Zn depresses Cu absorption and vice versa). Administration of ferrous sulfate with enteral nutrition can result in zinc deficiency.[14]

8.3 EFFECT OF INFLAMMATORY RESPONSE ON MICRONUTRIENT STATUS

8.3.1 VITAMINS

Serum levels of various vitamins decrease with the inflammatory response, though the clinical significance of this is unclear.[15] For example, in postoperative patients, levels of vitamins A, C, and E are decreased.[16,17] Septic patients have high vitamin A excretion in the urine.[18] Levels of vitamins B_2, B_{12}, B_1, and folate are not affected by inflammation, so decreased levels may represent a true deficiency. However, there is no conclusive proof to indicate that additional supplementation is needed when the serum level of a specific vitamin declines.

8.3.2 TRACE ELEMENTS

Serum levels of various trace elements decrease in critical illness, as is well summarized by Berger.[19] Serum levels of Se, Cu, and Zn are decreased. This may be due to increased urinary or other losses and due to increased protein catabolism. Additionally, trace elements are sequestered away from the circulating blood.

8.4 TOXICITY OF MICRONUTRIENTS

8.4.1 VITAMINS

Toxicity from water-soluble vitamins is unlikely, and up to 100 times the RDA can be safely administered. Fat-soluble vitamin toxicity can occur, and it is generally recommended that a safe limit is 10 times the RDA. Serum levels of vitamins are not routinely measured in critical care. Several forms of vitamins, provitamins, active forms, and metabolites can be measured. The clinical significance of low levels is unclear, and supplementation may not increase the serum levels. Adverse reactions and toxicity of individual vitamins, where clinically relevant, and dosage recommendations are discussed subsequently.

TABLE 8.1
Micronutrient Functions and Recommended Intakes

Nutrient	Role	Cause of Deficient State	Clinical Manifestations of Deficient State	Toxicity/Adverse Effects	Recommendations
Vitamin A	Maintains mucosal integrity and wound healing. Fat-soluble vitamin with antioxidant activity.	GI losses, use of steroids.	Poor wound healing, diarrhea, poor epithelial cell regeneration, factor in bacterial translocation, impairs neutrophil function.	Excess amounts can lead to liver dysfunction and failure.	1mg/d or 3000 IU/d. Enteral nutrition formulas contain 2,600 to 5,200 IU/l, and enhanced formulas contain 4,500 to 12,000 IU/l. Amount needed to counteract steroid effects is 10,000 to 15,000 IU/d × 7 days.
Vitamin B_1	A cofactor for oxidation of pyruvate, alpha ketoacids, and branched-chain amino acids. Water soluble.	Alcoholism, high carbohydrate intake, as a component of "refeeding syndrome," iatrogenic (when TPN is given without thiamine).	TPN given without thiamine results in refractory metabolic (lactic) acidosis. Mental changes, confabulation, confusion and congestive heart failure, so-called wet beri beri.	None known	Give additional thiamine (100 mg/d) to patients at risk for deficiency, especially alcoholics and patients with preexisting malnutrition.
Vitamin B_6	Metabolism of amino acids and fatty acids, synthesis of heme and neurotransmitters. Water soluble.	Levels are decreased in renal failure.	Anemia, skin and mucosal changes, mental changes (depression, confusion).	Very high doses of over 2 g can cause convulsions.	RDA is 1.5 mg.
Vitamin B_{12}	Needed for the conversion of methyl folate to tetrahydrofolate, thus affecting DNA synthesis. Water soluble.	Due to adequate body reserves, a deficiency state in critically ill patients is unlikely. Exposure to nitrous oxide anesthesia can result in vitamin B_{12} deficiency.	Macrocytic anemia	None known	RDA is 2.4 µg. A single dose of 1 mg virtually saturates body stores for several months.

	Function	Causes of deficiency	Deficiency signs	Toxicity / adverse effects	Recommendations
Vitamin C	A nonenzymatic antioxidant that is also needed for collagen synthesis and wound healing. It is required for the synthesis of carnitine. Water soluble.	Increased requirements in burns. Abrupt cessation can lead to rebound scurvy.	Perifollicular petechiae, poor wound healing, and gingivitis.	Increases free Fe, which promotes bacterial proliferation and decreases bacteriocidal activity. Known to produce hyperoxaluria and renal calculi.	75 to 90 mg/d. Standard PN recommendation is 20 mg/d. Standard EN solutions contain 125 to 250 mg/l. Supplementation recommendations are 500 to 3000 mg/d. Enhanced formulas have 80 to 850 mg/l.
Vitamin D	Calcium and bone metabolism. Fat soluble.	Lack of sunlight, hepatic and renal insufficiency. Vitamin D levels decrease with stress, but the significance of this is not known.	Osteomalacia and osteoporosis are not relevant for critically ill patients. Prolonged inactivity can result in osteoporosis.	Hypercalcemia. Toxicity occurs only when intakes are in the range of 40,000 IU/d (1,000 μg/d), a situation unlikely to occur.	Paucity of data for recommending in critically ill patients. RDA is 5 μg (200 IU), present 1 l of EN formulas. Use active 1,25 dihydroxy form in renal or hepatic failure.
Vitamin E	Antioxidant, cofactor for selenium, membrane fluidity and integrity. Fat soluble.	Vitamin E levels decline with stress. The decrease seen when septic shock occurs in parallel with lipid peroxidation and may represent increased free radical activity.	None	Excess antagonizes vitamin A. High doses may adversely affect wound healing and may contribute to platelet dysfunction. It may also up-regulate proinflammatory cytokines. Doses as high as 3 g/d have been given without deleterious clinical effects.	RDA is 15 mg. Multivitamin preparations for PN contain 10 mg/dose. EN formulas have variable amounts: 25 to 50 mg/l. In critically ill patients, higher parenteral doses of 50 to 60 mg/d are recommended.
Vitamin K	Required in the hepatic production of serine proteases of the coagulation cascade. Fat soluble.	There are no storage forms. Alterations in microbiologic flora can diminish bacterial synthesis. Deficiencies occur rapidly in patients, especially when TPN void of vitamin K is administered.	Estimation of prothrombin time (PT) may not detect subclinical vitamin K deficiency states, which may become pronounced after surgery or resuscitation.	Rapid intravenous administration can result in hypotension. Excessive administration of vitamin K results in inability to anticoagulate patients adequately with warfarin.	RDA (150 μg) in enteral feeding. Multivitamin preparations have recently been reformulated to provide 150 μg/d.
Folic acid	Homocysteine metabolism. Water soluble.	Alcoholism, nitrous oxide exposure, dialysis, anti-epileptic drugs.	Macrocytic anemia, skin rash, increased serum homocysteine levels	None known	RDA is 400 μg present in EN and PN. One mg/day is needed in deficiency states, including dialysis.

(continued)

TABLE 8.1 (CONTINUED)
Micronutrient Functions and Recommended Intakes

Nutrient	Role	Cause of Deficient State	Clinical Manifestations of Deficient State	Toxicity/Adverse Effects	Recommendations
Niacin	An indirect role in oxidation through NAD+. Water soluble.	Alcohol abuse produces niacin deficiency. Isonicotinic acid hydrazine (INH), an antituberculosis medication, and 6-mercapto-purine, an anticancer drug, also produce niacin deficiency.	Deficiency is a chronic problem with pellagra, or dry skin, and associated with diarrhea, dermatitis, and dementia.	None known	RDA for niacin is 16 µg, adequate in most enteral formulas. Recommend 40 mg/d for PN. Some infused tryptophan gets converted to niacin. Niacin deficiency can also occur acutely in patients with severe GI problems. Supplemental niacin can rapidly reverse symptoms. No specific recommendations for critically ill patients.
Zinc	Zn content is the highest of any trace element except for Fe. Ninety-five percent of body Zn is intracellular. Functions in the formation of metalloenzymes, RNA conformation and membrane stabilization, and protein metabolism. Zn interacts with insulin and has important roles in the immune system.	Excessive GI losses, short bowel syndrome, trauma, burns, history of alcoholism, pancreatic insufficiency, renal insufficiency, high-dose steroids, HIV infection, malignancies. Simultaneous administration of ferrous salts with enteral feeding can precipitate Zn deficiency.	Skin rash involving elbows and knees, also called acrodermatitis enteropathica, characteristic rash around ala nasi, glucose intolerance, poor wound healing, abnormal hemostasis, immune dysfunction, loss of hair, altered taste (dysgeusia) and smell perception, diarrhea.	High doses of Zn result in immune dysfunction, as noted in text.	Parenteral, 2.5 to 4 mg/d. Additional amounts are as follows: 2 mg/d in acute catabolism, 12.2 mg/l of small bowel fluid losses, and 17.1 mg/kg of stool or ileostomy output. Enteral RDA is 15 mg. Additional doses are given when indicated.

	Function	Deficiency (causes)	Deficiency (manifestations)	Toxicity	Dosing
Selenium	Se has antioxidant functions. Its function is linked with that of vitamin E. Selenocysteine is in glutathione peroxidase. Se is also important for thyroid hormone production. Supplemental Se in trauma patients has been shown to normalize thyroxine (T4) and reverse T3 plasma levels. Se inhibits nuclear transcription factor κB expression, a key step in the development of inflammation.	Administration of Se-free TPN or EN, history of alcoholism, surgical resection of duodenum and proximal jejunum, especially when EN formulas deficient in Se are used.	Se deficiency manifests as congestive heart failure and arrhythmias. Involvement of peripheral muscles is manifested as myositis, with weakness and muscle cramps.	No report of Se toxicity due to nutritional support.	PN intake of 30 to 100 μg/d. The recommended enteral intake is 55 to 70 μg/d. Enteral formulas may also be deficient in bioavailable forms of Se. Se levels should be monitored in renal insufficiency and intake decreased if indicated. GI excretion of Se offers some protection against Se toxicity.
Iron	In association with hemoglobin, Fe is an oxygen carrier.	Fe deficiency is seen in critical illness as part of anemia, blood loss with microcytic anemia.	Low hemoglobin production, with possible hypoxia at the tissue level.	Free Fe is released in critical illness. Free Fe interferes with the reticuloendothelial system (RES), decreases macrophage activity, and promotes bacterial growth.	IV supplementation is not recommended in acute phase of illness, but enteral is recommended during recovery phase to support production of red cells. Diminished in renal failure, and IV supplementation may be useful.
Copper	Part of proteins; ferroxidase and ceruloplasmin. Component of metalloenzymes (SOD, cytochrome oxidase).	Seen most often in malnourished young children, in patients with disrupted gastric and small bowel anatomy.	Neutropenia, anemia, arrested maturation of myeloid cell line in bone marrow with megaloblastic changes. Bone spur formation, osteoporosis, and long bone fractures.	Red cell toxin, damages cell membranes and inhibits red cell enzymes. Manifests as hemolysis and GI disturbances. Accumulation of metal in liver and other organs, leading to death of hepatocytes.	RDA is for 1.0 to 1.5 mg for adolescents and adults and about 50 mcg/kg body weight in infants.
Manganese	Involved in sustaining several enzyme systems, most notably that of SOD.	Lack of proper diet, mostly seen in vegan and similar diets.	Impaired insulin production, altered lipid profile, deficient oxidant defense, and abnormal growth factor metabolism.	Decreased appetite and growth, reproductive failure. CNS abnormalities with inhaled form in miners.	RDA about 2 to 5 mg. Rarely of concern because EN and PN formulas with trace metals supply sufficient amounts.

TABLE 8.2
Suggested Composition of Parenteral Multivitamin and Trace Element Products for Adults

Vitamin/Trace Element	Unit of Measurement	Amount
A	mg (IU)	1.0 (~ 3000)
B_1 (thiamine)	mg	3.0
B_6 (pyridoxine)	mg	3.6
B_{12} (cyanocobalamin)	μg	5.0
C (ascorbic acid)	mg	100
D	μg[a] (IU)	5 (200)
E	mg[b] (IU)	6.7 (10)
Folic acid	μg	400
K	μg	150
Niacin	mg	40
Copper	mg	0.3–0.5
Manganese	μg	60–100
Selenium	μg	20–60
Zinc	mg	2.5–5.0

Note: IU = international units.

[a] As cholecalciferol.

[b] As di-alpha tocopherol.

Sources: Mirtallo, J.M., Parenteral formulas, in *Patenteral Nutrition*, 3rd ed., Rombeiau, J.L., Rolandelli, R.H., Eds. W.B. Saunders, Philadelphia, 2001, 124; American Medical Association, *JAMA*, 241, 2051, 1979; ASPEN Board of Directors and Clinical Guidelines Task Force, *J. Parenter. Enteral Nutr.*, 26, 1, Supplement, 1SA, 2002; and Fuhrman, P.M. and Herrmann, V.M., in *Nutritional Considerations in the Intensive Care Unit*, American Society for Parenteral and Enteral Nutrition, Silver Springs, MD, 2002, 51–60.

8.4.2 TRACE ELEMENTS

In the doses recommended for clinical use, toxicity of Zn and Se has not been reported. Depression of immune responses from high doses (150 mg/d) of Zn administered for six weeks orally has been shown.[20] Up to 100 mg of Zn per day administered parenterally over 24 h is well tolerated.[21] Se is safe up to 400 μg/d administered parenterally.[23]

8.5 THE ROLE OF MICRONUTRIENTS IN THE TREATMENT OF THE OXIDATIVE STRESS STATE IN CRITICAL ILLNESS

8.5.1 INTRODUCTION

Critically ill patients are prone to various levels of physiologic and biochemical stress. The acute phase of critical illness is typified by a systemic inflammatory response that can be either a cause, a comorbid condition, or a consequence of critical illness. This systemic inflammatory response causes a catabolic state in the patient that can best be described as a parasitic condition. It has been stressed throughout this book that an essential tool in our present armamentarium to care for critically ill patients includes providing the appropriate combination of macronutrients in an attempt to reverse some of the catabolic processes that occur. Micronutrient replacement also plays a significant role in the management of critical illness. As demonstrated in Table 8.1 and the preceding

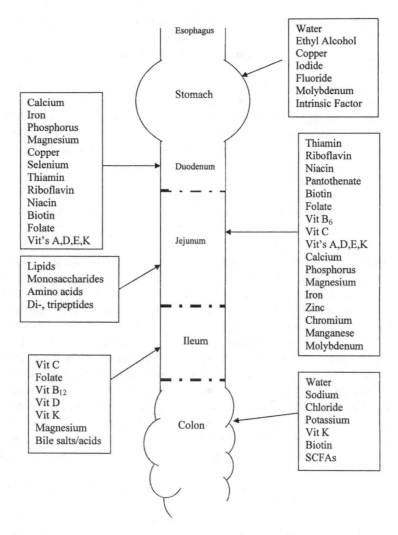

FIGURE 8.1 Nutrient absorption in the gastrointestinal tract.

text, micronutrients act to maintain and stabilize many of the homeostatic processes and enzymatic reactions required to sustain life.

However, there has been increasing data in the literature that the prolonged inflammatory response in the critically ill patient leads to an imbalance between pro-oxidant and antioxidant mechanisms in the patient, leading to an oxidative stress state. This results in the production of large quantities of reactive oxygen species (ROS). The effects of this oxidative stress state have also been shown to respond to treatment with antioxidants, many of which are the same micronutrients utilized in the daily care of the critically ill patient.

8.5.2 Oxidative Stress State

The inflammatory response to critical illness leads to release of numerous proinflammatory and anti-inflammatory cytokines. The overall effect is that inflammatory cells, including neutrophils and macrophages, release ROS. These substances interact with cellular molecules, such as proteins, DNA, and lipids, causing damage to cell membranes, structural proteins, and cellular enzyme systems (leading to organ dysfunction) and prolonging the inflammatory response (leading to organ dysfunction and failure).[22,23] This overabundance of ROS can overwhelm the endogenous antioxidant mechanisms in the host and lead to a rapid depletion of these antioxidants, leaving the host at risk for further injury with repeated attacks from the ROS.[24-26]

Specifically, the mechanisms leading to the formation of ROS include:

- Up-regulation during sepsis of the mitochondrial transport chain, with overproduction of O_2^- as a product of the interaction between oxygen and semiubiquinone.[27]
- In activated neutrophils and macrophages during severe sepsis, the NADPH oxidase enzyme system is a predominant pathway for significant production of ROS.
- Major vascular, cardiac, and organ transplant surgery has been demonstrated to activate the xanthine oxidase enzyme as a consequence of ischemia and reperfusion. This enzyme system is responsible for the formation of ROS during these set conditions.
- Cellular apoptosis or accelerated death and lysis releases certain metallic ions, such as iron and copper, which in turn act as cofactors in enzyme systems, converting hydrogen peroxide into more caustic and damaging hydroxyl radicals.[28]

Proof of an increased oxidative stress state is difficult to obtain based solely on measured levels of ROS, due to their short half-life.[28] Rather, evidence for an increased oxidative stress state in critically ill patients is seen indirectly through the measurement of the byproducts of ROS with cellular molecules. Hence, these patients demonstrate elevated levels of such substances as thiobarbituric acid–reacting substances (TBARs: byproducts of the interactions of lipids with ROS), DNA, and proteins. Also, there will be a concurrent depletion of endogenous antioxidant stores noted (TRAP: total radical trapping antioxidant parameter).[29-32] Several studies have demonstrated that an increased oxidative stress state occurs mostly in patient with sepsis, septic shock, acute respiratory failure, and acute respiratory distress syndrome.[33,34] Elevated TBAR levels have been found in patients with SIRS and multiple organ dysfunction syndrome, and elevated TBARs in patients with MDOF (as opposed to patients without MDOF) with a correlation of these levels with the Sequential Organ Failure Assessment score.[32] Other studies have documented an elevation of lipid–ROS byproducts and an increase in endogenous antioxidant enzyme activity and demonstrated a decrease in TRAP in patients with critical illness, yet improvement with resolution of the inflammatory process in survivors paralleling vitamin C and E levels in plasma, and no improvement in patients who were nonsurvivors.[35,36]

8.5.3 ENDOGENOUS ANTIOXIDANT ACTIVITY

Endogenous mechanisms act in a network-like fashion to neutralize the production of ROS in an attempt to ablate the deleterious effects of these agents. Intracellular glutathione acts as one of the major antioxidant buffers. Nonenzymatic ROS scavengers also include commonly occurring molecules, such as utate, ubiquinone, bilirubin, and vitamins such as ascorbic acid (vitamin C), β-carotene, and α-tocopherol (vitamin E). Once vitamin E is oxidized, vitamin C and glutathione play a role in reducing the vitamin E back to its active form.

Enzymatic systems then act in concert to detoxify ROS further. Thus, superoxide dismutase (SOD) converts O_2^- to H_2O_2; catalase and glutathione peroxidase convert H_2O_2 to water and alcohols. These enzyme systems are inducible and dependent on minerals such as selenium, copper, zinc, and manganese as important in cofactors in these enzymatic reactions.

Currently, recommendations exist for the supplementation of micronutrients in the nutritional support, either enteral or parenteral, of hospital patients. This list was recently modified to include recommendations for critically ill patients.[8]

8.5.4 MICRONUTRIENT REPLACEMENT IN CRITICAL ILLNESS

The previous sections discussed the etiology of an oxidative stress state in the critically ill patient and how research data have demonstrated an increase in the byproducts of oxidized cellular

TABLE 8.3
Micronutrients in Critical Illness

Micronutrient	RDA	Standard Dose Recommended PN	Recommended EN	Supplementation (per day)	Enhanced EN Formulas
Vitamin A	1 mg	1.0 mg	0.9–1.0 mg	PN: 3.5 mg EN: 8.6 mg	1.5–4.0 mg/l
Vitamin C	75–90 mg	200 mg	125–250 mg/l	500–3000 mg	80–844 mg/l
Vitamin E (α-tocopherol)	15 mg	10 mg	25–50 mg/l	PN: 400 mg EN: 40–1000 mg	40–212 mg/l
Vitamin K	150 μg	150 μg	40–135 μg		
Iron	10–15 mg	0 mg	12–20 mg/l		
Selenium	50–100 μg	20–60 μg	20–70 μg/l	100–400 μg	77–100 μg/l
Zinc	15 mg	2.5–5.0 mg	11–19 mg/l	10–30 mg	15–24 mg/l

Note: EN: enteral nutrition; PN: parenteral nutrition. 1 IU of vitamin A = 0.344 μg.

Sources: From Fuhrman, P.M. and Herrmann, V.M., in *Nutritional Considerations in the Intensive Care Unit*, Shikora, S.A., Martindale, R.G., Schwartberg, S.D., Eds., American Society for Parenteral and Enteral Nutrition, Silver Springs, MD, 2002, 51–60.

molecules. The literature has also demonstrated a decline in endogenous antioxidant activity in critically ill patients. Clearly, this situation could lend itself to a goal-directed therapy in which beneficial effects may be demonstrated.

The goal of this therapy would be to provide the necessary factors to replenish the endogenous antioxidants at appropriate levels to counteract the toxic effects of ROS and to supply these factors through the most appropriate route. Numerous studies have indicated that prophylactic supplementation of antioxidants has demonstrated benefits for the patient. See Table 8.3 for recommended doses of select micronutrients during critical illness.

Most of the studies recently performed have dealt with the use of antioxidants as "premedications" in surgical procedures in which significant ischemia and reperfusion injuries can occur. One study demonstrated improvement in creatinine values and clearance in kidney transplantation surgery when an infusion of multivitamins was delivered prior to reperfusion of the kidney.[37] Another study rated an oxidative stress index, looking at myocardial tissue samples before and after cross-clamping of the aorta. The oxidative stress index was elevated in the control group, but in the group pretreated with vitamins A and E, 100% protection against oxidative stress was found.[38] These studies clearly indicate an advantage to micronutrient supplementation prior to an inflammatory insult.

Fewer studies have addressed direct outcome benefits in patients with established critical illness and inflammation before any supplementation can be provided. The development of sepsis and ARDS seems to be favored by an oxidative stress state in the early stages of the disease, and replacement with recommended amounts of micronutrients may be an issue of too little too late.[31,39]

A recent study compared the beneficial effects between two groups of critically ill patients with a mean APACHE II score of 33. Both groups received isocaloric, isonitrogenous enteral formulas. The experimental group feeds were supplemented with vitamins A, E, and C. Blood samples were taken for measurement of antioxidant levels and products of lipid oxidation, and 28-day outcomes were evaluated. There was no difference in ultimate outcome between groups, although the study was not powered to demonstrate small differences. Vitamin levels became slowly elevated during treatment in the supplemented group, and there appeared to be improved resistance to lipid perox-idation.[25]

Other studies have demonstrated benefits of antioxidant supplementation. In a study of 98 patients with ARDS, vitamins E and A in enteral formulas were well absorbed in the experimental group and their TRAP and TBAR products did not change compared to controls, indicating a beneficial effect from the supplemented diet.[40] Likewise, clinical outcome variables demonstrated improved PaO_2/FiO_2 ratios and fewer days of mechanical ventilation in patients receiving this formula.[41] In a large-scale study of 301 critically ill trauma patients, a supplemented diet with 1000 mg of Vitamin C IV and 3000 IU/d enterally demonstrated elevated levels of these vitamins. Comparison of this group with a control group of 294 trauma patients also showed a relative risk reduction of multiple organ failure, fewer ventilator days of care, and shorter length of stay in the ICU.[42] Similar studies have demonstrated beneficial effects from supplementation of trace minerals in critically ill patients in similar settings.[26]

8.6 SUMMARY

Nutritional support of the critically ill patient is a key component of therapy. Although great pains are taken to provide adequate carbohydrate, lipid, and protein combinations, the role of micronutri-ents (trace minerals and vitamins) must not be overlooked.

A growing body of literature indicates that critical illness provides a setting for the formation of ROS as a result of the activation of various mechanisms. At the same time, this overproduction of ROS overwhelms endogenous mechanisms, leading to depletion in nonenzymatic and enzymatic antioxidant activity. This situation leads to an oxidative stress state that will ultimately cause damage of cellular molecules and structural proteins, resulting in cell death, organ dysfunction, and organ failure, with prolongation of critical illness and diminished survival.

Clinical evidence has defined a role for the prophylactic use of antioxidant vitamins and trace minerals to avoid the deleterious effects of ischemia and reperfusion injury in cardiac, vascular, and organ transplantation surgery. A growing body of evidence is just now being developed that also demonstrates benefits of antioxidant supplementation for patients already diagnosed with critical illness. Yet several questions still need to be answered about the amount (routine recom-mended replacement amounts vs. higher amounts), route of replacement (enteral vs. parenteral), and timing of replacement (is early in the course of ICU admission good enough or is this too late, and should replacement be considered at time of admission?). Further research continues in this field.

8.7 RECOMMENDATIONS FOR SUPPLEMENTATION

8.7.1 WHO NEEDS SUPPLEMENTATION?

All critically ill patients need micronutrient supplementation as soon as nutritional support is initiated enterally or parenterally. It is also possible to supply these micronutrients directly via the intravenous fluids of patients who are not yet at goal enteral or parenteral nutrition.

8.7.2 TIMING

The largest increases in ROS production occurs early in the course of acute illness. Likewise, decreased serum levels of micronutrients are seen in this period. In burns, early administration of micronutrients has been shown to be beneficial.[43–45] It is therefore logical to conclude that micro-nutrient supplementation should begin early in the course of acute illness to offset the deleterious effects of ROS. During the first five to seven days, the emphasis is on antioxidant supplementation. After this period, routine micronutrient supplementation is provided.

8.7.3 ROUTE

In critically ill patients, the intravenous route is the only reliable method by which micronutrients can be administered. Very few clinical trials have used the enteral route for micronutrient supplementation in critically ill patients. This has been studied in trauma and burns.[46,47] Absorption by the enteral route in critically ill patients is unpredictable, due to hemodynamic instability, bowel edema, and alterations in blood supply.[48] Vitamin E absorption is reduced in critically ill patients.[49] Interactions between various micronutrients in normal individuals, discussed earlier, are even more complex in critically ill patients. Thus, micronutrients are initially administered intravenously, either as a component of total parenteral nutrition or separately. If and when enteral feeding is initiated and tolerated, micronutrient supplementation can be provided enterally.

8.7.4 DOSE

Although firm conclusions and recommendations are not available, we believe that additional modest doses of vitamins A (10,000 IU/d), E (50 to 60 IU/d), and C (500 mg/d) will benefit critically ill patients.

8.7.5 MONITORING

Though serum levels can be used to detect deficiencies, they are not easy to obtain in most hospitals and may not reflect a true deficiency. There are no reliable laboratory indicators for vitamins and trace elements to determine adequacy of supplementation. Functional end points, such as using enzyme assays (alkaline phosphatase for Zn and glutathione peroxidase for Se) are also not reliable.

8.8 CONCLUSION

We have attempted to provide some general and safe guidelines for the use of vitamins in critically ill patients. The information available is, at best, incomplete. However, this discussion should assist the clinician to make individual choices in the management of critically ill patients, specifically regarding the use of micronutrients.

The routine inclusion or supplementation of standard doses of vitamins and trace elements with enteral and parenteral nutritional support is accepted. The data on antioxidant supplementation in critically ill patients are evolving, but this supplementation is considered safe.

REFERENCES

1. Vrees, M.D. and Albina, J.E., Metabolic response to illness and its mediators, in *Clinical Nutrition: Parenteral Nutrition*, Rombeau, J.L., and Rolandelli, R.H., Eds., W.B. Saunders, Philadelphia, 2000, 21.
2. Solomons, N.W. and Ruz, M., Trace element requirements in humans: an update, *J. Trace Elem. Exp. Med.*, 11, 177, 1998.
3. Nutrition Advisory Group, Multivitamin preparations for parenteral use, *J. Parenter. Enteral Nutr.*, 3, 1979.
4. American Medical Association, Dept. of Foods and Nutrition, Guidelines for essential trace element preparations for parenteral use: a statement by an expert panel, *JAMA*, 241, 2051, 1979.
5. Elia, M., Changing concepts of nutrient requirements in disease: implications for artificial nutritional support, *Lancet*, 5, 1279, 1995.
6. Schorah, C.J., Downing, C., Piripitsi, A., et al., Total vitamin C, ascorbic acid and dehydroascorbic acid concentrations in plasma of critically ill patients, *Am. J. Clin. Nutr.*, 63, 760, 1996.
7. Food and Drug Administration (FDA), *Parenteral Multivitamin Products: Drugs for Human Use: Drug Efficacy Study Implementation*, Amendment, Federal Register, 65(77), 21200–21201, 2000.

8. ASPEN Board of Directors and Clinical Guidelines Task Force, Guidelines for the use of parenteral and enteral nutrition in adult and pediatric patients, *J. Parenter. Enteral Nutr.*, 26(1), Supplement, 1SA, 2002.

9. Fuhrman, P.M. and Herrmann, V.M., Micronutrients in critical illness, in *Nutritional Considerations in the Intensive Care Unit*, Shikora, S.A., Martindale, R.G., Schwaitzberg, S.D., Eds., American Society for Parenteral and Enteral Nutrition, Silver Spring, MD, 2002, 51–60.

10. Sriram, K. and Sridhar, R., Gastroduodenal decompression and simultaneous nasoenteral nutrition: extracorporeal gastrojejunostomy, *Nutrition,* 12(6), 440, 1996.

11. Sriram, K., Gergans, G., and Badger, H., Vitamin B_{12} (cobalamin) absorption via feeding jejunostomy, *J. Am. Coll. Nutr.,* 8(1), 75, 1989.

12. Goldberg, L.S. and Fudenberg, H.H., Effect of pH on the vitamin B_{12}-bindin capacity of intrinsic factor, *J. Lab. Clin. Med.*, 73, 469, 1969.

13. Demling, R.H. and De Biasse, M.A., Micronutrients in critical illness, *Crit. Care Clin.*, 11, 651, 1995.

14. Kenny, F., Sriram, K., and Hammond, J., Clinical zinc deficiency during adequate enteral nutrition, *J. Am. Coll. Nutr.*, 8(1), 83, 1989.

15. Galloway, P., McMillan, D.C., and Sattar, N., Effect of the inflammatory response on trace element and vitamin status, *Ann. Clin. Biochem.,* 37, 289, 2000.

16. Louw, J.A., Werbeck, A., Louw, M.E.J., et al., Blood vitamin concentrations during the acute-phase response. *Crit. Care Med.,* 20, 934, 1992.

17. Agarwal, N., Norkus, E., Gacia, C., et al., Effect of surgery on serum antioxidant vitamins, *J. Parenter. Enteral Nutr.*, 20 (Suppl.), 32S, 1996.

18. Cruickshank, A.M., Telfer, A.B., and Shenkin, A., Thiamine deficiency in the critically ill, *Intens. Care Med.*, 14, 384, 1988.

19. Berger, M.M. and Chiolero, R.L., Key vitamins and trace elements in the critically ill, in *Nutrition and Critical Care*, Cynober, L., Moore, F.A., Eds., Nestle Nutrition Workshop Series Clinical & Performance Program, 2003, 8, 1999.

20. Chandra, R.K., Excessive intake of zinc impairs immune responses, *JAMA*, 252, 1443, 1984.

21. Baumgartner, T.G., Ed., *Clinical Guide to Parenteral Micronutrition.* 3rd ed., Fujisawa, Chicago, 1997.

22. Halliwell, B., Free Radicals, antioxidants, and human disease: curiosity, cause or consequence? *Lancet*, 344, 721, 1994.

23. Bielsalski, H.K., The role of antioxidants in nutritional support, *Nutrition*, 16, 578, 2000.

24. Goodyear-Bruch, C., Pierce, J.D., Oxidative stress in critically ill patients, *Am. J. Crit. Care*, 11, 543, 2002.

25. Preiser, J.C., Van Gossum, A., Barré, J., et al., Enteral feeding with a solution enriched with antioxidant vitamins A, C, and E enhances resistance to oxidative stress. *Crit. Care Med.*, 28, 3828, 2000.

26. Berger, M.M., Cavadini, C., Chiolero, R., et al., Influence of larger amounts of trace elements on recovery after major burns, *Nutrition*, 10, 327, 1994.

27. Brealey, D., Brand, M., and Hargreaves, I., Association between mitochondrial dysfunction and severity and outcome of septic shock, *Lancet*, 360, 219, 2002.

28. Lovat, R., Preiser, J.C., Antioxidant therapy in intensive care, *Curr. Opin. Crit. Care*, 9, 266, 2003.

29. Therond, P., Bonnefont-Rousselot, D., Davit-Spraul, A., et al., Biomarkers for oxidative stress: an analytical approach, *Curr. Opin. Nutr. Metabol. Care*, 3, 373, 2000.

30. Goode, H.F., Cowley, H.C., Walker, B.E., et al., Decreased antioxidant status and increased lipid peroxidation in patients with septic shock and secondary organ dysfunction, *Crit. Care Med.*, 23, 646, 1995.

31. Metnitz, P.G., Bartens, C., Fischer, M., et al., Antioxidant status is patients with acute respiratory distress syndrome. *Intens. Care Med.*, 25, 180, 1999.

32. Motoyama, T., Okamoto, K., Kukita, I., et al., Possible role of increased oxidative stress in multiple organ failure after systemic inflammatory response syndrome, *Crit. Care Med.*, 31, 1048, 2003.

33. Baiouali, A.B., Aube, H., Maupoil, V., et al., Plasma lipid peroxidation in critically ill patients: importance of mechanical ventilation, *Free Radicals Biol. Med.*, 16, 223, 1994.

34. Takeda, K., Shimada, Y., Amano, M., et al., Plasma lipid peroxides and alpha-toropherol in critically ill patients, *Crit. Care Med.,* 12, 957, 1984.

35. Alonso de Vega, J.M., Diaz, J., Serrano, E., et al., Oxidative stress in critically ill patients with systemic inflammatory response syndrome, *Crit. Care Med.*, 30, 1782, 2002.

36. Tsai, K., Hsu, T., Kong, C., et al., Is the endogenous peroxyl radical scavenging capacity of plasma protective in systemic inflammatory response in humans? *Free Radicals Biol. Med.*, 28, 926, 2000.
37. Rabl, H., Khoschsorur, G., Colombo, T., et al., A multivitamin infusion prevents lipid peroxidation and improves transplantation performance, *Kidney Int.*, 43, 912, 1993.
38. Milei, J., Ferreira, R., Grana, D.R., and Boveris, A., Oxidative stress and mitochondrial damage in coronary artery bypass graft surgery: effect of antioxidant treatments, *Comprehensive Therapy*, 27, 108, 2001.
39. Punz, A., Nanobashvili, J., Fuegl, A., et al., Effect of α-tocopherol pretreatment on high-energy metabolites in rabbit skeletal muscle after ischemia/reperfusion, *Clin. Nutr.*, 17, 85, 1998.
40. Nelson, J.L., DeMichele, S.J., Pacht, E.R., et al., Enteral nutrition in ARDS study group: effect of enteral feeding with eicosapentaenoic acid, gamma-linolenic and antioxidants on antioxidant status in patients with acute respiratory distress syndrome, *J. Parenter. Enteral Nutr.*, 27, 98, 2003.
41. Gadek, J.E., DeMichele, S.J., Karlstad, M.D., et al., Effect of enteral feeding with eicosapentaenoic acid, gamma-linolenic acid, and antioxidants in patients with acute respiratory distress syndrome: enteral nutrition in ARDS study group, *Crit. Care Med.,* 27, 1409, 1999.
42. Nathens A.B., Neff M.J., Jurkovich G.J., et al., Randomized, prospective trial of antioxidant supplementation in critically ill surgical patients, *Ann. Surg.*, 236, 814, 2002.
43. Tanaka, H., Matsuda, T., Miyagantani, Y. et al., Reduction of resuscitation fluid volumes in severely burned patients using ascorbic acid administration, *Arch. Surg.,* 135, 326, 2000.
44. Angswrum, M.W.A., Schottdorf, J., Schopohl, J., et al., Selenium replacement in patients with severe systemic inflammatory response syndrome improves clinical outcome, *Crit. Care Med.,* 27, 1807, 1999.
45. Berger, M.M., Spertini, F., Shenkin, A., et al., Trace element supplementation modulates pulmonary infection rates after major burns: a double-blind placebo-controlled trial, *Am. J. Clin. Nutr.,* 68, 365, 1998.
46. Porter J.M., Ivatury, R.R., Azimuddin, K., et al., Antioxidant therapy in the prevention of organ dysfunction syndrome and infectious complications after trauma: early results of a prospective randomized study, *Am. Surg.*, 65, 478, 1999.
47. Pochon, J.P. and Kloti, J., Zinc and copper replacement therapy in children with deep burns, *Burns*, 5, 123, 1979.
48. Berger, M.M., Berger-Gryllaki, M., Wiesel, P.H., et al., Gastrointestinal absorption after cardiac surgery, *Crit. Care Med.*, 28, 2217–2223, 2000.
49. Seeger, W., Wiegler, A., and Wolf, H.R.D., Serum alpha-tocopherol levels after high-dose enteral vitamin E administration in patients with acute respiratory failure, *Intens. Care Med.*, 13, 395, 1987.

9 Fluid, Electrolyte, and Acid–Base Requirements

Maria R. Lucarelli, Lindsay J. Pell, Mary Beth Shirk, and Jay M. Mirtallo
The Ohio State University Medical Center

CONTENTS

9.1 INTRODUCTION

Critically ill patients manifest a multitude of fluid, electrolyte, and acid–base disturbances. Specialized nutrition support in the form of enteral tube feeding or parenteral nutrition may be associated with these disorders either by being a primary cause or by being the major mode of treatment. As such, the clinician providing nutrition support must know basic and advanced concepts of fluid, electrolyte, and acid–base balance. The purpose of this chapter is to summarize the etiology,

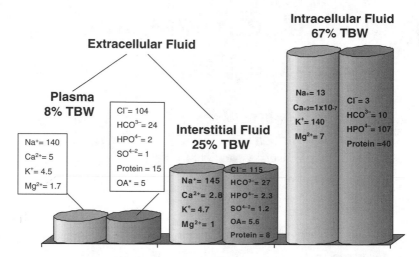

FIGURE 9.1 Distribution and composition of body fluids. TBW: total body water; OA: organic acids. (Adapted from Whitmire SJ, in *Contemporary Nutrition Support Practice: A Clinical Guide,* WB Saunders, Philadelphia, 1998, 128; and Ohs MS, Uribarri J, in *Modern Nutrition in Health and Disease,* 9th ed. Williams and Wilkins, Baltimore, 1999, 107. With permission.)

symptoms, and treatments of fluid, electrolyte, and acid–base disorders commonly observed in the intensive care patient receiving nutrition support.

9.2 BODY FLUID COMPARTMENTS

Maintenance of fluid and electrolyte homeostasis is necessary for normal cell function, and the human body has an incredible ability to compensate for excessive fluid and electrolyte losses and intake. Figure 9.1 illustrates the distribution of fluid and electrolytes of the body. In the critically ill patient, the balance may be challenged, at times to such an extreme that the body is unable to compensate. Early recognition and treatment of such abnormalities by critical care practitioners can avoid morbidity and mortality.

9.3 EFFECTS OF STARVATION AND CRITICAL ILLNESS ON FLUID AND ELECTROLYTE STATUS

During periods of prolonged starvation, there is a loss of lean tissue mass, water, and minerals. Up to 150 g of lean muscle is lost daily during simple starvation, resulting in the release of 15 to 20 mmol of potassium and 110 ml of water from the intracellular to the extracellular fluid (1). Stress or injury increases the lysis of lean tissue and may result in as much as 1.2 g of phosphorus, 60 mmol of potassium, and 450 ml of water loss per day (1). These deficits predispose the patient to acute electrolyte abnormalities, fluid retention, and dysfunction of various organ systems. As such, nutrition support in the presence of severe malnutrition may lead to acute electrolyte shifts and fluid retention, which are well known symptoms of refeeding syndrome (RFS) (2). For parenteral nutrition (PN) patients, RFS has been associated with severe complications of hypophosphatemia in patients being refed after severe weight loss (3). The effects of RFS on fluid, electrolytes, and organ function, however, are much more comprehensive than those of hypophosphatemia. Solomon and Kirby proposed a definition and components of the refeeding syndrome as the metabolic and physiologic consequences of the depletion, repletion, and compartmental shifts and interrelationships of the following: phosphorus, potassium, magnesium, glucose metabolism,

TABLE 9.1
Electrolyte Composition and Osmolality of Common IV Fluids

IV Fluid	Glucose (G/l)	Osmolality (mOsm/l)	Sodium (mEq/l)	Chloride (mEq/l)	Potassium (mEq/l)	Lactate (mEq/l)	Calcium (mEq/l)
Dextrose 5% in water (D5W)	50	252	0	0	0	0	0
Lactated Ringer's solution (LR)	0	273	130	109	4	28	2.7
0.9% Sodium chloride (NS)	0	308	154	154	0	0	0
0.45% Sodium chloride (1/2 NS)	0	154	77	77	0	0	0

vitamin deficiency, and fluid resuscitation (3). As such, the nutritional status of the patient must be considered when determining fluid and electrolyte requirements and when diagnosing and managing electrolyte disorders.

9.4 REQUIREMENTS FOR FLUID AND ELECTROLYTES

In patients receiving nutrition support, the enteral nutrition (EN) or PN fluid becomes the patient's major source, if not the primary source, of fluid and electrolytes. The critically ill patient may have conditions that alter tolerance of fluid and electrolytes, so these parameters are frequently monitored. During patient assessment, adjustment of the electrolyte content of PN or the fluid content of EN or PN is often considered. Therefore, the fluid volume and electrolyte composition of nutrition support is based on normal nutritional requirements and adjustments are based on patient clinical condition and overall response to the fluids and electrolytes being administered.

9.4.1 FLUID

Normal requirements for water are 30 to 40 ml/kg or 1 to 1.5 ml/Kcal provided in nutrition support. Adjustments are usually required for those patients with cardiac, renal, and hepatic dysfunction. Critically ill patients need fluid in adequate amounts to maintain blood pressure, urine output, and perfusion to vital organs. Nutrition support fluids are only one of many sources of fluids infused in these patients. Other sources include parenteral maintenance fluids (Table 9.1), parenteral medications, blood products, and fluids from renal replacement therapy. These fluids are important to consider when the need for fluid restriction is present. Where appropriate, fluid restriction may be accomplished by limiting the volume of drug infusions and maintenance IV solutions so that the fluid for nutrition support may be spared. In some cases, the electrolyte content of PN can be adjusted to include the electrolytes previously provided by IV fluids so that the IV fluid may be discontinued.

9.4.2 ELECTROLYTES

Electrolyte requirements are based on three conditions:

- Replacement of a deficit
- Normal nutritional needs
- Recognition and appropriate replacement of extraneous fluid losses

TABLE 9.2
Etiology of Common Electrolyte Deficiencies

Electrolyte	Cause of Deficiency
Sodium	Loss from skin, GI system, lungs
	Kidney: diuretic use, renal damage, adrenal insufficiency
Potassium	Starvation; loss from skin, bile, lower GI, or fistula
	Kidney: diuretic use, alkalosis, amphotericin
Bicarbonate	Diarrhea, pancreas, or small bowel loss; mineralocorticoid deficiency
	Kidney: renal tubular acidosis
Chloride	Loop diuretics, gastric loss, intestinal loss
Magnesium	Starvation, intestinal loss due to malabsorption or diarrhea, alcoholism, laxative abuse, diuretics, cyclosporine
Phosphorus	Starvation, alkalosis, glucose administration, diabetic ketoacidosis, gastrointestinal losses, use of Al-containing antacids

9.4.2.1   Replacement of a Deficit

Conditions that predispose to electrolyte deficiency are listed in Table 9.2. With severe malnutrition, the deficits may be intracellular and may not be apparent from serum chemistries. If renal function is adequate, normal serum levels may be maintained, even though significant cellular deficits are developing. For example, there may be as much as a 40% total body deficit of magnesium before it is demonstrated as a low serum level (4). Therefore, patients with severe malnutrition are at high risk of electrolyte deficiencies, some of which only become manifest or symptomatic when nutrition support is initiated. Because nutrition support increases the demand of these electrolytes, there are some circumstances in which the electrolyte disorder should be corrected prior to initiating the nutrient infusion, for example, hypokalemia (serum K < 2.7 mEq/l), hypophosphatemia (serum phosphorus < 2 mg/dl), and hypochloremic metabolic alkalosis (serum carbon dioxide content > 50 mEq/l or arterial blood gas pH > 7.50).

9.4.2.2   Normal Nutritional Needs

Rudman et al. (5) demonstrated that a proper proportion of electrolytes per gram of nitrogen administered is required to promote repletion of lean body mass. In this investigation, a ratio of phosphorus 0.8 g, sodium 3.9 mEq, potassium 3 mEq, chloride 2.5 mEq, and calcium 1.2 mEq per gram of nitrogen was required to achieve positive nitrogen balance and improve lean body mass rather than fat or water mass. These data support the concept that electrolytes are required for nutritional purposes irrespective of renal, liver, or cardiac function and serve as the basis for the normal requirements for EN and PN (Table 9.3) (6,7).

9.4.2.3   Recognition and Appropriate Replacement of Extraneous Fluid Losses

Deficits in fluid, electrolyte, and acid or base may occur in critically ill patients, resulting from large amounts of extraneous fluid outputs. Extraneous fluid outputs are those that are not normally present (e.g., ostomy, fistula, or nasogastric drainage; high urine output; or diarrhea) and are in volumes in excess of that which can be managed without some form of intravenous replacement fluid. Generally, volume losses < 600 ml/d in patients with normal renal function can be tolerated with minimal adjustments in intravenous fluid content (e.g., addition of potassium or magnesium to a maintenance IV solution or adjustment of the sodium, potassium chloride, or acetate content of PN). When this volume is exceeded, a parenteral replacement fluid is required to be administered

TABLE 9.3
Daily Electrolyte Requirements

Electrolyte	Enteral RDA/AI Reference Value	Parenteral
Sodium	500 mg (22 mEq/kg)	1–2 mEq/kg
Potassium	2 g (51 mEq/kg)	1–2 mEq/kg
Chloride	750 mg (21 mEq/kg)	As needed to maintain acid–base balance with acetate
Magnesium	420 mg (17 mEq/kg)	8–20 mEq
Calcium	1200 mg (30 mEq/kg)	10–15 mEq
Phosphorus	700 mg (23 mg/kg)	20–40 mmol

TABLE 9.4
Electrolyte Content of Extraneous Fluid Loss

Source	Electrolyte Content of Fluid Loss (mEq/l)				
	Sodium	Hydrogen	Potassium	Chloride	Bicarbonate
Gastric	40–65	90	10	100–140	—
Pancreatic	135–150		5–10	60–75	70–90
Bile	128–160		4–12	90–120	30
Intestinal (jejunum)	95–120		5–15	80–130	10–20
Intestinal (ileum)	110–130		10–20	90–110	20–30
Diarrhea	90–120		5–10	75–120	5–40

TABLE 9.5
Electrolyte Replacement for Extraneous Fluid Loss

Source	Major Electrolyte Lost	Parenteral Replacement Fluid
Gastric	Hydrogen (acid), chloride	0.9% sodium chloride 0.45% sodium chloride if receiving acid-suppression therapy
Pancreatic	Sodium, bicarbonate	Lactated Ringer's with added bicarbonate
Biliary and small bowel	Sodium, chloride, bicarbonate	Lactated Ringer's
Diarrhea	Sodium, potassium, chloride, bicarbonate	Lactated Ringer's or lactated Ringer's with added bicarbonate

such that the fluid and electrolytes in the extraneous output are replaced. To ensure proper replacement, the electrolyte content of the fluid being lost should be known (Table 9.4) and a replacement fluid should be selected that is similar in electrolyte content (Table 9.5). Lactated Ringer's should be used with caution in critically ill patients with low perfusion states. These patients may be prone to a lactic acidosis due to anaerobic glucose oxidation and the lactate dose provided by the IV solution. Other fluids, such as 0.45% sodium chloride, may need to be modified by adding sodium or potassium acetate in order to provide a source of bicarbonate.

9.5 FLUID AND SODIUM DISORDERS

9.5.1 HYPONATREMIA

Abnormally low sodium values are commonly encountered, with an estimated incidence of 1% in all hospitalized patients and an incidence of 14% in the critically ill (8,9). Hyponatremia is defined as serum sodium levels < 135 mmol/l, though clinically significant hyponatremia usually occurs at levels < 130 mmol/l. In evaluating patients with hyponatremia, it is important to assess tonicity. Hyponatremia may occur in hypotonic, normotonic, and hypertonic states. Pseudohyponatremia, seen in patients with hyperlipidemia or hyperproteinemia, reflects a decreased sodium in whole plasma while the sodium concentration in plasma water remains constant. Hyperglycemia is the most common setting of hypertonic hyponatremia because increased plasma glucose results in a shift of water from the intracellular to extracellular space in response to the osmolar effect of glucose. In hyperglycemic states, the serum sodium is expected to decrease 1.6 mmol/l for every 100 mg/dl rise in serum glucose (10).

In the hospitalized patient, the syndrome of inappropriate antidiuretic hormone (SIADH) is the most common cause of hyponatremia (11). Clinically, the patient appears euvolemic but is total body water overloaded because there is inappropriate concentration of the urine. Spot urine sodium values are elevated (> 20 mmol/l), with a corresponding elevated urine osmolality (> 100 mOsm/l) (12). This results in hypotonic hyponatremia. SIADH can be seen in patients with central nervous system disease, malignancy, and lung disease, and with the administration of some drugs, including diuretics, antidepressants, and analgesics.

Other causes of hypotonic hyponatremia (Figure 9.2) must be considered in the critically ill patient. In patients who are volume depleted, one must consider both renal and extrarenal salt wasting. Most commonly, this occurs in the setting of dehydration, diuretic use, vomiting, or diarrhea. Hyponatremia can also occur in edematous patients, such as those with heart failure or liver failure as a result of increased extracellular water.

Clinical manifestations of hyponatremia include malaise, headache, seizures, coma, and even death. The rate at which the decreased sodium develops contributes to the degree of signs and symptoms a patient will demonstrate. That is, the more rapid the decline in serum levels, the more symptomatic a patient may become. Treatment is aimed at the underlying mechanism. Hypovolemic patients can usually be treated with isotonic saline. In the settings of symptomatic normovolemic or hypervolemic hyponatremia, hypertonic saline infusions, in conjunction with furosemide-induced diuresis, can be attempted. This must be performed under close monitoring of the serum sodium levels. Correction of the serum sodium should be 1 to 2 mmol/l/h with a goal of < 8 mmol/l/d to avoid the potential complication of the osmotic demyelination syndrome (13). In all patients with hyponatremia, access to free water should be limited.

9.5.2 HYPERNATREMIA

Hypernatremia, defined as a serum sodium of > 145 mmol/l, has been estimated to occur at a frequency of 6% in the intensive care unit (ICU) (14). This is despite the often daily monitoring of fluid and electrolytes. Hypernatremia that develops during a patient's ICU stay has been linked to an increase in overall mortality compared to patients that present with elevated serum sodium levels (14). Hypernatremia denotes an imbalance between body water and sodium in the body. In the hospital setting, this is usually a combination of patient's lack of access to free water and excessive loss of hypotonic fluids (i.e., gastrointestinal and respiratory fluid loss). This is compounded by inappropriate fluid prescriptions, sodium bicarbonate administration, medications, and hypertonic parenteral nutrition.

Clinical manifestations include lethargy, altered mental status, irritability, hyperreflexia, and spasticity. If the rise in serum sodium occurs rapidly, it can lead to rapid brain shrinkage and intracranial hemorrhage. Management of hypernatremia involves addressing the underlying cause

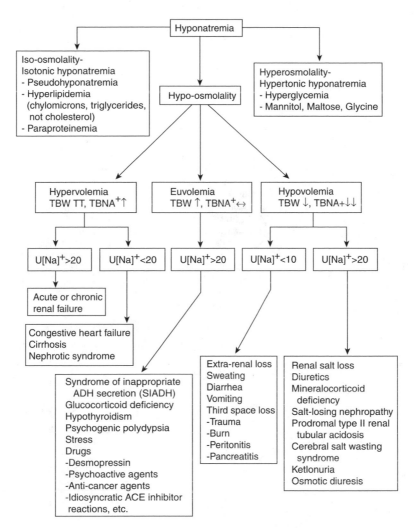

FIGURE 9.2 Etiology of hyponatremia. (Reprinted from Weiss-Guillet EM, Takala J, Jakob SM, *Best Pract. Res. Clin. Endocrinol. Metab.* 2003, 17, 623–651. With permission.)

and restoring the water balance. Patients with hypernatremia will require hypotonic fluid administration. This is best accomplished via the enteral route. If this is not possible, hypotonic fluids can be given intravenously. The rate of correction depends on how rapidly the hypernatremia developed. If the rise in sodium is rapid, serum sodium levels can be returned to normal rapidly without sequela. However, if the rate of rise of the serum sodium was slow or is unknown, the rate of correction should be no more than 0.5 mmol/l/h to avoid cerebral edema (15).

9.6 ELECTROLYTE DISORDERS

9.6.1 POTASSIUM

Hypokalemia and hyperkalemia occur commonly in hospitalized patients (16). Both conditions can lead to cardiac arrhythmias and even death. This is particularly important in the critically ill patient, because many of these patients have underlying cardiovascular disease and other risk factors for cardiac arrythmias. As such, hypokalemia and hyperkalemia may increase the morbidity and mortality of these patients.

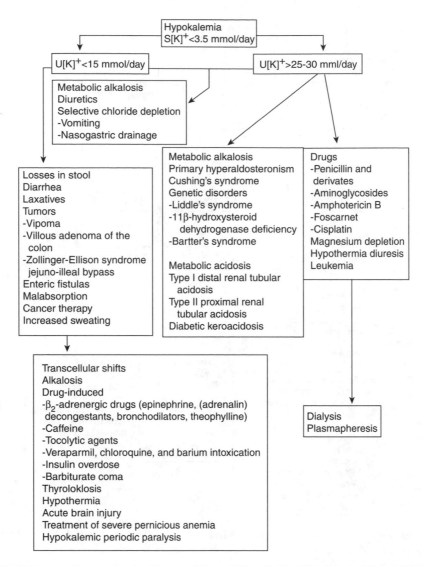

FIGURE 9.3 Etiology of hypokalemia. (Reprinted from Weiss-Guillet EM, Takala J, Jakob SM, *Best Pract. Res. Clin. Endocrinol. Metab.* 2003, 17, 623–651. With permission.)

Hypokalemia is the result of one of three mechanisms (Figure 9.3):

- Decreased intake
- Increased loss, as seen in nasogastric suctioning, diarrhea, and diuresis
- Transcellular shifts as a result of medications (i.e., beta-adrenergic drugs and insulin)

Treatment of hypokalemia is best accomplished by the oral route to avoid hyperkalemia, because the most common cause of hyperkalemia is physician-ordered potassium supplements (17). We have developed a potassium replacement protocol in our ICU for patients with intact renal function. We have found replacement doses of 80 mEq of oral or intravenous potassium in patients with no potassium in the maintenance IV fluids to be safe and effective in correcting episodes of hypokalemia. These data are currently in progress for publication (18). In cases of cardiac arrythmias, severe myopathy, and paralysis, intravenous potassium replacement may be warranted. It should be remembered that magnesium deficiency often coexists with potassium deficiency and that magnesium replacement is necessary in this setting to achieve potassium repletion.

Hyperkalemia is defined as a serum potassium of > 5 mEq/l and is seen less commonly than hypokalemia. At potassium levels > 6.0 mEq/l, life-threatening arrythmias can occur. Hyperkalemia results from impaired renal excretion, drug effect, or impaired potassium entry into the cell, or it can be factitious (i.e., hemolysis, severe leukocytosis/thrombocytosis, fist clenching during venipuncture). Renal insufficiency is present in 80% of clinical episodes of hyperkalemia (17).

Clinically, hyperkalemia is usually silent but can result in cardiac conduction abnormalities. The earliest sign is peaking of the T waves followed by widening of the QRS. Slow idioventricular rhythms, ventricular fibrillation, or cardiac standstill can occur.

Treatment to lower serum potassium levels should be initiated when serum levels are > 6.0 mEq/l or cardiac conduction abnormalities are present (17). Intravenous calcium can reverse these abnormalities and should be given in this setting. Glucose and insulin administration can be used to encourage transcellular shift in the potassium. This is a temporizing measure that can be used until therapy to remove potassium from the body is initiated. Sodium polystyrene (Kayexalate) can be given to bind potassium in the colon. Hemodialysis can be undertaken for rapid removal of potassium. Any offending agents should be removed. The mainstay of management is to reduce dietary potassium intake.

9.6.2 MAGNESIUM

Many of the conditions associated with hypokalemia can result in decreased serum magnesium levels. Magnesium is affected by dietary intake, gastrointestinal absorption, and renal loss. Magnesium wasting can occur with volume expansion or diuresis, because magnesium reabsorption by the kidneys is dependent on urine volume. Renal tubular damage and many drugs can contribute to magnesium wasting. The most common drugs to cause hypomagnesemia include ethanol, diuretics, aminoglycosides, amphotericin, and foscarnet. It is often accompanied by hypocalcemia, hypokalemia, and metabolic alkalosis.

Hypomagnesemia occurs in 60 to 65% of the critically ill (19). Clinically, patients can present with symptoms of weakness, dizziness, tremors, paresthesias, and seizures, as well as cardiac arrythmias. Because hypokalemia and hypocalcemia are often present, the clinical symptoms can overlap.

Treatment includes therapy directed at the underlying problem, if possible, and oral or parenteral administration of magnesium. In cases of asymptomatic hypomagnesemia, the oral route is preferred in divided doses. Diarrhea may become problematic and limit the amount that can be given orally. In patients with symptomatic hypomagnesemia, parenteral infusions of 1 to 2 mEq/kg body weight (parenteral source is magnesium sulfate, which provides 8.12 mEq Mg per gram of salt) are given over 8 to 24 hours (20).

Hypermagnesemia is rare and usually iatrogenic, resulting from intake in PN or in magnesium-containing antacids or laxatives. Patients with renal insufficiency and the elderly are at highest risk (21,22).

Clinical manifestations include nausea, vomiting, altered mental status, muscle weakness, paralysis, respiratory depression, and hypotension. Treatment includes discontinuing magnesium intake. Intravenous calcium can be given in life-threatening cases. Hemodialysis can also be employed for magnesium removal, usually in cases where there is coexisting renal failure.

9.6.3 CALCIUM

The body goes to extreme measures to maintain calcium homeostasis. It is willing to sacrifice its skeleton and dentition to maintain normocalcemia. This alone is an indication of the critical role calcium plays in human physiology. Calcium is essential for muscle contraction, neural conduction, bone strength, and proper function of the coagulation cascade. The actions of three hormones (parathyroid hormone [PTH], calcitonin, and activated vitamin D or $1,25[OH]_2VitD_3$) and three organs (kidney, bone, and small intestine) are integrated to regulate the body's content of calcium, one of the body's most abundant ions (Figure 9.4). Ninety-eight percent of the body's calcium is stored in the bone. Less than 1% of the total body calcium exists in the extracellular fluid, and nearly half of that 1% exists in a bound, inactive form. It is the remaining 0.5%, the unbound, or ionized, serum calcium, that is responsible for most of the physiologic actions of calcium.

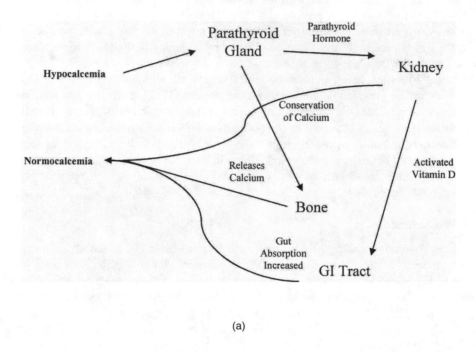

(a)

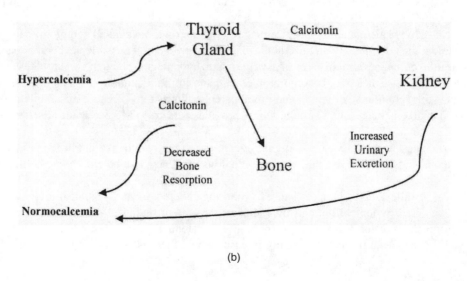

(b)

FIGURE 9.4 Regulation of calcium homeostasis. (a) Response to hypocalcemia. (b) Response to hypercalcemia.

The incidence of hypocalcemia in the ICU is reported to be up to 90% for total calcium and 50% for ionized (23). Causes of hypocalcemia are diverse and include:

- Insufficient action of PTH or $1,25(OH)_2VitD_3$ and an impaired ability to mobilize skeletal calcium
- Hypomagnesemia, because adequate magnesium is required for PTH release and its action
- Increases in calcium chelation
- Parathyroidectomy
- Pancreatitis

Chelation as a cause of hypocalcemia is common in the ICU because of the greater frequency of citrated packed red blood cell (PRBC) transfusions. Citrate, which is also used as an anticoagulant for continuous renal replacement therapies in the ICU, binds calcium and results in a decrease in effective serum levels. Other causes of hypocalcemia specific to the critically ill are not well understood. In a study evaluating hypocalcemia in septic ICU patients, Lind et al. found that bone resorption was not attenuated, nor was there an increase in urinary excretion of calcium; the authors proposed that hypocalcemia in septic patients is related to the inflammatory response (24).

Hypocalcemia is more likely to be symptomatic if it develops acutely. Tetany, paresthesias, circumoral numbness, decreased myocardial contractility, bradycardia, hypotension, psychosis, and confusion are a few of the common symptoms of hypocalcemia. Most of these symptoms have multifactorial causes, particularly in the critically ill patient, and a thorough assessment should include a calcium level (Figure 9.5). When interpreting low serum calcium levels, one must first ask, "Is it real?" Recall that slightly less than half of the serum calcium is protein bound and that it is the unbound form of calcium that is active. Low total serum calcium levels need not be treated if the unbound, or ionized, portion is within the normal range. But often it is the total, not the unbound, calcium measurement that is available. Factors affecting the ionized fraction include albumin available for binding (each 1g/dl decrease of serum albumin results in a decrease of total serum calcium by 0.8 mg/dl) and serum pH (alkalosis decreases ionized calcium by increasing the protein binding of calcium; acidosis increases available ionized calcium). For critically ill patients, these factors are highly variable. Although ionized calcium can be predicted from total calcium when all other factors affecting its binding are considered, in the critically ill patient this method has not been shown to be reliable; therefore, the most accurate method for measuring calcium in this setting is the ionized calcium (25).

As with all electrolyte abnormalities, the cause of hypocalcemia should be identified and corrected. For example, if hypocalcemia is accompanied by hypomagnesemia, treatment of hypomagnesemia must be initiated; otherwise, attempts to correct the calcium will be unsuccessful. If hypocalcemia is a result of hyperphosphatemia, attempts to correct the hyperphosphatemia should be undertaken prior to replacing with calcium, and replacement should be delayed until serum phosphate has fallen below 6 mg/dl (26).

Hypocalcemia is typically symptomatic if total calcium is < 7 to 8 mg/dl or if the ionized calcium is < 2.8 mg/dl (0.7 mmol/l) (27,28). A replacement threshold of 3.2 mg/dl (0.8 mmol/l) in the critically ill patient has been proposed; mild degrees of hypocalcemia (ionized calcium < 0.8 mmol/l) are typically well tolerated and often not acutely replaced (25). Patients with symptomatic hypocalcemia and those with corrected serum levels of 7.5 mg/dl (1.875 mmol/l) or less should be treated with parenteral calcium until the symptoms cease.

Calcium gluconate is the preferred injectable product, because calcium chloride is extremely hyperosmolar and irritating to the veins. Calcium chloride 10%, however, provides more elemental calcium per volume than does calcium gluconate 10% injectable solution (27.2 mg/ml vs. 9.4 mg/ml). Chronic, asymptomatic, mild hypocalcemia should be treated enterally (26). Available calcium products are listed in Table 9.6.

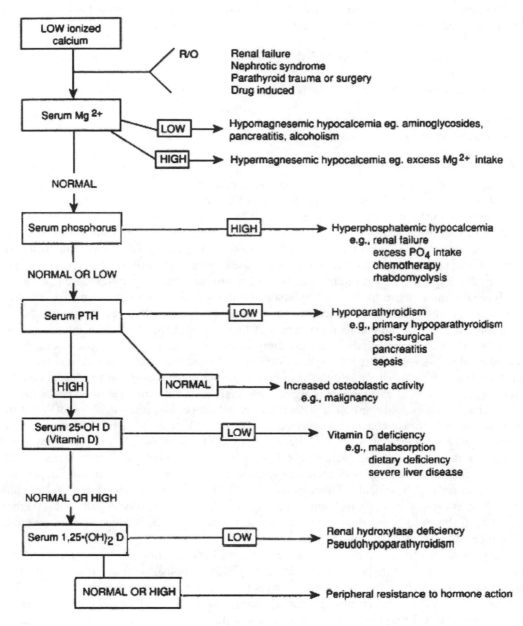

FIGURE 9.5 Evaluation of hypocalcemia. (Reprinted from Zaloga GP, Chernow B, in *Pharmacologic Approach to the Critically Ill Patient*, 3rd ed., Lippincott, Williams & Wilkins, Baltimore, 1994, 784. With permission.)

Hypercalcemia does not occur as frequently as hypocalcemia in the critically ill patient. The primary causes of hypercalcemia include malignancy, hyperparathyroidism, and increased calcium intake. Mild hypercalcemia is generally asymptomatic (up to 12 mg/dl or 3 mmol/l). Initial symptoms may include fatigue, weakness, anorexia, constipation, and depression. Levels > 12 mg/dl can result in confusion, hallucinations, and somnolence. High calcium levels can cause acute pancreatitis, and levels of 16 mg/dl or greater can result in stupor or coma. The therapeutic intervention undertaken should reflect the severity of the clinical manifestation. Treatment includes

TABLE 9.6
Agents for Calcium Replacement

Product	Dose Form	Elemental Calcium Content
Calcium acetate (Phos-Lo®)	667 mg tablet/capsule	8.5 mEq or 169 mg
	333.5 mg capsule	4.2 mEq or 84.5 mg
Calcium carbonate tablets (Tums®, various)	500 mg tablets, chewable	10 mEq or 200 mg
	650 mg tablet	13 mEq or 260 mg
	1000 mg tablet	20 mEq or 400 mg
	1250 mg tablet	25 mEq or 500 mg
	1.25 g/5 ml	25 mEq or 500 mg/5 ml
Calcium citrate (Citracal®, various)	950 mg chewable tablet	10.6 mEq or 211 mg
Calcium gluconate	500 mg tablet	2.25 mEq or 45 mg
Calcium chloride for injection	10% solution, 1 g/10 ml	13.6 mEq or 273 mg
Calcium gluconate for injection	10% solution, 1 g/10 ml	4.65 mEq or 93 mg

aggressive hydration, a loop diuretic (such as furosemide) to increase urinary excretion, and agents directed at bone resorption, such as calcitonin and bisphosphonates.

9.6.4 PHOSPHORUS

Phosphorous is a vital electrolyte, particularly in the ICU patient. It is the source for the high-energy bonds of adenosine triphosphate (ATP), which supplies energy for all physiologic functions. In addition, it is required for the proper synthesis of 2,3-diphosphoglycerate in red blood cells, a substance required for normal oxygen delivery to tissues. Phosphorous thus facilitates electrolyte transport, muscle contractibility, and the metabolism of protein, carbohydrates, and fat.

Phosphate is the body's most abundant intracellular anion. Almost all plasma phosphorous exists as either free or protein-bound phosphate. Approximately 85% of phosphorous is in the bones and about 14% in the body's soft tissues, leaving only 1% of total body phosphorous in the ECF. Homeostasis is maintained via interactions of hormones and organs, as with calcium. The exchange between the ECF and other forms of phosphorus is relatively slow.

Hypophosphatemia results from poor gastrointestinal absorption, significant intracellular shifts, or excessive loss of phosphate via the kidneys. True hypophosphatemia takes 4 to 8 weeks to develop. Patients particularly at risk for severe hypophosphatemia include chronic alcoholics and patients with diabetic ketoacidosis.

Seizures, chest and muscle pain, red blood cell hemolysis, and numbness and tingling occur with acute hypophosphatemia. Chronic depletion can result in bone stiffness, lethargy, memory loss, bruising, and bleeding. In critical illness, shifts in the oxygen dissociation curve resulting from hypophosphatemia can result in significant pulmonary compromise.

Replacement protocols for phosphorus supplementation provide a weight-based replacement for phosphorus levels of < 2 mg/dl (29) or < 3 mg/dl (30). It has been suggested to adjust the dose for renal function and to replace phosphorus until a level above 2 mg/dl is achieved (29). Phosphate maintenance replacement following initiation of the protocol is recommended, although it is for a brief period of time.

A point of debate is the recommended infusion time for phosphate-containing products. Recommendations range from at a rate of 7.5 mmol/h (29) to 0.64 mM/kg over up to 12 hours, which equates to a rate of 3.7 mmol/h for a 70 kg patient (30). Our preference is to infuse 15 mmol of phosphorus over 2 h.

Potassium phosphate injection is included in the list of high-alert medications of the Institute for Safe Medication Practices (ISMP). Confusion surrounds the injectable phosphate products due

TABLE 9.7
Agents for Phosphorous Replacement

Product	Phosphorus		Potassium		Sodium	
	mg	mmol	mg	mEq	mg	mEq
K-Phos Neutral Tablet®	250	8	45	1.1	298	13
Neutra-Phos Powder® (75 ml reconstituted)	250	8	278	7.125	164	7.125
Neutra-Phos K Powder® (75 ml reconstituted)	250	8	556	14.25	0	0
Uro-KP-Neutral Tablet®	250	8	49.4	1.27	250.5	10.9
Fleets Phosphosoda® (per 5 ml)	640	20.5	0	0	552	24
Skim milk (per quart)	1000	32	1600	40	552	24
Sodium phosphate for injection	3 mmol phosphate and 4 mEq sodium/ml					
Potassium phosphate for injection	3 mmol phosphate and 4.4 mEq potassium/ml					

to the dose terminology — mmoles and mEqs for the products. One of ISMP's safety recommendations is always to order phosphate products in both millimoles of phosphate and mEqs of potassium (or sodium). ISMP also featured two oral phosphate products, K-Phos Neutral® and Neutra-Phos K® on the "Look-alike/sound-alike drug names" list. Neutra-Phos K® contains a significant amount of potassium, and K-Phos Neutral® does not. The report included a case in which a patient received the incorrect product following hospital discharge and later required readmission to the hospital as a result of the error (31,32). Caution should be exercised when prescribing, dispensing, or administering any phosphate product (Table 9.7).

Hyperphosphatemia in the ICU is most often the result of renal insufficiency but can also be due to the release of phosphorus from intracellular fluid following the lysis of red blood cells or injury to skeletal muscle. Symptoms of hyperphosphatemia are commonly associated with the resultant hypocalcemia; the primary complication of hyperphosphatemia is metastatic calcification of calcium phosphate in soft tissues, blood vessels, and organ parenchyma. The risk of metastatic calcification is increased when the phosphorus and calcium product exceeds 70, that is, inorganic phosphorus (mg/dl) × total calcium (mg/dl) exceeds 70 (33).

If hyperphosphatemia is acute and life threatening, hemodialysis should be considered. Both dextrose and insulin cause an intracellular shift of phosphate into cells and can be administered for an immediate response. Phosphate excretion can be increased with a saline infusion. In the more chronic setting, phosphate-binding salts can be used. Agents such as calcium carbonate, calcium acetate, sevelamer, and aluminum hydroxide are effective.

9.7 ACID–BASE DISORDERS

Acid–base disorders are common in critically ill patients and can cause alterations in physiologic function that have a deleterious effect on a patient's medical condition. Prompt identification and appropriate management of these disorders are essential to patient care. This section discusses the principles of acid–base regulation, pathophysiology of the common acid–base disorders, and treatment strategies in the critically ill patient.

An acid is a substance that donates hydrogen ions (H^+), and a base is a substance that accepts hydrogen ions. The balance between acid and base determines the pH, which is representative of the hydrogen ion concentration. The normal pH of blood is 7.35 to 7.45. Lower pH values indicate acidemia; higher values are indicative of an alkalemic state.

Acidosis is defined as a process that decreases the pH of the blood, and alkalosis is a process that increases the pH. There are three processes that occur within the body to regulate acid–base balance in an attempt to maintain the pH within or close to its normal range. The first is chemical buffering. A *buffer* is a substance that can both accept and donate hydrogen ions. When a buffer is present in a solution, addition of acid or base to a solution will have a blunted effect on the pH. Three buffers serve to regulate acid–base balance: carbonic acid/bicarbonate, protein, and inorganic phosphate. Of these three, the carbonic acid/bicarbonate buffer is the most important. Buffering acts very quickly, and its effects are immediate (34).

The other two physiologic mechanisms for acid–base balance are compensatory responses. *Compensation* is defined as the physiologic changes that occur within the body to shift the pH toward a normal value in response to a primary acidosis or alkalosis. Respiratory compensation involves changes in the depth and rate of ventilation to control CO_2 excretion. This type of compensation is rapid and takes place within minutes of the disorder's onset. Metabolic or renal compensation is a much slower process than respiratory compensation, because it involves alterations in renal acid excretion, bicarbonate reabsorption, and bicarbonate generation. These changes can take 6 to 24 hours to take effect (34).

Acid–base disorders can be divided into simple and mixed disorders. In a *simple* disturbance, there is only a single acid–base process and its expected compensation. *Mixed* disturbances consist of more than one primary acid–base disorder. The pH is determined by the magnitude of each individual disturbance. There are four types of simple acid–base disorders. These are defined by the direction of the pH deviation from normal (acidosis vs. alkalosis) and the primary abnormality that exists (metabolic vs. respiratory). Hence, the four disorders are referred to as metabolic acidosis, metabolic alkalosis, respiratory acidosis, and respiratory alkalosis. Each of these disorders will be discussed in greater detail later in this chapter.

The assessment and diagnosis of acid–base disorders involves arterial blood gases (ABGs), serum electrolytes, history and clinical signs and symptoms, and a review of the patient's medications and nutrition. The ABG is used to determine both oxygenation status and acid–base condition. The components of an ABG report are pH, partial pressure of oxygen (PaO_2), oxygen saturation (SaO_2), partial pressure of carbon dioxide ($PaCO_2$), and bicarbonate (HCO_3^-). Normal ABG values are found in Table 9.8.

The components of the ABG can be assessed one at a time in a stepwise fashion, starting with pH, followed by $PaCO_2$ and HCO_3^-. Table 9.9 provides the values that would be expected in each of the four types of simple acid–base disorder. It also indicates the expected compensation for each disorder. If the actual compensation is greater or less than expected, a mixed acid–base abnormality exists (35).

The consequences of acidosis involve numerous organ systems. The cardiovascular system may undergo arteriolar dilatation, decreased cardiac contractility and cardiac output, and predisposition to arrhythmias. In addition, patients can experience central nervous system (CNS) depression, hyperventilation, and GI symptoms such as nausea and vomiting. Hyperglycemia can result from insulin resistance, and hyperkalemia often occurs secondary to a shift in intracellular potassium to the extracellular fluid (36).

TABLE 9.8
Normal Arterial Blood Gas Values

pH	7.40 (7.35–7.45)
PaO_2	80–100 mmHg
SaO_2	95%
$PaCO_2$	35–45 mmHg
HCO_3^-	22–26 mEq/l

Source: From Palevsky PM, Matzke GR, in *Pharmacotherapy: A Pathophysiologic Approach*, 5th ed., McGraw-Hill, New York, 995–1013, 2002.

TABLE 9.9
Arterial Blood Gas Interpretation

Disorder	pH	Primary Change	Compensatory Response	Expected Compensation
Metabolic acidosis	Decreased	↓ HCO_3^-	↓ pCO_2	pCO_2 decreases by 10–13 mmHg for each 10 mEq/l decrease in HCO_3^-
Metabolic alkalosis	Increased	↑ HCO_3^-	↑ pCO_2	pCO_2 increases by 6–7 mmHg for each 10 mEq/l increase in HCO_3^-
Respiratory acidosis	Decreased	↑ pCO_2	↑ HCO_3^-	Acute: HCO_3^- increases by 1 mEq/l for each 10 mmHg increase in pCO_2 Chronic: HCO_3^- increases by 3–4 mEq/l for each 10 mmHg increase in HCO_3^-
Respiratory alkalosis	Increased	↓ pCO_2	↓ HCO_3^-	Acute: HCO_3^- decreases by 2 mEq/l for each 10 mmHg decrease of pCO_2 Chronic: HCO_3^- decreases by 5 mEq/l for each 10 mmHg decrease in pCO_2

Source: Adapted from Shapiro JI, Kaehny WD, in *Renal and Electrolyte Disorders*, 6th ed. Lippincott Williams & Wilkins, Philadelphia, 2003, 115–153.

Like acidosis, alkalosis has detrimental physiologic effects. These include arteriolar vasoconstriction, decreased myocardial and cerebral perfusion, arrhythmias, hypoventilation, and low serum concentrations of potassium, magnesium, phosphorus, and ionized calcium (37).

9.7.1 METABOLIC ACIDOSIS

Metabolic acidosis occurs when serum pH is decreased secondary to a decrease in the serum bicarbonate concentration. Metabolic acidosis can be classified as either anion gap or non–anion gap acidosis. The anion gap measures the difference between the unmeasured anions (proteins, sulfates, phosphates, organic anions) and the unmeasured cations (magnesium, calcium, potassium) in the serum and can be determined using the following equation:

$$\text{Anion gap} = [Na^+] - ([Cl^-] + [HCO_3^-]) \tag{9.1}$$

Serum albumin is one of the unmeasured anions. Therefore, hypoalbuminemia (which is often seen in critically ill patients) may cause a decreased anion gap, even if no acid–base disorder is present (35). Because the total concentration of cations and anions must be equal in the serum, increases in the anion gap indicate accumulation of unmeasured anions in the serum. The normal value for anion gap is 9 mEq/l (range of 3 to 11 mEq/l), and a value of 17 to 20 mEq/l or greater reflects an increase in unmeasured serum anions. The presence or absence of an increased anion gap can assist in determining the cause of a metabolic acidosis. Increased anion gap acidosis is seen when bicarbonate losses are replaced by an anion other than chloride (i.e., phosphates, sulfates, or organic anions). This occurs in conditions such as lactic acidosis, ketoacidosis, renal failure, excessive electrolyte administration, dehydration, and toxic ingestion of methanol, ethylene glycol, and salicylates. Normal anion gap acidosis is also referred to as *hyperchloremic acidosis* because of its association with increased serum chloride, which has replaced depleted bicarbonate. This type of acidosis is seen with diarrhea, renal tubular acidosis with renal wasting of bicarbonate and excessive exogenous chloride administration.

When metabolic acidosis is present, the body compensates by increasing its respiratory rate, which in turn increases CO_2 excretion. The result is a decrease in $PaCO_2$. Respiratory compensation typically starts within 15 to 30 minutes of the onset of metabolic acidosis, but its full compensatory effects are not seen for 12 to 24 hours. This compensation occurs such that for every 1 mEq/l decrease of bicarbonate, the $PaCO_2$ decreases by 1 to 1.3 mmHg (Table 9.9).

Treatment of metabolic acidosis should first be aimed at correcting the underlying cause (Table 9.10). In addition, resuscitation and adequate ventilation are of immediate concern. Pharmacologic alkali therapy can be used to moderate the acidosis until the underlying cause is adequately treated or endogenously corrected. The available alkalinizing agents include sodium bicarbonate (which should generally be avoided in lactic acidosis and other acidotic conditions associated with tissue hypoxia due to its propensity to increase CO_2 production), tromethamine (THAM), and dichloroacetate (34). For patients receiving PN, the acetate content in the formulation should be increased and the chloride content decreased (particularly in hyperchloremic patients) (35).

9.7.2 METABOLIC ALKALOSIS

Metabolic alkalosis presents as increased arterial pH associated with increased serum bicarbonate. Metabolic alkalosis can be caused by excessive loss of H^+ via the GI tract (nasogastric suctioning, vomiting, secretory diarrhea) or kidneys (diuretic use). Other causes include volume depletion, high-dose penicillin therapy, excess mineralocorticoid activity, and organic anion administration (lactate from lactated Ringer's solution, acetate from PN, and citrate from blood transfusion). Finally, inappropriate alkali therapy for respiratory acidosis can lead to metabolic alkalosis. Patients with normal kidney function are able to maintain acid–base balance, even in the presence of factors that are known to cause metabolic alkalosis. However, there are two renal mechanisms that result in maintenance of metabolic alkalosis. The first occurs with diuretic use and GI losses and is characterized by volume depletion and chloride loss. Metabolic alkalosis of this type is referred to as *sodium chloride–responsive alkalosis*. The second metabolic alkalosis is sodium chloride resistant and is most often associated with excess mineralocorticoid activity and associated hypokalemia.

The body's compensation for metabolic alkalosis is hypoventilation, which leads to an increase in $PaCO_2$ within hours. For every 10 mEq/l increase in bicarbonate, the $PaCO_2$ increases by 6 to 7 mmHg (Table 9.9).

The treatment of sodium chloride–responsive metabolic alkalosis should first be directed at correcting the factor that is maintaining the alkalosis, followed by a correction of the causative factors (Table 9.10). Administration of sodium chloride– and potassium chloride–containing IV fluids will replenish both chloride and fluid. Patients with volume overload or an inability to tolerate a volume load may receive acetazolamide. This agent is a carbonic anhydrase inhibitor, which inhibits the reabsorption of bicarbonate by the kidneys. Acetazolamide also causes increased potassium and phosphorus excretion, so these electrolytes must be monitored and replaced as necessary. In severe or refractory cases of metabolic alkalosis, acidifying agents may be considered. These include hydrochloric acid, arginine monohydrochloride, and ammonium chloride (34). Hemodialysis using a low-bicarbonate dialysate can also expedite correction of metabolic alkalosis.

Sodium chloride–resistant metabolic alkalosis is rarely life threatening and can often be managed by reducing or eliminating the cause of mineralocorticoid excess. Approaches to achieve this goal include decreasing corticosteroid dosages or changing to a corticosteroid with less mineralocorticoid activity in patients receiving these agents. For those individuals with an endogenous source of mineralocorticoid excess, a potassium-sparing diuretic (spironolactone, triamterene, amiloride) may be administered or aggressive potassium repletion may be undertaken.

9.7.3 RESPIRATORY ACIDOSIS

Respiratory acidosis is primary CO_2 retention that decreases the serum pH and results from the pulmonary system's failure to excrete CO_2 normally. Because metabolic compensation is slow and does not occur for at least 12 to 24 hours after the onset of the disturbance, respiratory acidosis can be divided into two categories: acute and chronic. *Acute respiratory acidosis* occurs over

TABLE 9.10
Etiology-Specific Treatment of Acid–Base Disorders

Disorder	Etiology	Treatment
Metabolic acidosis	Methanol or ethylene glycol ingestion	Forced diuresis
		Alkali replacement
		Thiamine and pyrixodine supplementation
		Ethanol or fomepizole administration
		Hemodialysis
	Lactic acidosis	Correct underlying cause
		Ensure adequate tissue oxygenation
		Mechanical ventilation
		Fluid repletion
		Inotropic drugs
		Avoid vasoconstricting agents
	Diabetic ketoacidosis	Insulin
		Fluid, sodium, and potassium replacement
		Alkali therapy not advisable unless pH < 7.10 or hypotension is refractory to fluid repletion
	Alcoholic ketoacidosis	Fluid repletion with 5% dextrose in 0.9% sodium chloride
		Replace phosphorus, magnesium, and potassium as needed
		Benzodiazepines may be required for prevention of delirium tremens
	Administration of non-alkali-containing IV fluids	Add bicarbonate to the IV fluid
	GI bicarbonate losses	Correct GI pathology
		Oral or IV alkali replacement
		Correct associated losses of fluid and electrolytes (sodium and potassium)
	Renal failure	Increase bicarbonate or acetate in dialysate
		Oral alkali replacement over several days, followed by maintenance alkali regimen
	Type I RTA (distal)	Alkali therapy
		Potassium replacement usually not necessary if alkali therapy is effective
	Type II RTA (proximal)	Large doses of alkali
		Potassium replacement
		Vitamin D for prevention of bone disorders
	Type IV RTA (hyperkalemic)	Treat hyperkalemia
		Low-dose alkali therapy may be necessary
Metabolic alkalosis	GI acid losses	Administer H2 blocker or proton pump inhibitor to reduce gastric acid secretion
		Administer antiemetics for vomiting
	Villous adenomas	Surgical removal
	Chloride-responsive with volume depletion	Administer IV normal saline
		Potassium replacement to correct concomitant hypokalemia

(continued)

TABLE 9.10 (CONTINUED)
Etiology-Specific Treatment of Acid–Base Disorders

Disorder	Etiology	Treatment
Metabolic alkalosis (continued)	Chloride-responsive with volume overload	Administer potassium chloride
		Administer acetazolamide or a potassium-sparing diuretic (spironolactone, triamterene, amiloride) if diuresis is indicated
	Chloride-resistant due to primary hyperaldosteronism or Cushing's syndrome	Administer a potassium-sparing diuretic
		Surgical removal of adrenal tumor if present
	Excessive black licorice ingestion	Discontinue licorice ingestion
		May administer potassium-sparing diuretics until alkalosis corrects
Respiratory acidosis	Upper airway obstruction	Immediate oxygenation
		Airway suctioning for secretion removal
	Impaired alveolar gas exchange	Immediate oxygenation
		Antibiotic therapy for pneumonia
		Diuresis for pulmonary edema
	Obstructive airway disease	Immediate oxygenation
		Inhaled bronchodilator for bronchospasm
	Disorders of the respiratory muscles and chest wall	Immediate oxygenation
		Consider inspiratory aids or assisted ventilation
	Inhibition of central respiratory control	Immediate oxygenation
		Reversal of narcotic agents with naloxone
	Chronic obstructive pulmonary disease	Smoking cessation
		Bronchodilators
		Inhaled or oral corticosteroids
Respiratory alkalosis	Anxiety/pain	Provide reassurance and nonpharmacologic pain control
		Treat with appropriate pain and antianxiety medication
	Mechanical hyperventilation	Decrease tidal volume
		Decrease respiratory rate
	Voluntary hyperventilation	Reassurance
		Rebreathing into paper bag
		Treat underlying psychological stress
		Consider sedative agents
		Consider beta-adrenergic antagonists
	Salicylate toxicity	Provide airway protection and stabilization
		Contact poison control center for information about gastric lavage or activated charcoal administration
		Fluid replacement
		Potassium repletion
		Consider hemodialysis in severe cases

minutes to hours and does not allow enough time for metabolic compensation. Causes of this type of disturbance include severe pulmonary disease, neuromuscular conditions that affect control of ventilation, and incorrect mechanical ventilator settings. In addition, the administration of PN with greater than 50% of nonprotein calories provided by glucose can result in drastic increases in CO_2 production and consequently lead to respiratory acidosis. *Chronic respiratory acidosis* is seen when the increase in $PaCO_2$ and hypoxia occurs to a non–life-threatening degree, allowing time for metabolic compensation to occur. Conditions that are often associated with chronic respiratory acidosis include chronic obstructive pulmonary disease and disorders involving restriction of the chest wall or lung.

The body's immediate response to acute respiratory acidosis is chemical buffering via the carbonic acid/bicarbonate mechanism. As a result of this buffering, the serum bicarbonate increases by 1 mEq/l for each 10 mmHg increase in $PaCO_2$. When respiratory acidosis persists beyond 12 to 24 hours, metabolic compensation occurs in the form of increased renal bicarbonate reabsorption, increased hydrogen ion secretion, and ammoniagenesis. This compensation causes an increase of serum bicarbonate of 3–4 mEq/l for every 10 mmHg rise in $PaCO_2$ (Table 9.9).

The treatment of acute respiratory acidosis consists of providing immediate adequate oxygenation, which may require intubation and mechanical ventilation. In addition, airway secretions should be adequately removed. The underlying cause must then be addressed. Specifically, patients receiving nutrition support should be assessed for overfeeding because this can cause excess CO_2 production (Table 9.10). Alkali therapy is rarely necessary and may in fact decrease the patient's respiratory drive or cause a metabolic alkalosis. Patients with a severe respiratory acidosis with hemodynamic compromise may require careful administration of sodium bicarbonate or tromethamine.

Patients with chronic respiratory acidosis may experience respiratory decompensation with precipitating conditions such as infection, oxygen therapy, or narcotic use. As with acute respiratory acidosis, the primary intervention is provision of adequate oxygenation. However, it is imperative to realize that, at baseline, these patients have a lower PaO_2 and higher $PaCO_2$ than patients without chronic lung disease. Therefore, the respiratory drive is dependent on hypoxemia, not hypercarbia, and oxygen administration can eliminate the drive to breathe.

9.7.4 RESPIRATORY ALKALOSIS

Respiratory alkalosis is a primary decrease in $PaCO_2$ caused by increased excretion of CO_2 by the lungs. This may occur via central or peripheral stimulation of respiration, mechanical ventilation, or voluntary hyperventilation. Metabolic CO_2 production may also be increased by stress or excess carbohydrate administration (as may occur with PN).

The body's most rapid response to acute respiratory alkalosis occurs through the carbonic acid/bicarbonate buffer system, which takes only minutes to exert its full effect. For each 10 mmHg drop in $PaCO_2$, the serum bicarbonate concentration decreases by 2 mEq/l. If the respiratory alkalosis is still present six hours after its onset, subsequent metabolic compensation will begin. The renal response is to increase bicarbonate elimination and decrease bicarbonate production. This compensation leads to a decrease in bicarbonate by 5 mEq/l per 10 mmHg decrease in $PaCO_2$ (Table 9.9).

Identification and correction of the underlying cause are the initial steps in treatment of respiratory alkalosis (Table 9.10). Patients who are awake and alert can breathe into a paper bag to increase the $PaCO_2$ in inspired air. If severe hypoxemia occurs, oxygen therapy should be initiated. In more severe cases (pH > 7.60), complications such as seizures and arrhythmias may be seen. If this is the case, mechanical ventilation, accompanied by sedation and possible neuromuscular blockade, may be necessary. For patients who are already undergoing mechanical ventilation, consider the possibility that the ventilator settings are the cause of the alkalosis and need to be adjusted.

9.8 ELECTROLYTE COMPATIBILITY WITH ENTERAL OR PARENTERAL NUTRITION

Electrolyte disorders are common in nutrition support patients. As such, electrolyte replacement is considered via nutrition support fluids and access devices. This coadministration with nutritional fluids creates issues of compatibility and sterility.

For enteral nutrition, most organizations use a closed system to avoid inadvertent contamination that may result in clinical infections if infused into the patient. With a closed enteral nutrition delivery system, electrolytes may not be added to the formula without opening the system and creating the possibility of contamination. Compatibility of oral liquid electrolyte products with enteral nutrition fluids must also be considered. Liquid formulations of potassium chloride, magnesium, and phosphorus are not compatible with enteral nutrition products (38). These medications should not be infused with enteral nutrition. If compatibility of the electrolyte product is not known, in general, syrups cause coagulation of enteral nutrition products and should be avoided. The best practice of administering electrolytes via enteral feeding tubes is to turn off the tube feeding, flush the catheter with 10 to 30 ml of fluid, administer the electrolyte, flush the catheter, and then resume the tube feeding. Another concern of electrolyte replacement is with gastrointestinal tolerance. Potassium chloride is very hyperosmolar (3000 to 3500 mOsm/kg) and may cause abdominal discomfort and diarrhea if administered in an undiluted form. Magnesium citrate and milk of magnesia are 1000 and 1250 mOsm/kg, respectively, and sodium phosphate (Fleet's phospho soda) is 2250 mOsm/kg. It is recommended that these formulations be diluted prior to administration (39). Other formulations contain sorbitol, which may also cause GI distress.

Compatibility of electrolyte additives in PN is a continual concern. Some of the additives are conditionally compatible (interactions and precipitation are dependent on electrolyte concentration, final PN pH, order of admixture into PN, and environmental temperature and light during dispensing, distribution, and storage). Calcium salts are reactive compounds and readily form insoluble products with phosphorus, oxalate, and bicarbonate. The formation of the insoluble product, dibasic calcium phosphate, is an incompatibility of calcium and phosphorus in PN. Many factors influence the solubility of calcium and phosphorous, including high concentrations of calcium and phosphorus, decreased amino acid concentrations, increased environmental temperature, increased PN formulation pH, and hang time prolonged beyond 24 hours (40). In 1994, an FDA safety alert addressed two deaths and two near-fatal injuries associated with the infusion of an incompatible mixture of calcium phosphate (41). To avoid problems with calcium phosphate compatibility, it is recommended to use only the gluconate salt for PN admixture, to follow the proper sequence for electrolyte addition to PN during compounding, and not to exceed maximal compatible doses of calcium and phosphorus. Also, "borderline" doses should be avoided by considering separate infusions of calcium, phosphorus, or both when higher-than-normal doses are required. Calcium may also react with bicarbonate in PN formulations. As such, bicarbonate is contraindicated, especially because acetate salts of potassium and sodium are effective sources of bicarbonate that are compatible in PN. Electrolytes administered separately from PN may be coinfused if compatible (Table 9.11).

9.9 SUMMARY

Fluid, electrolyte, and acid–base disorders are a frequent concern to the clinician providing nutrition support to the intensive care patient. The underlying condition of the patient, along with its treatment, often results in derangements in fluid, electrolyte, and acid–base status. The clinical significance and management of these disorders (Table 9.12) is important to providing optimal nutrition support. The principles and concepts addressed in this chapter are commonly used by the clinician providing nutrition support to the critically ill patient.

TABLE 9.11
Electrolyte Compatibility with PN

PN Type	2-in-1	3-in-1
Calcium gluconate	C	C
Hydrochloric acid	C	I
Magnesium sulfate	C	I
Potassium chloride	C	C
Potassium/sodium phosphate	I	I

Note: C = compatible, I = Incompatible.

TABLE 9.12
Clinical Significance and Management of Electrolyte Disorders

Electrolyte Disorder	Threshold of Clinical Significance	Treatment Approach
Hyponatremia	Clinical symptoms Usually sodium < 130	Treat underlying disorder Water restriction (< 1–2 l/d) Saline infusion with goal 8 mmols/l/d correction (13) Diuretics can increase free water excretion but should be used cautiously In hypertonic hyponatremia, treat increased glucose Can consider 3% saline in cases of severe hyponatremia (< 110) and central nervous system symptoms Careful monitoring of sodium
Hypernatremia	Clinical symptoms Serum sodium > 158	Correction should be < 0.5 mmol/l/h (15) Hypotonic saline infusion Hypovolemic patients should be given saline to stabilize hemodynamics, then proceed with hypotonic saline solutions In central diabetes insipidus, Desmopressin 2–4 mcg IV Careful monitoring of sodium
Hypokalemia	Clinical symptoms Serum K+ < 3.5 mEq/l in patient with cardiovascular disease	ECG monitoring Oral potassium replacement preferred Intravenous potassium rate should not exceed 20 mEq/h and serum potassium rechecked after 60 mEq (17)
Hyperkalemia	Clinical symptoms Serum K+ > 6.5 mEq/l	Confirm laboratory finding Discontinue any potassium or potassium-containing agents Nonemergent Loop diuretic increases renal excretion; effects last up to 2 h Sodium polystyrene sulfonate (Kayexalate) ion exchange resin; effects last 1–3 h Hemodialysis/peritoneal dialysis; effects last 48 hours Emergent Calcium antagonizes cardiac conduction abnormalities; onset 5 min; duration 1 h Bicarbonate causes transcellular shift; onset 15–30 min; duration 1–2 h Insulin causes transcellular shift; onset 15–60 min; duration 4–6 h Albuterol causes transcellular shift; onset 15–30 min; duration 2–4 h

(continued)

TABLE 9.12 (CONTINUED)
Clinical Significance and Management of Electrolyte Disorders

Electrolyte Disorder	Threshold of Clinical Significance	Treatment Approach
Hypomagnesemia	Clinical symptoms Magnesium < 1.0 mg/dl	Oral replacement preferred in asymptomatic individuals Symptomatic patients consider parenteral administration 1–2 mEq/kg of magnesium over 8–24 h; rapid infusion can lead to renal magnesium wasting
Hypermagnesemia	Clinical symptoms	Discontinue magnesium intake Intravenous calcium for life-threatening circumstances Hemodialysis
Hypocalcemia (25)	Clinical symptoms 3.2 mg/dl (0.8 mmol/l) ionized calcium < 2.5 mg/dl urgently	Symptomatic patients parenteral administration of 1–2 g calcium gluconate IVPB over 10 min, then 1–2 mg/kg/h of elemental calcium until serum calcium normalizes, then decrease rate based on patient response Replace serum magnesium and phosphorus Oral calcium replacement when stable Consider addition of vitamin D (calcitriol) 0.25 mcg po daily
Hypercalcemia (25)	Clinical symptoms Calcium > 12 mg/dl ionized calcium > 6 mg/dl	Discontinue calcium intake Correct underlying cause Aggressive hydration (approximately 200 ml/h 0.9% sodium chloride) Loop diuretic (e.g., furosemide 20–40 mg IVP) Calcitonin 1–2 units/kg IV, SC every 12 h up to 8 units/kg every 6 h (onset in 6–10 h; unreliable response) Bisphosphonates (e.g., pamidronate 60–90 mg IV infusion over 2–24 h; onset 4–7 d) Hemodialysis with low calcium bath for life-threatening cases
Hypophosphatemia (25)	Clinical symptoms iPhos < 2.5 mg/dl iPhos < 1 mg/dl urgently	IV if symptomatic IV administration rates are highly variable (0.3–4 mg/kg/h) Evaluate need for magnesium replacement Oral causes diarrhea in large doses Replace for 5–7 days to replace stores, then maintenance dose of 1200 mg/d orally or 1000 mg/d intravenously
Hyperphosphatemia (25)	Laboratory evidence Symptomatic from hypocalcemia	Discontinue phosphate intake Correct underlying cause 0.9% sodium chloride infusion (250–500 ml/h) Acetazolamide (500 mg every 6 hours) Enteral phosphate binders (e.g., aluminum hydroxide, calcium acetate, or sevelamer) Hemodialysis for life-threatening cases

REFERENCES

1. Moore FD, Brennan MF. Surgical injury: body composition, protein metabolism and neuroendocrinology. In: Ballinger WF, Collins JA, Ducker WR, et al., eds. *Manual of Surgical Nutrition.* Philadelphia: WB Saunders, 1975, 169–222.
2. Marinella MA. Refeeding syndrome: implications for the inpatient rehabilitation unit. *Am. J. Phys. Med. Rehabil.* 2004, 83: 65–68.
3. Solomon SM, Kirby DF. The refeeding syndrome: a review. *J. Parenter. Enteral. Nutr.* 1990, 14: 90–97.
4. Juan D. Clinical review: the clinical importance of hypomagnesemia. *Surgery.* 1982, 91: 510–517.

5. Rudman D, Millikan WJ, Richardson TJ, Bixler TJ, Stackhouse J, McGarrity WC. Elemental balances during intravenous hyperalimentation of underweight adult subjects. *J. Clin. Invest.* 1975, 55, 94–104.

6. ASPEN Board of Directors and the Clinical Guidelines Task Force. Guidelines for the use of parenteral and enteral nutrition in adult and pediatric patients. *J. Parenter. Enteral Nutr.* 2002, 26: 1SA–138SA.

7. National Advisory Group on Standards and Practice Guidelines for Parenteral Nutrition. Safe practices for parenteral nutrition formulations. *J. Parenter. Enteral Nutr.* 1998, 22: 49–66.

8. Al Salman J, Kemp D, Randall D. Hyponatremia. *West. J. Med.* 2002, 176: 173–176.

9. Bennani SL, Abouqal R, Zeggwagh AA, Madani N, Abidi K, Zekraoui A, et al. [Incidence, causes and prognostic factors of hyponatremia in intensive care]. *Rev. Med. Interne.* 2003, 24: 224–229.

10. Katz MA. Hyperglycemia-induced hyponatremia: calculation of expected serum sodium depression. *N. Engl. J. Med.* 1973, 289: 843–844.

11. Peixoto AJ. Critical issues in nephrology. *Clin. Chest Med.* 2003, 24: 561–581.

12. Fried LF, Palevsky PM. Hyponatremia and hypernatremia. *Med. Clin. North Am.* 1997, 81: 585–609.

13. Adrogue HJ, Madias NE. Hyponatremia. *N. Engl. J. Med.* 2000, 342: 1581–1589.

14. Polderman KH, Schreuder WO, Strack van Schijndel RJ, Thijs LG. Hypernatremia in the intensive care unit: an indicator of quality of care? *Crit. Care Med.* 1999, 27: 1105–1108.

15. Kahn A, Brachet E, Blum D. Controlled fall in natremia and risk of seizures in hypertonic dehydration. *Intens. Care Med.* 1979, 5: 27–31.

16. Gennari FJ. Hypokalemia. *N. Engl. J. Med.* 1998, 339: 451–458.

17. Gennari FJ. Disorders of potassium homeostasis: hypokalemia and hyperkalemia. *Crit. Care Clin.* 2002, 18: 273–288, vi.

18. Lucarelli MR, Pell L, Hoffmann S, and Shirk MB. Potassium replacement protocol in medical intensive care unit patients. 2004. Unpublished work.

19. Wong ET, Rude RK, Singer FR, Shaw ST, Jr. A high prevalence of hypomagnesemia and hypermagnesemia in hospitalized patients. *Am. J. Clin. Pathol.* 1983, 79: 348–352.

20. Agus ZS, Wasserstein A, Goldfarb S. Disorders of calcium and magnesium homeostasis. *Am. J. Med.* 1982, 72: 473–488.

21. Clark BA, Brown RS. Unsuspected morbid hypermagnesemia in elderly patients. *Am. J. Nephrol.* 1992, 12: 336–343.

22. Schelling JR. Fatal hypermagnesemia. *Clin. Nephrol.* 2000, 53: 61–65.

23. Zaloga GP. Hypocalcemia in critically ill patients. *Crit. Care Med.* 1992, 20: 251–262.

24. Lind L, Carlstedt F, Rastad J, Stiernstrom H, Stridsberg M, Ljunggren O, et al. Hypocalcemia and parathyroid hormone secretion in critically ill patients. *Crit. Care Med.* 2000, 28: 93–99.

25. Zaloga GP, Chernow B. Divalent ions: calcium, magnesium, and phosphorus. In: Chernow B, ed. *Pharmacologic Approach to the Critically Ill Patient.* 3rd ed. Baltimore: Lippincott, Williams & Wilkins, 1994, 777–804.

26. Bushinsky DA, Monk RD. Electrolyte quintet: calcium. *Lancet.* 1998, 352: 306–311.

27. Weiss-Guillet EM, Takala J, Jakob SM. Diagnosis and management of electrolyte emergencies. *Best Pract. Res. Clin. Endocrinol. Metab.* 2003, 17: 623–651.

28. Vanek VW. Assessment and management of fluid and electrolyte abnormalities. In: Shikora SA, Martindale RG, Schwaitzberg SD, eds. *Nutritional Considerations in the Intensive Care Unit.* Dubuque, IA: Kendall/Hunt, 2002, 79–100.

29. Guidelines for phosphorus supplementation in adults. *Formulary.* 1998, 33: 263.

30. Clark CL, Sacks GS, Dickerson RN, Kudsk KA, Brown RO. Treatment of hypophosphatemia in patients receiving specialized nutrition support using a graduated dosing scheme: results from a prospective clinical trial. *Crit. Care Med.* 1995, 23: 1504–1511.

31. *Look-alike/Sound-alike Drug Names and Other Product-Related Issues.* ISMP Medication Safety Alert. 2002.

32. *ISMP's list of high-alert medications.* ISMP Medication Safety Alert. 2003.

33. Brenner R, Brenner BM. Disturbances of renal function. In: Braunwald E, Fauci A, Kasper D, et al., eds. *Harrison's Principles of Internal Medicine.* 15th ed. New York: McGraw-Hill Professional, 2001, 1535–1541.

34. Palevsky PM, Matzke GR. Acid–base disorders. In: DiPiro JT, Talbert RL, Yee GC, Matzke GR, Wells BG, Posey LM, eds. *Pharmacotherapy: A Pathophysiologic Approach.* 5th ed. New York: McGraw-Hill, 2002, 995–1013.

35. Vanek VW. Assessment and management of acid–base abnormalities. In: Shikora SA, Martindale RG, Schwaitzberg SD, eds. *Nutritional Considerations in the Intensive Care Unit*. Dubuque, IA: Kendall/Hunt , 2002, 101–109.

36. Adrogue HJ, Madias NE. Management of life-threatening acid–base disorders. First of two parts. *N. Engl. J. Med.* 1998, 338: 26–34.

37. Adrogue HJ, Madias NE. Management of life-threatening acid–base disorders. Second of two parts. *N. Engl. J. Med.* 1998, 338: 107–111.

38. Johnson DR, Nyffeler MS. Drug–nutrient considerations for enteral nutrition. In: Merritt RJ, et al., eds. *The ASPEN Nutrition Support Practice Manual*. Silver Spring, MD: ASPEN, 1998: 6-1–6-20.

39. Dickerson RN, Melnik G. Osmolality of oral drug solutions and suspensions. *Am. J. Hosp. Pharm.* 1988, 45: 832–834.

40. Niemiec PW Jr., Vanderveen TW. Compatibility considerations in parenteral nutrient solutions. *Am. J. Hosp. Pharm.* 1984, 41: 893–911.

41. Lumpkin MM. Safety alert: hazards of precipitation associated with parenteral nutrition. *Am. J. Hosp. Pharm.* 1994, 51: 1427–1428.

42. Shapiro JI, Kaehny WD. Pathogenesis and management of metabolic acidosis and alkalosis. In: Schrier RW, ed. *Renal and Electrolyte Disorders*. 6th ed. Philadelphia: Lippincott Williams & Wilkins, 2003, 115–153.

43. Whitmire S. Fluids and electrolytes. In: Gottschlich MM, Matarese LE, eds. *Contemporary Nutrition Support Practice: A Clinical Guide*. Philadelphia: WB Saunders, 1998, 128.

44. Ohs MS, Uribarri J. Electrolytes, water, and acid–base balance. In: Shils ME, Olson J, Shike M, Ross AC, eds. *Modern Nutrition in Health and Disease*. 9th ed. Baltimore: Williams and Wilkins, 1999, 107.

10 Fiber (Prebiotics) and Probiotics: Prevention of ICU Infections with Bioecological Control and Symbiotic Treatment

Stig Bengmark
University College London (UCL), London University

CONTENTS

10.1 INTRODUCTION

To a large extent, modern medicine has failed in its ambition to control both acute and chronic diseases. Acute diseases, defined as medical and surgical emergencies such as myocardial infarction, stroke, and severe pancreatitis and those related to advanced medical and surgical treatments, such as stem cell transplantation or advanced surgical operations, have an unacceptably high morbidity and comorbidity. Furthermore, the world suffers an epidemy of chronic diseases of a dimension never seen before, and these diseases are now like a prairie fire spreading to so-called developing countries. Chronic diseases, including such diseases as cardiovascular and neurodegenerative conditions, diabetes, stroke, cancers, and respiratory diseases, constitute 46% of the global disease burden and 59% of global deaths. Each year, approximately 35 million individuals die in conditions related to chronic diseases.[1] Similarly, the morbidity related to advanced medical and surgical treatments and emergencies, especially infectious complications, is also fast increasing. Sepsis presently increases in the U.S. by 1.5% per year and constitutes the tenth most common cause of death in that country.[2]

Each year, severe, often life-threatening infections occur in the U.S. in approximately 751,000 individuals, and approximately 215,000 (29%) of these individuals will die.[2,3] ICU mortality realistically is higher than officially reported: Vincent et al. recently reported that estimates of intensive care unit (ICU) mortality are most likely conservative, because deaths of ICU patients are often attributed to the original condition.[4] More than half of the patients with life-threatening infections (51%), or 383,000, are treated in ICUs and about 130,000 are managed at intermediary-type care units with facilities for ventilation. The extra treatment cost is calculated to be $22,100 per case, and the annual cost in the U.S. alone for this treatment is at the level of about $17 billion.[3]

10.2 INTERRELATED CONDITIONS

The two seemingly disparate groups — those suffering chronic conditions and those developing posttreatment and ICU morbidity — are in many aspects related. Both types of condition seem to be expressions of a failing innate immune system. To a large extent, it is also patients with imminent or obvious chronic diseases who are affected by significantly increased surgical and ICU morbidity. In fact, about half of the patients affected by sepsis are in the age group over 65 years, and 48% of the patients are neutropenic.[5] Both groups of diseases are characterized by exaggerated immune response with profound, although somewhat different, changes in both acute-phase proteins and cytokine response.[6]

The reaction of the body to acute physical and psychological stress is similar, irrespective of the cause: microbial invasion, allergic reaction, surgical operation, trauma, burn, tissue ischemia, tissue infarction, strenuous exercise, childbirth, or mental trauma. The body's reaction to stress is often referred to as *acute-phase response* (APR). The common clinical symptoms of APR are fever, chills, somnolence, and anorexia, which are accompanied by profound changes in plasma proteins, especially in so-called acute-phase proteins (APPs) but also in lipids, minerals, hormones, cytokines, coagulation factors, and cellular components of the blood. Similar reactions are observed in patients with subclinical or obvious chronic diseases: arteriosclerosis, Alzheimer's, cancer, coronary heart disease, diabetes, chronic liver disease, chronic renal disease, rheumatoid arthritis, and many other chronic diseases. Elevations in acute-phase proteins, cytokines, and other signal molecules, although less pronounced, are regularly observed during weeks and months even before the patients clinically manifest disease.

The dominant clinical manifestations of what can be called chronic-phase response (CPR) are, however, somewhat different from those of APR and consist mainly of anorexia, asthenia, anemia, decline in food intake, fatigue, muscle wasting, depressed mood, and often clinically manifest mental depression. Although the extent of changes observed differs between APR and CPR,

TABLE 10.1
Conditions of Acute and Chronic Phase Response

APR and CPR

    General hypermetabolism with higher resting energy expenditure
    Increased hepatic gluconeogenesis
    Increased glucose turnover and decreased muscle glucose uptake
    Hyperlipidemia
    Adipose tissue lipolysis
    Increased production of nonesterified fatty acids
    Increased whole-body protein turnover
    Increased hepatic protein synthesis
    Decreased muscle amino-acid uptake
    Insulin resistance
    Increased production of cytokines
    Increased endotoxin in blood
    Elevated levels of catecholamines, cortisol, and glucagon

Sources: From Simons, J.P., Schools A.M., Buurman, W.A., Wouters, E.F., *Clin. Sci.* 97, 215, 1999; and Preston, T., Slater, C., McMillan, D.C., et al., *J. Nutr.* 128, 1355, 1998.

Table 10.1 lists common conditions for both. The changes in plasma proteins, lipids, minerals, hormones, cytokines, and cellular components of blood are somewhat different. In APR, the increase in cytokines and acute-phase proteins is instant and reaches very high levels within a few hours, but is often more or less over within 10 to 14 days; in CPR, cytokines and APPs remain at levels that are not so high, but are clearly increased, over months and years. While in APR, APP production constitutes approximately 30% of the body's total protein synthesis; it is only about 5% in CPR.[8] Increase in C-reactive protein is prominent in APR, whereas increase in fibrinogen dominates in CPR.[8]

10.2.1 EXAGGERATED IMMUNE RESPONSE — THE CAUSE?

Individuals affected by metabolic syndrome (MS), a condition often affecting and preceding chronic diseases, seem to respond to stress with an exuberant acute or chronic superinflammation, manifested by exaggerated and prolonged release of proinflammatory cytokines, such as IL-6, and acute phase proteins, such as C-reactive protein, but also plasminogen activator inhibitor 1 (PAI-1) — see reference for more information.[6] IL-6 and PAI-1 are often regarded as prognosticators of outcome both in acute conditions, such as after operation or trauma, myocardial infarction, or pancreatitis, and in semichronic or chronic inflammatory conditions, such as arthritis, mental depression, or Alzheimer's. The overwhelming IL-6 response (e.g., prolonged or extreme elevations of circulating IL-6) seen in patients suffering from conditions such as infection, burns, or trauma is strongly associated with severe exacerbation of the disease, such as acute respiratory distress syndrome (ARDS) and multiple organ failure (MOF).[9] The effect of overwhelming acute-phase response on outcome is well demonstrated in a study in human liver transplantation; all patients who had a sixfold or larger increase in the cytokines TNFα and IL-6 during the later phase of the operation developed sepsis in subsequent postoperative days.[10]

    Among the changes observed in overexuberant acute-phase response are augmented endothelial adhesion of polymorphonuclear (PMN) cells, increased production of intracellular adhesion molecule-1 (ICAM-1) and priming of the PMNs for an oxidative burst, release of proinflammatory platelet activating factor (PAF), and, associated with this, a delay in PMN apoptosis.[9] Visceral adipocytes are, compared to subcutaneous fat cells, known to secrete many more free fatty acids but also three times as much IL-6 and PAI-1 per gram of tissue, observations that well explain the high risk of disease in visceral obesity.[11,12] The load of these and other molecules on the liver can vary a thousand times or more because the amount of fat in the abdomen varies among individuals from a few milliliters to about six liters in persons with gross obesity.[13]

10.2.2 NEURO–ENDOCRINE CONTROL OF STRESS OF APR/CPR

The neuro–endocrine control on resistance to disease is important. Glial cells are embryologically and functionally related to macrophages and have the capacity to synthesize and secrete a whole range of cytokines, such as IL-1, IL-2, IL-4, IL-6, and TNFα. In stress and other critical conditions, do these cytokines have pronounced effects on the hypothalamic–pituitary–adrenal (HPA) axis and the function of the involved organs? Cytokines such as IL-1, IL-6, and TNFα are known to stimulate hypothalamic synthesis and secretion of corticotropin-releasing hormone, vasopressin, and other hormones known to have profound regulatory effects. In acute conditions, activation in the CNS of cytokines will lead to symptoms such as anorexia, drowsiness, depressed mood, sleepiness, coma, and increased body temperature and, in chronic conditions such as neurodegenerative diseases, will contribute to the destruction of neurons, cell death, and dementia.

The glial cells respond to the same stimuli as macrophages, and fatty infiltration of or other challenges to these cells, especially in the hypothalamic region, contribute to an exaggerated and prolonged immune response. One of the main functions of the HPA response seems to be to control and prevent overexuberant acute- (and chronic-) phase and immune responses. This also explains why principal immunoregulatory organs, such as Peyer's patches, lymph nodes, thymus, and spleen, are abundantly supplied with sympathetic and parasympathetic autonomic nerves.[15] Vasoactive intestinal peptides, secreted by nerves in the Peyer's patches, regulate the traffic of immunocompetent cells through the small bowel wall and control the immune function of the gut.[16]

10.3 THE GUT — AN IMPORTANT IMMUNOLOGICAL ORGAN

The disease *per se* — but also nutrition and drugs supplied, changes in physical activity, sleep, mood, age, gender, circadian rhythm, and body temperature — will heavily influence lymphocyte function, production of immunoglobulins, and resistance to disease. It is not always realized that about 80% of the total immunoglobulin-producing cells of the body are localized in lamina propria of the gut and that large amounts of immunoglobulins, especially IgA, are released daily into the gut lumen.[16] The synthesis of IgA is highly dependent on T-cells, and several cytokines produced by activated lymphocytes influence different steps in the IgA differentiation pathway.[17] Transforming growth factor-β (TGF-β) in mice has been found to be the crucial "switch" factor, but other cytokines, such as IL-2, IL-5, and IL-10, are also involved — see reference for more information.[18]

10.4 IATROGENIC SUPPRESSION OF RESISTANCE TO DISEASE

Multiple external and internal factors contribute to reduced resistance to disease and to immunoparesis, especially in predisposed individuals. Also, some clinical measures can add to this condition. It is especially important in this type of care that every single treatment is based on solid scientific evidence. We must admit that several measures, common in perioperative and ICU management, seem not to be supported by scientific evidence, as required in modern medicine. Some such measures might also negatively affect the innate immune system, reduce resistance, and contribute to secondary morbidity. These treatments, often instituted at a time when the demand for scientific evidence was not as strict as it is today, should be reevaluated. Some treatments, when studied, might have well documented beneficial effects — but might also be accompanied by significant negative consequences that exceed the observed beneficial effects. Among these measures to study further are:

- Excessive and prolonged antibiotic treatment
- Inhibition of salivation
- Inhibition of gastrointestinal secretions
- Prophylactic nasogastric decompression
- Routine postoperative drainage of body cavities
- Preoperative bowel preparation and postoperative enemas
- Extensive transfusion with old stored blood
- Overloading with nutrients, or hyperalimentation

10.4.1 EXCESSIVE AND PROLONGED USE OF ANTIBIOTICS

Many, if not most, modern pharmaceuticals seem to have a negative influence on immune function and resistance to disease. As an example, it has been known for more than 50 years that supply of antibiotics increases susceptibility to new infections.[19] It has also been shown that administration of antibiotics results in suppression of various macrophage functions, demonstrated by chemiluminescence response, chemotactic motility, and bactericidal and cytostatic ability.[20,21] Also, many other commonly used drugs might have similar effects, although these have not been properly studied. Numerous clinical studies show clearly that appropriately timed, short-term, most often "single shot" prophylaxis is as effective as multiple-dose prophylaxis and should not have the same negative consequences on the immune system as are obtained with prolonged treatments.[22–24] Restriction of prolonged treatment has long been recommended, but clinical policy is difficult to change. Antibiotics are still heavily overprescribed in connection with surgery as well as for ICU patients.[25]

10.4.2 INHIBITION OF SALIVATION

The amount of GI secretion in an adult is as much as 10 l/d; saliva is about 2.5 l, and another 2.5 l are gastric secretions. These secretions are extremely rich in immunosupportive factors, such as immunoglobulins, lactoferrin, lysozyme, fibronectin, and mucin, but they are also an important source of healing factors, such as epidermal growth factor. Removal of the salivary gland function leads to gastric and intestinal ulcer formation, poor healing of wounds and ulcers, and poor regeneration of organs, especially of the liver. From an immunological point of view, a practice that stimulates these secretions, instead of inhibiting them, should be preferred whenever possible, especially in the very sick and critically ill — see references for more information.[26–28] Unfortunately, most drugs, especially those commonly used in ICUs, have strong antisecretory effects. For more information, including a list of drugs, see Bengmark.[26]

10.4.3 INHIBITION OF GI SECRETIONS

Low gastric pH is a prerequisite for gastric nitric pump oxide (NO) production, a function that is totally eliminated by the supply of H_2 blockers and proton inhibitors. Maintenance of gastric NO production is of the utmost importance for maintaining GI motility and mucosal and splanchnic blood flow, and for elimination of pathogens in the stomach.[29–31] Furthermore, normal gastric acid production is essential for absorption of several vitamins and antioxidants, including vitamin C and glutathione. In the absence of a low pH, the stomach will become a reservoir for pathogens, which are regurgitated into the lungs and frequently cause chest infections.[32] Use of H_2 blockers and proton pump inhibitors might have been useful to prevent peptic ulcers in patients on total parenteral nutrition, but with today's aggressive and early enteral feeding, this practice is totally unnecessary and often counterproductive.[26–28,33] Routine use of H_2 blockers or proton pump inhibitors in enterally fed postoperative and ICU patients cannot be regarded as based on scientific evidence.[33–35]

10.4.4 Prophylactic Nasogastric Decompression

The use of nasogastric decompression — introduced by Mayo in order to prevent nausea, vomiting, and abdominal distension; to decrease postoperative ileus and wound complications; and to protect enteric anastomoses — has been forcefully questioned for more than 50 years but is still commonly used.[36–39] Use of nasogastric decompression will seemingly delay return of adequate bowel function but, what is more severe, will contribute significantly to septic complications. Several controlled studies have clearly confirmed that routine nasogastric decompression can be omitted without any negative consequences.[39–42] Even if a slight gastric distention might occur, it will resolve spontaneously, without any active measures, with no serious consequences observed. Even if a no-drainage policy might lead to an increased incidence of gastric distention, no other negative consequences will be seen, and insertion of drainage should usually not be needed.[43–46] A meta-analysis based on 26 trials (a total of 3964 patients) concluded that routine nasogastric decompression is not supported by scientific evidence.[47] Fever, atelectasis, and pneumonia are significantly less if patients are managed without nasogastric tubes.[47] Gastric distention should normally be no contraindication to continuation of tube feeding, and high residual volumes should not automatically lead to cessation of tube feeding. Instead, the symptoms will soon disappear and the residual volume soon decrease if tube feeding is continued.[48–51]

10.4.5 Postoperative Drainage of Body Cavities

Little evidence supports routine use of postoperative drainage of body cavities. Drainage tubes serve as much as an entrance for microbes as an outlet of fluid accumulations. Most body cavities, especially the abdomen, have excellent capacity for absorption of fluids, especially blood, unless the fluids are infected or mixed with body fluids like urine and bile. Most studies suggest that there is no need for abdominal drainage in biliary and gastric surgery. Some controlled studies also suggest advantages of a no-drainage policy in liver and pancreatic surgery. Several randomized studies have documented clear benefits of a no-drainage policy in colonic surgery. This is especially true for appendicitis, where use of drains has been associated with an *increased* rate of complications, especially adhesion formation. There is presently little evidence to support the use of drains that connect body cavities with the patient's exterior. As suggested by a recent review, the only valid conclusion at present is that high-quality clinical studies are necessary in order to provide solid, evidence-based recommendations for the use of drainage devices.[52] This is especially true in visceral surgery.

10.4.6 Preoperative Bowel Preparation

Intact intestinal flora are needed for the production, release, and absorption of important nutrients in the lower GI tract, but also for prevention of infection, stimulation of anastomotic healing, and prevention of excessive peritoneal adhesion formation. All of these important processes seem to be negatively influenced by both antibiotic treatment and lavage/bowel preparation. Aggressive bowel preparation and postoperative supply of a fiber-free diet have detrimental effects on the expression of important biological factors, such as transforming growth factor-beta 1 and pro-collagen type I, which are both important to intestinal healing.[53]

Long-term results of bowel surgery and the postoperative morbidity have remained unchanged in recent decades.[54] The practice of bowel preparation has seemingly not improved the situation. Even if it is suggested that careful bowel preparation might not enhance microbial translocation, there are still several other important reasons for omission of extensive bowel preparation.[55] Experience from some recent studies demonstrates that bowel preparation can safely be omitted.[56–58] A recently published meta-analysis found no evidence that bowel preparation reduces anastomotic leaks or prevents other complications.[59] Instead, accumulating experimental and clinical evidence indicates that bowel preparation, as usually practiced today, might be harmful and that reduced morbidity and considerable cost savings can be expected from modification of the practice.[60–62] One modification, which is biologically correct and might prove successful, is to use symbiotic treatment a few days before surgery (see Section 10.7). In addition, such a practice might contribute to less anastomotic dehiscences, infections, and reduced adhesion formation.

10.4.7 TRANSFUSION WITH OLD STORED BLOOD

Cellular debris (or, as documented in experimental studies, homogenized cells) are strong inducers of coagulation and thrombosis. We observed some 35 years ago that extensive disseminated intravascular coagulation and fibrinolysis occurs after intraportal or intravenous infusion of hemolyzed blood.[63–65] Similar changes are also seen in organs affected by hypoxia, as in intestinal or liver ischemia, or by increased levels of alcohol in the blood.[66,67] Blood transfusion has constantly been shown to be a major risk factor for postinjury MOF.[68–70] Trauma does often occur in alcohol-intoxicated persons, who also suffer severe shock and poor organ perfusion, and often are the object of extensive blood transfusions. Removal of old blood cells and restoration of tissues in organs damaged by ischemia and alcohol intoxication constitute an enormous burden on the reticulo–endothelial system, which results in immunoparalysis and increased sensitivity to infections. A strong association between the number of units transfused during the first six hours, the age of the stored blood transfused, and subsequent development of MOF was recently demonstrated.[70] Plenty of evidence shows that, whenever possible, fresh blood should be used for initial resuscitation of trauma patients but also when larger amounts of blood transfusion are needed.

10.4.8 OVERLOADING WITH NUTRIENTS (HYPERALIMENTATION)

Not long ago, overloading nutrients, called *hyperalimentation*, was regarded as key to success in the care of the critically ill; this is no longer so. Today, overfeeding macronutrients is considered much more dangerous than underfeeding, at least during the first few weeks following surgery, trauma, or onset of critical illness. A whole series of negative metabolic consequences is described following overfeeding, and the degree of impairment of both glucose and lipid metabolism seen in the ICU is reported to be significantly related to both the severity of illness and its outcome.[71,72] Increased amounts in the blood of free fatty acids (FFAs) are significantly and strongly associated with impaired immune functions. The endothelial cells seem to play a key role because they are responsible for the transport of nutrients, such as FFAs and glucose, to the underlying cells. This function is impaired by the inflammatory response *per se* and by various toxins and microbes, but also by high levels of FFAs.[73,74] Elevated serum FFAs have also been shown to inhibit T lymphocyte signaling, and FFA clearance through insulin infusion has been demonstrated to improve neutrophil function significantly, as observed in diabetic cardiac surgery patients.[75,76]

We observed some 35 years ago that high serum levels of fat and liver steatosis constitute poor risks in liver resection; a similar observation was recently made for liver transplant patients.[77–79] Most likely, this observation should also be valid for other types of extensive surgery, independent of whether the impaired fat metabolism and steatosis are induced by lifestyle, constitute a manifestation of metabolic syndrome, or are induced by overloading of calories, as is often the case in total parenteral nutrition (TPN).

10.5 OFTEN NEGLECTED MEASURES

Using supply of nutrients to modulate the inflammatory response and maximize the function of the immune system and the resistance to diseases is becoming increasingly accepted as an effective tool. Enteral nutrition (EN) is documented to improve outcome in critically ill and surgical patients. Proper nutrition is also an important tool to prevent chronic illnesses. Various nutrients have been shown to preserve and augment different aspects of cellular immunity and to modify the production of inflammatory mediators.[80] Much remains to be done before all the possibilities of immuno-modulatory nutrition are fully understood and practiced. However, some measures have proved effective:

- Aggressive perioperative enteral nutrition
- Tight blood glucose control
- Rich supply of antioxidants
- Rich supply of prebiotic fibers
- Maintenance of flora and supplementation of probiotic bacteria

10.5.1 Aggressive Perioperative Enteral Nutrition

The inflammatory response is immediate; all attempts to control the response must therefore also be immediate. Recent studies have demonstrated that immediate postoperative feeding is safe and prevents an increase in gut mucosal permeability. Early enteral feeding contributes to a positive nitrogen balance, reduce the incidence of septic complications and postoperative ileus, and accelerate restitution of pulmonary performance, body composition, and physical performance.[81–84] An important observation is that delaying institution of EN for more than 24 hours results in a significantly increased intestinal permeability and significantly higher incidence of MOF, compared to immediate enteral supply of nutrition.[85] Uninterrupted oral/enteral supply of nutrients the night before surgery, during surgery, and immediately thereafter might support the immune system even further and increase resistance to complication.

10.5.2 Tight Control of Blood Glucose

Hyperglycemia is known as a significant marker of in-hospital mortality that predisposes to infectious complications.[86,87] As an example, hyperglycemia predicts myocardial infarction in patients under hypertensive treatment.[88] Strict glucose control has been known for some time to reduce the incidence of wound infection in open heart surgery;[89] however, it was not until recently that strict glucose control has been widely adopted by modern ICU and postoperative care. Until recently, the state of the art was to feed critically ill patients and not provide exogenous insulin until blood glucose levels were up to 12 mmol/l (220 mg/dl). However, studies using strict glucose control (to below 6.1 mmol/l) have convincingly shown a decrease in blood stream infections by 46%, acute renal failure and need of hemofiltration by 41%, critical illness polyneuropathy by 44%, red cell transfusions by 50%, and mortality by 34%.[90,91] Equally important is the information that even small elevations of blood glucose (to 8 to 10 mmol/l) impairs gut motility and function and contributes to induction and prolongation of ileus.[92] This is another important reason for strict blood glucose control in the critically ill patient.

10.5.3 Supply of Antioxidants

Antioxidant have numerous beneficial effects in the postoperative and ICU patient.[93] Among the effects are:

- Direct antioxidant effects
- Anti-inflammatory effects
- Antibacterial effects
- Antithrombotic effects
- Anticarcinogenic effects
- Vasodilatory effects

The benefits of routine supply of megadoses of various antioxidants, especially flavonoids, to surgical and ICU patients are as yet almost unexplored. It is well known that the tissue and blood concentrations of pro-oxidants are almost invariably high and the levels of various antioxidants and micronutrients low — often extremely low — in critically ill patients. For example, total vitamin C and ascorbic acid are reported to be less than 25% of normal values in ICU patients.[94] A recently published study, performed mainly with trauma patients, reports a 19% reduction in pulmonary morbidity and a 57% lower incidence of MOF in the group receiving supplementation with α-tocopherol and ascorbate.[95] The benefit of antioxidant supplementation to surgical and ICU patients is also supported by other studies (for a review, see Chapter 8).[96]

Glutathione is an important antioxidant, synthesized by the body and supplied by food, mainly fruits and vegetables. Glutathione in serum is significantly decreased after surgery and in critically ill patients in general, and low blood levels of glutathione are associated with impaired lymphocyte and neutrophil functions. In the critically ill patient, glutamine constitutes an important source of fuel, especially for the small bowel enterocytes, but it is also a necessary substrate for the production of glutathione.[97] In experimental studies, supply of glutamine has been shown to reduce cytokine release, organ damage, and mortality and to counteract glutathione and lymphocyte depletion in Peyer's patches.[98,99] Significant clinical results, such as reductions in morbidity, mortality, and length of hospital stay, are obtained by glutamine supply in critically ill patients.[100] These benefits can also be expected from supply of glutamine-rich fruits and vegetables, which are fermented by flora or supplied probiotics in the lower GI tract.

10.5.4 SUPPLY OF PLANT FIBERS

Plant fibers are favored substrates for microbial fermentation in the lower digestive tract but also have their own strong bioactivities. Few studies on supply of plant fibers in connection with surgery and the critically ill are to be found in the medical literature. A most interesting controlled study, published some ten years ago, reports significant reduction in postoperative morbidity after supply of glucan (beta 1-3 polyglucose): nosocomial infections were reduced from 65 to 14% and mortality from 30 to 5%.[101] Most other recent studies in acute medicine have dealt mainly with the combined supply of probiotics and fibers (prebiotics). Experimental and clinical observations support that prebiotics have the following functions:[102,103]

- Provide nutrients and energy for the consumer
- Provide nutrients and energy for the flora
- Provide resistance against invading pathogens
- Maintain water and electrolyte balance
- Maintain mucosal growth
- Maintain mucosal function

The best fibers are undoubtedly those provided by eating fresh, uncooked, and otherwise unprepared fruits and vegetables. However, this is rarely possible for the critically ill patient. The more the fibers are processed, the more they have lost some of their potency. It is important to remember that the fibers supplied with commercial nutrition solutions are commonly hydrolyzed. This means that they are been made devoid of important antioxidants, various phytochemicals, glutathione, and other, rather unstable molecules such as glutamine. For that reason, it is recommended that extra fibers should be supplemented. By using a mix of several different fibers, it should be possible to supply 20 to 30 g/d, even to the critically ill. Often-used prebiotics are various oligosaccharides, such as fructooligosaccharides (FOS), trans-galactosaccharides, and lactulose. Oligosaccharides are especially rich in foods such as bananas, artichokes, leeks, onions, garlic, asparagus, and chicory. Larger molecules, such as oat fibers (beta-glucans), pectins, and resistant starch, are extremely effective fibers and should also be supplemented in the critically ill. These fibers are usually supplied as powders that can be diluted with water or acid fruit juices, such as pineapple juice, and fed through feeding tubes or mixed with mashed fruits, such as kiwis, apples, pears, or bananas, and eaten.

10.5.5 SUPPLEMENTING FLORA

A significant reduction of the commensal flora occurs very early in the disease process and is induced by the disease and the stress *per se* but also by pharmaceutical treatment. A significant reduction in anaerobic bacteria, and particularly lactobacilli, is observed in both the small intestine and the colon as early as six to eight hours after induction of experimental pancreatitis.[104] This reduction in beneficial flora pattern is almost instantly followed by significant increases in the number of various potentially pathogenic microorganisms (PPMs), such as *Escherichia coli*. Dramatic increases in mucosal barrier permeability (lumen to blood) and in endothelial permeability (blood to tissue) are observed and accompanied by increased microbial translocation and growth of PPMs, in both the mesenteric lymph nodes and the pancreatic tissue.[104–106] For obvious ethical reasons, few systematic studies have been done in patients, but there is much support for the assumption that patients who have undergone major operations and patients who suffer major trauma or are treated with modern antibiotics suffer a considerable reduction in the beneficial flora and a significant overgrowth of PPMs. Early supplemented beneficial bacteria, so-called probiotics, are reported to counteract such negative effects. From experimental and clinical observations, it can be concluded that supplied probiotics exhibit several important bioactivities, which should be of special benefit to the critically ill:[102,103]

- Reduce or eliminate potentially pathogenic microorganisms (PPMs)
- Reduce or eliminate various toxins and mutagens from the intestinal content
- Modulate innate and adaptive immune defense mechanisms
- Promote apoptosis
- Release numerous nutrients, antioxidants, growth factors, and coagulation and other factors from consumed fibers

10.6 A DUAL DIGESTIVE SYSTEM

Humans and animals have two separate and hugely different digestive systems:

- One based on digestion by secretions from eukaryotic cells, especially those located in the upper gut: saliva, pancreatic, and gastrointestinal secretions
- Another, equally important but much more complex and less understood, based on enzymatic fermentation by prokaryotic cells and microbes, occurring mainly in the lower gastrointestinal tract

Normally, the main substrates for GI fermentation will come from consumed fruit and vegetables, fibers indigestible by eukaryotic enzymes in the upper GI tract; this is why they reach the lower GI tract almost totally undigested. In the lower GI tract, extra energy and, more importantly, numerous nutrients, vitamins, antioxidants, coagulation factors, growth factors, signal substances, etc., are released and made available to the body. The human body contains approximately 65,000 genes, which should be compared to the 300,000 to 2 million genes in the GI flora.[107] This information provides an indication of the size and enormous complexity of the flora-driven digestive system. One can assume many more substances are released and absorbed in the lower ileum and the large bowel than in higher levels of the GI tract.

10.6.1 Mucosal Homeostasis

Many factors contribute to a satisfactory mucosal function, such as the following:[102,103]

- Satisfactory enteral supply of nutrients
- Satisfactory enteral supply of antioxidants
- Intact intestinal barrier
- Tolerant immunity
- "Normal" (not exaggerated) cytokine response
- "Normal" (not increased) PPM virulence
- Rich preventive flora
- Maintained mucosal repair

It has been suggested that, to a large extent, optimal health and well-being depend on the availability and "exact" balance, homeostasis, of the approximately two million different molecules that are said to constitute the human body. Some of these molecules are *essential* (e.g., must be obtained by eating); others become essential in critical conditions with increased demands and therefore are usually called *semiessential*. The largest number of consumed molecules is most likely released through action of prokaryotic enzymes and absorbed in the lower GI tract. Our paleolithic ancestors received a much richer and more variable supply of nutrients because they ate from more than 500 plants and, as a consequence, had significantly more abundant and richer flora. Modern humans have, in sharp contrast to our ancestors, chosen to obtain about 90% of their nutrition from as few as 17 plants and more than 50% of their caloric and protein need from only eight cereal grains. The reduced variability of typical modern Western foods, in combination with modern methods for conservation and preparation of foods, shows an obviously reduced access to nutrients and antioxidants. The flora of modern humans are, most likely as a consequence of this reduced access, restricted both in volume and in richness compared to that of our ancestors. And it is even worse in the critically ill, due to the disease and the drugs provided — but more than anything to the artificial nutrition provided to the sickest patients.

10.7 COMBINATION OF PRO- AND PREBIOTICS EQUALS SYMBIOTICS

Supplementing enteral nutrition with both fiber and lactic acid bacteria (LAB) has the potential to enhance the immune system further and provide protection from infectious complications. It is my personal conviction that fiber and LAB should be provided to surgical patients though feeding tubes continuously before, during, and immediately after surgery or, in the case of trauma or medical emergency, immediately upon arrival at the hospital. It is important to use a mixture of several bioactive fibers, and it is especially important to choose lactic acid bacteria with well documented bioactivities. Genetically, there is a great difference among the various bacteria called lactic acid bacteria (LAB); the difference from one LAB to another can be greater than the difference between a fish and a human. Most of the LAB used by the milk industry have limited or no ability to ferment strong bioactive fibers such as inulin or phlein, no ability to adhere to human mucus, or no low antioxidant capacity and, most importantly, no ability to survive the acidity of stomach and the bile acid content of the small intestine. Stronger clinical effects thus cannot be expected from the use of LAB such as yogurt bacteria, usually chosen mainly for palatability.

Most of the LAB suggested for use in ICU patients were originally identified on plants. Most experience obtained from studies of ICU patients comes from studies using two symbiotic combinations or mixtures of pre- and probiotics:

- A one LAB–one fiber composition, produced though fermentation of oatmeal with a specific *L. plantarum* strain 299.[108]
- A four LAB–four fiber composition, called Symbiotic 2000®, consisting in a mixture of 10^{10} (and more recently a composition with 10^{11} called Symbiotic 2000 forte®) of four different LAB — *Pediococcus pentosaceus* 5-33:3, *Leuconostoc mesenteroides* 32-77:1, *Lactobacillus paracasei* subsp paracasei 19, and *Lactobacillus plantarum* 2362 — combined with 10 g of fibers: 2.5 g of each of four fermentable fibers — betaglucan, inulin, pectin, and resistant starch.[109,110] It is a common practice to supply two sachets per day (i.e., 20 g fiber and 88 resp 880 billion [forte version] of LAB).

The most recent experience is summarized in the following sections.

10.7.1 ACUTE PANCREATITIS

Patients with severe acute pancreatitis were randomized to receive daily, during the first 7 days and administered through a nasojejunal tube, either a freeze-dried preparation containing live *Lb plantarum* 299 in a dose of 10^9 together with a substrate of oat fiber, or a similar but heat-inactivated preparation.[111] The study was interrupted when, on repeat statistical analysis, significant differences in favor of one of the two groups were obtained, which occurred after a total of 45 patients had entered the study. At that time, 22 patients had received treatment with live and another 23 with the heat-killed *Lb plantarum* 299. Infected pancreatic necrosis and abscesses were seen in 1/22 (4.5%) in the live LAB group vs. 7/23 (30%) in the heat-inactivated group (p = 0.023). The only patient in the lactobacillus group who developed infection, a urinary infection, did so on the 15th day (i.e., at a time when he had not received treatment for eight days). The length of stay was also considerably shorter in the live LAB group (13.7 days vs. 21.4 days), but the limited size of the material did not allow statistical significance to be reached.

10.7.2 ABDOMINAL SURGERY

Lb plantarum 299, in a dose of 10^9 and 15 gram of oat and inulin fiber, was used in a study in extensive abdominal surgical operations. The patient material consisted mainly in liver, pancreatic, and gastric resections, equally distributed among the three groups. Three groups were compared:[112]

- Live LAB and fiber
- Heat-inactivated LAB and fiber
- Standard enteral nutrition

Each group consisted of 30 patients. The 30-day sepsis rate was 10% (3/30 patients) in the two groups receiving either live or heat-inactivated LAB, compared to 30% (9/30 patients) in the group on standard enteral nutrition (p = 0.01). The largest difference was observed in the incidence of pneumonia:

- Live LAB and fiber: 2 patients
- Heat-killed LAB and fiber: 1 patient
- Enteral nutrition only: 6 patients

The beneficial effects of symbiotic treatment were seemingly most pronounced in gastric and pancreatic resections, the sepsis rate was:

- Live LAB: 7%
- Heat-inactivated LAB: 17%
- Standard enteral nutrition: 50%

The same pattern was observed for noninfectious complications:

- Live LAB: 13% (4/30)
- Heat-inactivated LAB: 17% (5/30)
- Standard enteral nutrition only: 30% (9/30)

The supply of antibiotics to the live LAB–treated patients was significantly less (p = 0.04). Also, the mean length of antibiotic treatment was considerably shorter:

- Live LAB: 4 ± 3.7 days
- Heat-killed LAB: 7 ± 5.2 days
- Standard enteral nutrition: 8 ± 6.5 days

No differences were observed in length of hospital stay. No significant differences could be observed in hemoglobin, leukocytes, CRP, BUN, bilirubin, albumin, total lymphocyte count, CD45 RA, CD45 RO, CD4, CD8, r in NK cells, or CD4/CD8 ratio.

10.7.3 LIVER TRANSPLANTATION

A prospective randomized study with the same one LAB–one fiber preparation was performed in 95 liver transplant patients by the same group of investigators.[113] Three groups of patients were studied:

- SDD — Selective digestive tract decontamination four times daily for six weeks (n = 32)
- LLP— *Lb plantarum* 299 in a dose of 10^9 plus 15 g of oat and inulin fibers (n = 31) supplied postoperatively for 12 days
- HLP — Identical to LLP, but with heat-killed *Lb plantarum* 299 (HLP) (n = 32)

Identical enteral nutrition was supplied to all patients from the second postoperative day. The numbers of postoperative infections were SDD 23, HLP 17, and LLP 4. Signs of infections occurred in SDD 48% (15/32), in HLP 34% (11/32), and in LLP 13% (4/31), p = 0.017, respectively. The most dominating infections were cholangitis, occurring in SDD in 10, HLP in 8, and LLP in 2 patients, respectively, and pneumonia, observed in SDD in 6, in HLP in 4, and in LLP in 1 patient, respectively. The most often isolated microbes were *Enterococci*: in 8 SDD, 8 HLP, and 1 LLP in 1 patient, respectively, closely followed by *Staphylococci*: in 6 SDD, 3 HLP, and 1 LLP patient, respectively. No *E. coli* or *Klebsiella* infections were seen in the LLP group. The numbers of patients requiring hemodialysis were 8 SDD, 4 HLP, and 2 LLP patients. The numbers of reoperations were 6 SDD, 2 HLP, and 4 LLP. There were no deaths. The stay in ICU, the hospital stay, and length of time on antibiotic therapy were shorter in the LLP group but did not reach statistical significance. The CD4/CD8 ratio was higher in the LLP group than in the other two groups (p = 0.06).

The same investigators have continued their efforts to reduce the septic morbidity in liver transplantation.[114] In a subsequent study, the four LAB–four fiber combination (Symbiotic 2000) was tried.[109,110] In a double-blind randomized study, 33 patients were supplied Symbiotic 2000 and another 33 patients only the four fibers in Symbiotic 2000. The treatment began on the day before surgery and continued for 14 days after surgery. During the first postoperative month, only one patient in the Symbiotic 2000–treated group (3%) showed signs of infection (urinary infection), compared to 17/33 (51%) in the patients supplied only the four fibers. The use of antibiotics was also significantly reduced in the symbiotic-treated group.

10.7.4 OTHER CONDITIONS

Probiotic or symbiotic treatment is also effective in other acute and chronic conditions. This is especially well studied in acute and chronic diarrhea.[115,116] Significant effects have also been observed when applied to prevent allergy, reduce *Helicobacter* infections, counteract negative manifestations of HIV, reduce symptoms in irritable bowel syndrome (IBS) and inflammatory bowel disease (IBD), and improve the condition of and prevent sepsis in patients with chronic kidney failure and on dialysis treatments.[117–124] Symbiotic treatment is reported to reduce serum fibrinogen and LDL cholesterol significantly when supplied to patients with moderately elevated cholesterol.[125] Recent observations of effects in patients with chronic liver disease are interesting and could be of importance for the management of patients on a waiting list for liver transplantation. The *in vitro* TNFα production in response to stimulation by endotoxin or *Staph aureus* enterotoxin B (SEB) was reduced by a median 46% (range: 8 to 67%), in comparison to presupplementation levels in 8/11 (72.7%) cirrhotic patients supplied Symbiotic 2000.[126]

The anti-infectious and anti-inflammatory effects of symbiotic treatment in chronic liver disease are further supported by a double-blind controlled study of 55 patients with chronic liver disease, not yet published.[127] Three groups of patients were studied:

- Symbiotic 2000 (n = 20)
- Only the fibers of Symbiotic 2000 (n = 20)
- Placebo (nonfermentable, nonabsorbable fiber) (n = 15)

A significant increase from 7.37 ± 047 to 9.64 ± 0.34 ($p < 0.05$) in the LAB flora was observed in the LAB-supplied group but not in the other two groups. The pH was significantly reduced from a level between 6.5 and 7 in the placebo group to the level of 5 to 5.5 in the two treatment groups. Statistically significant decreases in *E. coli*, *Staphylococcus,* and *Fusobacterium* ($p < 0.001$, $p < 0.01$ and $p < 0.05$) were observed in the two treatment groups but not in the placebo group. No differences due to treatment could be observed in the *Pseudomonas* and *Enterococcus* flora. Ammonia was significantly reduced in the Symbiotic 2000–supplied group (60.5 ± 2.9 to 38.6 ± 3.9) and in the fiber-supplied group (63.6 ± 3.9 to 41.5 ± 5.2) but not in the placebo group (60.5 ± 2.9 to 58.6 ± 3.9). The levels of endotoxin fell significantly in the two treatment groups but not in the placebo-treated group. The reduction in the levels of ALT is remarkable: it decreased from 252 ± 182 to 84 ± 65 ($p < 0.01$) in the Symbiotic 2000–treated group and to 110 ± 86 ($p < 0.05$) in the fiber-supplemented group, but not in the placebo group. Significant improvements in psychometric tests and in the degree of encephalopathy were also observed in the two treatment groups.

10.8 FUTURE ASPECTS

During my long career as a surgeon, I have always been frustrated by the high rate of septic complications, especially occurring in connection with extensive surgery. Since the early 1960s, I performed extensive surgery to the liver and the pancreas. Like most other surgeons of that time, I tried a perioperative and postoperative antibiotic umbrella in the hope of reducing septic manifestations. However, on a follow-up in the mid-1980s we detected that, for unknown reasons, one-third of patients had never received any prophylactic antibiotics at all. The infection rate of the total material was, as in most similar published materials, about 33%. However, to our great surprise, no infections had occurred among the patients who had not received antibiotics. This observation interested me in exploring the role of the commensal flora but also in developing techniques to refunctionalize the lower gastrointestinal tract in order to reestablish the function of the microflora in sick patients. At that time, I did not imagine that, some 20 years later, symbiotics would be regarded as a realistic, sometimes superior, alternative to antibiotics. Nor did I foresee that, some years later, pre-, pro-, and symbiotics would be considered an important tool to combat endemic diseases such as diabetes, atherosclerosis, and cancer.

Resistance to disease is a key factor in the preservation of health. The innate immune system, with its various components — traditional immune cells; epithelial, endothelial, and mesothelial cells; the glial cells; and flora — is extremely sensitive to external influence and especially to variations in the supply of nutrients and antioxidants. As mentioned earlier, about 80% of the various components are located in the digestive system and the abdominal cavity. The perioperative management of the abdominal cavity in general, and particularly the nutrition given, is of great importance to the outcome. Humans living in rural areas and consuming large amounts of fresh fruits, vegetables, and various types of fermented foods have an extremely low incidence of chronic diseases and are also resistant to morbidity in connection with trauma and surgical operations. As a consequence of lifestyle, the flora of their digestive tract are both large (approximately 2 kg bacteria) and rich (> 500 species). In fact, the bodies of such individuals will harbor about 20 times more microbial/karyotic cells than human/eukaryotic cells. These flora are significantly reduced in persons living a Western lifestyle. Important fiber-fermenting bacteria — such as *Lactobacillus plantarum, Lact. rhamnosus,* and *Lact. paracasei* ssp. *paracasei,* but also other LAB, such as *Lactobacillus acidophilus* and *Leuconostoc* — have often disappeared in the commensal flora of North Americans and Europeans. For example, *Lactobacillus plantarum* is reported to exist in only about 25% of omnivorous North Americans, in contrast to two-thirds of the mainly vegetarian North American Seventh Day Adventists.[128] A study of healthy European (Swedish) volunteers found *Lactobacillus plantarum, Lact. rhamnosus,* and *Lact. paracasei* ssp. *paracasei* to be the most common *Lactobacillus* flora both at the rectal and oral mucosa, occurring in 52%, 26%, and 17% of the individuals, respectively.[129] Other LAB, such as *Lact. reuteri, Lact. fermentum, Lact. acidophilus, Lact. oris,* and *Lact. vaginalis,* were only found occasionally.

Persons living a rural lifestyle similar to that of our paleolithic ancestors also have a rich protective flora in other parts of the body: the skin (200 g), vagina (20 g), lungs (20 g), mouth (20 g), nose (10 g), and eyes (1 g).[130] It is likely that these flora also have significant health-promoting functions. It is well known that persons with infective and inflammatory manifestations in the vagina do well on treatment with lactobacillus preparations. It has been observed that the incidence of diaper dermatitis is significantly reduced in children supplemented with LAB.[131] It is also interesting that two recent reports suggest that consumption of LAB-containing drinks prevents formation of biofilm and removes both yeast and bacteria from prostheses (in this case, silicon rubber voice prostheses) suggesting that an LAB-containing gel or cream could be effective in preventing catheter-related infections.[132,133] I would not be surprised if, one day, eye or nose drops with lactobacilli or even inhalation of lactobacillus will be shown to be effective in combating allergic, inflammatory, and infectious conditions in the respiratory tract and the eyes. Supply of lactobacillus has proved effective in reducing allergy.[134,135] Hopefully, it will be increasingly tried in prevention and treatment of various endemic chronic diseases.

10.9 PRACTICE POINTS

- Efforts should be made to preserve salivation and gastrointestinal secretions in the critically ill, because these secretions are important for optimal innate immune system function.
- H_2 blockers, proton pump inhibitors, and other antisecretory drugs should be avoided to the extent possible, especially if the patient is on enteral nutrition.
- If not possible before, attempts should be made to start supply immediately after an operation, acute medical illness, or trauma.

- If possible, insert a feeding tube into the jejunum the day before surgery and feed aggressively during the night before and after surgery. Continue with reduced speed during and immediately after surgery.
- Avoid extensive mechanical bowel preparations.
- Avoid, to the extent possible, use of all sorts of drains.
- If large transfusion volumes are necessary, make efforts to provide fresh blood.
- Maintain a strict control of blood sugar (below 6.1 mmol/l).
- Immunosuppressed patients benefit from pretreatment with probiotics and fiber several days before surgery, when possible.
- Attempts should always be made to provide a maximum of plant fibers: whenever possible as fresh fruits and vegetables, otherwise as supplements.
- Efforts should be made to provide several plant fibers to optimize the tolerability of the fibers supplied and the availability of substrate for fermentation and subsequent release of important nutrients, antioxidants, coagulation, and other factors.
- Fibers provided in enteral nutrition solutions are most often hydrolyzed and void of many important antioxidants and nutrients. Whenever possible, supplementation with fruits and vegetables or fibers such as pectins, betaglucans, oligosaccharides, and resistant starch should be provided as separate supplements.
- Use several fibers to increase tolerance. Strive to supply up to 20 to 30 g a day.
- Probiotic bacteria have, apart from eventual flatulence, no side effects and can safely be used in immunocompromised patients.
- Critically ill patients, especially those receiving antibiotics, suffer from a reduced commensal flora and reduced mucosal and barrier function. Such patients can be expected to benefit from a rich daily supply of probiotic bacteria.
- For clinical purposes, only pre- and probiotics with documented strong bioactivities should be chosen. The majority of lactic acid bacteria do not survive the acidity of the stomach or bile acid content of the small intestine.

REFERENCES

1. World Health Organization. Process for a global strategy on diet, physical activity and health. WHO, Geneva, February 2003.
2. Angus, D.C., Wax, R.S. Epidemiology of sepsis: an update. *Crit. Care Med.* 29, 109, 2001.
3. Angus, D.C., Linde-Zwirble, W.T., Lidicker, J., et al. Epidemiology of severe sepsis in the United States: analysis of incidence, outcome and associated costs of care. *Crit. Care Med.* 29, 1303, 2001.
4. Vincent, J.-L., Abraham, E., Annane, D., et al. Reducing mortality in sepsis: new directions. *Crit. Care* 6 (Suppl. 3), S1, 2002.
5. Schwartz, M.N. Hospital-acquired infections: diseases with increasingly limited therapies. *Proc. Natl. Acad. Sci. USA* 91, 2420, 1994.
6. Bengmark, S. Nutritional modulation of acute and "chronic" phase response. *Nutrition* 17, 489, 2001.
7. Simons, J.P., Schools A.M., Buurman, W.A., Wouters, E.F. Weight loss and low body cell mass in males with lung cancer: relationship with systemic inflammation, acute-phase response, resting energy expenditure, and catabolic and anabolic hormones. *Clin. Sci.* 97, 215, 1999.
8. Preston, T., Slater, C., McMillan, D.C., et al. Fibrinogen synthesis is elevated in fasting cancer patients with an acute phase response. *J. Nutr.* 128, 1355, 1998.
9. Biffl, W.L., Moore, E.E., Moore, F.A., Barnett, C.C. Interleukin-6 delays neutrophil apoptosis via a mechanism involving platelet-activating factor. *J. Trauma, Injury, Infection Crit. Care* 40, 575, 1996.
10. Sautner, T., Függer, R., Götzinger, P., et al. Tumour necrosis factor-α and interleukin-6: early indicators of bacterial infection after human orthotopic liver transplantation. *Eur. J. Surg.* 161, 97, 1995.
11. Alessi, M.C., Peiretti, F., Morange, P., et al. Production of plasminogen activator inhibitor 1 by human adipose tissue: possible link between visceral fat accumulation and vascular disease. *Diabetes* 46, 860, 1997.

12. Fried, S.K., Bunkin, D.A., Greenberg, A.S. Omental and subcutaneous adipose tissues of obese subjects release interleukin-6: depot difference and regulation by glucocorticoid. *J. Clin. Endocrinol. Metabol.* 83, 847, 1998.

13. Thomas, E.L., Saeed, N., Hajnal, J.V., et al. Magnetic resonance imaging of total body fat. *J. Appl. Physiol.* 85, 1778, 1998.

14. Felten, D.L., Felten, S.Y., Carlson, S.L., et al. Noradrenergic and peptinergic innervation of lymphoid tissue. *J. Immun.* 135 Suppl., 755, 1985.

15. Ottaway, C.A. Vasoactive intestinal peptide and immune function. In *Psychoneuroimmunology.* 2nd ed. Ader R, Felten DL, Cohen N, eds. Academic Press, San Diego, 1991, 225.

16. Brandtzaeg, P., Halstensen, T.S., Kett, K., et al. Immunobiology and immunopathology of human gut mucosa: humoral immunity and intraepithelial lymphocytes. *Gastroenterol.* 97, 1562, 1989.

17. Kiyono, H., McGhee, J.R. T helper cells for mucosal immune responses. In *Handbook of Mucosal Immunology.* Ogra P.L., Mestecky J., Lamm M.E., et al., eds. Academic Press, Orlando, FL, 1994, 263.

18. Brandzaeg, P. Molecular and cellular aspects of the secretory immunoglobulin system. *APMIS* 103, 1, 1995.

19. Freter, R. The fatal enteric cholera infection in guinea pig achieved by inhibition of normal enteric flora. *J. Infect. Dis.* 97, 57, 1955.

20. Roszkowski, K., Ko, K.L., Beuth, J., et al. Intestinal microflora of BALB/c-mice and function of local immune cells. *Zeitschr. F. Bakteriol. Hyg.* 270, 270, 1988.

21. Pulverer, G., Ko, H.L., Roszkowski, W., et al. Digestive tract microflora liberates low molecular weight peptides with immunotriggering activity. *Zentralbl. F. Bakteriol.* 272, 318, 1990.

22. Peiper, C., Seelig, M., Treutner, K.H., Schumpelick, V. Low-dose, single-shot perioperative antibiotic prophylaxis in colorectal surgery. *Chemother.* 43, 54, 1997.

23. Kriaras, I., Michalopoulos, A., Turina, M., Geroulanos, S. Evolution of antimicrobial prophylaxis in cardiovascular surgery. *Eur. J. Cardiothorac. Surg.* 18, 440, 2000.

24. Kirton, O.C., O'Neill, P.A., Kestner, M., Tortella, B.J. Perioperative antibiotic use in high-risk penetrating hollow viscus injury: a prospective randomized, double-blind, placebo-control trial of 24 hours versus 5 days. *J. Trauma* 49, 822, 2000.

25. Goossens, H., Peetermans, W., Sion, J.P., Bossens, M. "Evidence-based" perioperative antibiotic prophylaxis policy in Belgian hospitals after a change in the reimbursement system. *Ned. Tijdschr. Geneesk.* 14, 1773, 2001.

26. Bengmark, S. Gut and the immune system: enteral nutrition and immunonutrients. In *SIRS, MODS and MOF — Systemic Inflammatory Response Syndrome, Multiple Organ Dysfunction Syndrome, Multiple Organ Failure — Pathophysiology, Prevention and Therapy,* Baue, A.E., Faist, E., Fry, D., eds. Springer, New York, 2000, 420–436.

27. Bengmark, S. Pre-, pro-, and symbiotics. *Curr. Opin. Nutr. Metab. Care* 4, 571, 2001.

28. Bengmark S. Use of pro-, pre- and symbiotics in the ICU: future options. In *Nutritional Considerations in the Intensive Care Unit: Science, Rationale and Practice.* Shikora S.A., Martindale R.G., Schwaitzberg S.D., eds. Kendall/Hunt, Dubuque, IA, 2002, 381–399.

29. Lundberg, J.O.N., Weitzberg, E., Lundberg, J.M., Alving, K. Intragastric nitric oxide production in humans: measurement in expelled air. *Gut* 35, 1543, 1994.

30. Duncan, C., Dougall, H., Johnston, et al. Chemical generation of nitric oxide in the mouth from the enterosalivary circulation of dietary nitrates. *Nature Med.* 1, 546, 1995.

31. Heyland, D., Mandell, L.A. Gastric colonization by Gram-negative bacilli and nosocomial pneumonia in the intensive care unit patients. *Chest* 101, 187, 1992.

32. Gomes, G.F., Pisani, J.C., Macedo, E.D., Campos, A.C. The nasogastric feeding tube as a risk factor for aspiration and aspiration pneumonia. *Curr. Opin. Clin. Nutr. Metab. Care* 6, 32, 2003.

33. McDonald, W.S., Sharp, C.W., Deitch, E.A. Immediate enteral feeding in burn patients is safe and effective. *Ann. Surg.* 214, 177, 1991.

34. Donowitz, G.L., Page, M.L., Mileur, B.L. Alteration of normal gastric flora in critical care patients receiving antacid and cimetidine therapy. *Infect. Control* 7, 23, 1986.

35. Ben-Menachem, T., Fogel, R., Patel, R.V., et al. Prophylaxis for stress-related gastric hemorrhage in the medical intensive care unit: a randomized controlled, single-blind study. *Ann. Int. Med.* 121, 568, 1994.

36. Savassi-Rocha, P.R., Conceicao, S.A., Ferreira, J.T., et al. Evaluation of the routine use of the naso-gastric tube in digestive operation by a prospective controlled study. *Surg. Gynecol. Obstet.* 174, 317, 1992.

37. Gerber, A., Robert, F.A., Smith, L.L. The treatment of paralytic ileus without the use of gastrointestinal suction. *Surg. Gynecol. Obstet.* 107, 247, 1958.

38. Gerber, A. An appraisal of paralytic ileus and the necessity for postoperative gastrointestinal suction. *Surg. Gynecol. Obstet.* 117, 294, 1958.

39. Farris, J.M., Smith, K. An evaluation of temporary gastrostomy: a substitute for nasogastric suction. *Ann. Surg.* 144, 475, 1956.

40. Mehnert, I.H., Brown, M.J., Woodward, B., et al. A clinical evaluation of postoperative nasal gastric suction. *Surg. Gynecol. Obstet.* 109, 607, 1959.

41. Thomas, G.I., Metheny, D., Lundmark, V.O. Vagotomy without post-operative nasogastric suction. *Northwest. Med.* 60, 387, 1961.

42. Barnes, A.D., Williams, J.A. Stomach drainage after vagotomy and pyloroplasty. *Am. J. Surg.* 113, 494, 1967.

43. Burg, R., Geigle, C.F., Faso, J.M., et al. Omission of routine gastric decompression. *Dis. Colon Rectum* 21, 98, 1978.

44. Sitges-Serra, A., Cabrol, J., MaGubern, J., et al. A randomized trial of gastric decompression after truncal vagotomy and anterior pylorectomy. *Surg. Gynecol. Obstet.* 158, 557, 1980.

45. Schwartz, C.I., Heyman, A.S., Rao, A.C. Prophylactic nasogastric tube decompression: is its use justified? *Southern Med. J.* 88, 825, 1995.

46. Petrelli, N.J., Stulc, J.P., Rodrigues-Bigas, M., et al. Nasogastric decompression following elective colorectal surgery. *Am. Surg.* 59, 632, 1993.

47. Cheatham, M.L., Chapman, W.C., Key, S.P., et al. A meta-analysis of selective versus routine naso-gastric decompression after elective laparotomy. *Ann. Surg.* 221, 469, 1995.

48. Rombeau, J.L., Jacobs, D.O. Nasoenteric tube feeding. In *Enteral Nutrition and Tube Feeding.* Rombeau J.L., Caldwell M.D., eds. Saunders, Philadelphia, 1998, 261–274.

49. Norton, J.A., Otta, L.G., McClain, C., et al. Intolerance to enteral feeding in brain-injured patients. *J. Neurosurg.* 68, 62, 1988.

50. McClave, S.A., Snider, H.L., Lowen, C.C., et al. Use of the residual volume as a marker for enteral feeding intolerance: prospective blinded comparison with physical examination and radiographic findings. *J. Parenter. Enteral Nutr.* 16, 99, 1992.

51. Cook, D.J., Fuller, H.D., Guyatt, G.H., et al. Gastrointestinal bleeding in the critically ill: stress ulcer prophylaxis is not for everyone. *N. Engl. J. Med.* 330, 377, 1994.

52. Dominguez-Fernandez, E., Post, S. Abdominal drainages (in German). *Der Chirurg* 74, 91, 2003.

53. Buckmire, M., Parquet, G., Seeburger, J.L., et al. Effect of bowel preparation and a fiber-free liquid diet on expression of transforming growth factor and procollagen in colonic tissue preoperatively and postoperatively. *Dis. Colon Rectum* 41, 1273, 1998.

54. Rabeneck, L., El-Serag, H.B., Davila, J.A., Sandler, R.S. Outcomes of colorectal cancer in the United States: no change in survival (1986–1997). *Am. J. Gastroenterol.* 98, 471, 2003.

55. Kale, T.I., Kuzu, M.A., Tekeli, A., et al. Aggressive bowel preparation does not enhance bacterial translocation, provided the mucosal barrier is not disrupted: a prospective, randomized study. *Dis. Colon Rectum* 41, 636, 1998.

56. Santos Jr., J.C., Batista, J., Sirimarco, M.T., et al. Prospective randomized trial of mechanical bowel preparation in patients undergoing elective colorectal surgery. *Br. J. Surg.* 81, 1673, 1994.

57. Burke, P., Mealy, K., Gillen, P., et al. Requirement for bowel preparation in colorectal surgery. *Br. J. Surg.* 81, 907, 1994.

58. Zmora, O., Mahajna, A., Bar-Zakai, B., et al. Colon and rectal surgery without mechanical bowel preparation: a randomized prospective trial. *Ann. Surg.* 237, 363, 2003.

59. Guenaga, K.F., Matos, D., Castro, A.A., et al. Mechanical bowel preparation for elective colorectal surgery. *Cochrane Database Syst. Rev.* 2, CD001544, 2003.

60. Feres, O., Monteiro dos Santos Jr., J.C., Andrade, J.I. The role of mechanical bowel preparation for colonic resection and anastomosis: an experimental study. *Int. J. Colorectal. Dis.* 16, 353, 2001.

61. Platell, C., Hall, J. What is the role of mechanical bowel preparation in patients undergoing colorectal surgery? *Dis. Colon Rectum* 41, 872, 1998.

62. Nessim, A., Wexner, S.D., Agachan, F., et al. Is bowel confinement necessary after anorectal reconstructive surgery? A prospective, randomized, surgeon-blinded trial. *Dis. Colon Rectum* 42, 16, 1999.
63. Bengmark, S., Hafström, L.O., Korsan-Bengtsen, K. A trial to produce intravascular coagulation by infusion of connective-tissue homogenate and erythrocyte haemolysate: a comparative study. *Br. J. Surg.* 56, 619, 1969.
64. Bengmark, S., Hafström, L.O., Korsan-Bengtsen, K. A trial to produce disseminated intravascular coagulation with intravenous infusion of homologous haemolysate and serum in cats. *Acta Chir. Scand.* 138, 453, 1972.
65. Bengmark, S., Hafström, L.O., Korsan-Bengtsen, K. Effects of intraportal infusion of autologous hemolysate on blood coagulation factors and fibrinolysis in the cat. *Am. J. Surg.* 124, 647, 1972.
66. Hafström, L.O., Korsan-Bengtsen, K., Bengmark, S. Changes in blood clotting and fibrinolysis after liver ischemia in pigs. *Am. J. Surg.* 127, 300, 1974.
67. Zoucas, E., Bergqvist, D., Göransson, G., Bengmark, S. Effect of acute ethanol intoxication on primary haemostasis, coagulation factors and fibrinolytic activity. *Eur. Surg. Res.* 14, 33, 1982.
68. Sauaia, A., Moore, F.A., Moore, E.E., et al. Early predictors of postinjury multiple organ failure. *Arch. Surg.* 129, 39, 1994.
69. Moore, F.A., Moore, E.E., Sauaia, A. Blood transfusion: an independent risk factor for postinjury multiple organ failure. *Arch. Surg.* 132, 620, 1997.
70. Sauaia, A., Moore, F.A., Moore, E.E., et al. Multiple organ failure can be predicted as early as 12 hours after injury. *J. Trauma* 45, 291, 1998.
71. Klein, C.J., Stanek, G.S., Wiles, C.E. Overfeeding macronutrients to critically ill adults: metabolic complications. *J. Am. Diet. Assoc.* 98, 795, 1998.
72. Lind, L., Lithell, H. Impaired glucose and lipid metabolism seen in intensive care patients is related to severity of illness and survival. *Clin. Intens. Care* 5, 100, 1994.
73. Steinberg, H.O., Tarshoby, M., Monestel, R., et al. Elevated circulating free fatty acid levels impair endothelium-dependent vasodilation. *J. Clin. Invest.* 100, 1230, 1997.
74. Pleiner, J., Schaller, G. Mittermayer, F., et al. FFA-induced endothelial dysfunction can be corrected by vitamin C. *J. Clin. Endocrinol. Metab.* 87, 2913, 2002.
75. Stulnig, T.M., Berger, M., Roden, M., et al. Elevated free fatty acid concentrations inhibit T lymphocyte signaling. *FASEB J.* 14, 939, 2000.
76. Rassias, A.J., Marrin, C.A.S., Arruda, J., et al. Insulin infusion improves neutrophil function in diabetic cardiac surgery patients. *Anesth. Analg.* 88, 1011, 1999.
77. Almersjö, O., Bengmark, S., Engevik, L., et al. Serum lipids after extensive liver resection in man. *Acta Hepatosplenol.* 15, 1, 1968.
78. Bengmark, S. Liver steatosis and liver resection. *Digestion* 2, 304, 1968.
79. Marchesini, G., Forlani, G. NASH: from liver disease to metabolic disorders and back to clinical hepatology. *Hepatology* 35, 497, 2002.
80. Calder, P.C. Immunonutrition. *BMJ* 327, 117, 2003.
81. Carr, C.S., Ling. K.D.E., Boulos, P., Singer, M. Randomised trial of safety and efficacy of immediate postoperative enteral feeding in patients undergoing gastrointestinal resection. *BMJ* 112, 869, 1996.
82. Bisgaard, T., Kehlet, H. Early oral feeding after elective abdominal surgery: what are the issues? *Nutrition* 18, 944, 2002.
83. Basse, L., Raskov, H.H., Hjort-Jakobsen, D., et al. Accelerated postoperative recovery programme after colonic resection improves physical performance, pulmonary function and body composition. *Br. J. Surg.* 89, 446, 2002.
84. Kehlet, H., Holte, K. Review of postoperative ileus. *Am. J. Surg.* 182, Suppl, S3, 2001.
85. Kompan, L., Kremzar, B., Gadzijev, E., Prosek, M. Effects of early enteral nutrition on intestinal permeability and the development of multiple organ failure after multiple injury. *Intens. Care Med.* 25, 129, 1999.
86. Umpierrez, G.E., Isaacs, S.D., Bazargan, N., et al. Hyperglycemia: an independent marker of in-hospital mortality in patients with undiagnosed diabetes. *J. Clin. Endocrinol. Metabol.* 87, 978, 2002.
87. McCowen, K.C., Malhotra, A., Bistrian, B.R. Stress-induced hyperglycemia. *Crit. Care Clin.* 17, 107, 2001.

88. Dunder, K., Lind, L., Zethelius, B., Lithell, H. Increase in blood glucose concentration during hypertensive treatment as a predictor of myocardial infarction: population based cohort study. *BMJ* 326, 681, 2003.

89. Zerr, K.J., Furnary, A.P., Grunkemeier, G.L., et al. Glucose control lowers the risk of wound infection in diabetes after open heart operations. *Ann. Thorac. Surg.* 63, 356, 1997.

90. Van den Berghe, G., Wouters, P., Weekers, F., et al. Intensive insulin therapy in critically ill patients. *N. Engl. J. Med.* 345, 1359, 2001.

91. Mesotten, D., Van den Berghe, G. Clinical potential of insulin therapy in critically ill patients. *Drugs* 63, 625, 2003.

92. Rayner, C.K., Jones, K.L., Samson, N., Horowitz, M. Relationship of upper gastrointestinal motor and sensory function with glycemic control. *Diabetes Care* 24, 371, 2001.

93. Middleton Jr., E., Kandaswami, C., Theoharides, T.C. The effects of plant flavonoids on mammalian cells: implications for inflammation, heart disease, and cancer. *Pharmacol. Rev.* 52, 673, 2000.

94. Schorah, C.J., Downing, C., Piripitsi, A., et al. Total vitamin C, ascorbic acid, and dehydroascorbic acid concentrations in plasma of critically ill. *Am. J. Clin. Nutr.* 63, 760, 1996.

95. Nathens, A.B., Neff, M.J., Jurkovich, G.J., et al. Randomized, prospective trial of antioxidant supplementation in critically ill surgical patients. *Ann. Surg.* 236, 814, 2002.

96. Baines, M, Shenkin, A. Use of antioxidants in surgery: a measure to reduce postoperative complications. *Curr. Opin. Nutr. Metab.* 5, 665, 2002.

97. Cao, Y., Feng, F., Hoos, A., Klimberg, V.S. Glutamine enhances gut glutathione production. *J. Parenter. Enteral Nutr.* 22, 224, 1998.

98. Wischmeyer, P.E., Kahana, M., Wolfson, R., et al. Glutamine reduces cytokine release, organ damage, and mortality in a rat model of endotoxemia. *Shock* 16, 398, 2001.

99. Manhart, N., Vierlinger, K., Spittler, A., et al. Oral feeding with glutamine prevents lymphocyte and glutathione depletion of Peyer's patches in endotoxemic mice. *Ann. Surg.* 234, 92, 2001.

100. Kelly, D., Wischmeyer, P.E. Role of L-glutamine in critical illness: new insights. *Curr. Opin. Nutr. Metab.* 6, 217, 2003.

101. de Fellippe, J., da Rocha e Silva, M., Maciel, F.M.B., et al. Infection prevention in patients with severe multiple trauma with the immunomodulator beta 1-3 polyglucose (glucan). *Surg. Gynecol. Obstet.* 177, 383, 1993.

102. Bengmark S. Aggressive perioperative and intraoperative enteral nutrition: strategy for the future. In *SIRS, MODS and MOF — Systemic Inflammatory Response Syndrome, Multiple Organ Dysfunction Syndrome, Multiple Organ Failure — Pathophysiology, Prevention and Therapy*, Baue A.E., Faist E., Fry D., eds. Springer, New York, 2000, 365–380.

103. Bengmark, S. Pre-, pro-, and symbiotics in clinical enteral nutrition, In Old Herborn University Monographs.

104. Andersson, R., Wang, X., Ihse, I. The influence of abdominal sepsis on acute pancreatitis in rats: a study on mortality, permeability, arterial blood pressure and intestinal blood flow. *Pancreas* 11, 365, 1995.

105. Leveau, P., Wang, X., Soltesz, V., et al. Alterations in intestinal permeability and microflora in experimental acute pancreatitis. *Int. J. Pancreatol.* 20, 119, 1996.

106. De Souza, L.J., Sampietre, S.N., Figueiredo, S., et al. Bacterial translocation during acute pancreatitis in rats (in Portuguese, with English summary). *Rev. Hosp. Clin. Fac. Med. S. Paolo* 51, 116, 1996.

107. Hooper, L.V., Midtvedt, T., Gordon, J.I. How host–microbial interactions shape the nutrient environment of the mammalian intestine. *Annu. Rev. Nutr.* 22, 283, 2002.

108. Johansson, M.L., Molin, G., Jeppsson, B., et al. Administration of different lactobacillus strains in fermented oatmeal soup: *in vivo* colonization of human intestinal mucosa and effect on the indigenous flora. *Appl. Environ. Microbiol.* 59, 15, 1993.

109. Kruszewska, K., Lan, J., Lorca, G., et al. Selection of lactic acid bacteria as probiotic strains by *in vitro* tests. *Microecol. Ther.* 29, 37, 2002.

110. Ljungh, Å., Lan, J.-G., Yamagisawa, N. Isolation, selection and characteristics of *Lactobacillus paracasei* ssp *paracasei* isolate F19. *Microb. Ecol. Health Dis.* 3, Suppl, 4, 2002.

111. Oláh, A., Belágyi, T., Issekutz, Á., et al. Early enteral nutrition with specific lactobacillus and fibre reduces sepsis in severe acute pancreatitis. *Br. J. Surg.* 89, 1103, 2002.

112. Rayes, N., Hansen, S., Boucsein, K., et al. Early enteral supply of fibre and lactobacilli vs. parenteral nutrition: a controlled trial in major abdominal surgery patients. *Nutrition* 18, 609, 2002.

113. Rayes, N., Hansen, S., Seehofer, D., et al. Early enteral supply of *Lactobacillus* and fibre vs. selective bowel decontamination (SBD): a controlled trial in liver transplant recipients. *Transplantation* 74, 123, 2002.

114. Rayes, N., Seehofer, D., Theruvath, T., et al. Combined perioperative enteral supply of bioactive pre- and probiotics abolishes postoperative bacterial infections in human liver transplantation: a randomised, double-blind clinical trial. In press.

115. Huang, J.S., Bousvaros, A., Lee, J.E., et al. Efficacy of probiotic use in acute diarrhea in children: a meta-analysis. *Dig. Dis. Sci.* 47, 2625, 2002.

116. D'Souza, A.L., Rajkumar, C., Cooke, J., Bulpitt, C. Probiotics in prevention of antibiotic associated diarrhoea: meta-analysis. *Br. Med. J.* 324, 1361, 2002.

117. Kalliomaki, M., Salminen, S., Arvilommi, H., et al. Probiotics in primary prevention of atopic disease: a randomized placebo-controlled trial. *Lancet* 357, 1076, 2002.

118. Felley, C., Corthesy-Theulaz, I., Blanco, R.J., et al. Favourable effects of an acidified milk (La-1) on *Helicobacter pylori* gastritis in man. *Eur. J. Gastroenterol. Hepatol.* 13, 25, 2001.

119. Cunningham-Rundles, S., Ahrne, S., Bengmark, S., et al. Probiotics and immune response. *Am. J. Gastroenterol.* 95, Suppl. 1, S22, 2000.

120. Niedzielin, K., Kordecki, H., Birkenfeld, B. A controlled, double-blind, randomised study on the efficacy of *Lactobacillus plantarum* 299 in patients with irritable bowel syndrome. *Eur. J. Gastroentrol. Hepatol.* 13, 1143, 2001.

121. Shanahan, F. Probiotics and inflammatory bowel disease: from fads and fantasy to facts and future. *Br. J. Nutr.* 88 Suppl. 1, S5, 2002.

122. Marteau, P., Seksik, P., Jian, R. Probiotics and intestinal effects: a clinical perspective. *Br. J. Nutr.* 88 Suppl. 1, S51, 2002.

123. Simenhoff, M.L., Dunn, S.R., Zollner, G., et al. Biomodulation of the toxic and nutritional effects of small bowel bacterial overgrowth in end-stage kidney disease using freeze-dried *Lactobacillus acidophilus*. *Miner. Electrolyt. Metab.* 22, 92, 1006, 1996.

124. Hida, M., Aiba, Y., Sawamura, S., et al. Inhibition of the accumulation of uremic toxins in the blood and their precursors in feces after oral administration of Lebenin®, a lactic acid bacteria preparation, to uremic patients undergoing hemodialysis. *Nephron* 74, 349, 1994.

125. Bukowska, H., Pieczul-Mroz, J., Jastrzebska, M., et al. Decrease in fibrinogen and LDL-cholesterol levels upon supplementation of diet with *lactobacillus plantarum* in subjects with moderately elevated cholesterol. *Atherosclerosis* 137, 437, 1009, 1999.

126. Riordan, S.M., Skinner, N., Nagree, A., et al. Peripheral blood mononuclear cell expression of Toll-like receptors and relation to cytokine levels in cirrhosis. *Hepatology* 37, 5, 1154–1164, 2003.

127. Mao, H.C., personal communication.

128. Finegold, S.M., Sutter, V.L., Mathisen, G.E. Normal indigenous intestinal flora. In *Human Intestinal Microflora in Health and Disease*, Hentges D.J., ed. Academic Press, New York, 1983.

129. Ahrné, S., Nobaek, S., Jeppsson, B., et al. The normal *Lactobacillus* flora of healthy human rectal and oral mucosa. *J. Appl. Microbiol.* 85, 88, 1998.

130. Gustafsson, B. *The Future of Germ-Free Research*. Alan R. Liss, New York, 1985.

131. Hoyos, A.B. Reduced incidence of necrotizing enterocolitis associated with enteral administration of *Lactobacillus acidophilus* and *Bifidobacterium Infantis* to neonates in an intensive care unit. *Int. J. Infect. Dis.* 3, 197, 1999.

132. Buscher, H.J., Free, R.H., Van Weissenbruch, R., et al. Preliminary observations on influence of diary products on biofilm removal from silicon rubber voice prostheses *in vitro*. *J. Dairy Sci.* 83, 641, 1999.

133. van der Mei, H.C., Free, R.H., Elving, G.J., et al. Effect of probiotic bacteria on prevalence of yeasts in oropharyngeal biofilms on silicone rubber voice prostheses *in vitro*. *J. Med. Microbiol.* 49, 713, 2000.

134. Rosenfeldt, V., Benfeldt, E., Nielsen, S.D., et al. Effect of probiotic *Lactobacillus* strains in children with atopic dermatitis. *J. Allergy Clin. Immunol.* 111, 389, 2003.

135. Kalliomaki, M., Salminen, S., Poussa, T., et al. Probiotics and prevention of atopic disease: 4-year follow-up of a randomised placebo-controlled trial. *Lancet* 361, 1869, 2003.

11 Novel (Immune) Nutrients in Critical Illness

Joanna Lipp
University of Rochester

Harry C. Sax
University of Rochester School of Medicine and Dentistry

CONTENTS

11.1   INTRODUCTION

In recent years, the evolution of formulas containing pharmacologic doses of some nutrients has placed nutrition intervention beyond patient nourishment into the realm of disease prevention and treatment. Immunomodulary components are added to stimulate the immune response, increase wound healing, and, ultimately, decrease morbidity and mortality in the critically ill. The nutrients focused on are primarily glutamine, arginine, omega-3 fatty acids (FAs), and nucleotides. Few studies have been done on the effects of the individual nutrients in the critically ill human, and even fewer dose–response or kinetic studies have been undertaken. Most of the studies involving these nutrients in the critically ill patient population fall into one of two categories:

- Studies of tube feedings, most of which contain more than one immune-modulating agent
- Studies of parenteral glutamine

There is no agreement on exactly which combination or dose of nutrients is the "best" combination, and each enteral product marketed as "immune-enhancing" is different from every other product.

What does *immune-enhancing* actually mean? The normal inflammatory response to injury or infection increases fever and local blood flow, attracts immune cells to the site of injury, and activates those cells. Although some amount of inflammatory response is needed for appropriate immune function, excessive or chronic inflammatory response can lead to systemic inflammatory response syndrome (SIRS), adult respiratory distress syndrome (ARDS), chronic diseases such as rheumatoid arthritis, and possibly the wasting associated with AIDS or cancer.

Finally, determining which patients would benefit from having their immune responses altered, and to what extent, is unclear. In this chapter, we will review individual nutrients, then examine the multitude of studies involving immune-enhancing formulas.

11.2 GLUTAMINE

Glutamine is the most abundant amino acid in the plasma (1,2). The lung and skeletal muscle release glutamine into the plasma (1,2). Many major body systems utilize glutamine (1–3). The gut, kidney, and immune cells seem to have the highest utilization of glutamine, though the amount of glutamine that the human body or specific organs require is not known. Glutamine deficiency can occur after major trauma, major surgical stress, and in sepsis (4–8). Intracellular concentrations of glutamine in skeletal muscle fall in response to catabolic stress in septic patients, with survivors having higher muscle glutamine levels than nonsurvivors; blood levels did not correlate (4).

Glutamine participates in immune function in several ways (1,2). It may preserve the gut mucosal barrier and gut immune function, and it is a substrate for energy and for metabolic pathways involved in cell division, cytokine production, phagocytosis, and antioxidant production (9–11). Recent work has shown that glutamine is of equal significance to or greater significance than glucose as a fuel for immune cells, and the rate of utilization of both is high in both "resting" (8,9,12) and stimulated cells (9,12–14). Much of the glutamine used by immune cells is not fully oxidized but instead is shuttled into purine and pyrimidine synthesis, which is needed for the formation of DNA and RNA, supporting cell division and tissue regeneration (9).

Phagocytosis is the process by which cells of the immune system destroy foreign matter; this process involves releasing free radicals into the phagosome. Although it is not known what the immune system's response is to a low blood level of glutamine in the critical care patient, we know that, *in vitro*, phagocytosis is inefficient if there is a deficiency of glutamine in the culture medium (11).

If the cells had no protection against the free radicals they generate during phagocytosis, they would destroy themselves as well as the foreign matter they engulf. Glutathione is an intracellular antioxidant that is made in the cell from glutamate, cysteine, and glycine. Under various experimental conditions, the glutamate portion of the molecule can be derived from glutamine (15,16). Phagocytic cells devoid of glutathione become inactive a short time after phagocytosis, indicating that they were damaged by their own free radicals (17). Providing glutamine supplementation has been shown to improve glutathione levels in the gut (16) and liver (15).

Unfortunately, there is not a direct relationship between the blood level of glutamine and immune function (4). But what controls immune cells' use of glutamine is not known. Although the rate of glutamine metabolism in lymphocytes increases with increasing glutamine concentrations in the culture medium in the petri dish, what occurs in a critically ill patient is not as well characterized (8). Many factors, such as membrane transport and the functioning of certain enzymes, in addition to the blood level of glutamine, may affect the cells' rate of utilization of glutamine (8,9,12).

Several researchers have investigated the effect of glutamine supplementation on blood glutamine levels. Some of this work is with enteral glutamine, but most focuses on parenteral glutamine. The route of administration is important, because the kinetics and results are different, depending on the route. Hence, work done with parenteral glutamine does not seem to translate exactly to equivalent results when glutamine is used enterally.

Blood glutamine levels in bone marrow transplant patients receiving 0.285 vs. 0.57 g/kg/d glutamine in parenteral nutrition for 30 days were elevated but independent of dose (18). In summary, parenteral doses of glutamine of 12 to 40 g/d did not always return blood glutamine levels to normal in patients, though parenteral glutamine at a dose of about 40 g/d elevated blood glutamine levels in bone marrow transplant (BMT) patients (19). Only one study has examined the effect of glutamine supplementation on muscle glutamine levels, which is important in light of Roth's work on muscle glutamine and survival. In patients undergoing elective cholecystectomy, parenteral nutrition supplemented with a glutamine dose of 0.285 g/kg blunted the fall in muscle glutamine levels, compared to isonitrogenous, standard parenteral nutrition (6). Studies of enteral glutamine supplementation with doses in the range of 25 to 40 g/d show little or no increase in blood glutamine levels (20–22). The most commonly used dosing for enteral glutamine seems to be 0.5 g/kg/d.

Glutamine is relatively insoluble, heat labile, and unstable in solution. Because the processing may destroy glutamine, elemental and peptide-based products are likely to have less glutamine than formulas that contain intact proteins, unless glutamine has specifically been added (23). Glutamine is a component of protein, and all tube feedings that contain whole protein contain some glutamine. The glutamine content of most standard (non-glutamine-supplemented) tube feeding formulas is estimated to be in the range of 3 to 6 g/1000 kcal, though higher-protein formulas may contain a little more (23). The glutamine content of glutamine-supplemented formulas is about 10 to 15 g/1000 kcal. It may not be necessary to add free glutamine to enteral products. Protein-bound glutamine is effectively extracted by the GI tracts of healthy volunteers; however, the same may or may not be true in critical illness (24).

Glutamine is not a component of standard parenteral amino acid solutions in the United States, primarily because it is poorly soluble and unstable in solution or when warmed (18,25,26). However, glutamine-containing dipeptides may be a practical alternative. Parenteral glycylglutamine and alanylglutamine are both used by the body in a manner very similar to what would occur if each amino acid had been infused individually (27–29). Parenteral glutamine dipeptides are commercially available in Europe. Dipeptides are also being added to enteral formulas.

Some caution may be warranted with glutamine supplementation. Previous studies of the safety of parenteral glutamine have shown an increase in liver function tests (LFTs) in home parenteral nutrition patients who were switched to glutamine-supplemented parenteral nutrition (26). In addition, BMT patients who received glutamine-supplemented parenteral nutrition had a statistically significant increase in total bilirubin, though there was no definable adverse clinical outcome associated with it (19). Although no alteration in LFTs has been reported with enteral glutamine supplementation, LFTs should be monitored closely in patients receiving enteral glutamine supplementation until more research is done. It is also important to realize that the GI tract metabolizes glutamine into glutamate and ammonia, and enteral glutamine is now being used as an encephalapathy challenge for patients with liver insufficiency (30).

Little work has been done in the critically ill using enteral formulas that differ only in glutamine content. Jensen et al. studied 19 ICU patients, 10 of whom received a "high glutamine" elemental tube feeding; the controls received a feeding with a lower glutamine content (20). The amount of glutamine the patients received (g/d or g/kg body weight) was not specifically stated in the publication, but those on the high GLN formula probably received in the range of 30 to 35 g/d. Plasma glutamine levels rose in both groups and were not different between groups. The patients who received the higher-glutamine formula had an increased CD4/CD8 at day 5 compared to baseline; this difference disappeared by day 10. However, there was not a statistically significant difference overall in CD4/CD8 in those who received the higher amount of glutamine compared to those who received the lower amount of glutamine. Morbidity and mortality were not reported.

Houdijk also studied high- vs. low-glutamine enteral feedings (31). In 60 trauma patients, infectious morbidity during the first 15 days in ICU was the primary outcome. They found that those who received the higher amount of glutamine had less pneumonia, less bacteremia, less sepsis, and delayed onset of infectious complications (e.g., no significant infections in the first week for those who received the higher amount of glutamine). Despite what seem like clinically significant differences in infections, there were no differences in days on the ventilator, hospital length of stay (LOS), or mortality. Plasma glutamine rose more quickly in the group with the higher glutamine intake, but there was no difference in plasma glutamine after seven days. Those who received glutamine also had lower levels of soluble tumor necrosis factors. Likewise, Conejero found fewer infections, especially pneumonias, but no difference in morbidity, mortality, or length of stay in patients with SIRS who received glutamine supplementation (32).

Two studies of enteral glutamine have been done in patients with burns. Zhou et al. studied patients with 50 to 80% body surface area (BSA) burns without inhalation injury who received alanylglutamine to provide 0.35 g glutamine/kg body weight (33). They found hospital LOS to be shorter and healing time to be shorter in those who received the glutamine. Plasma glutamine levels improved in those who received the glutamine dipeptide but not in the control group. Garrel et al. provided 26 g glutamine/d to patients with burns of at least 20% body surface area, with or without inhalation injury (34). In this study, more than half of the patients in each group had < 40% BSA burn, and there was a slight preponderance toward more inhalation injury in the control group (37% in glutamine group, 45% in control group). This study is also confounded by the provision of a large percentage of the patients' nutrition as parenteral support. Garrel's group found that those who received glutamine did not have an improvement in blood glutamine levels, and although they had less bacteremia overall, there was no difference in Gram-negative vs. Gram-positive cultures. Those who received enteral glutamine also had a significantly lower mortality rate; however, this study should be interpreted with caution due to the high mortality rate in the control group: 63% (12/19 on intention-to-treat basis) with an average burn size of 42 ± 16%.

Parenteral glutamine, when given in addition to enteral nutrition in burn patients, reduced Gram-negative bacteremias and C-reactive protein (35). Wischmeyer randomized 26 patients with large burns (average 50% BSA) to receive 0.57 g glutamine/kg or isonitrogenous control intravenously. As with other studies of glutamine, despite decreases in some infectious data, there was not a statistically significant difference in mortality or length of stay, though those in the group that received IV glutamine had trends toward improvements in those outcomes.

Griffiths et al. studied outcomes in patients in an intensive care setting who could not tolerate enteral feedings (36). Patients were followed for six months. Patients were randomized to receive either standard parenteral nutrition or isonitrogenous glutamine-supplemented parenteral nutrition. On average, patients received about 20 g glutamine parenterally per day as long as they required parenteral nutrition. These patients were older (median age 65), and more than half were chronically ill prior to emergency admission to the ICU. There were few trauma patients overall, but there were more trauma patients in the glutamine group; nearly half of the control group developed renal failure. Those who received glutamine had a shorter time from ICU admission to death for the nonsurvivors; survivors who received glutamine had a longer length of stay overall, and although mortality for the first three weeks was not different between the groups, those who received glutamine had lower overall mortality at six months. Blood glutamine levels rose more quickly in those receiving glutamine-supplemented parenteral nutrition, but by seven days there was no difference in glutamine levels between the glutamine-supplemented patients and the controls.

Powell-Tuck et al. randomized 168 patients to glutamine-supplemented (20 g/d) vs. control parenteral nutrition and did not find any significant differences in morbidity, short-term or six-month mortality, or infectious complications (37). In this study, 40 to 45% of patients were ICU patients, and the remainder were apparently on the regular wards. The patients were from various services (primarily hematology and surgery, with some medicine and other services).

Although glutamine holds promise as an immune-enhancing agent, the data are not clear that supplementing glutamine in the critically ill improves outcomes. Generally, the few studies that have shown changes in immune parameters or outcomes have used parenteral glutamine; the exception seems to be Zhou's work with enteral alanylglutamine in burn patients.

11.3 ARGININE

Arginine, the major positively charged amino acid, holds a unique role in immunomodulation literature. Initial studies in arginine-deficient rodents showed significant thymic atrophy and was associated with reduced neutrophil and macrophage function. Supplementation with arginine reversed these effects (38,39). Arginine supports the production of nitric oxide (NO), an important component of smooth muscle relaxation and regulator of blood flow. The immunostimulatory effects were further studied by Alexander's group, who found improved survival in burned guinea pigs subjected to smoke inhalation. However, there appeared to be an inverted dose–response curve, in which both low and higher levels of arginine supplementation led to worse survival (0% ARG to 56% mortality, 1% ARG to 29% mortality, 2% ARG to 22% mortality, 4% ARG to 56% mortality) (40). Thus, the immunostimulatory effects of arginine can be exaggerated, raising the specter of SIRS induction (see Chapter 35).

Human studies have focused on the *in vitro* effects of arginine on human lymphocyte response and collagen synthesis. Barbul's groups have published a series of studies using oral supplementation of 17 g arginine per day, primarily in an elderly population. They have shown improved collagen deposition in subcutaneously implanted sponges, as well as increased peripheral lymphocyte response to mitogens. An elevation in IGF-1 is consistently seen, although the correlation to other immune metabolic effects is not clear (41–43). Arginine is a constituent of many of the immune-enhancing diets (IEDs). It is interesting that the high levels in some formulations may be ameliorated by relative inflammatory inhibiting compounds, such as the omega-3 PUFA.

Concern has been raised regarding the use of arginine in septic patients because the vasodilation associated with sepsis may be augmented by arginine through the NO pathway. Further, the issues of exacerbation of ARDS is not yet completely clear. On balance, the improved blood flow at the cellular level induced by arginine should support metabolic function, although reperfusion effects with the generation of free radicals is a theoretical concern. In a study of 220 critically ill patients, Caparros studied a diet enriched in arginine, fiber, and antioxidants to a standard enteral product. The supplemented group had lower incidence of catheter infections (44). There was no difference in other major septic complications, such as UTI, pneumonia, or bacteremia. Although there was no difference in mortality, subgroup analysis suggested improved six-month survival in medical patients treated with the experimental formula more than two days (76 vs. 67%). It seems unlikely such a short course would have any major metabolic effect.

On balance, arginine shows promise in reducing subsequent infections in hemodynamically stable, septic patients. It may induce further vasodilation and hypotension, although the heterogeneous nature of this subset of patients will make it difficult to identify specifically a single cause (45).

11.4 OMEGA-3 FATTY ACIDS

Two of the major n-3 FAs that appear in human tissues are 20:5n-3 (eicosapentanoic acid [EPA]), and 22:5n-3 (decosahexanoic acid [DHA]) (46). EPA and DHA are long-chain n-3 fatty acids currently of clinical interest for several reasons. DHA and EPA are thought to be beneficial for the infant brain and eyesight and are now added to some infant formulas (46,47). EPA can influence prostaglandin synthesis, which can alter immune response, and EPA and DHA are added to some enteral formulas for the critically ill.

Humans can make long-chain fatty acids of the n-6 and n-3 families once the 18 carbon precursors are provided (48) (Figure 11.1). Linoleic acid, an n-6 FA, is the precursor for arachadonic acid (ARA), and α-linolenic acid, an n-3 FA, is the precursor for EPA. Linoleic acid and α-linolenic acid share, and compete for, desaturation and elongation enzymes to transform them into longer-chain PUFAs. Although α-linolenic acid can be converted into longer-chain PUFAs, most undergo β-oxidation completely to carbon dioxide and water, or can undergo intermediate oxidation to precursors of DHA (46). The metabolic pathways and controls that transform α-linolenic acid into long-chain compounds are complex (49). In general, conversion of α-linolenic acid to EPA is a very inefficient process and is affected by age, gender, and either the absolute amount of n-6, the absolute amount of long chain n-3, or the ratio of n-6 to n-3 in the diet (46,50,51).

Supplying preformed EPA and DHA circumvents these metabolic controls, and this becomes important when one considers the n-3 FA source in nutritional formulations for the critically ill. Some vegetable oils (rapeseed [canola] and soybean) are good sources of α-linolenic acid, but most vegetable oils contain few n-3 fats, and they do not contain the long-chain n-3 FAs EPA and DHA (52).

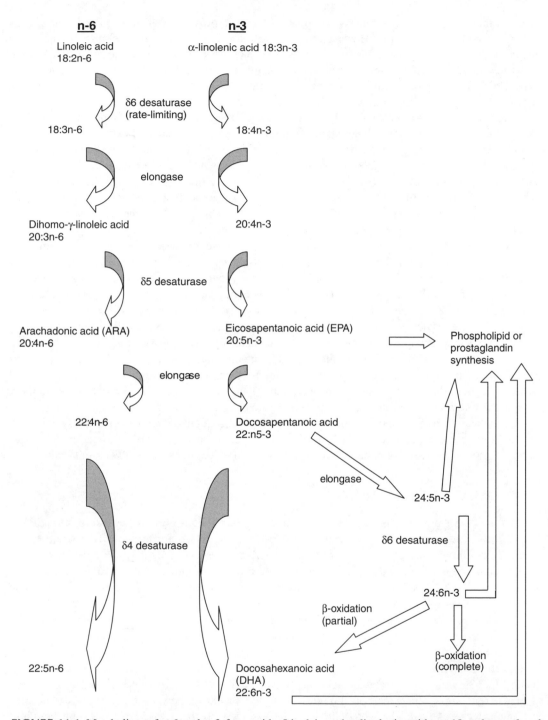

FIGURE 11.1 Metabolism of n-6 and n-3 fatty acids. Linoleic and α-linolenic acid are 18-carbon n-6 and n-3 precursors for longer-chain FAs. Longer-chain FAs of interest are ARA, EPA, and DHA. The n-6 and n-3 FAs compete for many of the same enzymes. EPA moves from peroxisome to endoplasmic reticulum for either phospholipid synthesis or elongation; the resulting 24:6n-3 can either move to the mitochondria for β-oxidation or be degraded to DHA. Also, EPA inhibits metabolism of linoleic acid to ARA. (Compiled from Sprecher H., Chen, Q., and Yin, F.Q., *Lipids*, 34, S153, 1999; and Holub, B.J., *Can. Med. Assoc. J.*, 166, 608, 2002.)

TABLE 11.1
n-3:n-6 Ratios of Immune-Enhancing Products

Product	n-3 : n-6
Immune-Aid	1.0 : 2.18
Impact	1.0 : 1.47
Option One	1.0 : 0.86
Oxepa	1.0 : 2.0

Note: Only products that contain n-3 from a marine source are included.

Oils from certain deep-ocean or cold-water fish are high in n-3 FAs, especially EPA and DHA. Although some products list canola oil as a source of n-3 FA, the source for EPA and DHA in most nutritional products for the critically ill is fish oils. "Fish oil" is a nonspecific term, and fish oils are approximately 30 to 37% n-3 (including all carbon lengths, not just EPA and DHA) (48,53); Manheden oil is approximately 13% EPA and 8% DHA (53).

The typical American diet provides about 1 to 3 g α-linolenic acid per day and 0.10 to 0.15 g EPA plus DHA per day (approximately 0.15% of dietary fat intake) but 12 to 15 g n-6 per day, such that the n-3:n-6 ratio of the typical American diet is about 1.0:8.0 (54). Commercially available "immune-enhancing" enteral products that have fish oil as a source of n-3 have n:3-n:6 ratios of 1.0:0.86 to 1.0:2.18 (based on 55) (Table 11.1). No studies have been done in the critically ill to determine whether there is an optimum ratio, but an n-3:n-6 ratio of 1:3 has been proposed (56).

The FA composition of the diet dictates the FA composition of the plasma membrane, which in turn influences membrane fluidity, receptors and their functions, and the activation of intracellular signaling pathways (48). Both ARA and EPA can be released from the cell membranes by phospholipase A_2 and then can be metabolized either via the cyclooxygenase pathway, to produce prostaglandins and thromboxanes, or via the 5-lipoxygenase pathway, to produce leukotrienes (48,57). The prostaglandins and thromboxanes derived from ARA are of the 2 series, whereas those derived from EPA are of the 3 series; leukotrienes from ARA are of the 4 series, and leukotrienes from EPA are of the 5 series. If the diet is high in n-6 FA and low in n-3 FA, cell membranes are correspondingly high in n-6; hence, ARA is usually the precursor for eicosanoids (57). These metabolites, when derived from n-6 FAs, are more biologically active in the inflammatory process than if the parent compound is n-3. However, the inflammatory process is very complex, and n-6- and n-3-derived substances participate in both up-regulation and down-regulation to some degree (Figure 11.2).

The FAs released into the cell by phospholipases can be used for prostaglandin synthesis, as discussed earlier, or can act directly as second messengers to alter both intracellular and extracelluar events. PGE_2 increases intracellular cAMP levels and prevents the increase in intracellular calcium that is an early event in T cell activation; it also inhibits the production of IL_2 and IL_2 receptors, which in turn alter protein kinase C activation (48). Long-chain n-3 FAs decrease many cytokines (IL-1, IL-2, IL-4, IL-6, TNF-α, INF-γ), monocyte and lymphocyte adhesion, neutrophil chemotaxis, and C-reactive protein (48,58). Fatty acids can act as secondary messengers to activate protein kinase C (48). Different isoforms of protein kinase C can be affected by different long-chain fatty acids (48), accounting for different biological effects of the different fatty acids, including changes in gene expression that may alter the redox status of the cell (58). Ultimately, the production of eicosanoids, cytokines, and other cellular activities, including gene expression, can be altered by plasma and cell membrane fatty acids (48), which are altered by dietary long-chain fatty acids.

Thus, the theory is that patients with up-regulated inflammatory processes (autoimmune diseases, sepsis, SIRS, ARDS) should be given fewer omega-6 FAs and more omega-3 FAs so that

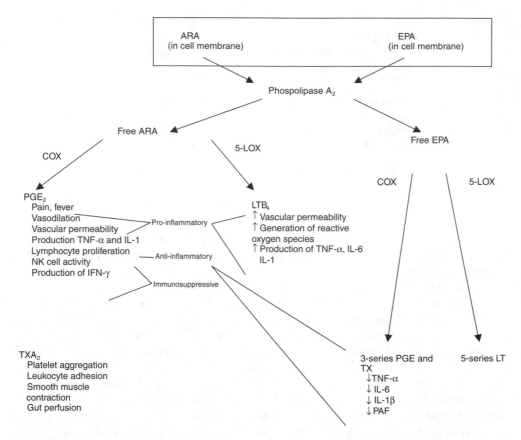

FIGURE 11.2 Metabolism of arachadonic acid (ARA) and eicosapentanoic acid (EPA) into prostaglandins. Both ARA and EPA in the cell membrane can be metabolized by the cyclooxygenase (COX) and 5-lipoxygenase (5-LOX) pathways. Metabolism of ARA results in prostaglandins (PGE) of the 2 series, leukotrienes (LT) of the 4 series, and thromboxanes (TX) of the A_2 series; most (but not all) of which are considered proinflammatory or immunosuppressive. Examples of some the prostaglandins and their functions (including whether they are considered proinflammatory, anti-inflammatory, or immunosuppressive) are depicted. Metabolism of EPA results in many similar prostagladins, but they are of the 3 series for PGEs and the 5 series for LTs. The EPA-derived prostaglandins are generally considered less inflammatory than their ARA-derived counterparts. Free ARA and EPA in the plasma may also serve as substrates for these pathways. (Compiled based on information in Alexander, J.W., *Nutrition*, 14, 627, 1998; and Calder, P.C., in *Nutrition and Critical Care*, Nestle Nutrition Workshop Series Clinical and Performance Program, 2003.)

fewer inflammatory cytokines are produced. Animal studies of n-3 FAs using endotoxemia/SIRS models have shown decreased production of ARA-derived eicosanoids, decreased catabolic response parameters (decreased fever, acidosis, weight loss, lung edema), maintenance of splanchnic blood flow, and decreased mortality (57). Several studies have recently been done with IV omega-3 lipids in human patients. These studies showed that patients who received 0.2 g fish oil/kg/d had some alterations in immune function but no differences in coagulation factors or platelet function (57). Although there were no differences in infection rates or mortality, ICU LOS and total hospital LOS were shortened (57).

A number of small clinical trials in humans have been done with enteral doses of 1.0 to 6.0 g/d of omega-3 FAs, with study time frames of weeks to years. The studies have shown decreased disease progression in IgA nephropathy, lower rejection rates and increased graft survival in renal transplant, decreased subjective complaints and medication requirements in rheumatoid arthritis, and decreased disease activity and reduction or discontinuation of steroid use in patients with ulcerative colitis (59). However, omega-3 FA supplementation showed no benefit in patients with lupus nephritis, Crohn's disease, psoriasis, or atopic dermatitis (59).

In one trial in critically ill humans, a primary variable was the amount of omega-3 FAs. This study was done on patients with ARDS and used enteral feedings with 4.55 g EPA/l and 0.49 g DHA/l, with an n:3–n:6 ratio of 1.0:1.75 (60). The study formula also differed from the control formula in the content of α-linolenic acid, vitamin E, vitamin C, taurine, and carnitine. Patients (n = 146) with "illnesses known to be associated with ARDS" were randomized, and if they had pulmonary compromise with P_aO_2/F_iO_2 < 250 torr but > 100 torr and neutrophil count > 10% on broncheolar lavage, they were entered in the study. Enteral nutrition was continued for a minimum of 3 days; the goal was to complete at least 7 days of enteral feeding, at a caloric minimum of 75% of BEE × 1.3. Conventional modes of ventilation with standard I:E ratios were used. Plasma phospholipids were checked upon study entry, between day 3 and day 5, and again between day 6 and day 8. Outcome variables included time of mechanical ventilation and days in the ICU. Patients were not well matched for gender (control 40% male, study 65% male), and nearly one-third of randomized patients were deemed "unevaluable" due to early extubation. Fifteen percent of patients (15/98) overall were extubated between day 4 and day 7 of the study, with 12/17 study patients, but only 3/16 control patients, extubated during this time. Fewer patients in the study group developed additional organ failures during the treatment period. Those in the study group had shorter ICU stays (decrease of 3 to 4 days, intent-to-treat analysis), but mortality was not different between the groups. The authors state that there were significant (p < 0.001) increases in EPA in the plasma of patients fed the study diet, but plasma levels *per se* are not reported; diagrams in the report suggest EPA rose from about 0.5% of plasma phospholipid at baseline to over 7%. No differences in adverse events were reported.

Another study, of burn patients, compared two low-fat diets (15% calories as fat), one of which contained 50% of the fat as fish oil, to a control diet that was 35% fat and high in omega-6 (61). Protocol at the institution where the study was conducted is to use a combination of parenteral and enteral nutrition, and patients in all groups received more calories parenterally than enterally. In this small study, the patients in both low-fat groups had better outcomes than the patients in the control group, with fewer pneumonias and shorter time to heal when calculated in days per percent burn. This study does not support the use of omega-3 fatty acids in burn patients in the doses studied to date.

Dosing, timing, and adverse effects of n-3 FAs on the critically ill are being researched. Because some studies of omega-3 use in ICU patients have shown improved outcomes in short periods of time, the mechanism of action may be one that does not actually require incorporation of these FAs into the cell membrane. Based on Gadek's study, plasma FA concentrations can change in as little as three days with enteral supplementation, and red cells may begin to change composition after five days of enteral supplementation (60). It may not be necessary for omega-3 fatty acids to be incorporated into the membranes to alter eicosanoid and cytokine responses — free FAs in the plasma may be sufficient. Dupont et al. suggest that a parenteral physical mixture containing 10% fish oil showed "substantial incorporation" of EPA into membrane phospholipids of white blood cells and platelets in as little as five hours (62). Even though the percentage of EPA in plasma phospholipids increased in healthy women who took 2.4 g EPA per day for 28 days, the percentage of arachadonic acid hardly decreased (63). This might suggest that the amount of long-chain n-3 in the diet is more important than the n:3–n:6 ratio, though this has not been researched.

Also, the optimal dose of omega-3 FA is not known — some studies in healthy volunteers suggest immunosuppression with very high intakes of fish oils, especially in states of low antioxidant status (57). One study suggested the greatest reduction in TNF-α occurs at 1.0 g/EPA plus DHA, with cytokine production higher at 2.0 g/d (64). Intakes of 3 to 4 g combined EPA and DHA per day result in mild increases in bleeding times (54).

11.5 DIETARY NUCLEOTIDES

Yeast RNA is an important component in the support of T cell function and immune competence. As is common in much nutritional research, this work sprang from investigations of dietary manipulation to increase graft survival after organ transplantation. This work has been promulgated in a series of animal studies by Van Buren and Kulkarni. They showed that a nucleotide-free diet would prolong allograft survival through manipulation of T lymphocyte function (65,66). They then showed that RNA could improve host response to candidiasis, a major pathogen in critically ill patients (67). Further, nucleotide synthesis may be an important component of the maintenance of enterocyte proliferation in response to arginine and glutamine, other major components of immune-enhancing diets (68). Finally, there is great interest in nucleotides to reverse the immune suppression seen in astronauts during long periods of weightlessness, as would be necessary with colonization of space (69). Although there are no studies using isolated nucleotide supplementation in critically ill patients, nucleotides appear to be synergistic with other immunonutrients.

11.6 IMMUNE-ENHANCING FORMULAS

Because nosocomial infections are a major concern in the critically ill and may significantly contribute to mortality, length of ICU stay, and length of overall hospital stay, it is hoped that immune enhancing diets (IEDs) will decrease the incidence of such infections and thus decrease these outcomes. This section will review some of the work done in this area, first in the critically ill or trauma situation, then in surgical patients.

A study by Bower et al. compared the use of one such formula (Impact®) containing n-3 PUFA, arginine, and nucleotides with a common-use formula in 296 critically ill patients whose precipitating event was either trauma, operation, or new onset of infection that required ICU admission (70). The study question was whether feeding the IED from within 48 hours of the "precipitating event" through day 7 of ICU stay would decrease hospital LOS. Patients were stratified by age and whether they had sepsis or SIRS. The goal was that by 96 hours after ICU admission, patients received a minimum of 60 cc/h of either formula, plus additional calories to meet their needs based on indirect calorimetry. On average, feedings were started 1.5 days after the precipitating event, and 200 of 279 patients were "successfully" fed by 96 hours. At day 7 of the study, the investigators were "free to provide whatever feeding was felt to be appropriate for the remainder of the hospitalization." The two formulas were not isonitrogenous, and therefore neither were the feeding regimens of the two groups; however, this difference in nitrogen intake was considered not to be a factor in the overall results. Data from some randomized patients were not analyzed because patients did not meet entrance criteria or did not receive feedings.

Of those who were fed, on an intent-to-treat basis, there was no significant difference in mortality or LOS, though there was a trend toward higher mortality in those who received the IED (23/147 vs. 10/132), especially for those stratified as septic (11/44 vs. 5/45). Most deaths in septic patients were due to multiple organ failure. There was a nonsignificant trend toward shorter LOS in those who received the IED (21 vs. 26 days). The authors did a *post hoc* subgroup analysis and concluded that, in a subgroup of patients who were septic and received a certain amount of feeding, those receiving the IED had decreased length of both ICU and overall hospital stays, as well as decreased use of antibiotics. Based on their subgroup analysis results, the authors concluded that the experimental formula decreased the probability of an infection that resulted from a high illness severity score and had an indirect benefit of reducing the length of stay by decreasing the probability of such infections (70). One should keep in mind that there was a higher mortality rate in the group of patients who received the experimental formula, especially those who were stratified as septic.

Kudsk et al. randomized patients who had suffered severe traumas (ATI > 25) to either an IED (Immune-Aid®) or isonitrogenous standard high-protein enteral diet (Promote with Casec) (71). There were 17 patients in the Immune-Aid group and 18 patients in the control group, and feedings were started about 1.5 days after admission and continued for 9 to 10 days. Immune-Aid is high in arginine, contains free glutamine, and claims to have omega-3 fatty acids, but the type of omega-3 in Immune-Aid is probably not functional in the critically ill. The authors also followed a third group, which served as unfed controls; these patients were not randomized to be unfed, they were patients who would have been eligible for the study but for some reason did not have enteral access. The authors state the "two patients died in the treatment group and were dropped from the study"; otherwise, no data on mortality are provided. Patients on the IED had fewer septic complications, including fewer intra-abdominal abscesses, and shorter overall hospital LOS, but trends toward shorter ICU LOS and fewer days on the ventilator did not reach significance.

Atkinson et al. randomized 398 "general ICU" patients with APACHE II score > 10 to either an IED (Impact) or isonitrogenous, intact-nutrient control feed, stratified by volume of feed received, with mortality as the primary endpoint (72). Patients were heterogeneous — some were trauma victims, some were surgical patients, and some were medical patients. Feeds were started within 48 hours (primarily through nasogastric tubes), goal feeds were 32 kcal/kg ideal body weight, and whatever feeding the patient was randomized to was continued until discharge from the ICU. Analyses were done on both intention-to-treat ($n = 390$) and volume-of-feed bases (any amount, $n = 369$; ≥ 2.5 l feed in 72 h, $n = 101$). Patients in the "successfully" fed group (≥ 2.5 l/72 h) received 17 to 19 kcal/kg ideal body weight. Data from patients who died were censored. Mortality was high, but equivalent, in both groups (48% Impact, 44% control) on an intention-to-treat basis, and tended slightly higher in the Impact group for those who were successfully fed (42% Impact, 37% control, NS). Patients in the "successfully fed" group who received Impact had statistically significantly shorter ICU and hospital LOS and fewer days on the ventilator, but Kaplan–Meier plots appear to show a higher early mortality for those who received Impact. When deaths were censored, the differences in LOS became nonsignificant.

Two studies have been done in patients with burns — one by Gottschlich et al. and one by Saffle et al. (73,74). Gottschlich's study compared three diets (73):

- Group 1 was a standard, moderate-fat diet.
- Group 2 was a modular IED that was low in fat overall and contained approximately 5 g n-3/l and 6 g arginine/l.
- Group 3 was a standard, high-fat diet.

The study showed those on the IED had a decrease in wound infections (based on wound culture results, not clinical significance), but no difference in days on the ventilator or other infectious complications. The study also showed a decrease in hospital LOS per % burn for those on the IED, but this was calculated for survivors only; there is no information on LOS on an intent-to-treat basis. There was no difference in mortality between the groups on the IED and the standard, moderate-fat diet, but those on the standard higher-fat diet (group 3) had a trend toward more deaths. A caveat here is that there were more patients with inhalation injury in group 3, which could have increased the mortality rate in this group.

In contrast, the study by Saffle et al. did not find any benefits to using the IED on burn patients (74). The authors suggest that there may not have been enough of a difference between the IED and the control diet; they state the control diet contains a similar amount of n-3 fats to the experimental diet, leaving them to suggest that the arginine content is the only truly different factor. However, the source of n-3 FA in the control diet was canola oil. As pointed out Section 11.4, 18-carbon n-3 PUFA have a low rate of conversion to EPA and DHA, and 18-carbon n-3s have little, if any, physiologic effect that we know of, so the n-3 content of the control formula is probably of little consequence. It may be worth observing that Gottschlich's study was done primarily with children, whereas Saffle's was done with adults.

One study has shown trends toward adverse effects of immune-altering feedings in the critically ill trauma patient. Mendez et al. used an experimental enteral diet that contained 6.6 g arginine/l and approximately 1.5 g/l n-3 from canola oil, or a control diet that was a standard commercial product (Osmolite HN with added protein) (75). Patients began enteral nutrition within three days of admission and received either the standard or test diet for at least five days. Outcome variables were:

- Mortality
- Incidence of ARDS
- Infection rates
- Pneumonia rates
- Length of ICU stay
- Number of days on the ventilator
- Overall LOS

Fifty-nine patients were enrolled, but only 43 were deemed evaluable. There were no statistical differences in outcomes between groups. However, there were trends toward more infections overall, including more pneumonias, longer overall LOS, longer ICU stay, and more days on the ventilator in those receiving the immune-altering formula. There was also more ARDS in the group who received the immune-altering diet, but most cases of ARDS in both groups were diagnosed before the start of the enteral feedings. This study is criticized for the inordinately large percentage of patients with ARDS, especially in the group that received the immune-altering enteral feeding. Some immune parameters were also studied, and it appeared that the immune responses of those who received the immune-altering enteral feeding returned to normal faster than those who received the standard feeding; in particular, monocyte PGE_2 was significantly higher in those who received the immune-altering diet. In this study, like Saffle's study, the source of n-3 fatty acids was canola oil, which is not efficiently converted to EPA, so the diets probably realistically differed only in arginine content. No work has been done on FA conversion in the critically ill, and, unfortunately, this study did not document any blood EPA levels.

Weimann et al. studied an immune-enhancing formula (Impact) that contained arginine, fish oils, and nucleotides after severe trauma ($n = 16$) vs. an isocaloric, isonitrogenous control feed ($n = 13$) (76). Twenty-nine patients were evaluable; patients in the immune-enhancing feed group had a trend toward more abdominal trauma (8/16 vs. 4/13), which, in this small study, did not reach statistical significance. Primary endpoints were SIRS and multiple organ failure (MOF); secondary endpoints were mortality, infection rates, and hospital LOS. Patients were fed gastrically and did not receive feedings overnight. Patients also received parenteral nutrition with IV MCT to meet caloric goals when enteral feeding did not reach target. On average, patients received 561 ml/d of feedings. Patients who received the IED had fewer days of SIRS per patient (8.3 ± 6.3 vs. 13.3 ± 6.7) and lower MOF scores on some days. There was no difference in infection rates, pneumonia rates, days on the ventilator, hospital LOS, or mortality between the two groups. So there seems to be no clear advantage to the immune-modulating diet in patients with severe trauma.

A study by Galban et al. randomized 181 hemodynamically stable, infected ICU patients to get an IED (Impact) vs. standard enteral nutrition; the most common infection upon study entry was pneumonia (57% of experimental patients, 69% of control patients) (77). Five patients were excluded after randomization. Treating physicians were not blinded to which feeding the patients received. Calories were prescribed based on ideal body weight and a fixed stress factor (1.3) for all patients; feedings were started by 36 hours after the diagnosis of sepsis and were scheduled to reach goal rate by day 4 of the study. Outcome variables were acquired infections, mortality, and ICU LOS. Total number of acquired infections was the same for both groups, though there were more acquired bacteremias in the control group (22%) than in the experimental group (8%). As well as having more bacteremias, the control group had a higher mortality rate (32%) than those who received the IED (19%). Subgroup analysis suggests the mortality advantage of the IED was most pronounced for those patients with an APACHE II score of 10 to 15. Of those who died, 59%

of those on the IED and 57% of those on the control diet died of MOF. ICU LOS and days on the ventilator were not different between groups.

In a meta-analysis, Heyland et al. state that immune-enhancing diets offer no advantages with regard to mortality or infections for the critically ill and, in fact, suggest that there may be an increased rate of death among those who get the IED (78). They analyzed 22 trials and approximately 200 patients. Immunonutrition led to a nonsignificant increased risk of mortality (RR 1.10, CI 0.93 to 1.31) but a significantly decreased risk of infectious complications (RR 0.66, CI 0.54 to 0.80). Heyland's group focused on the arginine content of the IEDs and suggested that the formulas with the higher arginine content (Impact, Immune-Aid) were the most efficacious. Most of the studies in the critically ill or trauma patients used Impact, which also contains n-3 fatty acids from fish oil (EPA and DHA); only one study used Immune-Aid, which contains n-3 from canola oil. Of interest is that the studies with the highest quality score showed both an increase in mortality risk and a decrease in infectious complications. The implication is that once infection-induced severe SIRS has developed, further immunostimulation is potentially harmful. In general, the data do not seem to support the use of IEDs in trauma or critical illness.

Any attempt at mediating the inflammatory response is most likely to be successful if the modulating agent is on board at the time of the insult. By the same token, maintenance of intracellular glutamine stores prior to insult and catabolism could reduce lean body mass loss. The ideal group to allow this type of study is patients undergoing major elective surgery. Unlike trauma patients, who tend to be healthy at the time of injury, patients with malignancy or in need of major GI or vascular surgery are already at increased risk. Even if they do not manifest weight loss, they will have a major, controlled traumatic insult that induces catabolism and raises the risk of infectious and wound complications. Buzby's classic study on the use of preoperative parenteral nutrition showed only benefit, with a reduction in wound complications in the most malnourished patients (79). This was offset by increased infectious complications in the less malnourished. One hypothesis is that, in retrospect, because significant calories were given as n-6 PUFAs, immunosuppression took place. The further issue of enteral vs. parenteral nutrition will not be addressed here.

Heys performed a meta-analysis of the use of immunonutrition in patients with both critical illness and cancer (80). He found an overall odds ratio of 0.47 (CI 0.30 to 0.73) for the development of major infectious complications in those patients receiving immune nutrition. This finding was repeated for the subgroup of patients with GI cancers. Nosocomial pneumonias and overall mortality were not affected. Perhaps due to the decreased infectious complications, patients receiving target IED had a short length of hospital stay of 2.5 days (CI 4.0 to 1.0 days).

Since publication of the meta-analysis, several papers have studied perioperative nutritional support, both with and without immunomodulating nutrients. Tepaske randomized 50 elderly patients who were to undergo CABG to an IED containing arginine, RNA, and n-3 PUFA or an isocaloric, isonitrogenous diet without immune-enhancing agents and with only n-6 PUFA (81). Patients consumed the diets for a minimum of five days preoperatively. The IED patients had increased delayed hypersensitivity *in vitro* and lower infectious complications. Length of stay and mortality were unchanged.

Braga entered almost 200 malnourished, elective surgical patients into three groups (82):

- "Standard" enteral feeds immediately postoperative
- Standard feeds both pre- and postoperatively
- An IED, both pre- and postoperatively

The operations were primarily gastric and pancreatic, with the remainder esophageal and colorectal. The group receiving perioperative IED had fewer infections and a shorter LOS than the group receiving the postoperative, standard diet. The perioperatively fed but nonenhanced diet was intermediate between the other two for infectious complications but also had a decreased LOS compared to control. This study emphasizes the importance of not only correcting preoperative deficits, but also of "loading" with immune-modulating nutrients prior to the insult.

Braga shortly thereafter published a study limited to colorectal cancer patients (83). It is unclear whether some patients from the previous study were included. The groups were slightly different:

- IED before and after surgery
- IED only preop
- Isocaloric isonitrogenous IED only preop
- No pre- or postop supplements

Diet was studied when GI function returned. Gut microperfusion was quantified intraoperatively, standard *in vitro* measures of macrophage response were assayed, and infectious complications were followed. The groups receiving immunomodulating nutrients, including arginine, had increased gut perfusion and decreased postoperative infectious complications (12% preop, 10% periop, 32% conventional preop, 35% standard). This was seen to support the concept of preemptive immunomodulation.

11.7 CONCLUSION

Immunonutrition is a broad category of interventions involving multiple nutrients targeting various end organs, with the most common immunomodulating nutrients being glutamine, arginine, and n-3 fatty acids. Immune-enhancing nutrients have been studied in various patient populations, with some surgical patients benefiting from these diets and many trauma or critically ill patients not showing any benefit from them. We may never see significant improvements in mortality; however, a reduction in infectious complications, leading to earlier discharge, may be an appropriate endpoint for use of these nutrients.

It is increasingly possible that these nutrients could be on board prior to planned surgeries or trauma or sepsis. For example, n-3 fatty acids are now prescribed under certain conditions for heart disease (84), as well as conditions such as rheumatoid arthritis, and because fish oils are available over the counter, many people may be taking them. DHA and EPA are now also added to some infant formulas and functional foods such as n-3-enriched eggs. Glutamine and arginine are being touted to improve many conditions, such as general immune function and increased recovery after sporting events. With supplement use on the rise, it is becoming increasingly possible that the nutritional status and immune function of patients now are different from what they were even 10 years ago. Research continues into which nutrients, in what amounts, and in what time frame they should be given.

REFERENCES

1. Smith, R.J., Glutamine metabolism and its physiologic importance, *JPEN*, 14, 40S, 1990.
2. Lacey, J.M., and Wilmore, D.W., Is glutamine a conditionally essential nutrient? *Nutr. Rev.*, 48, 297, 1990.
3. Souba, W.W., Smith, R.J., and Wilmore, D.W., Glutamine metabolism by the intestinal tract, *JPEN*, 9, 608, 1995.
4. Roth, E., et al., Metabolic disorders in severe abdominal sepsis: glutamine deficiency in skeletal muscle, *Clin. Nutr.*, 1, 25, 1982.
5. Askanazi, J., et al., Muscle and plasma amino acids following injury: influence of intercurrent infection, *Ann. Surg.*, 192, 78, 1980.
6. Hammarqvist, F., et al., Addition of glutamine to total parenteral nutrition after elective abdominal surgery spares free glutamine in muscle, counteracts the fall in muscle protein synthesis, and improves nitrogen balance, *Ann. Surg.*, 209, 455, 1989.

7. Souba, W.W., and Austgen, T.R., Interorgan glutamine flow following surgery and infection, *JPEN*, 14, 90S, 1990.
8. Newsholme, E.A., and Parry-Billings, M., Properties of glutamine release from muscle and its importance for the immune system, *JPEN*, 14, 63S, 1990.
9. Ardawi, M.S.M., and Newsholme, E.A., Glutamine metabolism in lymphocytes and its importance in the immune response, *Essays Biochem.*, 21, 1, 1985.
10. Wallace, C., and Keast, D., Glutamine and macrophage function, *Metabolism*, 41, 1016, 1992.
11. Ogle, C.K., et al., Effect of glutamine on phagocytosis and bacterial killing by normal and pediatric burn patient neutrophils, *JPEN*, 18, 128, 1994.
12. Ardawi, M.S.M., and Newsholme, E.A., Glutamine metabolism in lymphoid tissues. In *Glutamine Metabolism in Mammalian Tissues*, Haussinger, D., and Sies, H. (eds.), Springer-Verlag, Berlin, 235–246, 1984.
13. Brand, K., et al., Metabolism of glutamine in lymphocytes. *Metabolism*, 38, Suppl. 1, 29, 1989.
14. Spolaris, Z., et al., Glutamine and fatty acid oxidation are the main sources of energy for Kupffer and endothelial cells, *Am. J. Physiol.*, 261, G185, 1990.
15. Hong, R.W., et al., Glutamine preserves liver glutathione after lethal hepatic injury, *Ann. Surg.*, 215, 114, 1992.
16. Harward, T.R., et al., Glutamine preserves gut glutathione levels during intestinal ischemia/reperfusion, *J. Surg. Res.*, 56, 351, 1994.
17. Roos, D., Weening, R.S., and Voetman, A.A., Protection of human neutrophils against oxidative damage, *Agents and Actions*, 10, 528, 1980.
18. Ziegler, T.R., et al., Safety and metabolic effects of L-glutamine administration in humans, *JPEN,* 14, 137S, 1990.
19. Ziegler, T.R., et al., Clinical and metabolic efficacy of glutamine-supplemented parenteral nutrition after bone marrow transplantation, *Ann. Intern. Med.*, 116, 821, 1992.
20. Jensen, G.L., et al., A double-blind, prospective, randomized study of glutamine-enriched compared with standard peptide-based feeding in critically ill patients, *Am. J. Clin. Nutr.*, 64, 615, 1996.
21. Long, C.L., et al., Impact of enteral feeding of a glutamine-supplemented formula on the hypoaminoacidemic response in trauma patients, *J. Trauma*, 40, 97, 1996.
22. Buchman, A.L., et al., Parenteral nutrition is associated with intestinal morphologic and functional changes in humans, *JPEN*, 19, 453, 1995.
23. Swails, W.S., et al., Glutamine content of whole proteins: implications for enteral formulas, *Nutr. Clin. Pract.*, 7, 77, 1992.
24. Boza, J.J., et al., Free and protein-bound glutamine have identical splanchnic extraction in healthy human volunteers, *Am. J. Gastrointest. Liver Physiol.*, 281, G267, 2001.
25. Hardy, G., et al., Stability of glutamine in parenteral feeding solutions, *Lancet*, 342, 186, 1993.
26. Hornsby-Lewis, L., et al., L-glutamine supplementation in home total parenteral nutrition patients: stability, safety, and effects on intestinal absorption, *JPEN*, 18, 268, 1994.
27. Furst, P., and Stehle, P., The potential use of parenteral dipeptides in clinical nutrition, *Nutr. Clin. Prac.*, 8, 106, 1994.
28. Lochs, H., et al., Splanchnic, renal, and muscle clearance of alanylglutamine in man and organ fluxes of alanine and glutamine when infused in free and peptide forms, *Metab.*, 39, 833, 1990.
29. Abumrad, N.N., et al., Possible sources of glutamine for parenteral nutrition: impact on glutamate metabolism, *Am. J. Physiol.*, 257, E228, 1989.
30. Romero-Gomez, M., et al., Altered response to oral glutamine challenge as prognostic factor for overt episodes in patients with minimal hepatic encephalopathy, *J. Hepatol.*, 37, 781, 2002.
31. Houdijk, A.P.J., et al., Randomized trial of glutamine-enriched enteral nutrition on infectious morbidity in patients with multiple trauma, *Lancet*, 352, 772, 1998.
32. Conejero R., et al., Effect of a glutamine-enriched enteral diet on intestinal permeability and infectious morbidity at 28 days in critically ill patients with systemic inflammatory response syndrome: a randomized, single-blind, prospective, multicenter study, *Nutrition*, 18, 716, 2002.
33. Zhou, Y.P., et al., The effect of supplemental enteral glutamine on plasma levels, gut function, and outcome in severe burns: a randomized, double-blind, controlled clinical trial, *JPEN*, 27, 241, 2003.

34. Garrel, D., et al., Decreased mortality and infectious morbidity in adult burn patients given enteral glutamine supplements: a prospective, controlled, randomized clinical trial, *Crit. Care Med.*, 31, 2444, 2003.

35. Wischmeyer, P.E., et al., Glutamine administration reduces Gram-negative bacteremia in severely burned patients: a prospective, randomized, double-blind trial versus isonitrogenous control, *Crit. Care Med.*, 29, 2075, 2001.

36. Griffiths, R.D., Jones, C., and Palmer, T.E.A., Six-month outcome of critically ill patients given glutamine-supplemented parenteral nutrition, *Nutrition*, 13, 295, 1997.

37. Powell-Tuck, J., et al., A double-blind, randomised, controlled trial of glutamine supplementation in parenteral nutrition, *Gut*, 45, 83, 1999.

38. Barbul, A., Arginine: biochemistry, physiology, and therapeutic implications, *JPEN*, 10, 227, 1986.

39. Efron D., Barbul A., The role of arginine in immunonutrition, *J. Gastroenter.*, 35S 12, 20–28, 2000.

40. Saito H., Tocki O., Wang S.L., Gonce S.J., Joffe S.N., Alexander J.W., Metabolic and immune effects of dietary arginine supplementation after burn, *Arch. Surg.*, 122, 784–789, 1987.

41. Witte M.D., Thornton F.J., Tantry V., Barbul A., L-Arginine supplementation enhances diabetic wound healing: involvement of nitric oxide and arginase pathways, *Metab. Clin. Exp.*, 51, 1269–1273, 2002.

42. Kirk S.J., Hurson M., Regan M.C., Holt O.R., Wasserkreg H.L., Barbul A., Arginine stimulates wound healing and immune function in elderly human beings, *Surg.*, 114, 155–159, 1993.

43. Williams J.Z., Abumrad N., Barbul A., Effect of specialized amino acid mixture on human collagen deposition, *Ann. Surg.*, 236, 369–374, 2002.

44. Caparros T., Lopez J., Grau T., Early enteral nutrition in critically-ill patients with a high protein diet enriched with arginine, fiber and antioxidants compared with standard high-protein diet: the effect on nosocomial infections and outcome, *JPEN*, 25, 299–309, 2001.

45. Carcillo, J.A., Does arginine become a "near" essential amino acid during sepsis? *Crit. Care Med.* 31, 657–659, 2003.

46. Brenna, T.J., Efficiency of conversion of α-linolenic acid to long chain n-3 fatty acids in man, *Curr. Opin. Nutr. Metab. Care,* 5, 127, 2002.

47. Redgrave T.G., Lipids in enteral nutrition, *Curr. Opin. Clin. Metab. Care*, 2, 147, 1999.

48. Alexander, J.W., Immunonutrition: the role of -3 fatty acids, *Nutrition*, 14, 627, 1998.

49. Sprecher H., Chen, Q., and Yin, F.Q., Regulation of the biosynthesis of 22:5n-6 and 22:6n-3: a complex intracellular process, *Lipids*, 34, S153, 1999.

50. Emken, E., Alpha-linoleic acid conversion to n-3 LC-PUFAs, *PUFA Newsletter,* www.pufanewsletter.com, 2003.

51. Chen W, and Yeh, S., Effects of fish oil in parenteral nutrition, *Nutrition*, 19, 275, 2003.

52. Krause, M.L., Arlin, M., Lipids. In *Krause's Food, Nutrition and Diet Therapy*, 8th ed. W.B. Saunders, Philadelphia, 1992.

53. Bimbo, A.P., The emerging marine oil industry, *JAOCS*, 64, 706, 1987.

54. Holub, B.J., Clinical nutrition: omega-3 fatty acids in cardiovascular care, *Can. Med. Assoc. J.*, 166, 608, 2002.

55. American Society of Parenteral and Enteral Nutrition, Consensus recommendations from the U.S. summit on immune-enhancing enteral therapy, *JPEN*, 25 Suppl., S63, 2001.

56. Tashiro, T. et al., n-3 versus n-6 polyunsaturated fatty acids in critical illness, *Nutrition*, 14, 551, 1998.

57. Calder, P.C., Lipids and the critically ill patient. In *Nutrition and Critical Care*, vol. 8, Cynober C.L., and Moore, F.A. (eds.), Nestle Nutrition Workshop Series Clinical and Performance Program, Southampton, U.K., 2003.

58. Calder P.C., and Deckelbaum, R.J., Dietary lipids: more than just a source of calories, *Curr. Opin. Nutr. Metab. Care* 2, 105, 1999.

59. Endres, S., et al., n-3 polyunsaturated fatty acids: update 1995, *Eur. J. Clin. Invest.*, 25, 629, 1995.

60. Gadek, J.E., et al., Effect of enteral feeding with eicosapentaoic acid, -linolenic acid, and antioxidants in patients with acute respiratory distress syndrome, *Crit. Care Med.*, 27, 1409, 1999.

61. Garrel D.R., et al., Improved clinical status and length of care with low-fat nutrition support in burn patients, *JPEN*, 19, 482, 1995.

62. Dupont, I.E., and Carpentier, Y.A., Clinical use of lipid emulsions, *Curr. Opin. Clin. Nutr. Metab. Care*, 2, 139, 1999.

63. Stark, K.D., et al., Fatty acid compositions of serum phospholipids of postmenopausal women: a comparison between Greenland Inuit and Canadians before and after supplementation with fish oil, *Nutrition*, 18, 627, 2002.

64. *PUFA Newsletter*, www.pufanewsletter.com, September 2003.

65. Van Buren, C.T., et al., Dietary nucleotides, a requirement for helper/inducer T lymphocytes, *Transplantation*, 40, 694, 1985.

66. Kulkarni, S.S., et al., Prolongation of cardiac allograft survival by pretreatment of recipient mice with donor blood or spleen cells plus cyclophosphamide, *Cellular Immunol.*, 47, 192, 1979.

67. Fanslow, W.C., et al., Effect of nucleotide restriction and supplementation on resistance to experimental murine candidiasis, *JPEN*, 12, 49, 1988.

68. Yamauchi, K., et al., Glutamine and arginine affect Caco-2 cell proliferation by promotion of nucleotide synthesis, *Nutrition*, 18, 329, 2002.

69. Kulkarni, A.D., Yamauchi, K., Hales, N.W., Ramesh, V., Ramesh, G.T., Sundaresan, A., Andrassy R.J., Pellis, N.R., Nutrition beyond nutrition: plausibility of immunotrophic nutrition for space travel, *Clin. Nutr.*, 21, 231, 2002.

70. Bower, R.H., et al., Early enteral administration of a formula (Impact) supplemented with arginine, nucleotides, and fish oil in intensive care unit patients: results of a multicenter, prospective, randomized, clinical trial, *Crit. Care Med.*, 23, 436, 1995.

71. Kudsk, K.A., et al., A randomized trial of isonitrogenous enteral diets after severe trauma: an immune-enhancing diet reduces septic complications, *Ann. Surg.*, 224, 531, 1996.

72. Atkinson, S., Sieffert, E., and Bihari, D.: A prospective, randomized, double-blind, controlled clinical trial of enteral immunonutrition in the critically ill, *Crit. Care Med.*, 26, 1164, 1998.

73. Gottschlich, M.M., et al., Differential effects of three enteral dietary regimens on selected outcome variables in burn patients, *JPEN*, 14, 225, 1990.

74. Saffle, J.R., et al., Randomized trial of immune-enhancing enteral nutrition burn patients, *J. Trauma*, 42, 793, 1997.

75. Mendez, C., et al., Effects of immune-enhancing diet in critically injured patients, *J. Trauma*, 42, 933, 1997.

76. Weimann, A., et al., Influence of arginine, omega-3 fatty acids and nucleotide-supplemented enteral support on systemic inflammatory response syndrome and multiple organ failure in patients after severe trauma, *Nutrition*, 14, 165, 1998.

77. Galban, C, et al., An immune-enhancing enteral diet reduces mortality rate and episodes of bacteremia in septic intensive care unit patients, *Crit. Care Med.*, 28, 643, 2000.

78. Heyland, D.K., et al., Should immunonutrition become routine in critically ill patients? A systematic review, *JAMA*, 268, 944, 2001.

79. Veterans Affairs Total Parenteral Nutrition Cooperative Study Group, Perioperative total parenteral nutrition in surgical patients, *NEJM*, 325, 525, 1991.

80. Heys, S.D, et al., Enteral nutritional supplementation with key nutrient in patients with critical illness and cancer: a metaanalysis of randomized controlled clinical trials, *Ann. Surg.*, 229, 467, 1999.

81. Tepaske, R., et al., Effect of preoperative oral immune-enhancing nutritional supplement on patients at high risk of infection after cardiac surgery: a randomised placebo-controlled trial, *Lancet*, 358, 696, 2001.

82. Braga, M., et al., Nutritional approach in malnourished surgical patients. *Arch. Surg.*, 137, 174–180, 2002.

83. Braga, M., et al., Perioperative oral arginine and omega-3 fatty acid supplementation improves the immunometabolic host response and outcome after colorectal resection for cancer, *Surgery*, 132, 805, 2002.

84. Krauss, R.M., et al., AHA Dietary Guidelines Revision 2000: a statement for healthcare professionals from the Nutrition Committee of the American Heart Association, *Circulation*, 102, 2284, 2000.

Section III

Delivery of Nutrition Support in the Critically Ill

12 Parenteral vs. Enteral Nutrition

Naren Gupta and Robert G. Martindale
Medical College of Georgia

CONTENTS

12.1 INTRODUCTION

Nutritional support has progressed tremendously since 1678, when Sir Christopher Wren used a quill and a pig bladder to inject wine and ale into dogs. However, specialized nutrition support showed little real progress until the 1950s, when the concept of intensive care units was conceived. With the development of these areas of intensive care came the inception of nutritional support of the ICU patient. In 1967, Dudrick et al. (1) demonstrated that a central venous cannula could be used to deliver a concentrated mixture of protein hydrolysate and glucose. Parenteral nutrition was refined and found extensive clinical use in the 1970s. Clinicians were enamored of total parenteral nutrition (TPN) until the 1980s and 1990s, when its disadvantages became apparent. At the same time, the benefits of using the enteral route to provide nutrition were being reported (2–5).

The 1990s saw an increasing utilization of enteral nutrition (EN) as literature supported its numerous benefits over TPN. The purported role of EN in modulating the immune system continues to occupy a central place in comparisons between EN and TPN. Indeed, leaders in the field consider the immunologic benefits of EN more important than delivering calories or improving the nitrogen balance (6).

The proposed advantages of EN in surgical and critically ill patients are now well described. They include attenuation of the metabolic response to stress (7–9), improved nitrogen balance (10–13), better glycemic control (14–17), increased visceral protein synthesis (18,19), increased gastrointestinal anastomotic strength (20), and increased collagen deposition (21). Other benefits of EN include decreased nosocomial infections (22), enhanced visceral blood flow (9,23–25), increased variety of nutrients available for delivery, and decreased risk of gastrointestinal bleeding (26–28). Cost–benefit analysis has also shown EN to be superior to TPN (13,17,29), though in the light of more aggressive enteral access techniques, this may have to be reevaluated. Many of the proposed physiologic benefits of EN are based on animal studies, with limited corroborating human data. The advantages of EN have been largely supported by prospective randomized trials (30,31), though conflicting data exists (17,32–37).

Total parenteral nutrition offers the obvious advantage that a functional gastrointestinal tract is not required. The parenteral route provides considerable ease in nutrient delivery, and, as shown in recent large series, the nutritional requirements are met more consistently (17,38). These "ease of delivery" advantages may be overshadowed by TPN's alleged disadvantages. The adverse effect of TPN on the mucosal barrier and gut-associated lymphoid tissue (GALT) (39–41) has been extensively investigated. Other adverse effects often associated with TPN are hepatic impairment, including steatosis, cholestasis, and cholelithiasis (42,43); systemic immunosuppression (44–46) or, conversely, a proinflammatory condition (47); venous thrombosis (48); and local complications at the venous access site (49).

There is little doubt that EN is the preferred method of nutrient delivery in patients with functioning gastrointestinal tracts. However, despite heroic attempts, the gastrointestinal tract may be insufficient for adequate nutrient delivery. Access difficulties remain (37), there is difficulty in achieving nutritional delivery goals, and up to 50% of patients are intolerant to enteral feeds (50,51). Complications of EN include jejunal necrosis (51–54), aspiration (55,56), and respiratory compromise (57). High gastric residuals, constipation, diarrhea, abdominal distension, vomiting, and the risk of gut ischemia have been described as additional limitations to EN (58–62). Home EN has a reported complication rate of 0.16 to 0.62 per patient-year, of which 41 to 55% are gastrointestinal (constipation, vomiting, and diarrhea being the commonest) and 19 to 29% are mechanical (extraction is the commonest) (63,64).

It must be kept in mind that nutritional support is just one of the many treatment variables affecting outcome. Timely and appropriate resuscitation, wound care, respiratory support, and infection control all have an important impact on outcome. These factors should be taken into account when formulating an optimal nutrition plan. Recommendations for nutritional support should include not only the quantity of nutrient and its composition, but also the timing of its institution and the route of delivery.

12.2 ROLE OF EN IN MAINTAINING STRUCTURE AND FUNCTION OF THE GI TRACT

Lack of luminal nutrients and ischemia both result in an alteration of intestinal barrier function. Rats maintained on TPN alone show as much as 50% loss in the mass of their proximal small bowel mucosa within a week, accompanied by an increase in permeability (65–67). Intestinal mucosal epithelial cells provide a mechanical barrier to pathogen entry and are an important part of the body's innate immune system. Increased permeability due to intravenous feeding is associated with increased bacterial translocation to the mesenteric lymph nodes in animals (68,69). Changes in interferon-gamma expression (70) and keratinocyte growth factor levels (71) may be some of the mechanisms responsible for the loss of the epithelial barrier associated with TPN. Another mechanism may be abnormalities of the *tight junctions*, which, in the fed state, prevent small molecules and pathogens from penetrating through the intercellular spaces between adjoining intestinal epithelial cells. Enteral nutrition reverses the TPN-associated loss of mucosal mass and increase in permeability in these animal models. Organ permeability and death rates in animals after 15 minutes of ischemia are also reduced with EN, compared to TPN (72).

Partial confirmation of these animal studies came from Buchman et al. (73), who showed that reductions of 10 to 15% in small bowel mucosal thickness occur in human TPN models. Other investigators have also shown a decrease in villous height, as well as an increase in intestinal permeability in nutritionally depleted patients (74). TPN is associated with greater jejunal mucosal atrophy in patients of chronic pancreatitis than is seen in those who are maintained on enteral feeds (75). After an injury, gut disuse and TPN are particularly liable to increase intestinal mucosal permeability. Enteral nutrition can prevent the increase in gut permeability seen in patients on TPN (13). Increased gut permeability due to TPN has been shown to increase systemic endotoxemia in humans (76). However, increased permeability and mucosal atrophy have not been proved conclusively to predispose to bacterial translocation in man (77), and bacterial translocation did not increase with TPN when compared to EN in a well designed study by Sedman et al. (78). The clinical significance of bacterial translocation itself is very controversial (79). Some argue that translocation occurs and is responsible for septic complications (77). Others propose that translocation increases septic complications but not mortality (80).

Enteral nutrition is proposed to maintain the immune function of the gut better than TPN does. Two-thirds of the mammalian immune cells reside in the GI tract. With 8.5×10^{10} Ig-producing cells (compared to 2.5×10^{10} for bone marrow, spleen, and lymph nodes combined) gut-associated lymphoid tissue (GALT) is the largest lymphoid organ in the body. There are four configurations of GALT:

- Single cells close to the epithelium (IELs)
- Collections in the lamina propria
- Aggregates in the form of Peyer's patches
- Mesenteric lymph nodes

By a process of continual sampling of intestinal contents and sensitization of inflammatory cells in the Peyer's patches, GALT is constantly exposed to inflammatory stimuli from intestinal contents yet maintains a level of tolerance to normal bacterial flora and antigens. The lamina propria is a unique constituent of the GALT because it is continually in a state of physiologic inflammation, populated by activated lymphocytes and plasma cells. This is important for the sustained production of secretory IgA (sIgA), which inhibits bacterial attachment to the mucosa and is a vital component of the local immune response. Gut disuse results in a decrease in sIgA secretion within five days (81), accompanied by an increased susceptibility to infections normally controlled by sIgA in mice (82).

GALT is also important for systemic immunity, because sensitized immune cells sourced from the GALT migrate to and maintain other mucosal-associated lymphoid tissues (MALT), specifically those associated with the bronchial tree (BALT). Loss of GALT mass due to gut disuse adversely affects the entire MALT system. Gut disuse combined with TPN in mice decreases immunity against respiratory viruses. Refeeding the gut restores the protection and improves viral clearance (83). Mice fed on TPN alone have persistent respiratory viral infections, compared to enterally fed animals (84). Trauma patients receiving EN have significantly less pneumonia and intra-abdominal abscesses than those receiving TPN.

In animal studies, TPN shrinks the Peyer's patches and decreases the CD4:CD8 cell ratio in the lamina propria. It diminishes extraintestinal cellular immune mechanisms (44) and is associated with defective pulmonary macrophage function in rats (85). Defective cellular immunity reverses when the animals are subsequently fed enterally.

Infants receiving long-term TPN have impaired bacteriocidal activity against coagulase-negative staphylococcus (86). Excessive caloric intake, with resultant hyperglycemia and hepatic steatosis, may contribute to TPN-induced systemic immune suppression. Excessive long-chain triglycerides in TPN cause reticulo-endothelial system dysfunction, excess PGE_2, and altered macrophage function. In addition, TPN formulas lack glutamine, an important immunonutrient. EN improves the host's ability to kill bacteria that do translocate (87). A reversal of some of these detrimental effects occurs when the neuropeptide bombesin is given intravenously along with parenteral nutrition (88,89). Possibly, enteroendocrine mechanisms that are affected by luminal nutrition play a role in maintaining the immune function of the GI mucosa by increasing mucin and IgA production and stimulating GALT function.

A TPN-induced decrease in mucosal immunity could increase the susceptibility to virulent pathogens, increasing bacterial adherence to mucosa and subsequent inflammation. This may also serve to prime neutrophils, promoting a systemic proinflammatory condition (47). Preinjury priming of neutrophils plays an important role in systemic inflammatory response syndrome and multiple organ dysfunction syndrome by augmenting the inflammatory response to a subsequent insult.

Feeding the gut improves survival and decreases lung and liver damage after ischemia/reperfusion injury in mice (72). Administration of EN improves gut function and improves the global immunosuppressive and inflammatory response, compared to TPN in patients with acute pancreatitis and in postsurgical patients (76,90). However, this association of TPN with intestinal immune dysfunction in humans is not universally accepted (91). Cerra et al. (92) showed no difference in either the mortality or incidence of multiorgan failure syndrome in 66 septic patients prospectively randomized to isocaloric, isonitrogenous EN or TPN.

Diminished visceral blood flow due to any global insult results in intestinal ileus. Ileus promotes microbial overgrowth and disturbs the normal gut ecology, which increases microbial translocation in humans (93). Ischemia-induced dysmotility can be prevented by providing nutrients intraluminally (94). Enteral feeding stimulates peristalsis and biliary secretion, rich in secretory IgA, which helps flush bacteria downstream and decreases bacterial adhesiveness. Early oral feeding within four hours after colorectal resection and anastomosis is associated with earlier flatus, bowel movements, and tolerance of diet than is observed in traditionally managed patients (95). It is hypothesized that, by maintaining or improving intestinal motility in the critical care or postoperative setting, EN will help maintain the relative sterility of the proximal gut, prevent bacterial overgrowth and excess endotoxin production, and thereby decrease translocation of microbes and absorption of their toxic byproducts. Burn patients fed enterally within 24 hours of injury show less endotoxin absorption from the gut than patients who are fed after 48 hours (96). EN prevents the increase in IgM endotoxin antibodies seen in patients of acute pancreatitis receiving TPN (76).

Enteral nutrition has also been shown to protect against hypoperfusion by increasing visceral and mucosal blood flow. In postoperative cardiac patients with hemodynamic compromise, the introduction of postpyloric EN increases cardiac index and splanchnic blood flow, without any adverse affects on the myocardium or systemic hemodynamics. At the same time, there is an increased absorption and utilization of nutrients (97). Early EN has recently been reported to preserve mucosal ATP levels and gut absorptive capacity (24). There may be a hyperemic response to the presence of luminal nutrients, which actually improves blood flow and oxygen delivery to all layers of the gut following EN, compared to a fasting gut, in the presence of shock. In animal models and human studies of burns, hemorrhagic shock, and septic shock, EN improves gut blood flow (98,99), gut motility (94), and outcomes (100,101).

Delivery of nutrients to the lumen may offer other benefits. Human intestinal cell cultures exposed to nutrients on the luminal surface as well as the vascular side show increased cell proliferation, motility, and enzyme production (102) when compared to cells exposed to nutrition only on the vascular side. Following major upper gastrointestinal surgery, there is an improvement of peripheral protein kinetics and utilization of nutrients when they are provided enterally, compared to isonitrogenous, isocaloric TPN (103). However, in some studies, this did not translate into actual improvement in visceral protein markers (11), postoperative muscle function, fatigue, weight loss, or body composition (21). In fact, enteral carbohydrate administration, which normally promotes hepatic glucose uptake, actually failed to do so in a small number of critically ill patients (104). Enteral delivery of nutrients may also fail to suppress endogenous glucose production and gluconeogenesis in this patient population (105).

EN's proposed benefits appear to extend to other organ systems. By maintaining renal blood flow, EN decreases renal injury resulting from rhabdomyolysis (106) and improves recovery in a rodent model of ischemia-induced acute renal failure when compared with isocaloric, isonitrogenous TPN (107). EN has also been reported to minimize liver injury and improve survival after hemorrhagic shock (108).

The etiology of feeding associated nonobstructed bowel necrosis (NOBN) during EN is unclear but is probably multifactorial. Underlying bowel injury, hyperosmolar feeds, poor splanchnic perfusion secondary to excessive vasoconstriction, poor local bowel perfusion due to bowel dilatation, aggressive advancement of feeds, bacterial toxins, the use of tube instead of needle jejunostomies, and even flushing the jejunostomy tube with tap water (54) have been implicated. There is no clear association between NOBN and EN use in the presence of hemodynamic instability; in fact, enteral feeds may be beneficial after hemorrhagic shock (108). In patients requiring inotropic support after cardiac surgery, EN is well tolerated and may even increase cardiac output and splanchnic blood flow (97,109). Neither is there an association with early EN and NOBN: several studies have pointed out the benefits of early EN without any reported episodes of NOBN (110–113).

There are no prospective, randomized studies to determine accurately the risk of NOBN due to EN. Retrospective data would suggest that the incidence of NOBN is 0.3% of all critically ill trauma patients receiving EN by any route (114) and 0.29% of all feeding jejunostomies (52). In a retrospective analysis of 2022 consecutive needle catheter jejunostomies for early EN, only 0.15% developed NOBN (115). Witzel tube jejunostomies may be associated with higher necrosis rates (1 to 2%) (116). NOBN seems to occur more in patients undergoing abdominal surgery. In nonsurgical patients, high-dose clonidine has been implicated. NOBN has even been reported with gastric tube feeding (117). Though it is a rare event, bowel perforation during EN has a mortality of over 85% (52), and therefore any signs of intolerance to feeds, emesis, diarrhea, cramplike abdominal pain, abdominal distension, fever, tachycardia, and especially hypotension and hypovolemia during EN must be viewed with due suspicion. The risk of NOBN seems greatest during the first 24 hours of starting feeds, but anecdotal evidence points to onset even after several days of successful enteral feeds. Daily abdominal exams prior to advancing feeds are strongly encouraged. Timely operative intervention can significantly improve outcome (118,119). Overall, up to 92% of patients are successfully fed through needle jejunostomies after major abdominal operations (120).

12.3 HUMAN STUDIES: ENTERAL VS. PARENTERAL

In 1984, Bauer et al. showed that nutritional parameters increased faster with EN than with TPN in 60 prospectively randomized postoperative patients (4). A study soon after showed that EN was associated with faster resolution of malabsorption than TPN in a small, prospective randomized study of infants with intractable diarrhea (121). However, several prospective randomized studies published at that time (32,122–124) and more recently (125) have shown no significant nutritional advantage of EN over isonitrogenous, isocaloric TPN. Kotler et al. looked at the effect of EN and TPN on 23 AIDS patients suffering from malabsorption (126). There were no differences in intestinal function or CD4+ lymphocyte numbers in the peripheral blood, though the TPN group consumed more total calories and this correlated with better weight gain.

In 1991, a large VA study (127) showed that preoperative TPN administered to surgical patients increased infectious morbidities compared to patients randomized to standard preoperative care. However, this trial has been criticized for a poorly selected patient population. Patients at low risk of malnutrition will show minimal benefit from any nutrition plan. In fact, in a *post hoc* analysis of the 50 malnourished patients in this trial, TPN actually showed some benefit in reducing the noninfectious complication rate. The TPN group was clearly given excessive calories (3300 kcal/d). The resultant hyperglycemia and other complications of overfeeding are potential confounding variables (128).

Brennan et al. (129) showed a significant increase in complications after major pancreatic resection for cancer in patients randomized to TPN, compared to standard care. A meta-analysis by Heyland et al. (130) of 26 trials with a total of 2211 critically ill and surgical patients compared TPN to standard care (intravenous hydration and oral feeds when tolerated). Though TPN had no overall affect on mortality and malnourished patients benefited with a lower complication rate, the subset of critically ill patients and studies of a higher methodological quality showed an increase in mortality and complication rates with TPN. However, the adverse effects of TPN could have been exaggerated by the fact that several studies included patients who were accepting oral diets and some studies provided inadequate TPN calories. Recently, Koretz et al. (131) reported a meta-analysis of 82 randomized, controlled trials that compared postoperative TPN with standard care and found that the TPN-fed patients had significantly more infectious complications. However, this meta-analysis included very few studies that looked specifically at malnourished patients, raising the question of whether nutritional support was justified at all in most of these studies.

In contrast, EN decreased complications in trials comparing it to standard postoperative care. Beier-Holgersen et al. (132) showed a significant decrease in postoperative infective complications with EN compared to placebo in a randomized, double-blind trial of 60 patients undergoing major abdominal surgery. In a meta-analysis of 11 prospective randomized trials with a total of 837 patients (133), there was a significant decrease in infectious complications and postoperative hospital stay in the early EN group (within 24 hours of surgery), compared to those receiving standard care: nil-by-mouth. The only adverse effect was an increase in vomiting. Singh et al. (134) showed a similar significant reduction in septic morbidity with EN compared to standard care in a prospective, randomized study of 43 patients with nontraumatic perforative peritonitis.

Studies showing that, compared to TPN, EN improves resistance to infection in humans came from Moore et al. in 1986 and 1989. Data from two prospective, randomized studies of patients (n = 75 and 59) with an abdominal trauma index greater than 15 and less than 40 showed that patients randomized to EN had reduced major septic complications (abdominal abscesses and pneumonia), compared to those randomized to no supplemental nutrition (11) or TPN (30). A study by the same author in a similar patient population showed a blunting of the hepatic stress response, with higher constitutive proteins and lower acute-phase proteins in the EN-fed patients than in the TPN fed (135). In a subsequent meta-analysis of eight prospective randomized trials comparing EN to TPN in a total of 230 high-risk surgical patients, Moore et al. found that EN-fed trauma patients had significantly fewer septic complications (22).

A report of findings from a prospective study of 98 patients of blunt and penetrating trauma with an abdominal trauma index of at least 15, randomized to either enteral or parenteral feeding within 24 hours of injury, was published in 1992 (31). Patients were fed formulas with almost identical amounts of fat, carbohydrate, and protein, though the TPN patients received 19.1 kcal/kg/d compared to 15.7 kcal/kg/d in the EN group. The enteral group sustained significantly fewer pneumonias, intra-abdominal abscesses, and line sepsis, and sustained significantly fewer infections per patient, as well as significantly fewer infections per infected patient. The beneficial effects were more in severely injured patients and in patients with penetrating injuries. There was no significant benefit in the less severely injured subgroup.

An Italian group of surgical oncologists and nutritionists led by Bozzetti et al. studied 317 malnourished gastrointestinal cancer patients in a multicenter prospective randomized trial of early EN or isonitrogenous, isocaloric TPN after elective surgery (136). There was a significant decrease in infectious complications (27% with TPN, 16% with EN) and hospital stay, as well as a tendency toward decreased mortality with EN-treated patients. This suggested a decrease in the deleterious systemic inflammatory and metabolic responses associated with TPN. However, there were more therapy-associated adverse effects attributable to EN. Significantly more EN patients could not tolerate treatment due to gastrointestinal adverse effects and were switched to TPN. Only 78% of EN patients actually received at least 50% of their calculated target caloric intake. These authors have been criticized for not including a control arm with no nutritional support (standard care), but they argue that in their study of malnourished patients, not providing any nutritional support would fly in the face of established recommendations for postoperative care (137,138). A meta-analysis of RCTs comparing EN, TPN, and standard care (no nutritional therapy) did in fact show that in malnourished patients, standard care had a worse outcome than TPN (37).

A study by Baigrie et al. (139), also found a trend of reduction in postoperative septic complications with EN, compared to TPN, in 97 patients prospectively randomized after major surgery. Braga et al. (17) were unable to show any overall difference in complication rates or mortality with EN in 257 gastrointestinal patients prospectively randomized to postoperative isonitrogenous, isocaloric EN or TPN. However, less than 80% of the EN patients reached nutritional goals within four days, significantly less than the TPN group. Gastrointestinal adverse effects to EN contributed to this difference, as well as to the eventual crossover of patients from the EN to the TPN groups.

Interestingly, the EN arm had significantly better intestinal oxygenation, earlier flatus, and earlier bowel movements than the TPN arm did. Subset analysis of malnourished patients showed that EN was beneficial, but not significantly better than TPN.

Significant nutritional and immune benefits of EN over TPN have been shown in randomized controlled trials in the setting of severe acute ulcerative colitis (140), liver transplantation (112), neurosurgery (19), and acute pancreatitis (16,141). In acute pancreatitis, the concept of early enteral feeds went against the established, if arbitrary dictum of NPO for ten days and TPN (142). However, early EN has been shown to decrease the rate of septic complications compared to TPN in these patients (143). In the presence of necrosis, EN combined with prophylactic antibiotics decreased the rates of septic complications, multiorgan failure, and mortality, compared to TPN and antibiotics (144). Windsor et al. (76) also showed that early EN reduced systemic inflammatory response syndrome, sepsis, and organ failure, compared to TPN, in acute pancreatitis.

Recently, several large meta-analyses of randomized controlled trials comparing enteral to parenteral nutrition have been published. Lipman et al. (35) found that the only benefit of EN was lower cost and probably reduced septic morbidity in acute abdominal trauma. However, this meta-analysis did not examine the quality of the studies it included, nor did it attempt to evaluate comprehensively the methodology of each study.

Subsequently, a more vigorous meta-analysis by Braunschweig et al. (37) included 27 prospective randomized studies comparing TPN vs. EN or TPN vs. standard care in a total of 1829 patients with compromised gastrointestinal function. Aggregate results showed that TPN was associated with a higher relative risk of infection, even accounting for catheter sepsis, than either the EN or standard care groups, especially in normally nourished populations. Hyperglycemia in the TPN-fed patients was reported in several of the studies that showed a benefit of EN over TPN, and this could have played a confounding role. In a subset analysis of studies with more malnourished patients, TPN showed significantly less mortality than standard care did. In that same subset, enteral feeding significantly increased the risk of mortality. Of note, several studies delivered inadequate nutrition to the EN patients because of tolerance issues. The authors hypothesized that inadequate nutritional delivery by EN caused the increased mortality in malnourished populations. Nutritional support complications were more in the EN group, unless catheter sepsis was included, in which case there were no significant differences.

A meta-analysis of trials comparing EN to TPN in patients with acute pancreatitis by Al-Omran et al. (145) showed a trend toward improved outcomes with EN but suffered from the usual failings of this genre: heterogeneity of inclusion criteria, therapeutic parameters, and study quality.

The evidence from the last 20 years of prospective randomized trials is seemingly contradictory. Many studies have been criticized for including patient populations who were at low risk of malnutrition with normal gastrointestinal function, and who therefore were not expected to show much benefit from any nutritional intervention. At the same time, several studies randomized patients to EN or aggressive advancement of feeds, despite known gastrointestinal dysfunction, and that could have led to a higher rate of nutritional support complications. Earlier studies delivered excessive calories to their TPN patients, causing hyperglycemia. Conversely, underfeeding with EN due to intolerance was frequently reported, and the resultant persistent calorie debt probably clouded the outcome (146).

In a study that attempted to determine the effect of underfeeding due to inadequate EN, Bauer et al. (147) prospectively randomized 120 patients to early EN plus placebo or early EN plus TPN. Retinol-binding protein and prealbumin increased significantly in the treatment group, and there was a reduction in hospital stay, though there was no difference in morbidity. The study failed to address the core issue of long-term underfeeding due to gastrointestinal dysfunction or intolerance to EN; patients in both groups tolerated similar mean amounts of EN, and treatment extended for seven days or less though outcome was measured at two years. Moreover, the majority (59%) of patients in the study were not malnourished and included patients who were anticipated to have only two or more days of inadequate oral intake.

A well designed, randomized prospective trial by Woodcock et al. (148) addressed some of the criticisms of patient selection in previous trials of EN vs. TPN and attempted to provide answers that could be used in a clinical setting. In this study, the clinical assessment of gastrointestinal function determined route of delivery in 562 patients who had at least seven days of inadequate oral intake, actual or anticipated. Patients assessed to have inadequate gastrointestinal function were given TPN, those assessed as having functional gastrointestinal tracts were given EN, and the 64 patients in which there was a reasonable doubt were randomized equally to TPN or EN. The study had few well nourished patients (11.2%). Invasive techniques of EN were not routinely initially employed. Clinical judgment of gastrointestinal function was accurate across all groups, though poorest in randomized EN patients. Significantly more patients on TPN got their target intake than did patients on EN, in both the nonrandomized and the randomized groups, and significantly fewer randomized than nonrandomized EN patients got their target caloric intake. There was no significant difference in the incidence of septic complications between EN and TPN in either the randomized or the nonrandomized groups, or in malnourished and well nourished subsets. Significantly more nonseptic delivery-related complications occurred in both EN groups than in the TPN groups. This study showed more mortality in the EN groups than in the TPN groups, reaching statistical significance in the nonrandomized groups. The authors attributed this to differences in patient populations between these two nonrandomized groups.

A large, multicenter, randomized trial powered to determine differences in outcomes like mortality between EN and TPN has yet to be conducted. In the absence of those data, meta-analyses are the best available evidence, despite the inherent shortcoming of study heterogeneity. Overall, EN does have metabolic and immune benefits over TPN, as reflected by a reduction in hyperglycemia and infectious complications in most studies. This may not translate into a reduction in mortality, but it is probably accompanied by a significant cost savings.

12.4 CLINICAL APPROACH

The literature reviewed previously clearly shows that both parenteral and enteral nutrition have specific detrimental and beneficial effects. The question is: how should we use each method to minimize the disadvantages and maximize the advantages of nutritional therapy in our most gravely ill patients? In patients with a functional gastrointestinal tract, the enteral route is undoubtedly superior because of its ability to maintain the immune system. In critically ill patients, greater success in achieving enteral tolerance has been reported by implementing a standardized protocol and may be further improved by feeding beyond the ligament of Treitz (149). Gastric feeding, however, has the advantage of earlier institution than small bowel feeding (150). Determining tolerance to EN is not always an easy task, especially in the ICU patient, where the abdominal exam may be confounded by paralysis, mechanical ventilation, bulky dressings, and the occasional open abdomen. However, distension, pain, increased gastric residuals and nasogastric output, diarrhea, and pneumatosis are all signs of intolerance.

Critically ill patients often suffer from gastrointestinal dysmotility, which is an important cause of intolerance to EN (151). Contributing factors include electrolyte imbalances, mechanical ventilation (152), burns, extensive abdominal trauma, spinal cord injury and pancreatitis (153), and increased intracranial pressure following a head injury (154). Surgical trauma activates resident macrophages within the intestinal muscularis, which release several proinflammatory cytokines, contributing to postoperative ileus (155). Other risk factors include medications (opiates, antidepressants, calcium channel blockers, ganglion blocking agents, sedatives, dopamine, clonidine, and anticholinergics), sepsis, abdominal compartment syndrome, hypovolemia, hyperglycemia, previous vagotomy, systemic sclerosis, and muscular disease (156). Patient overhydration, hemodynamic instability, inadequate gastric decompression, and overly aggressive feeding are all important contributing factors. To restore normal gastrointestinal motility, it is important to correct these, as well as any electrolyte imbalances, establish strict glucose control, and discontinue drugs that decrease motility, especially opiate narcotics. Prokinetic agents like erythromycin, neostigmine, metoclopramide, and octreotide may all be considered, though each has its disadvantages. Clinical trials of newer prokinetic agents are under way: these include the opiod receptor antagonist ADL 8-2698 (157) and the erythromycin derivatives ABT-229 and EM574 (158). The use of arginine, the precursor for nitric oxide, in EN may enhance perfusion and thereby increase motility (159,160). Because high-fat formulas with long-chain triglycerides increase dysmotility, tolerance can be improved with the use of relatively low-fat formulas or some of the newer enteral formulas that contain medium-chain triglycerides.

A key factor in successful EN is to start conservatively and advance only as tolerated. Critically ill patients require fewer calories than was previously believed. It is now apparent that 20 to 30 kcal/kg/d is adequate in the ICU setting, a marked decrease from the past goals of 40 to 50 kcal/kg/d. In fact, enteral delivery of only 15 to 30% of the usual caloric intake is believed to be enough to maintain both the GALT and the gut barrier function, with the consequent local and systemic immunologic benefits (44,161,162). In a prospective randomized trial in which 53 patients with acute pancreatitis required nutritional support, the jejunal-fed patients had shorter hospital stays, significantly faster progression to oral diets, and significantly fewer complications (hyperglycemia, septic complications, catheter-related infections) than those receiving TPN, despite getting fewer calories (49% compared to 85% of the goal of 25 to 30 kcal/kg/d) (29). Contraindications to enteral feeding include continuing emesis, obstruction, major upper gastrointestinal bleeds, inaccessibility, and hemodynamic instability. A dietitian with the experience and patience to place the tube in the small intestine may better address accessibility issues than the use of expensive fluoroscopic equipment (163).

Guidelines for nutritional support in critically ill patients have been formulated based on an analysis of the existing data (164). Nutritional support should be initiated within 24 to 48 hours, using a standard, polymeric enteric formula fed postpylorically. Aspiration precautions, including feeding in a semirecumbent posture and elevation of the head of the bed, should be observed. Using an algorithmic approach optimizes success with EN. This includes starting at a target rate of 10 to 15 ml/h, advancing feeds based on gastric residual volumes and a clinical exam, and taking the steps outlined earlier to optimize gastrointestinal motility. EN should progress to 80% of target caloric intake (25 to 30 kcal/kg/d) within 72 hours and to 100% soon after. If EN cannot be advanced to meet these goals, the balance of the target should be supplemented with TPN. The patient should receive EN challenges every 12 hours in an effort to increase the enteral delivery and to wean him or her off TPN. If the gut is not available or EN is not tolerated, nutritional support should be instituted with TPN, while continuing EN challenges every 12 hours wherever appropriate. Enriching TPN with immunonutrients (glutamine) and neurohumoral enteric products like cholecystokinin, neurotensin, bombesin, etc., may serve to support the immune system to some degree in these patients (165). Hypocaloric dosing, using fewer long-chain triglycerides and intensive insulin therapy to keep strict glycemic control (blood glucose between 80 and 110 mg%), will help minimize the adverse metabolic effects of TPN. The implementation of such an evidence-based algorithm has been shown to improve patient outcomes in the intensive care setting (166).

The combination of clinical selection based on an assessment of gastrointestinal function and, whenever appropriate, early enteral feeding begun gradually with parenteral supplementation to maintain caloric support is a feasible, safe alternative, yielding the best outcomes in the critically ill.

REFERENCES

1. Dudrick SJ, Wilmore DW, Vars HM, Rhoads JE. Long-term total parenteral nutrition with growth, development, and positive nitrogen balance. *Surgery* 1968, 64: 134–142.
2. Chrysomilides SA, Kaminski MV, Jr. Home enteral and parenteral nutritional support: a comparison. *Am. J. Clin. Nutr.* 1981, 34: 2271–2275.

3. Kudsk KA, Stone JM, Carpenter G, Sheldon GF. Enteral and parenteral feeding influences mortality after hemoglobin-*E. coli* peritonitis in normal rats. *J. Trauma* 1983, 23: 605–609.

4. Bauer E, Graber R, Brodtke R, Lunstedt B, Seifert J. [Nutrition physiologic, immunologic and clinical parameters in prospective randomized patients by enteral or parenteral nutrition therapy following large intestine operations]. *Infusionsther Klin. Ernahr.* 1984, 11: 165–167.

5. Hull S. Enteral versus parenteral nutrition support: rationale for increased use of enteral feeding. *Zeitschrift fur Gastroenterologie* 1985, 23: 55–63.

6. Bengmark S. Enteral nutrition in HPB surgery: past and future. *J. Hepatobiliary Pancreat. Surg.* 2002, 9: 448–458.

7. Taylor SJ, Fettes SB, Jewkes C, Nelson RJ. Prospective, randomized, controlled trial to determine the effect of early enhanced enteral nutrition on clinical outcome in mechanically ventilated patients suffering head injury. *Crit. Care Med.* 1999, 27: 2525–2531.

8. Fong YM, Marano MA, Barber A, et al. Total parenteral nutrition and bowel rest modify the metabolic response to endotoxin in humans. *Ann. Surg.* 1989, 210: 449–456; discussion 456–457.

9. Gianotti L, Nelson JL, Alexander JW, Chalk CL, Pyles T. Post injury hypermetabolic response and magnitude of translocation: prevention by early enteral nutrition. *Nutrition* 1994, 10: 225–231.

10. Chiarelli A, Enzi G, Casadei A, Baggio B, Valerio A, Mazzoleni F. Very early nutrition supplementation in burned patients. A*m. J. Clin. Nutr.* 1990, 51: 1035–1039.

11. Moore EE, Jones TN. Benefits of immediate jejunostomy feeding after major abdominal trauma: a prospective, randomized study. *J. Trauma* 1986, 26: 874–881.

12. Hasse JM, Blue LS, Liepa GU, et al. Early enteral nutrition support in patients undergoing liver transplantation. *J. Parenter. Enteral Nutr.* 1995, 19: 437–443.

13. Carr CS, Ling KD, Boulos P, Singer M. Randomised trial of safety and efficacy of immediate postoperative enteral feeding in patients undergoing gastrointestinal resection. *BMJ* 1996, 312: 869–871.

14. Vernet O, Christin L, Schutz Y, Danforth E, Jr., Jequier E. Enteral versus parenteral nutrition: comparison of energy metabolism in healthy subjects. *Am. J. Physiol.* 1986, 250: E47–E54.

15. Magnusson J, Tranberg KG, Jeppsson B, Lunderquist A. Enteral versus parenteral glucose as the sole nutritional support after colorectal resection: a prospective, randomized comparison. *Scand. J. Gastroenterol.* 1989, 24: 539–549.

16. McClave SA, Greene LM, Snider HL, et al. Comparison of the safety of early enteral vs parenteral nutrition in mild acute pancreatitis. *J. Parenter. Enteral Nutr.* 1997, 21: 14–20.

17. Braga M, Gianotti L, Gentilini O, Parisi V, Salis C, Di Carlo V. Early postoperative enteral nutrition improves gut oxygenation and reduces costs compared with total parenteral nutrition. *Crit. Care Med.* 2001, 29: 242–248.

18. Kudsk KA, Minard G, Wojtysiak SL, Croce M, Fabian T, Brown RO. Visceral protein response to enteral versus parenteral nutrition and sepsis in patients with trauma. *Surgery* 1994, 116: 516–523.

19. Suchner U, Senftleben U, Eckart T, et al. Enteral versus parenteral nutrition: effects on gastrointestinal function and metabolism. *Nutrition* 1996, 12: 13–22.

20. Moss G, Greenstein A, Levy S, Bierenbaum A. Maintenance of GI function after bowel surgery and immediate enteral full nutrition. I. Doubling of canine colorectal anastomotic bursting pressure and intestinal wound mature collagen content. *J. Parenter. Enteral Nutr.* 1980, 4: 535–538.

21. Schroeder D, Gillanders L, Mahr K, Hill GL. Effects of immediate postoperative enteral nutrition on body composition, muscle function, and wound healing. *J. Parenter. Enteral Nutr.* 1991, 15: 376–383.

22. Moore FA, Feliciano DV, Andrassy RJ, et al. Early enteral feeding, compared with parenteral, reduces postoperative septic complications: the results of a meta-analysis. *Ann. Surg.* 1992, 216: 172–183.

23. Bengmark S, Gianotti L. Nutritional support to prevent and treat multiple organ failure. *World J. Surg.* 1996, 20: 474–481.

24. Kozar RA, Hu S, Hassoun HT, DeSoignie R, Moore FA. Specific intraluminal nutrients alter mucosal blood flow during gut ischemia/reperfusion. *J. Parenter. Enteral Nutr.* 2002, 26: 226–229.

25. Gosche JR, Garrison RN, Harris PD, Cryer HG. Absorptive hyperemia restores intestinal blood flow during *Escherichia coli* sepsis in the rat. *Arch. Surg.* 1990, 125: 1573–1576.

26. Cook D, Heyland D, Griffith L, Cook R, Marshall J, Pagliarello J. Risk factors for clinically important upper gastrointestinal bleeding in patients requiring mechanical ventilation. Canadian Critical Care Trials Group. *Crit. Care Med.* 1999, 27: 2812–2817.

27. Raff T, Germann G, Hartmann B. The value of early enteral nutrition in the prophylaxis of stress ulceration in the severely burned patient. *Burns* 1997, 23: 313–318.

28. Laggner AN, Lenz K. [Prevention of stress ulcer in intensive care patients]. *Wien Med. Wochenschr.* 1986, 136: 596–599.

29. Abou-Assi S, Craig K, O'Keefe SJ. Hypocaloric jejunal feeding is better than total parenteral nutrition in acute pancreatitis: results of a randomized comparative study. *Am. J. Gastroenterol.* 2002, 97: 2255–2262.

30. Moore FA, Moore EE, Jones TN, McCroskey BL, Peterson VM. TEN versus TPN following major abdominal trauma: reduced septic morbidity. *J. Trauma* 1989, 29: 916–922; discussion 922–923.

31. Kudsk KA, Croce MA, Fabian TC, et al. Enteral versus parenteral feeding: effects on septic morbidity after blunt and penetrating abdominal trauma. *Ann. Surg.* 1992, 215: 503–511; discussion 511–513.

32. Burt ME, Stein TP, Brennan MF. A controlled, randomized trial evaluating the effects of enteral and parenteral nutrition on protein metabolism in cancer-bearing man. *J. Surg. Res.* 1983, 34: 303–314.

33. Merkle NM, Wiedeck H, Herfarth C, Grunert A. [Immediate postoperative enteral tube feeding following resection of the large intestine: experiences with a controlled clinical study]. *Chirurg.* 1984, 55: 267–274.

34. Hausmann D, Mosebach KO, Caspari R, Rommelsheim K. Combined enteral-parenteral nutrition versus total parenteral nutrition in brain-injured patients: a comparative study. *Intens. Care Med.* 1985, 11: 80–84.

35. Lipman TO. Grains or veins: is enteral nutrition really better than parenteral nutrition? A look at the evidence. *J. Parenter. Enteral Nutr.* 1998, 22: 167–182.

36. Heyland DK, MacDonald S, Keefe L, Drover JW. Total parenteral nutrition in the critically ill patient: a meta-analysis. *JAMA* 1998, 280: 2013–2019.

37. Braunschweig CL, Levy P, Sheean PM, Wang X. Enteral compared with parenteral nutrition: a meta-analysis. *Am. J. Clin. Nutr.* 2001, 74: 534–542.

38. Gianotti L, Braga M, Gentilini O, Balzano G, Zerbi A, Di Carlo V. Artificial nutrition after pancreaticoduodenectomy. *Pancreas* 2000, 21: 344–351.

39. Tanaka S, Miura S, Tashiro H, et al. Morphological alteration of gut-associated lymphoid tissue after long-term total parenteral nutrition in rats. *Cell Tissue Res.* 1991, 266: 29–36.

40. Khan J, Iiboshi Y, Nezu R, et al. Total parenteral nutrition increases uptake of latex beads by Peyer's patches. *J. Parenter. Enteral Nutr.* 1997, 21: 31–35.

41. Janu P, Li J, Renegar B, Kudsk KA. Recovery of gut-associated lymphoid tissue and upper respiratory tract immunity after parenteral nutrition. *Ann. Surg.* 1997, 225: 707–715; discussion 715–717.

42. Quigley EM, Marsh MN, Shaffer JL, Markin RS. Hepatobiliary complications of total parenteral nutrition. *Gastroenterology* 1993, 104: 286–301.

43. Kaufman SS. Prevention of parenteral nutrition-associated liver disease in children. *Pediatr. Transplant* 2002, 6: 37–42.

44. Shou J, Lappin J, Minnard EA, Daly JM. Total parenteral nutrition, bacterial translocation, and host immune function. *Am. J. Surg.* 1994, 167: 145–150.

45. Kudsk KA, Li J, Renegar KB. Loss of upper respiratory tract immunity with parenteral feeding. *Ann. Surg.* 1996, 223: 629–635; discussion 635–638.

46. King BK, Kudsk KA, Li J, Wu Y, Renegar KB. Route and type of nutrition influence mucosal immunity to bacterial pneumonia. *Ann. Surg.* 1999, 229: 272–278.

47. Fukatsu K, Lundberg AH, Hanna MK, et al. Route of nutrition influences intercellular adhesion molecule-1 expression and neutrophil accumulation in intestine. *Arch. Surg.* 1999, 134: 1055–1060.

48. Lokich JJ, Bothe A, Jr., Benotti P, Moore C. Complications and management of implanted venous access catheters. *J. Clin. Oncol.* 1985, 3: 710–717.

49. Reimund JM, Arondel Y, Finck G, Zimmermann F, Duclos B, Baumann R. Catheter-related infection in patients on home parenteral nutrition: results of a prospective survey. *Clin. Nutr.* 2002, 21: 33–38.

50. Jones TN, Moore FA, Moore EE, McCroskey BL. Gastrointestinal symptoms attributed to jejunostomy feeding after major abdominal trauma: a critical analysis. *Crit. Care Med.* 1989, 17: 1146–1150.

51. Heyland D, Cook DJ, Winder B, Brylowski L, Van deMark H, Guyatt G. Enteral nutrition in the critically ill patient: a prospective survey. *Crit. Care Med.* 1995, 23: 1055–1060.

52. Schunn CD, Daly JM. Small bowel necrosis associated with postoperative jejunal tube feeding. *J. Am. Coll. Surg.* 1995, 180: 410–416.

53. Zetti G, Tagliabue F, Barabino M, Fontana S, Ceppi M, Samori G. Small bowel necrosis associated with postoperative enteral feeding. *Chir. Ital.* 2002, 54: 555–558.

54. Schloerb PR, Wood JG, Casillan AJ, Tawfik O, Udobi K. Bowel necrosis caused by water in jejunal feeding. *J. Parenter. Enteral Nutr.* 2004, 28: 27–29.

55. Heyland DK, Drover JW, MacDonald S, Novak F, Lam M. Effect of postpyloric feeding on gastro-esophageal regurgitation and pulmonary microaspiration: results of a randomized controlled trial. *Crit. Care Med.* 2001, 29: 1495–1501.

56. McClave SA, DeMeo MT, DeLegge MH, et al. North American Summit on Aspiration in the Critically Ill Patient: consensus statement. *J. Parenter. Enteral Nutr.* 2002, 26: S80–S85.

57. Watters JM, Kirkpatrick SM, Norris SB, Shamji FM, Wells GA. Immediate postoperative enteral feeding results in impaired respiratory mechanics and decreased mobility. *Ann. Surg.* 1997, 226: 369–377; discussion 377–380.

58. Seron Arbeloa C, Avellanas Chavala M, Homs Gimeno C, Larraz Vileta A, Laplaza Marin J. [Descriptive analysis of the nutritional support in a polyvalent intensive care unit: complications of enteral nutrition]. *Nutr. Hosp.* 1999, 14: 217–222.

59. Montejo JC. Enteral nutrition-related gastrointestinal complications in critically ill patients: a multi-center study. The Nutritional and Metabolic Working Group of the Spanish Society of Intensive Care Medicine and Coronary Units. *Crit. Care Med.* 1999, 27: 1447–1453.

60. Jorba R, Fabregat J, Borobia F G, Torras J, Poves I, Jaurrieta E. Small bowel necrosis in association with early postoperative enteral feeding after pancreatic resection. *Surgery* 2000, 128: 111–112.

61. Mentec H, Dupont H, Bocchetti M, Cani P, Ponche F, Bleichner G. Upper digestive intolerance during enteral nutrition in critically ill patients: frequency, risk factors, and complications. *Crit. Care Med.* 2001, 29: 1955–1961.

62. Braga M, Gianotti L, Gentilini O, Liotta S, Di Carlo V. Feeding the gut early after digestive surgery: results of a nine-year experience. *Clin. Nutr.* 2002, 21: 59–65.

63. Gomez Candela C, Cos Blanco A, Garcia Luna PP, et al. [Complications of enteral nutrition at home: results of a multicenter trial]. *Nutr. Hosp.* 2003, 18: 167–173.

64. Gomez Candela C, Cos Blanco AI, Iglesias Rosado C, et al. [Home enteral nutrition: annual report 1999. NADYA-SENPE Group]. *Nutr. Hosp.* 2002, 17: 28–33.

65. Johnson LR, Copeland EM, Dudrick SJ, Lichtenberger LM, Castro GA. Structural and hormonal alterations in the gastrointestinal tract of parenterally fed rats. *Gastroenterology* 1975, 68: 1177–1183.

66. Levine GM, Deren JJ, Steiger E, Zinno R. Role of oral intake in maintenance of gut mass and disaccharide activity. *Gastroenterology* 1974, 67: 975–982.

67. Saito H, Trocki O, Alexander JW, Kopcha R, Heyd T, Joffe SN. The effect of route of nutrient administration on the nutritional state, catabolic hormone secretion, and gut mucosal integrity after burn injury. *J. Parenter. Enteral Nutr.* 1987, 11: 1–7.

68. Alverdy JC, Aoys E, Moss GS. Total parenteral nutrition promotes bacterial translocation from the gut. *Surgery* 1988, 104: 185–190.

69. Deitch EA, Xu D, Naruhn MB, Deitch DC, Lu Q, Marino AA. Elemental diet and IV-TPN-induced bacterial translocation is associated with loss of intestinal mucosal barrier function against bacteria. *Ann. Surg.* 1995, 221: 299–307.

70. Yang H, Kiristioglu I, Fan Y, et al. Interferon-gamma expression by intraepithelial lymphocytes results in a loss of epithelial barrier function in a mouse model of total parenteral nutrition. *Ann. Surg.* 2002, 236: 226–234.

71. Yang H, Wildhaber B, Tazuke Y, Teitelbaum DH. 2002 Harry M. Vars Research Award. Keratinocyte growth factor stimulates the recovery of epithelial structure and function in a mouse model of total parenteral nutrition. *J. Parenter. Enteral Nutr.* 2002, 26: 333–340; discussion 340–341.

72. Fukatsu K, Zarzaur BL, Johnson CD, Lundberg AH, Wilcox HG, Kudsk KA. Enteral nutrition prevents remote organ injury and death after a gut ischemic insult. *Ann. Surg.* 2001, 233: 660–668.

73. Buchman AL, Moukarzel AA, Bhuta S, et al. Parenteral nutrition is associated with intestinal morphologic and functional changes in humans. *J. Parenter. Enteral Nutr.* 1995, 19: 453–460.

74. Hadfield RJ, Sinclair DG, Houldsworth PE, Evans TW. Effects of enteral and parenteral nutrition on gut mucosal permeability in the critically ill. *Am. J. Respir. Crit. Care Med.* 1995, 152: 1545–1548.

75. Groos S, Hunefeld G, Luciano L. Parenteral versus enteral nutrition: morphological changes in human adult intestinal mucosa. *J. Submicrosc. Cytol. Pathol.* 1996, 28: 61–74.

76. Windsor AC, Kanwar S, Li AG, et al. Compared with parenteral nutrition, enteral feeding attenuates the acute phase response and improves disease severity in acute pancreatitis. *Gut* 1998, 42: 431–435.

77. O'Boyle CJ, MacFie J, Dave K, Sagar PS, Poon P, Mitchell CJ. Alterations in intestinal barrier function do not predispose to translocation of enteric bacteria in gastroenterologic patients. *Nutrition* 1998, 14: 358–362.

78. Sedman PC, MacFie J, Palmer MD, Mitchell CJ, Sagar PM. Preoperative total parenteral nutrition is not associated with mucosal atrophy or bacterial translocation in humans. *Br. J. Surg.* 1995, 82: 1663–1667.

79. Van Leeuwen PA, Boermeester MA, Houdijk AP, et al. Clinical significance of translocation. *Gut* 1994, 35: S28–S34.

80. MacFie J. Enteral versus parenteral nutrition: the significance of bacterial translocation and gut-barrier function. *Nutrition* 2000, 16: 606–611.

81. Li J, Kudsk KA, Gocinski B, Dent D, Glezer J, Langkamp-Henken B. Effects of parenteral and enteral nutrition on gut-associated lymphoid tissue. *J. Trauma* 1995, 39: 44–51; discussion 51–52.

82. Kudsk KA. Current aspects of mucosal immunology and its influence by nutrition. *Am. J. Surg.* 2002, 183: 390–398.

83. Renegar KB, Small PA, Jr. Immunoglobulin A mediation of murine nasal anti-influenza virus immunity. *J. Virol.* 1991, 65: 2146–2148.

84. Johnson CD, Kudsk KA, Fukatsu K, Renegar B, Zarzaur BL. Route of nutrition influences generation of antibody-forming cells and initial defense to an active viral infection in the upper respiratory tract. *Ann. Surg.* 2003, 237: 565–573.

85. Shou J, Lappin J, Daly JM. Impairment of pulmonary macrophage function with total parenteral nutrition. *Ann. Surg.* 1994, 219: 291–297.

86. Okada Y, Klein NJ, van Saene HK, Webb G, Holzel H, Pierro A. Bactericidal activity against coagulase-negative staphylococci is impaired in infants receiving long-term parenteral nutrition. *Ann. Surg.* 2000, 231: 276–281.

87. Gianotti L, Alexander JW, Nelson JL, Fukushima R, Pyles T, Chalk CL. Role of early enteral feeding and acute starvation on postburn bacterial translocation and host defense: prospective, randomized trials. *Crit. Care Med.* 1994, 22: 265–272.

88. Zarzaur BL, Wu Y, Fukatsu K, Johnson CD, Kudsk KA. The neuropeptide bombesin improves IgA-mediated mucosal immunity with preservation of gut interleukin-4 in total parenteral nutrition-fed mice. *Surgery* 2002, 131: 59–65.

89. Li J, Kudsk KA, Hamidian M, Gocinski BL. Bombesin affects mucosal immunity and gut-associated lymphoid tissue in intravenously fed mice. *Arch. Surg.* 1995, 130: 1164–1169; discussion 1169–1170.

90. Braga M, Vignali A, Gianotti L, Cestari A, Profili M, Carlo VD. Immune and nutritional effects of early enteral nutrition after major abdominal operations. *Eur. J. Surg.* 1996, 162: 105–112.

91. Buchman AL, Mestecky J, Moukarzel A, Ament ME. Intestinal immune function is unaffected by parenteral nutrition in man. *J. Am. Coll. Nutr.* 1995, 14: 656–661.

92. Cerra FB, McPherson JP, Konstantinides FN, Konstantinides NN, Teasley KM. Enteral nutrition does not prevent multiple organ failure syndrome (MOFS) after sepsis. *Surgery* 1988, 104: 727–733.

93. MacFie J, O'Boyle C, Mitchell CJ, Buckley PM, Johnstone D, Sudworth P. Gut origin of sepsis: a prospective study investigating associations between bacterial translocation, gastric microflora, and septic morbidity. *Gut* 1999, 45: 223–228.

94. Grossie VB, Jr., Weisbrodt NW, Moore FA, Moody F. Ischemia/reperfusion-induced disruption of rat small intestine transit is reversed by total enteral nutrition. *Nutrition* 2001, 17: 939–943.

95. Stewart BT, Woods RJ, Collopy BT, Fink RJ, Mackay JR, Keck JO. Early feeding after elective open colorectal resections: a prospective randomized trial. *Aust. N.Z. J. Surg.* 1998, 68: 125–128.

96. Peng YZ, Yuan ZQ, Xiao GX. Effects of early enteral feeding on the prevention of enterogenic infection in severely burned patients. *Burns* 2001, 27: 145–149.

97. Revelly JP, Tappy L, Berger MM, Gersbach P, Cayeux C, Chiolero R. Early metabolic and splanchnic responses to enteral nutrition in postoperative cardiac surgery patients with circulatory compromise. *Intens. Care Med.* 2001, 27: 540–547.

98. Kazamias P, Kotzampassi K, Koufogiannis D, Eleftheriadis E. Influence of enteral nutrition-induced splanchnic hyperemia on the septic origin of splanchnic ischemia. *World J. Surg.* 1998, 22: 6–11.

99. Purcell PN, Davis K, Jr., Branson RD, Johnson DJ. Continuous duodenal feeding restores gut blood flow and increases gut oxygen utilization during PEEP ventilation for lung injury. *Am. J. Surg.* 1993, 165: 188–193; discussion 193–194.

100. Gianotti L, Alexander JW, Gennari R, Pyles T, Babcock GF. Oral glutamine decreases bacterial translocation and improves survival in experimental gut-origin sepsis. *J. Parenter. Enteral Nutr.* 1995, 19: 69–74.

101. Zaloga GP, Roberts P, Black KW, Prielipp R. Gut bacterial translocation/dissemination explains the increased mortality produced by parenteral nutrition following methotrexate. *Circ. Shock* 1993, 39: 263–268.

102. Perdikis DA, Basson MD. Basal nutrition promotes human intestinal epithelial (Caco-2) proliferation, brush border enzyme activity, and motility. *Crit. Care Med.* 1997, 25: 159–165.

103. Harrison LE, Hochwald SN, Heslin MJ, Berman R, Burt M, Brennan MF. Early postoperative enteral nutrition improves peripheral protein kinetics in upper gastrointestinal cancer patients undergoing complete resection: a randomized trial. *J. Parenter. Enteral Nutr.* 1997, 21: 202–207.

104. Tappy L, Berger M, Schwarz JM, et al. Hepatic and peripheral glucose metabolism in intensive care patients receiving continuous high- or low-carbohydrate enteral nutrition. *J. Parenter. Enteral Nutr.* 1999, 23: 260–267; discussion 267–268.

105. Schwarz JM, Chiolero R, Revelly JP, et al. Effects of enteral carbohydrates on *de novo* lipogenesis in critically ill patients. *Am. J. Clin. Nutr.* 2000, 72: 940–945.

106. Roberts PR, Black KW, Zaloga GP. Enteral feeding improves outcome and protects against glycerol-induced acute renal failure in the rat. *Am. J. Respir. Crit. Care Med.* 1997, 156: 1265–1269.

107. Mouser JF, Hak EB, Kuhl DA, Dickerson RN, Gaber LW, Hak LJ. Recovery from ischemic acute renal failure is improved with enteral compared with parenteral nutrition. *Crit. Care Med.* 1997, 25: 1748–1754.

108. Bortenschlager L, Roberts PR, Black KW, Zaloga GP. Enteral feeding minimizes liver injury during hemorrhagic shock. *Shock* 1994, 2: 351–354.

109. Berger MM, Berger-Gryllaki M, Wiesel PH, et al. Intestinal absorption in patients after cardiac surgery. *Crit. Care Med.* 2000, 28: 2217–2223.

110. Galban C, Montejo JC, Mesejo A, et al. An immune-enhancing enteral diet reduces mortality rate and episodes of bacteremia in septic intensive care unit patients. *Crit. Care Med.* 2000, 28: 643–648.

111. Gadek JE, DeMichele SJ, Karlstad MD, et al. Effect of enteral feeding with eicosapentaenoic acid, gamma-linolenic acid, and antioxidants in patients with acute respiratory distress syndrome. Enteral Nutrition in ARDS Study Group. *Crit. Care Med.* 1999, 27: 1409–1420.

112. Caparros T, Lopez J, Grau T. Early enteral nutrition in critically ill patients with a high-protein diet enriched with arginine, fiber, and antioxidants compared with a standard high-protein diet: the effect on nosocomial infections and outcome. *J. Parenter. Enteral Nutr.* 2001, 25: 299–308; discussion 308–309.

113. Atkinson S, Sieffert E, Bihari D. A prospective, randomized, double-blind, controlled clinical trial of enteral immunonutrition in the critically ill. Guy's Hospital Intensive Care Group. *Crit. Care Med.* 1998, 26: 1164–1172.

114. Marvin RG, McKinley BA, McQuiggan M, Cocanour CS, Moore FA. Nonocclusive bowel necrosis occurring in critically ill trauma patients receiving enteral nutrition manifests no reliable clinical signs for early detection. *Am. J. Surg.* 2000, 179: 7–12.

115. Myers JG, Page CP, Stewart RM, Schwesinger WH, Sirinek KR, Aust JB. Complications of needle catheter jejunostomy in 2022 consecutive applications. *Am. J. Surg.* 1995, 170: 547–550; discussion 550–551.

116. Holmes JH, Brundage SI, Yuen P, Hall RA, Maier RV, Jurkovich GJ. Complications of surgical feeding jejunostomy in trauma patients. *J. Trauma* 1999, 47: 1009–1012.

117. Frey C, Takala J, Krahenbuhl L. Non-occlusive small bowel necrosis during gastric tube feeding: a case report. *Intens. Care Med.* 2001, 27: 1422–1425.

118. Lawlor DK, Inculet RI, Malthaner RA. Small-bowel necrosis associated with jejunal tube feeding. *Can. J. Surg.* 1998, 41: 459–462.

119. Andersen DR, Christensen LT. [Small bowel necrosis associated with postoperative percutaneous jejunal tube feeding]. *Ugeskr. Laeger* 2003, 165: 2750–2751.

120. De Gottardi A, Krahenbuhl L, Farhadi J, Gernhardt S, Schafer M, Buchler MW. Clinical experience of feeding through a needle catheter jejunostomy after major abdominal operations. *Eur. J. Surg.* 1999, 165: 1055–1060.

121. Orenstein SR. Enteral versus parenteral therapy for intractable diarrhea of infancy: a prospective, randomized trial. *J. Pediatr.* 1986, 109: 277–286.

122. Muggia-Sullam M, Bower RH, Murphy RF, Joffe SN, Fischer JE. Postoperative enteral versus parenteral nutritional support in gastrointestinal surgery: a matched prospective study. *Am. J. Surg.* 1985, 149: 106–112.

123. Fletcher JP, Little JM. A comparison of parenteral nutrition and early postoperative enteral feeding on the nitrogen balance after major surgery. *Surgery* 1986, 100: 21–24.

124. Adams S, Dellinger EP, Wertz MJ, Oreskovich MR, Simonowitz D, Johansen K. Enteral versus parenteral nutritional support following laparotomy for trauma: a randomized prospective trial. *J. Trauma* 1986, 26: 882–891.

125. Borzotta AP, Pennings J, Papasadero B, et al. Enteral versus parenteral nutrition after severe closed head injury. *J. Trauma* 1994, 37: 459–468.

126. Kotler DP, Fogleman L, Tierney AR. Comparison of total parenteral nutrition and an oral, semielemental diet on body composition, physical function, and nutrition-related costs in patients with malabsorption due to acquired immunodeficiency syndrome. *J. Parenter. Enteral Nutr.* 1998, 22: 120–126.

127. Perioperative total parenteral nutrition in surgical patients. The Veterans Affairs Total Parenteral Nutrition Cooperative Study Group. *N. Engl. J. Med.* 1991, 325: 525–532.

128. Nordenstrom J, Thorne A. Benefits and complications of parenteral nutritional support. *Eur. J. Clin. Nutr.* 1994, 48: 531–537.

129. Brennan MF, Pisters PW, Posner M, Quesada O, Shike M. A prospective randomized trial of total parenteral nutrition after major pancreatic resection for malignancy. *Ann. Surg.* 1994, 220: 436–441; discussion 441–444.

130. Heyland DK, Montalvo M, MacDonald S, Keefe L, Su XY, Drover JW. Total parenteral nutrition in the surgical patient: a meta-analysis. *Can. J. Surg.* 2001, 44: 102–111.

131. Koretz RL, Lipman TO, Klein S. AGA technical review on parenteral nutrition. *Gastroenterology* 2001, 121: 970–1001.

132. Beier-Holgersen R, Boesby S. [Effect of early postoperative enteral nutrition on postoperative infections]. *Ugeskr. Laeger* 1998, 160: 3223–3226.

133. Lewis SJ, Egger M, Sylvester PA, Thomas S. Early enteral feeding versus "nil by mouth" after gastrointestinal surgery: systematic review and meta-analysis of controlled trials. *BMJ* 2001, 323: 773–776.

134. Singh G, Ram RP, Khanna SK. Early postoperative enteral feeding in patients with nontraumatic intestinal perforation and peritonitis. *J. Am. Coll. Surg.* 1998, 187: 142–146.

135. Moore EE, Moore FA. Immediate enteral nutrition following multisystem trauma: a decade perspective. *J. Am. Coll. Nutr.* 1991, 10: 633–648.

136. Bozzetti F, Braga M, Gianotti L, Gavazzi C, Mariani L. Postoperative enteral versus parenteral nutrition in malnourished patients with gastrointestinal cancer: a randomised multicentre trial. *Lancet* 2001, 358: 1487–1492.

137. Koretz RL. Enteral nutrition led to fewer postoperative complications than did parenteral feeding in gastrointestinal cancer. *ACP J. Club.* 2002, 136: 93.

138. Koretz RL. One if by gut and two if IV. *Gastroenterology* 2002, 122: 1537–1538; discussion 1538.

139. Baigrie RJ, Devitt PG, Watkin DS. Enteral versus parenteral nutrition after oesophagogastric surgery: a prospective randomized comparison. *Aust. N.Z. J. Surg.* 1996, 66: 668–670.

140. Gonzalez-Huix F, Fernandez-Banares F, Esteve-Comas M, et al. Enteral versus parenteral nutrition as adjunct therapy in acute ulcerative colitis. *Am. J. Gastroenterol.* 1993, 88: 227–232.

141. Kalfarentzos F, Kehagias J, Mead N, Kokkinis K, Gogos CA. Enteral nutrition is superior to parenteral nutrition in severe acute pancreatitis: results of a randomized prospective trial. *Br. J. Surg.* 1997, 84: 1665–1669.

142. Bank S, Singh P, Pooran N, Stark B. Evaluation of factors that have reduced mortality from acute pancreatitis over the past 20 years. *J. Clin. Gastroenterol.* 2002, 35: 50–60.

143. Olah A, Pardavi G, Belagyi T, Nagy A, Issekutz A, Mohamed GE. Early nasojejunal feeding in acute pancreatitis is associated with a lower complication rate. *Nutrition* 2002, 18: 259–262.

144. Olah A, Pardavi G, Belagyi T. [Early jejunal feeding in acute pancreatitis: prevention of septic complications and multiorgan failure]. *Magy. Seb.* 2000, 53: 7–12.

145. Al-Omran M, Groof A, Wilke D. Enteral versus parenteral nutrition for acute pancreatitis. *Cochrane Database Syst. Rev.* 2003: CD002837.

146. Griffiths RD. Nutrition in intensive care: give enough but choose the route wisely? *Nutrition* 2001, 17: 53–55.

147. Bauer P, Charpentier C, Bouchet C, Nace L, Raffy F, Gaconnet N. Parenteral with enteral nutrition in the critically ill. *Intens. Care Med.* 2000, 26: 893–900.

148. Woodcock NP, Zeigler D, Palmer MD, Buckley P, Mitchell CJ, MacFie J. Enteral versus parenteral nutrition: a pragmatic study. *Nutrition* 2001, 17: 1–12.

149. Kozar RA, McQuiggan MM, Moore EE, Kudsk KA, Jurkovich GJ, Moore FA. Postinjury enteral tolerance is reliably achieved by a standardized protocol. *J. Surg. Res.* 2002, 104: 70–75.

150. Neumann DA, DeLegge MH. Gastric versus small-bowel tube feeding in the intensive care unit: a prospective comparison of efficacy. *Crit. Care Med.* 2002, 30: 1436–1438.

151. Adam S, Batson S. A study of problems associated with the delivery of enteral feed in critically ill patients in five ICUs in the U.K. *Intens. Care Med.* 1997, 23: 261–266.

152. Mutlu GM, Mutlu EA, Factor P. GI complications in patients receiving mechanical ventilation. *Chest* 2001, 119: 1222–1241.

153. Ritz MA, Fraser R, Tam W, Dent J. Impacts and patterns of disturbed gastrointestinal function in critically ill patients. *Am. J. Gastroenterol.* 2000, 95: 3044–3052.

154. Kao CH, ChangLai SP, Chieng PU, Yen TC. Gastric emptying in head-injured patients. *Am. J. Gastroenterol.* 1998, 93: 1108–1112.

155. Kalff JC, Turler A, Schwarz NT, et al. Intra-abdominal activation of a local inflammatory response within the human muscularis externa during laparotomy. *Ann. Surg.* 2003, 237: 301–315.

156. DeMeo MT, Mutlu EA, Keshavarzian A, Tobin MC. Intestinal permeation and gastrointestinal disease. *J. Clin. Gastroenterol.* 2002, 34: 385–396.

157. Taguchi A, Sharma N, Saleem RM, et al. Selective postoperative inhibition of gastrointestinal opioid receptors. *N. Engl. J. Med.* 2001, 345: 935–940.

158. Cowles VE, Nellans HN, Seifert TR, et al. Effect of novel motilide ABT-229 versus erythromycin and cisapride on gastric emptying in dogs. *J. Pharmacol. Exp. Ther.* 2000, 293: 1106–1111.

159. Rhoden D, Matheson PJ, Carricato ND, Spain DA, Garrison RN. Immune-enhancing enteral diet selectively augments ileal blood flow in the rat. *J. Surg. Res.* 2002, 106: 25–30.

160. Houdijk AP, Van Leeuwen PA, Boermeester MA, et al. Glutamine-enriched enteral diet increases splanchnic blood flow in the rat. *Am. J. Physiol.* 1994, 267: G1035–G1040.

161. Okada Y, Klein N, van Saene HK, Pierro A. Small volumes of enteral feedings normalise immune function in infants receiving parenteral nutrition. *J. Pediatr. Surg.* 1998, 33: 16–19.

162. Sax HC, Illig KA, Ryan CK, Hardy DJ. Low-dose enteral feeding is beneficial during total parenteral nutrition. *Am. J. Surg.* 1996, 171: 587–590.

163. Cresci G, Martindale R. Bedside placement of small bowel feeding tubes in hospitalized patients: a new role for the dietitian. *Nutrition* 2003, 19: 843–846.

164. Heyland DK, Dhaliwal R, Drover JW, Gramlich L, Dodek P. Canadian clinical practice guidelines for nutrition support in mechanically ventilated, critically ill adult patients. *J. Parenter. Enteral Nutr.* 2003, 27: 355–373.

165. Genton L, Kudsk KA. Interactions between the enteric nervous system and the immune system: role of neuropeptides and nutrition. *Am. J. Surg.* 2003, 186: 253–258.

166. Martin CM, Doig GS, Heyland DK, Morrison T, Sibbald WJ. Multicentre, cluster-randomized clinical trial of algorithms for critical-care enteral and parenteral therapy (ACCEPT). *CMAJ* 2004, 170: 197–204.

13 Nutrition during Low Flow States: Influence of Critical Illness on Gut Function and Microenvironment

Hank Schmidt and Robert G. Martindale
Medical College of Georgia

CONTENTS

13.1   INTRODUCTION

Over 100 years of surgical dogma has firmly entrenched the principle of delaying enteral feeding in patients in the postoperative or posttraumatic period, in favor of awaiting evidence of return of gut function. Recent prospective trials, however, have given this issue a high priority in clinical practice, spurring the development of a new standard of care for many ICU patients. A wealth of data now exists demonstrating the benefits of early enteral feeding for the critically ill. Few concepts have affected our ability to improve outcomes in critical care more than the evolution of our understanding of the gastrointestinal tract as the major component of the immune system. It now seems clear that stimulation of the gut-associated lymphoid tissue (GALT) through luminal delivery of nutrients is key to the preservation not only of gut mucosal immunity but the entire epithelial-based immune system.

13.2   GUT IMMUNITY

The concept of mucosal immunity as a component of the entire immune system was not widely recognized in critical care until careful examination of studies comparing enteral and parenteral nutrition. A series of studies summarized in a meta-analysis by Moore et al. in 1991 confirmed significantly lower rates of postoperative sepsis by provision of early enteral nutrition.[1] Patients without enteral nutritional support develop both functional and morphometric mucosal atrophy.[2]

Recent data also support the concept that nonluminal nutrient delivery translates into loss of immune function as a result of deficient functioning GALT. Gut-associated lymphoid tissue includes Peyer's patches, intraepithelial lymphocytes, and lymphoid cells of the lamina propria. In total, the GALT is estimated to compose approximately 70% of the body's immunologic function.[3] This tissue collectively plays a significant role in mucosal immunity, modulating responses to both infectious and resident bacterial flora. It is clear from descriptive studies that the immune function of the gut epithelium forms an important component of intestinal barrier function. Compromise to this barrier by one of several mechanisms, including nonluminal nutrient supply, has been hypothesized to be a predisposing factor in development of nosocomial infections. As mentioned earlier, prospective randomized clinical trials comparing enteral and parenteral nutrition in postinjury patients have demonstrated significantly lower rates of infectious complications when feeding the gut.[4,5] These outcomes are likely a reflection of the preservation of mucosal integrity, the GALT, as well as systemic immunity. In fact, numerous studies have supported the finding that TPN induces systemic immune suppression.[6,7]

13.3 ALTERED BARRIER FUNCTION

Considerable effort has been dedicated to defining the role of altered gut mucosal integrity in development of sepsis and multiorgan system failure in critically ill patients. However, in spite of consistent data on the benefits of enteral nutrition in critical illness, no consensus exists on the role of the gut in development of septic complications and multiple organ failure. In ICU patients, numerous insults, such as npo status, use of histamine-receptor antagonists, bowel preps, antibiotics, and ongoing ischemia during resuscitation or intervention, all contribute to loss of normal gut flora and permeability changes at the brush border. In spite of a host of laboratory data identifying bacterial or endotoxin translocation as a key factor in sepsis models, clinical evidence of this phenomenon is less convincing. Early bacterial translocation has been observed in burn patients; however, no study has correlated this phenomenon with multiorgan failure or mortality.[8] There does exist indirect evidence that translocation is an important factor in septic complications, most notably occurring in the conversion of sterile pancreatic necrosis to infected pancreatic necrosis by way of mesenteric lymph nodes.[9,10] The only study published in noncompromised bowel comparing bacterial translocation in patients receiving enteral vs. parenteral nutrition found no difference in prevalence of organisms harvested from mesenteric lymph nodes.[11] Therefore, it is clear that changes in permeability in the gut do occur and that intestinal bacteria and endotoxin do find their way into extraluminal tissue, but the role of this phenomenon in development of distant infection and multiorgan failure remains open to some debate.[12–14] Despite the attractive hypotheses and extensive animal data, no clinical studies to date have shown that bacterial translocation correlates with the incidence of septic complications, multiorgan failure, or mortality.

If altered gut barrier function and subsequent bacterial translocation were in fact the key inciting event leading to nosocomial infections and disseminated sepsis, then measures to control gut flora should influence infection rates in critically ill patients. Numerous clinical trials examining selective gut decontamination (SGD) have been performed since 1986. A recent meta-analysis of prospective clinical studies reported that SGD was effective in reducing rates of hospital-acquired pneumonias.[15] This therapy did not, however, influence mortality or development of multiorgan failure. Other meta-analyses of these trials have reached similar conclusions.[16,17]

13.4 HOST–LUMINAL MICROBE INTERACTIONS IN STRESS STATES

Until now, the focus of study on microenvironmental changes in ischemia–reperfusion injury has been predominantly on intestinal epithelia. Investigators are now assembling a fascinating body of knowledge surrounding high-level interactions between the native gut bacterial flora and the changing luminal surface environment in critical illness. Gut luminal microbes are altered by these host environmental cues, such that relative gut ischemia and resuscitation are responsible for local changes in catecholamine concentrations, pH, redox state, nutrient availability, and osmolality that affect bacterial growth and adherence.[38]

A number of subversive tactics used by bacteria to enhance microbial virulence and host infection have been documented. These strategies vary based on what the bacteria consider the microenvironmental "threat assessment." They include intracolony communication, modulation of virulence gene expression, biofilm generation, hypervariable genomics, and molecular mimicry to escape immune surveillance.[39,40] For example, upon "sensing" stressful host events, *E. coli* expresses receptors that allow adherence to the mucosa, inducing contact-dependent signal transduction pathways in the epithelial mucosa, resulting in disruption of tight junctions, cytokine release, cell apoptosis, and neutrophil release.

These elaborate microbial–host responses spawned the concept that promoting maintenance of the normal gut microflora might decrease the invasive tendency of the microbial population when presented with stressful host events. It is clear that numerous changes occur at the gut mucosal brush border in critically ill patients. It also seems apparent that these changes significantly impact development of further complications, incurring added morbidity and mortality. It is a non sequitur, then, that preservation of this gut luminal microenvironment is a high priority. Recently, a new interest has developed in pre- and probiotics and their importance in critical illness. Probiotics consist of live microbes that, when ingested, confer some benefit to the host organism as a result of microbial influence on human physiology.[37] Rapidly evolving concepts in this field suggest that maintenance of the luminal microenvironment may prevent normally nonpathogenic species from developing mucosal adherence and invasion. These opportunistic microbes may then modulate the inflammatory and immune response. Numerous bacterial and yeast species have been described that have dramatically different effects on the gastrointestinal system. For further discussion of this approach, see Chapter 10.

13.5 iNOS AND INTESTINAL REPERFUSION INJURY

Another important initiating factor in the alteration in mucosal permeability is felt to be ischemia and subsequent reperfusion of the gut. Common to many intensive care patients is the challenge of recovery after episodes of intestinal hypoperfusion, whether it be a result of surgery; hemorrhagic, cardiogenic, or septic shock; use of vasoactive drugs; or a mesenteric embolic event. Mesenteric circulation is subjected to a disproportionate response to shock by selective vasoconstriction of mesenteric arterioles and venous capacitance vessels essentially to autotransfuse the systemic circulation benefiting "vital" organs.[18,19] (See Figure 13.1.) We are now beginning to uncover a vast array of physiologic consequences of gut ischemia–reperfusion injury, impacting the inflammatory response at the mucosal level. Significant data have accumulated pointing to the inducible nitric oxide synthase (iNOS) as one of the major mediators of these mucosal changes.[20,21] Nitric oxide is a known inhibitor of gastrointestinal smooth muscle contractility and has recently been implicated in post ischemia–reperfusion-induced ileus in animal models.[22]

Other experiments have shown that inhibition of iNOS allows lower rates of bacterial translocation, prevention of increased mucosal permeability, and preservation of mucosal mitochondrial function in similar models of bacterial LPS challenge.[23] Inhibition of intestinal smooth muscle function, recruitment of neutrophils and macrophages, induction of proinflammatory cytokine release, increased membrane permeability, actin cytoskeletal rearrangement, and ATP wasting have all been ascribed to nitric oxide.[24] Nitric oxide production is augmented with leukocyte infiltration, causing vasodilation and elaboration of tissue damage by reactive oxygen metabolites. Concomitant acidosis in the setting of ischemia promotes conversion of nitric oxide to a damaging peroxynitrite anion. Animal data suggest that bacterial lipopolysaccharide from enteropathogenic organisms stimulates nitric oxide synthesis and cyclooxygenase-2 (COX-2). The increased COX-2 activity

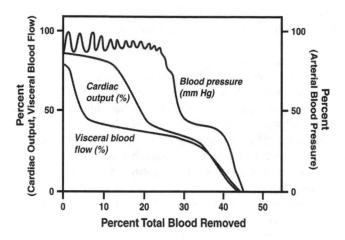

FIGURE 13.1 Mesenteric circulation is subjected to a disproportionate response to shock.

results in elaboration of prostaglandins, allowing complex regulation of gut epithelial resident macrophages by both agents (nitric oxide and prostaglandins).[25] Recently, an interesting hypothesis has been developed by studying a nitric oxide synthase (iNOS) knockout mouse model.[26] Deitch and colleagues[26] found that bacterial translocation measured by mesenteric lymph node analysis in mice on total parenteral nutrition was absent in the iNOS knockout. The exact mechanism and role of nitric oxide in gut mucosa remains unclear and is likely regulated by a complex orchestration of a number of mediators and enzyme systems. In general, nitric oxide is part of a befuddling paradox in human physiology in that it seems both to inhibit and to induce inflammation (Figure 13.2). It appears essential in its role as an effector of cellular immune response and an agent of homeostasis in stress states; however, nitric oxide is also a free radical and can purvey the deleterious effects of oxidizing proteins, lipids, and DNA.[27] Complete inhibition of iNOS in septic shock patients resulted in early closure of a multicenter randomized trial when preliminary review demonstrated a 10% higher mortality in the iNOS inhibitor group.[28] Recent work by Lee et al.[27] proposes an interesting model to resolve this paradox. These investigators observed that cytokines up-regulate iNOS mRNA; however, translation into protein is dependent on transport of arginine into the cell by specific membrane proteins. Therefore, extensive compartmentalization of nitric oxide pathways is facilitated by colocalization with a particular arginine transporter, providing a higher level of regulating iNOS activity.

Numerous studies have attempted to isolate a gut-derived factor inciting shock-induced acute respiratory distress syndrome. Gonzales et al.[29] find a novel approach to this question in a study in which the authors first used a rat hemorrhagic shock model to isolate lymph. Human pulmonary microvascular endothelial cells (HMVEC) in culture were then incubated with activated neutrophils and lymph. Not only was marked HMVEC death observed in the cells treated with lymph from the hemorrhage animals, but this effect was also abrogated by addition of an antibody to intercellular adhesion molecule (ICAM-1).[29] Several proinflammatory cytokines and their mediators, such as ICAM-1, E and P selectin, IL-8, IL-6, and beta2 integrin, are likely induced by gut ischemic insult and ultimately play a role in systemic end-organ damage.[30–33] Even our relatively limited knowledge of the intricacies of these signaling molecules has opened the door to new approaches for therapeutic manipulation in critical care. Animal data have demonstrated that, following mesenteric ischemia, novel methods of resuscitation attenuating nitric oxide generation definitively limit gut barrier dysfunction and propagation of systemic inflammatory indicators.[34,35] Hypertonic saline resuscitation caused a significant decrease in intestinal mucosa, pulmonary alveolar injury, and neutrophil sequestration. Likewise, a combination of the novel anti-inflammatory ethyl pyruvate with Ringer's solution used for resuscitation in a murine shock model significantly reduced permeability changes

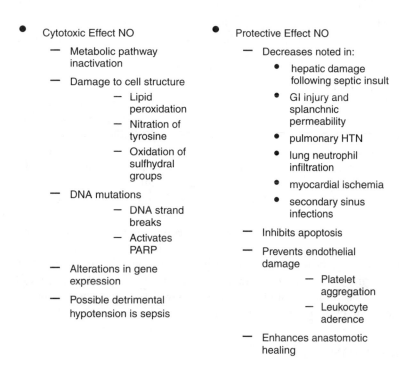

- Cytotoxic Effect NO
  - Metabolic pathway inactivation
  - Damage to cell structure
    - Lipid peroxidation
    - Nitration of tyrosine
    - Oxidation of sulfhydral groups
  - DNA mutations
    - DNA strand breaks
    - Activates PARP
  - Alterations in gene expression
  - Possible detrimental hypotension is sepsis

- Protective Effect NO
  - Decreases noted in:
    - hepatic damage following septic insult
    - GI injury and splanchnic permeability
    - pulmonary HTN
    - lung neutrophil infiltration
    - myocardial ischemia
    - secondary sinus infections
  - Inhibits apoptosis
  - Prevents endothelial damage
    - Platelet aggregation
    - Leukocyte aderence
  - Enhances anastomotic healing

FIGURE 13.2 Arginine paradox.

and bacterial translocation. A recent animal model of hemorrhagic shock indicates that resuscitation with improved oxygen-carrying blood substitutes may also be effective in controlling the degree of inflammation induced by injury.[36]

13.6 GUT DYSMOTILITY

A profound impact has been rendered on delivery of ICU care by the completion of over 22 prospective randomized trials, which have now verified the multiplicity of benefits of early enteral feeding in critically ill patient populations in terms of decreased morbidity and length of ICU and hospital stays. The major limiting factor in uniform application of this tactic, however, remains our inability to overcome gut dysmotility observed in critical illness.

A number of ongoing studies have recently enhanced our understanding of mechanisms underlying ileus after surgery and during sepsis.[41,42] A novel investigation by Kalff and colleagues now lends human data to previous animal models identifying an inflammatory cascade, triggered by resident macrophages that had migrated to the muscularis mucosa followed by some mechanical or metabolic stress. This migration then sets up an inflammatory cascade of events, leading to loss of normal motility.[43] The authors harvested human small bowel specimens at various times during abdominal surgery and found a time-dependent induction of a number of inflammatory cytokines in the muscularis externa (LFA-1, IL-6, IL-1beta, TNF-alpha, iNOS, and COX-2). Smooth muscle bath experiments verified enhanced contractility during incubation with iNOS and COX-2 inhibitors. Most studies evaluating the effects of sepsis on gut motility have used single large doses of endotoxin or single events, which lead to overwhelming sepsis (i.e., cecal ligation and puncture). In contrast to the single-dose models, Bruins et al. have developed a clinically relevant pig model to evaluate the effects of prolonged hyperdynamic endotoxemia.[44] In this model, which very closely resembles the human septic patient, the investigators found low-dose, continuous endotoxin infusion accelerated the migrating motor complex (MMC) along the entire jejunum. Despite the accelerated MMC, the animals tolerated enteral feeding without compromise of hemodymanics.

Numerous clinical trials have also focused their efforts on eliminating delayed recovery of normal gastrointestinal function. Of note, administration of enteral naloxone to block local opioid receptors in mechanically ventilated, nonsurgical patients on fentanyl analgesia resulted in significant decreases in gastric tube reflux and frequency of pneumonia (34% vs. 56%).[45] This therapy had no effect on length of ICU stay, however. Another well known agent affecting gastrointestinal motility through stimulation of motilin receptors is the antibiotic erythromycin. In a recent prospective randomized trial of intravenous erythromycin therapy vs. placebo, critically ill patients on the drug demonstrated a slight improvement in tube feeding tolerance; however, no significant difference was observed in most clinical outcome variables measured.[46] Despite those listed previously and numerous other attempts at eliminating or minimizing gastrointestinal-related dysmotility in the ICU patient, none has been uniformly successful.

Yet another exciting area of recent study and clinical relevance to nutrition delivery in the ICU setting is the acute control of blood glucose concentration in intensive care patients. The report by Van den Berghe using "intensive insulin therapy" to keep blood glucose between 80 and 110 mg/dl was associated with significant reductions in infection rate, progression to sepsis, and mortality.[47] Glucose control is also a factor in modulating gastrointestinal motility, particularly in the upper tract. Both animal and human studies have documented a dose-dependent effect of hyperglycemia on antral motility.[48] Therefore, tight glucose control may also be an important factor for enhancing tolerance of early enteral feeding in critical illness.

13.7 CONCLUSION

Numerous clinical trials have now verified that early enteral feeding in critically ill patients is feasible. In general, benefits of this strategy include a decrease in infectious complications and shorter hospital stays. Likewise, enteral feeding allows better glycemic control and facilitates both mucosal and systemic wound healing. At the level of the intestinal tract, enteral nutrition promotes increased visceral blood flow and improved nutrient transport and mucosal preservation for both barrier function and immune surveillance. The most important factor in enteral feeding is likely the global benefit derived from immune system maintenance via stimulation of the GALT. Obviously, not all patients are candidates for enteral feeding, and some may fall into a category placing them at increased risk of complications in this setting. Patients with significant gut dysmotility primarily from postoperative ileus may require a delay in feeding while efforts are focused on return of gut function, avoiding predisposing factors such as electrolyte abnormalities, narcotics, and hyperglycemia. Inadequate gastric decompression may also be a key element in lack of tolerance of enteral feeding. We cannot overemphasize the point that patients enduring hemodynamic instability are far less likely to tolerate enteral nutrition until initial resuscitation is completed. An additional negative approach is overly aggressive enteral feeding to involve the colon. Initial rates of 10 to 20 ml/h are appropriate until tolerance is demonstrated; feedings may then be advanced to goal over the next 48 hours.

13.8 CLINICAL APPLICATIONS

Early enteral nutrition should now become the standard of care in critically ill patients. The work of Kozar et al. has noted that enteral feeding is well tolerated in severely ill patients using a standardized management protocol.[49] In order to maximize tolerance, we recommend the following:

- Quickly obtain enteral access via postpyloric feeding tube on admission to the ICU.
- Ensure that the patient demonstrates hemodynamic stability and has had adequate resuscitation.

- Begin enteral feeding slowly at 10 to 15 ml/h; advance every 8 to 12 hours to goal rate over 24 to 96 hours. Add free water flushes to maintain tube patency and to minimize parenteral fluid infusions.
- Maintain meticulous glycemic control, maintaining normal ranges.
- Frequently monitor and correct electrolytes.
- Minimize use of hypomotility agents such as narcotics, clonidine, psychotropics, and pressors.
- Adopt an opiate-sparing approach including preferential use of epidural anesthesia or analgesia, use of propofol as a sedative or hypnotic, and use of COX-2 inhibitors for pain control.
- Employ selective use of prokinetic agents to enhance enteral feeding tolerance.
- Consider combining enteral nutrition with TPN.

This armamentarium of tools, combined with an institutional protocol for enteral feeding, should significantly enhance success of enteral nutrition in maintaining critically ill patients. As our knowledge of and experience with immunomodulation through nutrition continues to expand, we can expect a greater understanding of these strategies to improve patient outcomes further in a variety of clinical settings.

REFERENCES

1. Moore FA, Feliciano DF, Andrassy JR, et al. Early enteral feeding compared with parenteral, reduces postoperative septic complications: the result of a meta-analysis. *Ann. Surg.* 1991, 216: 172–183.
2. Levine GM, Deren JJ, Steiger E, Zinno R. Role of oral intake in maintenance of gut mass and disaccharide activity. *Gastroenterol.* 1974, 67: 975–982.
3. Brandtzaeg, P, Halstensen TS, Krajci P, Kvale D, Rognum TO, Scott H, Sollid LM. Immunobiology and immunopathology of human gut mucosa: humoral immunity and intraepithelial lymphocytes. *Gastroenterol.* 1989, 97: 1562–1584.
4. Moore FA, Moore EE, Jones TN, McCroskey BL, Peterson VM. TEN versus TPN following major abdominal trauma: reduced septic morbidity. *J. Trauma* 1989, 29: 916–923.
5. Kudsk KA, Croce MA, Fabian TC, et al. Enteral versus parenteral feeding: effects on septic morbidity following blunt and penetrating abdominal trauma. *Ann. Surg.* 1992, 215: 503–513.
6. Kudsk KA, Li J, Renegar KB. Loss of upper respiratory tract immunity with enteral feeding. *Ann. Surg.* 1996, 223(6): 629–635.
7. Shou J, Lappin J, Daly JM. Impairment of pulmonary macrophage function with TPN. *Ann. Surg.* 1994 219(3): 291–297.
8. Nieuwenhuijzen GA, Goris JA. The gut: the "motor" of multiple organ dysfunction syndrome? *Curr. Opin. Clin. Nutr. Metab. Care* 1999, 2: 399–404.
9. Lehocky P, Sarr MG. Early enteral feeding in severe acute pancreatitis: can it prevent secondary pancreatic (super) infection? *Dig. Surg.* 2000, 17(6): 571–577.
10. Bengmark S. Aggressive peri- and intraoperative enteral nutrition: strategy for the future. In *Nutritional Considerations in the Intensive Care Unit: Science, Rationale, and Practice.* Shikora SA, Martindale RG, and Schwaitzberg SD, eds. 2002, ASPEN, Silver Spring, MD.
11. Sedman PC, MacFie J, Palmer MD, Mitchell CJ, Sagar PM. Preoperative total parenteral nutrition is not associated with mucosal atrophy or bacterial translocation in humans. *Br. J. Surg.* 1995, 82: 1663.
12. Kucharzik T, Lugering N, Rautenberg K, Lugering A, Schmidt MA, Stoll R, Domschke W. Role of M cells in intestinal barrier function. *Ann. N.Y. Acad. Sci.* 2000, 915: 171–183.
13. Isolauri E, Sutas Y, Kankaanpaa P, Arvilommi H, Salminen S. Probiotics: effects on immunity. *Am. J. Clin. Nutr.* 2001, 73(suppl.): 444S–450S.
14. O'Brien D, Nelson L, Stern L, Williams J, Kemp C, Wang Q, Tso P, Erwin C, Hasselgren P, Warner B. Epithelial permeability is not increased in rats following small bowel resection. *J. Surg. Res.* 2001, 97: 65–70.

15. Krueger W, Unertl K. Selective decontamination of the digestive tract. *Curr. Opin. Crit. Care* 2002, 8:139–144..

16. D'Amico R, Pifferi S, Leonetti C, Torri V, Tinazzi A, Liberati A. Effectiveness of antibiotic prophylaxis in critically ill adult patients: systematic review of randomised controlled trials. *Br. Med. J.* 1998, 316: 1275–1285.

17. Heyland DK, Cook DJ, Jaeschke R, Griffith L, Lee H, Guyat G. Selective decontamination of the digestive tract: an overview. *Chest* 1994, 105: 1221–1229.

18. Ceppa EP, Fuh KC, Bulkley GB. Mesenteric hemodynamic response to circulatory shock. *Curr. Opin. Crit. Care* 2003, 9(2): 127–132.

19. Jakob SM. Splanchnic blood flow in low-flow states. *Anesthesia & Analgesia* 2003, 96(4): 1129–1138.

20. Nadler EP, Ford HR. Regulation of bacterial translocation by nitric oxide. *Pediatr. Surg. Int.* 2000; 16(3): 165–168.

21. Fink MP. Nitric oxide and the gut: one more piece in the puzzle. *Crit. Care Med.* 1999, 27(2): 248–249.

22. Hassoun H, Weisbrodt N, Mercer D, Kozar R, Moody FG, Moore FA. Inducible nitric oxide synthase mediates gut ischemia/reperfusion-induced ileus only after severe insults. *J. Surg. Res.* 2001, 97: 150–154.

23. Unno N, Wang H, Menconi MJ, et al. Inhibition of inducible nitric oxide synthase ameliorates lipopolysaccharide-induced gut mucosal barrier dysfuncion in rats. *Gastroenterol.* 1997, 113: 1246–1257.

24. Fink MP. Intestinal epithelial hyperpermeability: update on the pathogenesis of gut mucosal barrier dysfunction in critical illness. *Curr. Opin. Crit. Care* 2003, 9(2): 143–151.

25. Hori M, Kita M, Torihashi S, Miyamoto S, Won KJ, Sato K, Ozaki H, Karaki H. Upregulation of iNOS by COX-2 in muscularis resident macrophage of rat intestine stimulated with LPS. *Am. J. Physiol.* 2001, 280: G930–G938.

26. Deitch EA, Shorshtein A, Houghton J, Lu Q, Xu D. Inducible nitric oxide synthase knockout mice are resistant to diet-induced loss of gut barrier function and intestinal injury. *J. Gastrointest. Surg.* 2002, 6: 599–605.

27. Lee J, et al. Translational control of inducible nitric oxide synthase expression by arginine can explain the arginine paradox. *PNAS*, 15, 2003, 100(8): 4843–4848.

28. Lopez A, Lorente J, Steingrub J et al. Multiple-center, randomized, placebo-controlled, double-blind study of nitric oxide synthase inhibitor 546C88: effect on survival in patients with septic shock. *Crit. Care Med.* 2004, 32(1): 21–30.

29. Gonzales RJ, Moore EE, Ciesla DJ, Nieto JR, Johnson J, Silliman C. Post-hemorrhagic shock mesenteric lymph activates human pulmonary microvascular endothelium for *in vitro* neutrophil-mediated injury: the role of intercellular adhesion molecule-1. *J. Trauma* 2003, 54(2): 219–223.

30. Fukatsu K, Kudsk KA, Zarzaur BL, Sabek O, Wilcox HG, Johnson CD. Increased ICAM-1 and beta2 integrin expression in parenterally fed mice after a gut ischemic insult. *Shock* 2002, 18(2): 119–124.

31. Nemeth ZH, Deitch EA, Szabo C, Hasko G. Pyrrolidinedithiocarbamate inhibits NF-kappaB activation and IL-8 production in intestinal epithelial cells. *Immunol. Lett.* 2003, 85(1): 41–46.

32. Jaeschke H. Molecular mechanisms of hepatic ischemia–reperfusion injury and preconditioning. *Am. J. Physiol.* 2003, 284: G15–G26.

33. Dayal SD, Hasko G, Lu Q, Xu DZ, Caruso JM, Sambol JT, Deitch EA. Trauma/hemorrhagic shock mesenteric lymph upregulates adhesion molecule expression and IL-6 production in human umbilical vein endothelial cells. *Shock* 2002, 17(6): 491–495.

34. Shi HP, Deitch EA, Da Xu Z, Lu Q, Hauser CJ. Hypertonic saline improves intestinal mucosa barrier function and lung injury after trauma-hemorrhagic shock. *Shock* 2002, 17(6): 496–501.

35. Sappington PL, Yang R, Delude RL, Fink MP. Delayed treatment with ethyl pyruvate (EP) ameliorates LPS-induced gut barrier dysfunction in mice. *Crit. Care Med.* 2002, 30(12) (suppl): A9.

36. Knudson MM, Lee S, Erickson V, Morabito D, Derugin N, Manley G. Tissue oxygen monitoring during hemorrhagic shock and resuscitation: a comparison of lactated Ringer's solution, hypertonic saline dextran, and HBOC-201. *J. Trauma* 2003, 54(2): 242–252.

37. Ishibashi N, Yamazaki S. Probiotics and safety. *Am. J. Clin. Nutr.* 2001, 73(suppl): 465S–470S.

38. Freestone PP, Haigh RD, Williams PH, et al. Stimulation of bacterial growth by heat-stable norepinephrine-induced autoinducers. *FEMS Microbiol. Lett.* 1991, 172: 53–60.

39. Alverdy JC, Laughlin RS, Wu L. Influence of the critically ill state on host-pathogen interactions within the intestine: gut derived sepsis redefined. *Crit. Care Med.* 2003, 31(2): 598–607.

40. Faguy D. Bacterial genomics: the controlled chaos of shifty pathogens. *Curr. Biol.* 2000, 10: R498–R501.

41. Ritz M, Fraser R, Tam W, Dent J. Impacts and patterns of disturbed gastrointestinal function in critically ill patients. *Am. J. Gastroenterol.* 2000, 95(11): 3044–3052.

42. Bauer AJ, Schwarz NT, Moore BA, Turler A, Kalff JC. Ileus in critical illness: mechanisms and management. *Curr. Opin. Crit. Care* 2002, 8(2): 152–157.

43. Kalff JC, Turler A, Schwarz NT, Schraut WH, Lee KKW, Tweardy DJ, Billiar TR, Simmons RL, Bauer AJ. Intra-abdominal activation of a local inflammatory response within the human muscularis externa during laparotomy. *Ann. Surg.* 2003, 237(3): 301–315.

44. Bruins MJ, Luiking YC, Soeters PB, Akkermans LMA, Deutz NEP. *Ann. Surg.* 2003, 237: 44–52.

45. Meissner W, Dohrn B, Reinhart K. Enteral naloxone reduces gastric tube reflux and frequency of pneumonia in critical care patients during opioid analgesia. *Crit. Care Med.* 2002, 31(3): 776–780.

46. Berne J, Norwood S, McAuley C, Vallina V, Villareal D, Weston J, McClarty J. Erythromycin reduces delayed gastric emptying in critically ill trauma patients: a randomized, controlled trial. *J. Trauma* 2002, 53(3): 422–425.

47. van den Berghe G, Wouters P, Weekers F, Vaerwaest C, Bruyninckx F, Schetz M, Vlasselaers D, Ferdinande P, Lauwers P, Bouillon R. Intensive insulin therapy in the critically ill patients. *NEJM* 2001, 345(19): 1359–1367.

48. Rayner CK, Samsom M, Jones KL, Horowitz M. Relationships of upper gastrointestinal motor and sensory function with glycemic control. *Diabetes Care* 2001, 24: 371–381.

49. Kozar RA, McQuiggan MM, Moore EE, Kudsk KA, Jurkovich GJ, Moore FA. Postinjury enteral tolerance is reliably achieved by a standardized protocol. *J. Surg. Res.* 2002, 104(1): 70–75.

14 Parenteral Nutrition Access for the Critically Ill

Troy F. Kimsey
Medical College of Georgia

CONTENTS

14.1 INTRODUCTION

Delivery of nutritional support is an essential component of caring for the critically ill patient. The pros and cons of enteral and parenteral nutrition have been discussed in previous chapters. This chapter will focus on the critically ill patient requiring total parenteral nutrition (TPN) and the factors involved in determining which access device and access site are most appropriate. TPN solutions are hypertonic and must be administered into high flow areas of the central venous circulation. For this reason, administering TPN would be more difficult without the advances made in central venous access over the past 50 years.

14.2 HISTORY

The first central venous catheter (CVC) was placed by Dr. Forssmann in 1929. Forssmann, a German urologist, placed a catheter into one of his peripheral veins, advanced the catheter into his right atrium, and confirmed the catheter's placement by radiography. Twenty years later, Dr. Aubaniac, a French surgeon, described percutaneously accessing the subclavian vein in order to resuscitate a patient [1], and in 1953 Dr. Seldinger described his technique of placing a catheter over a guidewire [2]. Dr. Dudrick was the first physician to describe administering parenteral nutrition through a central venous catheter. Dudrick placed a catheter into the subclavian vein with a percutaneous, infraclavicular approach and administered parenteral nutrition [3]. In 1973, Broviac, Cole, and Scribner developed a long-term, in-dwelling, right atrial Silastic catheter for administering home TPN [4]. This catheter was placed intravenously following a cutdown to the cephalic or internal jugular vein and was tunneled subcutaneously to the upper chest wall. It also contained a poly-ethylene terphthalate (Dacron) cuff in the subcutaneous tunnel adjacent to the exit site to reduce the risk of infection. In 1979, Dr. Hickman modified the Broviac catheter by increasing the internal diameter of the catheter [5]. Peripherally inserted central venous catheters (PICCs) were introduced in 1975 [6]; in 1982, the implantable central venous access device (chemoport or Port-A-Cath) was developed [7]. The latest advances in central venous catheters include improved biomaterials, additional lumina, split ports, antibiotic and anticoagulant impregnation, and fluoroscopic or ultra-sound guidance for catheter placement. These advances have enhanced our ability to use CVCs in the care of critically ill patients while reducing the number of catheter-related complications.

14.3 INDICATIONS FOR ACCESS

In the United States, physicians insert more than five million CVCs each year [8]. Although this chapter will focus on the need for central venous access for the administration of TPN, it is important to be familiar with other indications for central venous access (see Table 14.1). Several indications can be present in a critically ill patient that influence the type of catheter placed and the site selected for its placement. In this chapter, we will focus on the factors that influence catheter selection, site selection, technique of placement, catheter care, and the complications associated with placing and maintaining CVCs.

14.3.1 CATHETER CHARACTERISTICS

Advances in the different biomaterials used in manufacturing CVCs have greatly enhanced their usefulness and safety (see Table 14.2). The chemical structure and physical properties of these biomaterials determine their suitability for use in venous access. Pliability is an important physical property that affects the degree of difficulty in placing catheters. Pliable catheters can be technically difficult to place, whereas stiff catheters can cause injury to the patient during placement.

TABLE 14.1
Indications for Central Venous Access

Total parenteral nutrition
Need for hemodynamic monitoring
Continuous infusion therapy
Inability to obtain peripheral access
Long-term antibiotic therapy
Hemodialysis
Caustic chemotherapy
Intensive chemotherapy with anticipated transfusions

TABLE 14.2
Biomaterials Used in Central Venous Catheters

Polyurethane
Polyethylene
Polyvinyl chloride (PVC)
Polytetrafluoroethylene (PTFE)
Silicone elastomer (Silastic)

Additionally, catheters are not passive conduits. They elicit various responses from the patient and endogenous microorganisms, which influence the development of thrombosis, inflammation, and infection. The microscopic texture of catheters influences their thrombogenicity. Catheters that are smooth under scanning electron microscopy are thought to cause less thrombosis than rough catheters. The macromolecular structure of different biomaterials also promotes varying degrees of inflammation in the host [9,10]. The catheter's surface electrical charge influences bacterial adherence, because bacteria preferentially adhere to positively charged surfaces [11]. The ideal biomaterial would be smooth and appropriately pliable, without promoting bacterial adherence, thrombosis, or inflammation in the host.

Unfortunately, no such biomaterial currently exists. Polyurethane is a relatively stiff material that improves catheter placement, but it is pliable enough to provide some endothelial protection while indwelling [12]. Polyurethane is also smooth and causes less thrombosis and inflammation than other biomaterials [13]. Polyethylene is produced as high-density and low-density polymers. The low-density polyethylene polymers used in venous catheters cause significant chronic inflammation and are limited to use in acute catheters. In its native state, PVC is rigid, brittle, and unsuitable for venous access devices [14]. The addition of plasticizers has improved the flexibility of PVC catheters, making them more suitable for clinical use [15]. Unfortunately, these plasticizers cause platelet activation and surface fibrinogen adsorption, which correlates clinically with the increased incidence of thrombotic complications with these catheters [16,17]. Chronic implantation of PTFE catheters causes an inflammatory response that is typically followed by chronic fibrosis [18]. For this reason, PTFE is used more commonly in peripheral IV catheters and CVC introducers. Catheters made of PTFE and polyurethane cause fewer infectious complications than catheters made of PVC and polyethylene [19–21]. Silastic promotes less thrombosis, inflammation, and bacterial adherence than the other biomaterials [22,23]. For these reasons, it is the most common biomaterial used in chronic indwelling CVCs. It is, however, very pliable, making direct insertion technically difficult. Most Silastic catheters are inserted over a guidewire or through an introducer sheath.

In addition to the biomaterials used in manufacturing CVCs, catheter design also influences catheter selection. When selecting a CVC for administering parenteral nutrition in a critically ill patient, the need for additional intravenous fluids, medications, infusions, and hemodynamic monitoring must be considered. There are numerous catheters available today, with different designs for different needs (see Table 14.3). The Broviac catheter is a tunneled, single- or double-lumen CVC with a subcutaneous Dacron cuff. It has a small internal diameter and is designed for administering long-term TPN. Hickman modified the Broviac catheter by increasing the internal diameter of the catheter. Hickman catheters are now available as single-, double-, or triple-lumen catheters. The larger lumina facilitate administering TPN, drugs, fluids, and blood products, as well as obtaining blood draws. The Groshong catheter is a Silastic catheter with a three-way valve. The valve reduces the risk of air embolism and serves to prevent the reflux of blood, thereby eliminating the need for heparin flushes. A comparison study between Groshong and Hickman catheters demonstrated no significant difference in infectious or thrombotic complications, but it did demonstrate a higher catheter malfunction rate with the Groshong catheter [24]. Percutaneous, uncuffed CVCs are easier to place. They provide multiple lumina but are more temporary and lack a subcutaneous tunnel and cuff to protect against infections. Pulmonary artery catheters are helpful in hemodynamically unstable patients by providing measurements of different hemodynamic parameters. They do, however, require placement of a cordis sheath and have limited sites for intravenous access.

Peripherally inserted central catheters (PICCs) are inserted into a peripheral vein and advanced into a central vein. These catheters can be placed by the IV team or an interventional radiologist. PICCs are available as single- or double-lumen catheters and are useful for administering long-term home TPN or antibiotics.

TABLE 14.3
Characteristics of Different Catheter Types

Type of Catheter	Pros	Cons
Broviac	Decreased infection with tunneled catheter and Dacron cuff Single or double lumen	Narrow lumen, which limits the infusate
Hickman	Larger diameter than the Broviac catheter Single, double, or triple lumen	Refluxes blood, which requires heparin flushes Possible air embolism
Groshong	Three-way valve decreases the risk of air embolism and reflux	Increased malfunction rate
Percutaneous central catheter	Ease of placement with no subcutaneous tunnel Single, double, or triple lumen	More temporary than tunneled catheters Increased risk of infection
Pulmonary artery catheter	Ability to monitor hemodynamic parameters	Requires a cordis sheath Limited ports
Peripherally inserted central catheter	Ease of placement and removal	Limited usefulness — home TPN or antibiotics
Implantable central venous access device	No external component, with decreased risk of infection and easier maintenance	Requires surgical placement Requires trained personnel to access

Implantable central venous access devices (ICVADs) are also known as *chemoports* or *Port-A-Caths*. They have a CVC connected to a reservoir located in a subcutaneous pocket. Without the external component, these devices require less maintenance and are associated with a lower incidence of infectious complications [25–27]. They are, however, more difficult to place and require skilled personnel to access. Despite one study in which ICVADs were safely used for administering cyclic TPN [28], prolonged, repetitive access of these devices can potentially cause skin breakdown and an increase in infectious complications.

Catheters and cuffs impregnated with antimicrobial agents reduce the incidence of CRBSIs [15,29–32]; however, silver-impregnated cuffs left in place for more than 20 days have no impact on the incidence of CRBSIs [33,34]. Catheters coated with chlorhexidine–silver sulfadiazine on the external surface reduced the risk of CRBSIs, compared to noncoated catheters [30,35,36]. CVCs impregnated with minocycline–rifampin on the external and internal surfaces further reduced the risk of CRBSIs, compared to the first-generation chlorhexidine–silver sulfadiazine catheters [31]. A second-generation chlorhexidine–silver sulfadiazine with chlorhexidine on the internal surface and chlorhexidine–silver sulfadiazine on the external surface has now been developed. Preliminary studies showed prolonged antimicrobial activity [37], but further studies are needed to compare the minocycline–rifampin impregnated and second-generation chlorhexidine–silver sulfadiazine impregnated catheters.

14.3.2 SITE SELECTION

Several factors influence catheter site selection (see Table 14.4). Catheterization should not be attempted at sites with herpes zoster, bacterial infections, burns, malignancies, or rashes present at the access site. The subclavian vein should be avoided when possible in coagulopathic patients because of its location beneath the clavicle and the difficulty of obtaining adequate vascular compression. In morbidly obese patients, external landmarks can be obscured, making successful catheterization difficult. Hemodynamically unstable patients in need of pulmonary artery monitoring require a cordis sheath and pulmonary artery catheter. These devices can be placed at several sites, but the right internal jugular vein provides a straight course for the sheath and catheter. Accessing

TABLE 14.4
Considerations for CVC Site Selection

Comorbidities	Cutaneous lesions or wounds
	Coagulopathies
	Morbid obesity
	Hemodynamic instability
	Respiratory failure
	Renal failure
Anatomical	Previous surgery or scarring
	Skeletal deformities
	Aberrant vascular anatomy
	Venous occlusion
Site-Specific Risks	
Internal jugular vein	Increased risk of infection vs. subclavian vein
	Increased risk of thrombosis
Subclavian vein	Increased risk of pneumothorax
	Increased risk of hemothorax
Femoral vein	Increased risk of infection vs. subclavian vein
	Increased risk of arterial puncture
	Increased risk of puncture-site hematoma
	Increased risk of DVT

the subclavian vein is associated with a higher incidence of pneumothoraces [38–45] and should be avoided when possible in patients with respiratory compromise. In patients with renal failure, the subclavian vein should also be avoided to prevent subclavian vein stenosis or occlusion [45]. These complications prohibit arteriovenous fistula or graft placement, which may be needed in the ipsilateral upper extremity for long-term dialysis access. Previous surgery and scarring near an access site can distort normal anatomical landmarks and disrupt the underlying venous system. Skeletal deformities can also distort anatomical landmarks, prohibit proper positioning of the patient, and alter the underlying venous anatomy [40]. Patients with venous distension, edema, or a history of difficult access may have venous occlusion. Vascular studies should be obtained prior to attempting CVC placement in these patients.

Accessing the internal jugular, subclavian, and femoral veins has site-specific risks. The risk of pneumothorax and hemothorax are higher when accessing the subclavian vein, whereas the risk of arterial puncture and puncture-site hematoma are higher when accessing the femoral vein [38–45]. Although there have been no randomized trials comparing the relative risks of infection for different catheter sites, subclavian vein catheters have been associated with a lower incidence of infection than catheters placed in the internal jugular vein [29,46–49] or the femoral vein [38]. In addition, femoral venous catheters are associated with a higher incidence of deep venous thrombosis, compared to internal jugular and subclavian vein catheters [38,42,50–52]. Initially, subclavian vein catheters demonstrated a higher incidence of thrombosis than internal jugular vein catheters [44,53]. More recently, Timsit demonstrated a fourfold increase in the risk of thrombosis with internal jugular vein catheters, compared to subclavian vein catheters [54]. Each of these site-specific risks, as well as the patient's condition, comorbidities, and anatomy, must be considered when selecting the appropriate site for CVC placement.

14.3.3 TECHNIQUE OF PLACEMENT

Using proper technique for CVC placement reduces the risk of developing complications [55]. Although some technical considerations are site specific, most are broadly applied. Regardless of the site selected, proper technique requires good skin antisepsis, sterile-barrier precautions, and a thorough understanding of the equipment used.

Skin antisepsis and barrier protection during catheter placement have been studied. In the United States, povidone–iodine is the most commonly used skin antiseptic at insertion sites; however, there is a lower incidence of CRBSIs using 2% chlorhexidine gluconate, compared to 10% povidone–iodine or 70% alcohol [56,57]. For this reason, the guidelines for preventing intravascular catheter-related infections published by the Centers for Disease Control (CDC) recommend the use of a 2% chlorhexidine-based preparation but accept tincture of iodine or 70% alcohol as alternatives. The use of maximal sterile-barrier precautions, including a mask, hat, sterile gown, sterile gloves, and sterile drape, has also been associated with a lower incidence of CRBSIs [46,55]. Maximal sterile-barrier precautions should be used during the placement of all CVCs.

In addition to good skin antisepsis and sterile-barrier precautions, a thorough understanding of the equipment and the involved anatomy is critical during CVC placement. Catheterization of the internal jugular vein or subclavian vein requires a comprehensive knowledge of the anatomy of the neck, with its associated external landmarks. The internal jugular vein is located within the carotid sheath, just lateral and slightly anterior to the carotid artery. These vessels pass deep to the triangle formed by the sternal and clavicular heads of the sternocleidomastoid muscle and the clavicle. Three approaches to accessing the internal jugular vein are:

- The anterior route
- The middle (central) route
- The posterior route

The most common approach is the anterior route, which will be described here. With the patient in a slightly Trendelenburg position, the neck is prepared with an appropriate skin antiseptic (preferably 2% chlorhexidine solution) and draped using full sterile-barrier precautions. Local anesthetic is applied at the apex of the described triangle, and the access needle is advanced at a 45-degree angle from the apex of this triangle toward the ipsilateral nipple. Negative pressure is maintained on the syringe during insertion for the anticipated return of venous blood. Confirmation of venous blood includes return of nonpulsatile, dark blood, which can become difficult to differentiate from arterial blood in hypotensive, hypoxic patients. Once the internal jugular vein is successfully cannulated, the needle is secured in place and the syringe is removed. A guidewire is slowly advanced through the needle, and the catheter is placed over the guidewire using a modified Seldinger technique. Following catheter placement, each port is aspirated and flushed with heparin flush. The catheter is then secured in place. Preliminary data suggest sutureless securement devices may be associated with a lower incidence of CRBSIs, compared to suturing [58], but standard practice still involves suturing these catheters in place. Additional studies are needed to clarify this issue before recommendations can be made for a broad-based change in current practices.

The subclavian vein is a continuation of the axillary vein and courses just under the clavicle anterior to the subclavian artery. With the patient in a slightly Trendelenburg position, the neck and shoulder are prepared with an appropriate skin antiseptic and draped using full sterile-barrier precautions. Local anesthetic is applied just lateral to and including the periostium at the angle of the clavicle. With the practitioner's thumb on the angle of the clavicle and the first finger in the suprasternal notch, the access needle is inserted 1 to 2 cm lateral to the angle of the clavicle in the delto–pectoral groove and advanced toward the suprasternal notch in a plane parallel to the chest wall. When the needle reaches the angle of the clavicle, the needle is advanced just under the clavicle toward the suprasternal notch, maintaining the plane parallel to the chest wall. Negative pressure is maintained on the syringe during insertion. Once the subclavian vein is successfully cannulated, the catheter is advanced over a guidewire and secured in place, as described for internal jugular vein catheterization.

TABLE 14.5
Recommended Catheter Care

Use gauze or semipermeable transparent dressings
Use gauze dressings if drainage is present
Change dressings if they become damp, damaged, or contaminated
Do not use antibiotic creams or ointments, in order to prevent fungal infections and bacterial resistance

Catheterization of the femoral vein requires a good understanding of the vascular anatomy of the inguinal region. The femoral vessels are a continuation of the external iliac vessels and originate as these vessels pass under the inguinal ligament and into the groin. It is essential to understand the relationship of the femoral vein to its adjacent structures. The mnemonic *NAVeL* describes the structures in the groin from lateral to medial and includes the femoral *N*erve, femoral *A*rtery, femoral *V*ein, *e*mpty space, and *L*ymphatics. Knowing these relationships is essential, because the palpable femoral artery is the most reliable landmark when assessing the position of the femoral vein in the groin. Prior to preparing the skin and draping the field, the selected groin is adequately exposed. In obese patients with a significant pannus, this may require retracting the pannus using an assistant or tape. Following adequate exposure of the groin, the patient is placed in a slightly reverse Trendelenburg position. The groin is then prepared with an appropriate skin antiseptic and draped using full sterile-barrier precautions. The femoral artery is palpated carefully to define its medial and lateral boundaries. Local anesthetic is applied just medial to the femoral artery, below the inguinal crease. With control of the femoral artery, the access needle is slowly advanced at a 45-degree angle in a caudal-to-cephalad and slightly lateral-to-medial direction just medial to the femoral artery. Negative pressure is maintained on the syringe during insertion. When the femoral vein is successfully cannulated, the catheter is placed over a guidewire and secured in place, as described for internal jugular vein catheterization.

14.3.4 CATHETER CARE

In an effort to reduce the risk of catheter-related infections, several studies have focused on catheter care after placement (see Table 14.5). In one study, 2000 catheters were examined to evaluate the use of transparent dressings and their effect on catheter-related infections [20]. This study found no significant difference in the incidence of catheter-site colonization or phlebitis in catheters dressed with transparent dressings vs. gauze. Additionally, a meta-analysis of several studies assessing the risk of CRBSIs in patients with CVCs dressed with transparent dressings or gauze dressings demonstrated no significant difference between these two groups [59]. Current recommendations for catheter care include the use of sterile gauze or transparent, semipermeable dressings. Gauze dressings are preferred in the presence of drainage from the catheter site. In addition, all dressings should be replaced if they become damp, damaged, or contaminated. A multicenter study demonstrated a reduction in the risk of catheter colonization and CRBSIs using a chlorhexidine-impregnated sponge (Biopatch) at the site of short-term arterial access and CVCs; however, the CDC recommends not using topical antibiotic ointments and creams at catheter sites because of the increased risk of fungal infections and bacterial resistance [32,60].

14.4 COMPLICATIONS OF ACCESS

Complications associated with central venous access have been categorized in the literature as mechanical, infectious, thrombotic, acute, and late. In order to maintain a clinical focus, we will consider catheter-related complications as either acute or late complications. As with any procedure, an individual's level of experience in placing CVCs affects the risk of complications developing.

TABLE 14.6
Acute Complications of CVC
Placement

Pneumothorax
Hemothorax
Hydrothorax
Hemomediastinum
Hydromediastinum
Hematoma
Air embolism
Catheter embolism
Catheter misplacement

A physician who has placed fewer than 50 CVCs has twice the risk of developing a mechanical complication during placement of the catheter than a physician who has placed 50 or more CVCs [39,61]. Experience with CVC placement also improves the physician's consideration of catheter selection, site selection, proper technique, and catheter care following placement. These factors aid in reducing the risk of developing catheter-related infections and thrombosis.

14.4.1 ACUTE COMPLICATIONS

Acute complications occur at the time of catheter placement (see Table 14.6). They vary depending on the access site chosen and are typically the result of a technical error during catheter placement. The use of ultrasound guidance has reduced the number of mechanical complications associated with and the time required for placement of internal jugular venous catheters [62–67]. Studies evaluating the use of ultrasound during subclavian vein catheterization have had mixed results [63,68,69].

A pneumothorax occurs when the thoracic cavity is entered during attempted access of the subclavian or internal jugular vein. With penetration of the parietal and visceral pleura, air collects in the pleural space, causing partial or total collapse of the lung. The clinical course can vary from a small, asymptomatic pneumothorax to a life-threatening tension pneumothorax with cardiovascular collapse. An end-expiratory chest radiograph should be obtained. Free air will be seen outside of the lung within the pleural cavity. Small, asymptomatic pneumothoraces usually resolve with conservative management. Larger pneumothoraces require a tube thoracostomy.

A hemothorax can occur with perforation of the back wall of the subclavian vein or artery and the parietal pleura [70]. A chest radiograph demonstrates fluid in the pleural cavity, and pleurocentesis with return of bloody fluid confirms the diagnosis. Small, asymptomatic hemothoraces can also be managed conservatively with close observation. Symptomatic or larger hemothoraces require placement of a large-bore thoracostomy tube. Further surgical intervention is rarely indicated.

A hydrothorax occurs when the catheter tip is placed in the pleural space and fluids are administered. Thoracentesis is typically diagnostic and therapeutic with drainage of the hydrothorax. The CVC should be removed, and further intervention is rarely indicated.

Hemomediastinum and hydromediastinum occur following perforation of the innominate vein or superior vena cava, with bleeding or infusion of fluids into the mediastinum. Chest pain and widening of the mediastinum on chest radiograph suggest the diagnosis [71]. Immediate catheter removal is usually sufficient therapy. Rarely, the patient does not improve, and surgical repair through a median sternotomy is indicated.

Subcutaneous hematomas can develop following puncture or laceration injuries of the artery or vein at the access site. Direct pressure should be applied and is generally effective in the neck and groin. This can be difficult following injury to the subclavian vessels, because of their location under the clavicle. The development of an expanding hematoma, despite attempted compression, requires surgical exploration and repair. The rare development of arteriovenous fistulas and pseudo-aneurysms also requires surgical repair [72].

Catheter misplacement is reported in 6 to 8% of cases [73]. The desired location of the tip of internal jugular and subclavian vein catheters is immediately proximal to the superior vena cava–right atrial junction [74]. Misplacement proximally in a low flow area can cause irritation of the venous intima, with an increased risk of thrombus formation [75,76]. Misplacement distally in the heart can cause cardiac irritability, with dysrhythmias or cardiac injury. Migration of the catheter tip following placement has also been reported [77,78]. Migration or misplacement of the catheter tip in distal vessels should be identified and corrected promptly. Infusion of hyper-osmolar solutions into the distal vessels of the extremities or central nervous system can cause irreversible injury. Additionally, errant placement of a CVC within an adjacent artery can cause arterial injury, with an increased risk of bleeding, thrombosis, arterial dissection, arteriovenous fistulas, and pseudoaneurysms.

Air embolism is a rare complication caused when air enters the central venous system during catheter placement or manipulation. Air becomes trapped in the right ventricle and can cause a decrease in right ventricular outflow, with cardiovascular collapse and respiratory distress [79–81]. The classic physical finding is a millwheel, machinery-type murmur over the precordium. If air embolism is suspected, 100% oxygen should be administered. With the patient in a Trendelenburg, left lateral decubitus position, the air should be aspirated through the inserted catheter to restore right ventricular outflow.

Catheter embolism is a rare complication with current catheter placement systems. This complication was more common when catheters were placed through a needle introducer. With this system, the catheter was more frequently sheared off with embolization of the catheter segment. Although much less common with the newer catheter placement systems, fracture and embolization of long-term indwelling catheters are possible [82]. For this reason, catheters should be carefully examined following removal to ensure complete catheter removal. If suspected, catheter embo-lization can be confirmed with a radiograph and managed with retrieval by an interventional radiologist [83].

Less common mechanical complications are cardiac injury, thoracic duct laceration, and nerve injury. Transient dysrhythmias are not uncommon during guidewire placement and are typically corrected by withdrawing the guidewire. Flexible catheters are very unlikely to cause significant cardiac trauma, but large, rigid catheters can cause cardiac perforation with cardiac tamponade. This must be recognized immediately and treated with surgical repair. Thoracic duct laceration is rare during attempted access of the left internal jugular and subclavian veins. The lymphorrhea resulting from this injury can be managed conservatively and usually resolves with no further intervention. Nerve injuries can involve the brachial plexus following attempted access of the subclavian vein. These injuries are usually transient, but needles and catheters should be removed immediately and central venous access attempted at another site. Significant nerve sheath hemato-mas may require surgical decompression.

14.4.2 LATE COMPLICATIONS

For the purpose of this discussion, late complications will be defined as complications developing more than 72 hours after catheter placement. These complications develop primarily as a result of infection and thrombosis, but the previously discussed acute complications can also have a delayed onset and present as late complications (see Table 14.7). Many factors contribute to the development of late complications, including the patient's comorbidities, catheter type and characteristics, site of placement, and catheter care following placement. Each of these factors contributes to the risk of developing catheter-related infections and catheter-related thrombosis.

TABLE 14.7
Late Complications of CVC Placement

Infectious	Catheter-site infections
	Thrombophlebitis
	Catheter-related blood stream infections
	Sepsis
Thrombotic	Catheter occlusion
	Venous thrombosis
	Pulmonary embolism
Delayed onset of acute complications	Pneumothorax, hemothorax, hydrothorax, hemomediastinum, hydromediastinum, hematoma, air embolism, catheter embolism, catheter misplacement or migration

Infectious complications are the most frequently encountered catheter-related complications and can present as catheter site infections, thrombophlebitis, CRBSIs, and sepsis [84–87]. A CRBSI is defined as a clinical infection with isolation of the same organism from the blood stream and catheter segment, with no other source of infection present. In intensive care units in the United States, there are 15 million CVC days each year, with an average of 5.3 CVC-associated blood stream infections (BSIs) per 1,000 catheter days [88]. The financial impact of these infections is substantial, with an average cost of $34,000 to $56,000 per infection [89,90] totaling $296 million to $2.3 billion annually [36]. Risk factors for CRBSIs include recent bone marrow transplantation, previous blood stream infection, TPN administration, and outpatient intravenous infusion outside of the home. CRBSIs develop as a result of contamination of the catheter hub [91–95] or catheter site [46,96,97], with subsequent microbial adherence, growth within a biofilm, and passage into the bloodstream [98].

Much attention has recently been focused on this biofilm and its role in infections involving CVCs and other medical devices. *Staphylococcus aureus*, coagulase-negative staphylococci, *Candida albicans*, and aerobic Gram-negative bacilli are the most common organisms involved in catheter-related infections [99]. When these organisms attach to the surface of catheters and divide, they grow in towers and produce an extracellular matrix of polysaccharide material, creating a biofilm. The organization of these bacteria within the biofilm makes antibiotic penetration and phagocytic cell migration more difficult. In some cases, the extracellular matrix is able to neutralize antibiotics. With these organisms shielded and antibiotics neutralized, antibiotic therapy becomes compromised. Current microbial testing and determination of antibiotic sensitivities are performed with free-swimming or planktonic bacteria. These results may be misleading when attempting to treat catheter-related infections. Although the formation of a biofilm does not necessarily correlate with clinical catheter sepsis [100], the described characteristics of the biofilm allow these bacteria to become up to 1000 times more resistant to antibiotics than planktonic bacteria. For this reason, antibiotics have a greatly increased mean inhibitory concentration for organisms within a biofilm [101–107].

In the 1980s and 1990s, several authors published rates of only 30 to 65% for successfully salvaging catheters using conventional antibiotic regimens [108–111]. For this reason, the treatment of CRBSIs has historically involved catheter removal. In 1988, Messing described antibiotic lock therapy [112]. He placed a high concentration of antibiotics in the catheter for 12 hours and reported a catheter salvage rate of 91%. Multiple studies since its introduction have demonstrated catheter salvage rates of 92 to 100% using antibiotic lock therapy [113–116]. This therapy does not, however, alter the biofilm matrix, which allows persistence of this framework for subsequent bacterial ingrowth. Several experimental methods for eradicating the biofilm are being investigated but currently remain in preclinical trials [117,118]. For this reason, removal of the device remains the only definitive treatment for eradicating the biofilm when catheter-related infections remain a clinical concern.

Thrombotic complications are another source of late complications that compromise catheter function, increase healthcare costs, and adversely affect patients' outcomes. Thrombotic complications can present as catheter occlusion, venous thrombosis, and rarely as pulmonary embolism. Catheter occlusion and venous thrombosis cause 25 to 40% of all catheter-related complications [73,119–121] and contribute to the incidence of catheter-related infections [122,123]. Central venous catheters are thought to cause thrombosis through adsorption of fibrinogen and vitronectin, activation of the coagulation cascade, and activation of the complement system. The risk of thrombosis increases when patients are hypercoagulable, hypertonic solutions are infused, catheter size approaches vessel size, and catheterization is prolonged [74]. Hirsch demonstrated that one-third of the MICU patients he studied developed venous thrombosis within a median of seven days. Fifteen percent of these were associated with CVCs [124]. Catheter-related venous thrombosis can lead to pulmonary embolism. If this is suspected, an appropriate workup with V/Q scanning or spiral chest CT should be performed. When thrombosis is confirmed, an appropriate treatment plan with anticoagulation should be instituted. Catheters with surface-bound heparin have not reduced the incidence of catheter-related thrombosis; studies involving impregnated thrombolytic agents are pending. For current clinical practice, the use of softer catheters and heparin in the infusate lowers the incidence of catheter-related thrombosis [125,126].

14.5 CASE STUDY

A 54-year-old male underwent a low anterior colon resection for a rectal adenocarcinoma 12 cm from the anal verge. His initial postoperative course was stable, but he was unable to receive significant enteral nutrition secondary to a mild postoperative ileus. On postoperative day 5, the patient's condition worsened and studies revealed an anastomotic leak with an intra-abdominal abscess. He was taken back to the operating room for an abdominal washout, revision of the anastamosis, and formation of a loop ileostomy. Postoperatively, he remains hemodynamically stable but will need central venous access for intravenous fluid administration, lab draws, and initiation of TPN.

What are the potential acute and late complications of catheter placement? How do these potential complications affect your decisions involved in obtaining central venous access? What factors should you consider in choosing the type of catheter to insert and the site of insertion? What do studies show to help you determine the type of dressing to apply and whether antibiotic ointments should be applied to the catheter site following catheter placement?

REFERENCES

1. Aubaniac, R., [Subclavian intravenous injection: advantages and technique]. *Presse Med.*, 1952. 60(68): 1456.
2. Seldinger, S.I., Catheter replacement of the needle in percutaneous arteriography; a new technique. *Acta Radiol.*, 1953. 39(5): 368–376.
3. Dudrick, S.J., et al., Long-term total parenteral nutrition with growth, development, and positive nitrogen balance. *Surgery*, 1968. 64(1): 134–142.
4. Broviac, J.W., J.J. Cole, and B.H. Scribner, A silicone rubber atrial catheter for prolonged parenteral alimentation. *Surg. Gynecol. Obstet.*, 1973. 136(4): 602–606.
5. Hickman, R.O., et al., A modified right atrial catheter for access to the venous system in marrow transplant recipients. *Surg. Gynecol. Obstet.*, 1979. 148(6): 871–875.
6. Hoshal, V.L., Jr., Total intravenous nutrition with peripherally inserted silicone elastomer central venous catheters. *Arch. Surg.*, 1975. 110(5): 644–646.

7. Niederhuber, J.E., et al., Totally implanted venous and arterial access system to replace external catheters in cancer treatment. *Surgery*, 1982. 92(4): 706–712.

8. Raad, I., Intravascular-catheter-related infections. *Lancet*, 1998. 351(9106): 893–898.

9. Dougherty, S.H. and R.L. Simmons, Infections in bionic man: the pathobiology of infections in prosthetic devices. Part I. *Curr. Probl. Surg.*, 1982. 19(5): 217–264.

10. Dougherty, S.H. and R.L. Simmons, Infections in bionic man: the pathobiology of infections in prosthetic devices. Part II. *Curr. Probl. Surg.*, 1982. 19(6): 265–319.

11. Ashkenazi, S., E. Weiss, and M.M. Drucker, Bacterial adherence to intravenous catheters and needles and its influence by cannula type and bacterial surface hydrophobicity. *J. Lab. Clin. Med.*, 1986. 107(2): 136–140.

12. Sheth, N.K., et al., *In vitro* quantitative adherence of bacteria to intravascular catheters. *J. Surg. Res.*, 1983. 34(3): 213–218.

13. Krause, T.J., et al., Differential production of interleukin 1 on the surface of biomaterials. *Arch. Surg.*, 1990. 125(9): 1158–1160.

14. Maki, D.G., et al., An attachable silver-impregnated cuff for prevention of infection with central venous catheters: a prospective randomized multicenter trial. *Am. J. Med.*, 1988. 85(3): 307–314.

15. Kamal, G.D., et al., Reduced intravascular catheter infection by antibiotic bonding: a prospective, randomized, controlled trial. *JAMA*, 1991. 265(18): 2364–2368.

16. Kim, S.W., R.V. Petersen, and E.S. Lee, Effect of phthalate plasticizer on blood compatibility of polyvinyl chloride. *J. Pharm. Sci.*, 1976. 65(5): 670–673.

17. Baier, R.E. and R.C. Dutton, Initial events in interactions of blood with a foreign surface. *J. Biomed. Mater. Res.*, 1969. 3(1): 191–206.

18. Clowes, A.W., T.R. Kirkman, and M.M. Clowes, Mechanisms of arterial graft failure. II. Chronic endothelial and smooth muscle cell proliferation in healing polytetrafluoroethylene prostheses. *J. Vasc. Surg.*, 1986. 3(6): 877–884.

19. Sheth, N.K., et al., Colonization of bacteria on polyvinyl chloride and Teflon intravascular catheters in hospitalized patients. *J. Clin. Microbiol.*, 1983. 18(5): 1061–1063.

20. Maki, D.G. and M. Ringer, Evaluation of dressing regimens for prevention of infection with peripheral intravenous catheters: gauze, a transparent polyurethane dressing, and an iodophor-transparent dressing. *JAMA*, 1987. 258(17): 2396–2403.

21. Maki, D.G. and M. Ringer, Risk factors for infusion-related phlebitis with small peripheral venous catheters: a randomized controlled trial. *Ann. Intern. Med.*, 1991. 114(10): 845–854.

22. Peters, G., R. Locci, and G. Pulverer, Adherence and growth of coagulase-negative staphylococci on surfaces of intravenous catheters. *J. Infect. Dis.*, 1982. 146(4): 479–482.

23. Larsson, N., et al., Cannula thrombophlebitis: a study in volunteers comparing polytetrafluoroethylene, polyurethane, and polyamide-ether-elastomer cannulae. *Acta Anaesthesiol. Scand.*, 1989. 33(3): 223–231.

24. Pasquale, M.D., J.M. Campbell, and C.M. Magnant, Groshong versus Hickman catheters. *Surg. Gynecol. Obstet.*, 1992. 174(5): 408–410.

25. Ingram, J., et al., Complications of indwelling venous access lines in the pediatric hematology patient: a prospective comparison of external venous catheters and subcutaneous ports. *Am. J. Pediatr. Hematol. Oncol.*, 1991. 13(2): 130–136.

26. Mirro, J., Jr., et al., A comparison of placement techniques and complications of externalized catheters and implantable port use in children with cancer. *J. Pediatr. Surg.*, 1990. 25(1): 120–124.

27. Pegues, D., et al., Comparison of infections in Hickman and implanted port catheters in adult solid tumor patients. *J. Surg. Oncol.*, 1992. 49(3): 156–162.

28. Pomp, A., M.D. Caldwell, and J.E. Albina, Subcutaneous infusion ports for administration of parenteral nutrition at home. *Surg. Gynecol. Obstet.*, 1989. 169(4): 329–333.

29. Raad, I., et al., Central venous catheters coated with minocycline and rifampin for the prevention of catheter-related colonization and bloodstream infections: a randomized, double-blind trial. The Texas Medical Center Catheter Study Group. *Ann. Intern. Med.*, 1997. 127(4): 267–274.

30. Maki, D.G., et al., Prevention of central venous catheter-related bloodstream infection by use of an antiseptic-impregnated catheter: a randomized, controlled trial. *Ann. Intern. Med.*, 1997. 127(4): 257–266.

31. Darouiche, R.O., et al., A comparison of two antimicrobial-impregnated central venous catheters. Catheter Study Group. *N. Engl. J. Med.*, 1999. 340(1): 1–8.

32. Flowers, R.H., 3rd, et al., Efficacy of an attachable subcutaneous cuff for the prevention of intravascular catheter-related infection: a randomized, controlled trial. *JAMA*, 1989. 261(6): 878–883.

33. Dahlberg, P.J., et al., Subclavian hemodialysis catheter infections: a prospective, randomized trial of an attachable silver-impregnated cuff for prevention of catheter-related infections. *Infect. Control Hosp. Epidemiol.*, 1995. 16(9): 506–511.

34. Groeger, J.S., et al., A prospective, randomized evaluation of the effect of silver impregnated subcutaneous cuffs for preventing tunneled chronic venous access catheter infections in cancer patients. *Ann. Surg.*, 1993. 218(2): 206–210.

35. Veenstra, D.L., et al., Efficacy of antiseptic-impregnated central venous catheters in preventing catheter-related bloodstream infection: a meta-analysis. *JAMA*, 1999. 281(3): 261–267.

36. Mermel, L.A., Prevention of intravascular catheter-related infections. *Ann. Intern. Med.*, 2000. 132(5): 391–402.

37. Bassetti, S., et al., Prolonged antimicrobial activity of a catheter containing chlorhexidine-silver sulfadiazine extends protection against catheter infections *in vivo. Antimicrob. Agents Chemother.*, 2001. 45(5): 1535–1538.

38. Merrer, J., et al., Complications of femoral and subclavian venous catheterization in critically ill patients: a randomized controlled trial. *JAMA*, 2001. 286(6): 700–707.

39. Sznajder, J.I., et al., Central vein catheterization: failure and complication rates by three percutaneous approaches. *Arch. Intern. Med.*, 1986. 146(2): 259–261.

40. Mansfield, P.F., et al., Complications and failures of subclavian-vein catheterization. *N. Engl. J. Med.*, 1994. 331(26): 1735–1738.

41. Martin, C., et al., Axillary or internal jugular central venous catheterization. *Crit. Care Med.*, 1990. 18(4): 400–402.

42. Durbec, O., et al., A prospective evaluation of the use of femoral venous catheters in critically ill adults. *Crit. Care Med.*, 1997. 25(12): 1986–1989.

43. Timsit, J.F., et al., Use of tunneled femoral catheters to prevent catheter-related infection: a randomized, controlled trial. *Ann. Intern. Med.*, 1999. 130(9): 729–735.

44. Uldall, R., Subclavian cannulation for hemodialysis: the present state of the art. *Artif. Organs*, 1982. 6(1): 73–76.

45. Barrett, N., et al., Subclavian stenosis: a major complication of subclavian dialysis catheters. *Nephrol. Dial. Transplant*, 1988. 3(4): 423–425.

46. Mermel, L.A., et al., The pathogenesis and epidemiology of catheter-related infection with pulmonary artery Swan-Ganz catheters: a prospective study utilizing molecular subtyping. *Am. J. Med.*, 1991. 91(3B): 197S–205S.

47. Heard, S.O., et al., Influence of triple-lumen central venous catheters coated with chlorhexidine and silver sulfadiazine on the incidence of catheter-related bacteremia. *Arch. Intern. Med.*, 1998. 158(1): 81–87.

48. Richet, H., et al., Prospective multicenter study of vascular-catheter-related complications and risk factors for positive central-catheter cultures in intensive care unit patients. *J. Clin. Microbiol.*, 1990. 28(11): 2520–2525.

49. McKinley, S., et al., Incidence and predictors of central venous catheter related infection in intensive care patients. *Anaesth. Intensive Care*, 1999. 27(2): 164–169.

50. Joynt, G.M., et al., Deep venous thrombosis caused by femoral venous catheters in critically ill adult patients. *Chest*, 2000. 117(1): 178–183.

51. Mian, N.Z., et al., Incidence of deep venous thrombosis associated with femoral venous catheterization. *Acad. Emerg. Med.*, 1997. 4(12): 1118–1121.

52. Trottier, S.J., et al., Femoral deep vein thrombosis associated with central venous catheterization: results from a prospective, randomized trial. *Crit. Care Med.*, 1995. 23(1): 52–59.

53. Cimochowski, G.E., et al., Superiority of the internal jugular over the subclavian access for temporary dialysis. *Nephron.*, 1990. 54(2): 154–161.

54. Timsit, J.F., et al., Central vein catheter-related thrombosis in intensive care patients: incidence, risks factors, and relationship with catheter-related sepsis. *Chest*, 1998. 114(1): 207–213.

55. Raad, II, et al., Prevention of central venous catheter-related infections by using maximal sterile barrier precautions during insertion. *Infect. Control Hosp. Epidemiol.*, 1994. 15(4 Pt. 1): 231–238.

56. Maki, D.G., M. Ringer, and C.J. Alvarado, Prospective randomised trial of povidone-iodine, alcohol, and chlorhexidine for prevention of infection associated with central venous and arterial catheters. *Lancet*, 1991. 338(8763): 339–343.

57. Mimoz, O., et al., Prospective, randomized trial of two antiseptic solutions for prevention of central venous or arterial catheter colonization and infection in intensive care unit patients. *Crit. Care Med.*, 1996. 24(11): 1818–1823.

58. Yamamoto, A.J., et al., Sutureless securement device reduces complications of peripherally inserted central venous catheters. *J. Vasc. Interv. Radiol.*, 2002. 13(1): 77–81.

59. Hoffmann, K.K., et al., Transparent polyurethane film as an intravenous catheter dressing: a meta-analysis of the infection risks. *JAMA*, 1992. 267(15): 2072–2076.

60. Zakrzewska-Bode, A., et al., Mupirocin resistance in coagulase-negative staphylococci, after topical prophylaxis for the reduction of colonization of central venous catheters. *J. Hosp. Infect.*, 1995. 31(3): 189–193.

61. Fares, L.G., 2nd, P.H. Block, and S.D. Feldman, Improved house staff results with subclavian cannulation. *Am. Surg.*, 1986. 52(2): 108–111.

62. Teichgraber, U.K., et al., A sonographically guided technique for central venous access. *Am. J. Roentgenol.*, 1997. 169(3): 731–733.

63. Randolph, A.G., et al., Ultrasound guidance for placement of central venous catheters: a meta-analysis of the literature. *Crit. Care Med.*, 1996. 24(12): 2053–2058.

64. Gratz, I., et al., Doppler-guided cannulation of the internal jugular vein: a prospective, randomized trial. *J. Clin. Monit.*, 1994. 10(3): 185–188.

65. Troianos, C.A., D.R. Jobes, and N. Ellison, Ultrasound-guided cannulation of the internal jugular vein: a prospective, randomized study. *Anesth. Analg.*, 1991. 72(6): 823–826.

66. Denys, B.G., B.F. Uretsky, and P.S. Reddy, Ultrasound-assisted cannulation of the internal jugular vein: a prospective comparison to the external landmark-guided technique. *Circulation*, 1993. 87(5): 1557–1562.

67. Hatfield, A. and A. Bodenham, Portable ultrasound for difficult central venous access. *Br. J. Anaesth.*, 1999. 82(6): 822–826.

68. Lefrant, J.Y., et al., Pulsed Doppler ultrasonography guidance for catheterization of the subclavian vein: a randomized study. *Anesthesiology*, 1998. 88(5): 1195–1201.

69. Bold, R.J., et al., Prospective, randomized trial of Doppler-assisted subclavian vein catheterization. *Arch. Surg.*, 1998. 133(10): 1089–1093.

70. Borja, A.R., Current status of infraclavicular subclavian vein catheterization. *Ann. Thorac. Surg.*, 1972. 13(6): 615–624.

71. Ryan, J.A., Jr., et al., Catheter complications in total parenteral nutrition: a prospective study of 200 consecutive patients. *N. Engl. J. Med.*, 1974. 290(14): 757–761.

72. Clark, V.L. and J.A. Kruse, Arterial catheterization. *Crit. Care Clin.*, 1992. 8(4): 687–697.

73. Christensen, K.H., B. Nerstrom, and H. Baden, Complications of percutaneous catheterization of the subclavian vein in 129 cases. *Acta Chir. Scand.*, 1967. 133(8): 615–620.

74. Henriques, H.F., 3rd, et al., Avoiding complications of long-term venous access. *Am. Surg.*, 1993. 59(9): 555–558.

75. Langston, C.S., The aberrant central venous catheter and its complications. *Radiology*, 1971. 100(1): 55–59.

76. Raffensperger, J.G. and M.L. Ramenofsky, A fatal complication of hyperalimentation: a case report. *Surgery*, 1970. 68(2): 393–394.

77. Ouriel, K., et al., Migration of a permanent central venous catheter. *J. Parenter. Enteral Nutr.*, 1983. 7(4): 410–411.

78. Rasuli, P., D.I. Hammond, and I.R. Peterkin, Spontaneous intrajugular migration of long-term central venous access catheters. *Radiology*, 1992. 182(3): 822–824.

79. Flanagan, J.P., et al., Air embolus: a lethal complication of subclavian venipuncture. *N. Engl. J. Med.*, 1969. 281(9): 488–489.

80. Hoshal, V.L., Jr. and G.H. Fink, The subclavian catheter. *N. Engl. J. Med.*, 1969. 281(25): 1425.

81. Levinsky, W.J., Fatal air embolism during insertion of CVP monitoring apparatus. *JAMA*, 1969. 209(11): 1721–1722.

82. McMenamin, E.M., Catheter fracture: a complication in venous access devices. *Cancer Nurs.*, 1993. 16(6): 464–467.

83. Block, P.C., Transvenous retrieval of foreign bodies in the cardiac circulation. *JAMA*, 1973. 224(2): 241–248.

84. Bernard, R.W., W.M. Stahl, and R.M. Chase, Jr., Subclavian vein catheterizations: a prospective study. II. Infectious complications. *Ann. Surg.*, 1971. 173(2): 191–200.

85. Uldall, P.R., C. Joy, and N. Merchant, Further experience with a double-lumen subclavian cannula for hemodialysis. *Trans. Am. Soc. Artif. Intern. Organs*, 1982. 28: 71–75.

86. Eyer, S., et al., Catheter-related sepsis: prospective, randomized study of three methods of long-term catheter maintenance. *Crit. Care Med.*, 1990. 18(10): 1073–1079.

87. Wiener, E.S., et al., The CCSG prospective study of venous access devices: an analysis of insertions and causes for removal. *J. Pediatr. Surg.*, 1992. 27(2): 155–163; discussion 163–164.

88. National Nosocomial Infections Surveillance (NNIS) System report, data summary from October 1986–April 1998, issued June 1998. *Am. J. Infect. Control*, 1998. 26(5): 522–533.

89. Rello, J., et al., Evaluation of outcome of intravenous catheter-related infections in critically ill patients. *Am. J. Respir. Crit. Care Med.*, 2000. 162(3 Pt 1): 1027–1030.

90. Dimick, J.B., et al., Increased resource use associated with catheter-related bloodstream infection in the surgical intensive care unit. *Arch. Surg.*, 2001. 136(2): 229–234.

91. Sitges-Serra, A., J. Linares, and S. Capell, Catheter sepsis: the fourth mechanism. *J. Antimicrob. Chemother.*, 1985. 15(5): 641–642.

92. Sitges-Serra, A., J. Linares, and J. Garau, Catheter sepsis: the clue is the hub. *Surgery*, 1985. 97(3): 355–357.

93. Sitges-Serra, A., et al., A randomized trial on the effect of tubing changes on hub contamination and catheter sepsis during parenteral nutrition. *J. Parenter. Enteral Nutr.*, 1985. 9(3): 322–325.

94. Linares, J., et al., Pathogenesis of catheter sepsis: a prospective study with quantitative and semiquantitative cultures of catheter hub and segments. *J. Clin. Microbiol.*, 1985. 21(3): 357–360.

95. Raad, I., et al., Ultrastructural analysis of indwelling vascular catheters: a quantitative relationship between luminal colonization and duration of placement. *J. Infect. Dis.*, 1993. 168(2): 400–407.

96. Maki, D.G., C.E. Weise, and H.W. Sarafin, A semiquantitative culture method for identifying intravenous-catheter-related infection. *N. Engl. J. Med.*, 1977. 296(23): 1305–1309.

97. Maki, D.G., F. Jarrett, and H.W. Sarafin, A semiquantitative culture method for identification of catheter-related infection in the burn patient. *J. Surg. Res.*, 1977. 22(5): 513–520.

98. Habash, M. and G. Reid, Microbial biofilms: their development and significance for medical device-related infections. *J. Clin. Pharmacol.*, 1999. 39(9): 887–898.

99. Mermel, L.A., et al., Guidelines for the management of intravascular catheter-related infections. *Clin. Infect. Dis.*, 2001. 32(9): 1249–1272.

100. Ludwicka, A., et al., Attachment of staphylococci to various synthetic polymers. *Zentralbl. Bakteriol. Mikrobiol. Hyg.* [A], 1984. 256(4): 479–489.

101. Norman, J.C., et al., Intracorporeal (abdominal) left ventricular assist devices or partial artificial hearts: a five-year clinical experience. *Arch. Surg.*, 1981. 116(11): 1441–1445.

102. Park, K., F.W. Mao, and H. Park, The minimum surface fibrinogen concentration necessary for platelet activation on dimethyldichlorosilane-coated glass. *J. Biomed. Mater. Res.*, 1991. 25(3): 407–420.

103. Donlan, R.M., Biofilms and device-associated infections. *Emerg. Infect. Dis.*, 2001. 7(2): 277–281.

104. Donlan, R.M., Biofilm formation: a clinically relevant microbiological process. *Clin. Infect. Dis.*, 2001. 33(8): 1387–1392.

105. Costerton, J.W., P.S. Stewart, and E.P. Greenberg, Bacterial biofilms: a common cause of persistent infections. *Science*, 1999. 284(5418): 1318–1322.

106. Schierholz, J.M., et al., Antimicrobial substances and effects on sessile bacteria. *Zentralbl. Bakteriol.*, 1999. 289(2): 165–177.

107. Schierholz, J.M., J. Beuth, and G. Pulverer, Adherent bacteria and activity of antibiotics. *J. Antimicrob. Chemother.*, 1999. 43(1): 158–160.

108. Buchman, A.L., et al., Catheter-related infections associated with home parenteral nutrition and predictive factors for the need for catheter removal in their treatment. *J. Parenter. Enteral Nutr.*, 1994. 18(4): 297–302.

109. Press, O.W., et al., Hickman catheter infections in patients with malignancies. *Medicine* (Baltimore), 1984. 63(4): 189–200.

110. Flynn, P.M., et al., *In situ* management of confirmed central venous catheter-related bacteremia. *Pediatr. Infect. Dis. J.*, 1987. 6(8): 729–734.

111. Miller, S.J., et al., Antibiotic therapy of catheter infections in patients receiving home parenteral nutrition. *J. Parenter. Enteral Nutr.*, 1990. 14(2): 143–147.

112. Messing, B., et al., Antibiotic-lock technique: a new approach to optimal therapy for catheter-related sepsis in home-parenteral nutrition patients. *J. Parenter. Enteral Nutr.*, 1988. 12(2): 185–189.

113. Benoit, J.L., et al., Intraluminal antibiotic treatment of central venous catheter infections in patients receiving parenteral nutrition at home. *Clin. Infect. Dis.*, 1997. 24(4): 743–744.

114. Krzywda, E.A., et al., Treatment of Hickman catheter sepsis using antibiotic lock technique. *Infect. Control Hosp. Epidemiol.*, 1995. 16(10): 596–598.

115. McCarthy, A., et al., Central venous catheter infections treated with teicoplanin. *Eur. J. Haematol. Suppl.*, 1998. 62: 15–17.

116. Rao, J.S., et al., A new approach to the management of Broviac catheter infection. *J. Hosp. Infect.*, 1992. 22(2): 109–116.

117. Johnson, L.L., R.V. Peterson, and W.G. Pitt, Treatment of bacterial biofilms on polymeric biomaterials using antibiotics and ultrasound. *J. Biomater. Sci. Polym. Ed.*, 1998. 9(11): 1177–1185.

118. McLeod, B.R., et al., Enhanced bacterial biofilm control using electromagnetic fields in combination with antibiotics. *Methods Enzymol.*, 1999. 310: 656–670.

119. Lowell, J.A. and A. Bothe, Jr., Venous access. Preoperative, operative, and postoperative dilemmas. *Surg. Clin. North Am.*, 1991. 71(6): 1231–1246.

120. Riella, M.C. and B.H. Scribner, Five years' experience with a right atrial catheter for prolonged parenteral nutrition at home. *Surg. Gynecol. Obstet.*, 1976. 143(2): 205–208.

121. Sariego, J., et al., Major long-term complications in 1,422 permanent venous access devices. *Am. J. Surg.*, 1993. 165(2): 249–251.

122. Mohammad, S.F., Enhanced risk of infection with device-associated thrombi. *Asaio. J.*, 2000. 46(6): S63–S68.

123. Raad, II, et al., The relationship between the thrombotic and infectious complications of central venous catheters. *JAMA*, 1994. 271(13): 1014–1016.

124. Hirsch, D.R., E.P. Ingenito, and S.Z. Goldhaber, Prevalence of deep venous thrombosis among patients in medical intensive care. *JAMA*, 1995. 274(4): 335–337.

125. Fabri, P.J., et al., Incidence and prevention of thrombosis of the subclavian vein during total parenteral nutrition. *Surg. Gynecol. Obstet.*, 1982. 155(2): 238–240.

126. Padberg, F.T., Jr., et al., Central venous catheterization for parenteral nutrition. *Ann. Surg.*, 1981. 193(3): 264–270.

15 Enteral Feeding Access in the Critically Ill

Beth Taylor
Barnes-Jewish Hospital

John E. Mazuski
Washington University School of Medicine, Barnes-Jewish Hospital

CONTENTS

15.1 ENTERAL ACCESS DEVICES

The usefulness of enteral feeding for critically ill patients has been well documented [1–7]. Although there is debate over the type and amount of enteral feeding that is most beneficial, there is consensus that critically ill patients with a functioning gastrointestinal tract should be fed enterally if specialized nutritional support is thought to be warranted [2,8]. There is considerable debate, however, with regard to the techniques that should be used for enteral feeding in the critically ill patient and, specifically, what enteral access device is most appropriate for this patient. In order to answer these questions, a clear understanding of the enteral access devices presently available is needed. The selection of a specific device will be based, in part, on whether the patient will be fed into the stomach (prepyloric feeding) or the small bowel (postpyloric feeding), and whether the patient is likely to need short-term (< 4 weeks) or long-term (≥ 4 weeks) enteral access.

In this overview, we will first discuss the general characteristics of feeding devices and the methods of using them and then review the specific issues related to feeding device selection, based on duration of use and where the patient will be fed.

15.2 GENERAL CHARACTERISTICS OF ENTERAL ACCESS DEVICES

Enteral access devices vary markedly in the type of material used for their construction, their length and diameter, the presence of a stylet or guidewire, weighting of the tube, the presence of a Y-port, and the presence of more than one lumen.

15.2.1 CONSTRUCTION

Currently available adult feeding tubes are made of polyvinyl chloride, polyurethane, silicone, or a polyurethane–silicone mix material (see Table 15.1). Polyurethane, silicone, and the combination tubes are soft and made of nonreactive materials. Silicone tubes are the softest and may collapse when aspirating. Polyvinyl chloride is an inexpensive material, but in the presence of acid it may stiffen over time, leading to increased risks of nares irritation, cracking or breaking of the tube, or possible gastric perforation as the distal tip hardens. Foley catheters are made of latex, which may be irritating to the skin of some patients and dangerous to those with latex allergies [9]. Tubes designed for bedside, surgical, endoscopic, or fluoroscopic placement usually are completely radiopaque or have a radiopaque stripe to facilitate radiographic confirmation of their location.

15.2.2 TUBE SIZE — LENGTH AND DIAMETER

The length of the feeding tube is dictated both by the site of its insertion and by the desired site of feeding (see Table 15.1). Lengths can range from 6 in. for a gastrostomy tube to 60 in. for a nasojejunal tube. The shortest surgically implanted tubes are called *button* or *skin-level* tubes, but these are rarely placed acutely in the critically ill patient. Some surgically placed devices are

TABLE 15.1
Properties of Enteral Access Devices

Tube Type	Material	Length (inches)	French Size (fr)	Stylet or Guidewire	Y-Port
Nasogastric/Salem Sump	Polyvinyl chloride or silicone	36–48	12–20	No	No
Nasoenteric feeding tube	Polyurethane, silicone, or mixture	36–60	8–14	Yes/No	Yes/No
Percutaneous endoscopic gastrostomy (PEG)	Silicone or polyurethane	Cut to fit	14–24	No	Yes
Gastrostomy	Silicone or polyurethane	4–6	12–24	No	Yes
Jejunostomy	Silicone or polyurethane	6–10	8–14	No	Yes/No
Jejunostomy via PEG	Silicone or polyurethane	35–45	8–10	Yes	Yes/No
Needle jejunostomy	Silicone or polyurethane	6–10	8–10	Yes	No
Gastro-jejunostomy	Silicone or polyurethane	Jejunal length 35–45	G-port: 22–24 J-port: 8–10	Yes	Yes
MOSS gastrostomy	Silicone	18 to feeding tip	18	Yes	Yes

combination tubes that have a shorter gastric lumen for decompression and medication administration, and a longer jejunal limb for feeding purposes. Other gastrostomy tubes, especially those
implanted endoscopically, can accommodate a second jejunal tube inserted through the gastrostomy
and thereby function as a combination tube.

Besides having different lengths, tubes also differ with regard to diameter (see Table 15.1).
Usually the tube diameter is measured in French units, where one French unit equals 0.33 mm. In
general, for nasoenteric tubes, the smallest-diameter tube that allows optimal delivery of the
nutritional formula should be used. Smaller-diameter tubes are more comfortable for the patient
and less likely to produce sinusitis but are also more susceptible to clogging.

15.2.3 STYLETS

Stylets are often used to stiffen softer feeding tubes made of polyurethane or silicone to facilitate
insertion (see Table 15.1). Most stylets end in a blunt loop or a spring tip to decrease the risk of
tube puncture during placement. In addition, they do not extend completely to the end of the tube.
Most stylets have a flow-through design that allows air or water to be flushed through the tube
ports while the stylet is in place. In most tubes with stylets, the inner lumen is coated with a water-
soluble lubricant for ease of stylet removal.

15.2.4 Y-PORTS

Most nasoenteric feeding tubes have a Y-port on the end to facilitate flushing of the tube and
medication administration without having to disconnect the feeding administration set (see Table
15.1). Some feeding tubes have only a single port. In this case, a Y extension set can be added to
the end of the tube. The port may be designed to accommodate a feeding set, a syringe, or both.
The use of the Y-port is effective in minimizing contamination of the nutritional formulation. The
use of Y-ports occasionally causes some confusion with gastrostomy tubes, because a gastrostomy
tube with a Y-port might be misinterpreted as a gastrojejunal combination tube. To avoid this
misinterpretation, ports should be labeled as clearly as possible with respect to the purpose (e.g.,
gastrostomy port, for flushing only, etc.).

15.2.5 WEIGHTED VS. NONWEIGHTED FEEDING TIPS

Nasoenteric feeding tubes are available on the market with or without a tungsten weight (see
Table 15.1). Initially, it was thought that the weight would facilitate tube placement. However,
clinical trials have not clearly identified an advantage to the use of weighted tubes, and some studies
suggest that placement of a nasoenteric feeding tube into the small bowel is easier with nonweighted
tubes [10–12]. Ultimately, the decision whether to use a weighted or a nonweighted tube is a matter
of personal preference and should be based on the experience of those performing the procedure
on a routine basis. Choosing a feeding tube strictly based on cost or facility contract without
considering the clinicians' expertise is unlikely to result in any cost savings, because of increased
device wastage after unsuccessful deployments.

15.3 FEEDING METHODS AND EQUIPMENT

15.3.1 FEEDING METHODS

Enteral feedings can be infused either continuously or intermittently by two different methods. In
critically ill patients, feeding pumps should be used for all continuous feedings, so that the rate of
feeding can be adequately regulated. Intermittent feedings may be administered either by gravity,
using a gravity drip bag, or via a syringe to provide a bolus feeding. Critically ill patients rarely

tolerate large volumes via the syringe or bolus feeding method, but these patients will often tolerate a gravity feeding delivered over 20 to 40 minutes several times a day. (See Chapter 19.)

15.3.2 FEEDING SETS AND PUMPS

Feeding sets are designed for either gravity or pump feeding. Feeding sets are often preattached to the gravity or pump feeding bags and cannot be separated. The gravity feeding delivery sets have a roller clamp to help control the flow rate. Generally, the feeding sets designed for the continuous method are pump specific, which must be taken into consideration when contracting for these items. Most of the connectors on a feeding set will not attach to an intravenous needle or a leur connector, making it impossible to administer enteral feeding inadvertently into an intravenous line.

Enteral feeding containers come in different sizes and hold different volumes. In the hospital setting, they are generally changed every 24 hours. Closed-system containers are available that are prefilled with a specific volume. Theoretically, these should decrease the risk of contamination. However, use of these closed systems in the critically ill patient population may lead to increased wastage of enteral formulas. Enteral feedings are often withheld in the critically ill patient because of a change in the patient's clinical status or the need for the patient to undergo an invasive procedure. As for other hospitalized patients, any product that remains in the container after 24 hours should be discarded.

Several factors should be considered when selecting a pump for use in the intensive care setting. Most importantly, the pump should come with clear instructions and be simple to use. The pump should be quiet but have both audio and visual alarms to protect against overinfusion. The pump should provide accurate volumetric delivery and offer the ability to preset an intermittent dose or a continuous flow rate. Given space limitations in an ICU, a 24-hour battery and built-in intravenous pole clamp are also highly desirable.

15.4 INSERTION AND CARE OF FEEDING TUBES

The major differences between various types of enteral access devices are the following:

- Where the tip of the tube is located (stomach vs. small bowel)
- Whether the tube is inserted via the nasal or oral cavity directly into the gastrointestinal tract (for short-term access) or is surgically placed through the skin of the abdomen into the stomach or small bowel (for longer-term access)
- Whether the tube has different lumens and can be used to decompress the stomach while allowing feeding into the small bowel

Each tube type has potential advantages and disadvantages for the critically ill patient (see Table 15.2).

15.4.1 SHORT-TERM FEEDING TUBES

As previously mentioned, many critically ill patients will have a large-bore tube inserted nasally or orally for gastric decompression [13]. When the patient no longer requires gastric decompression, these tubes may be used for medication administration and enteral feeding. The disadvantage of these tubes is that they are uncomfortable and may become even more irritating to the patient over time as they harden. In addition, these larger, stiffer tubes are more likely to cause sinusitis or nasal necrosis [14,15]. Therefore, if a patient no longer requires gastric decompression, the larger-bore nasogastric tube should be replaced with a smaller-bore, more flexible nasoenteric tube for patient comfort and safety. These tubes can usually be successfully placed at the bedside by the staff nurse.

If a patient's condition precludes gastric feeding and only short-term access is needed, a nasoduodenal or nasojejunal tube can be utilized. Although usually placed transnasally, these tubes can be inserted transorally in patients with facial or sinus fractures. In general, the goal is to place the feeding tip at or beyond the ligament of Treitz, in order to decrease the risk of reflux of feedings into the stomach. Placement of these tubes by any method (endoscopic, fluoroscopic, or at the bedside) requires trained personnel.

15.4.1.1 Confirmation of Placement and Monitoring of Short-Term Feeding Access

Prior to utilization of any feeding tube placed at the bedside, radiographic confirmation of its location should be obtained. This virtually eliminates the risk of inadvertent administration of enteral feedings into the lungs, although it does not eliminate the initial risk of misplacement of the tube down the tracheobronchial tree [16–20]. In many mechanically ventilated, critically ill patients, the use of sedative and paralytic medications or the patient's underlying disease process itself impairs the normal reflexes protecting the airway and allows a nasoenteric tube to be inserted past the balloon of an endotracheal or tracheostomy tube without detection. Oral placement of the feeding tube is recommended in patients who have sustained craniofacial trauma, to reduce the risk of intracranial placement [21].

During blind bedside placement, several tools exist that can be utilized to aid in the correct placement of a nasoenteric tube into the gastrointestinal tract and its correct positioning into the stomach or small bowel. These tools include capnography, auscultation, and comparison of gastric and small bowel aspirates.

15.4.1.1.1 Capnography

Capnography is a common noninvasive technique used in critically ill patients to determine the adequacy of ventilation by measuring end-tidal carbon dioxide (CO_2). To use this technique for nasoenteric or nasogastric tube placement, it is only necessary to distinguish the presence or absence of a CO_2 waveform. An end-tidal CO_2 detector is attached to the end of the feeding tube for continuous monitoring during placement. Theoretically, the presence of an end-tidal CO_2 > 15 mm Hg, a respiratory waveform, or both implies inadvertent placement of the tube into the airway. The absence of these two findings suggests that the tube has been placed correctly and is not in the respiratory tract.

Some authors have found this technique to be highly sensitive. This finding was replicated in our institution, when the technique was used with placements of larger-bore nasogastric tubes [22,23]. However, we did have inadvertent placement of a nasojejunal tube into the airway, despite the fact that end-tidal CO_2 monitoring did not identify detectable CO_2 or a respiratory waveform. We hypothesize that this failure may have been due in part to the small diameter of the tube (10 French) or the total length of the nasoenteric tube and end-tidal CO_2 detector tubing combined. We presently do not advocate using this technique for nasoenteric tube placement.

15.4.1.1.2 Auscultation

Auscultation of air over the stomach and small bowel is a commonly used method for detecting placement of the feeding tube [24–26]. Sounds of air injected into the stomach are heard best in the midline or left upper quadrant regions. In the small bowel, these sounds are best heard in the right upper quadrant for the proximal duodenum and in the left flank area for the distal duodenum or proximal jejunum. Unfortunately, air injection in the thoracic cavity may be auscultated in the abdomen and misinterpreted as indicating correct placement of the tube into the stomach. A more sensitive technique of auscultation is to determine whether the location of the sound changes during tube advancement. Such a finding makes it unlikely that the tube has been inadvertently placed into the tracheobronchial tree.

TABLE 15.2
Advantages and Disadvantages

Tube Type	Access Duration	Placement Technique and Expertise Level	Advantages	Disadvantages and Risks	Patient Types
Nasogastric Salem Sump	Short-term	Bedside/RN	Large bore; less clogging; nasal or oral route; staff RN can replace if needed; used for decompression	Aspiration risk; patient discomfort; sinusitis; nasal necrosis	Normal gastric emptying; low risk of aspiration
Nasoenteric feeding tube — gastric or small bowel placement	Short-term	Bedside gastric placement/RN Bedside small bowel placement/trained RN, RD, MD Endoscopy, fluoroscopy/MD	Softer more flexible material for improved patient comfort; nasal or oral placement; patient can swallow "around" tube; if larger than 8 French, unlikely to clog with good flushing techniques; available for immediate use after placement verification	Cannot be used for decompression; sinusitis. If placed in stomach, may migrate easily into the small bowel; aspiration risk. If placed in small bowel, tube may "flip" back to stomach; may not be able to be placed in patients with altered anatomy.	Gastric — low risk of aspiration Small bowel — delayed gastric emptying, increased risk of aspiration secondary to condition or positioning
Percutaneous endoscopic gastrostomy (PEG) or fluoroscopically placed gastrostomy	Long-term	Endoscopy, fluoroscopy/MD	Large bore; low risk of clogging; may feed via intermittent or syringe method; may accommodate a small bowel feeding tube, if necessary	Hemorrhage; infection at insertion site; risk of peritonitis; may have to wait 24 hours to use; persistent gastrocutaneous fistula if tract does not close when removed. Cannot be placed if endoscopy unable to be done.	Normal gastric emptying, low risk of aspiration; need for long-term enteral feeding
Surgical gastrostomy	Long-term	Surgical/ MD	Large bore; low risk of clogging; may feed via intermittent or syringe method	Requires surgical placement; hemorrhage, infection at incision or insertion site; anesthetic complications; may have to wait 24 hours to use; persistent gastrocutaneous fistula if tract does not close when removed	Normal gastric emptying, low risk of aspiration; need for long-term enteral feeding; unable to place gastrostomy via endoscopic or fluoroscopic techniques

Percutaneous endoscopic jejunostomy (PEJ)	Long-term	Endoscopy/MD	Decreased risk of aspiration; can provide supplemental feeds at night; may use immediately post placement; bypasses the stomach if decreased gastric motility a problem	Hemorrhage; infection at insertion site; risk of peritonitis; may "flip" back into stomach; difficult to replace; cannot check residuals; requires continuous infusion; smaller bore; may occlude easily; persistent gastrocutaneous fistula if tract does not close when removed; cannot be placed if endoscopy unable to be done	Increased risk of aspiration, gastric motility disorders
Jejunostomy via PEG	Long-term	Endoscopy, fluoroscopy/MD	Decreased risk of aspiration; can provide supplemental feeds at night; may use immediately post placement; simultaneous gastric decompression and small bowel feeding possible	May be difficult to get tube in position, jejunal extension may "flip" back into stomach; requires continuous infusion; smaller bore; may occlude easily	Increased risk of aspiration, gastric motility disorders
Double-lumen gastro-jejunostomy	Long-term	Surgical/MD	Decreased risk of aspiration; can provide supplemental feeds at night; may use immediately post placement; simultaneous gastric decompression and small bowel feeding possible	Requires surgical placement; hemorrhage, infection at incision or insertion site; anesthetic complications; jejunal extension may "flip" back into stomach; small bore tube; may clog easily; unable to be replaced if inadvertently pulled; persistent gastrocutaneous fistula if tract does not close when removed	Increased risk of aspiration, motility disorders; endoscopic placement not feasible
Surgical jejunostomy	Long-term	Surgical/MD	Decreased risk of aspiration; can provide supplemental feeds at night; may use immediately post placement; bypasses the stomach if decreased gastric motility a problem	Requires surgical placement, hemorrhage, infection at incision or insertion site; anesthetic complications; small-bore tube may clog easily, unable to easily replace if inadvertently pulled	Increased risk of aspiration, motility disorders, gastric outlet obstruction or other anatomy precluding gastric placement

15.4.1.1.3 Aspiration

Aspiration of gastric and small bowel contents for color and pH testing is also used to determine tube placement [27–30]. Gastric fluid typically has a lower pH (3 to 4) than respiratory (6 to 8) and small bowel fluid (> 6). However, because many critically ill patients receive H_2 blockers or proton pump inhibitors to protect against bleeding from stress ulceration, they may have a higher gastric pH (5 to 7). Therefore, color and appearance of the aspirate may be more important than pH in determining placement. A small bowel aspirate is generally a clear, golden, syrupy fluid. If the stomach and small bowel aspirates are different in appearance and pH, the tip of the feeding tube is usually found to be within the small bowel.

Because nasogastric tubes may migrate into the small bowel, rechecking for correct tube placement should be performed on a routine basis. Inadvertent bolus feeding into the intestine instead of the stomach may result in diarrhea. A gastric pH should be rechecked prior to each bolus or intermittent feed. If the color or pH changes, an abdominal radiograph is ordered to determine where the tip of the tube is located. In patients with nasoenteric tubes, it is also advisable to check color and pH of small bowel aspirate at least one time per day in continuously fed patients, because the tip of the feeding tube can migrate back into the stomach.

Bilirubin concentrations of enteral aspirates have been evaluated as a method by which to monitor feeding tube location [31,32]. The bilirubin content of the small bowel should be higher than that of the stomach or lung. However, because commercially available bedside methods for measuring bilirubin are not yet available, this technique is not yet in common practice.

In order to compare gastric and small bowel aspirates, it must be possible to sample them. In our experience, aspirates can be obtained approximately 70% of the time. The success of obtaining an aspirate may depend on the number of exit holes at the end of the tube; successful aspiration of gastrointestinal contents is more likely using tubes that have more than one exit hole.

15.4.2 LONG-TERM FEEDING TUBES

A surgically implanted feeding tube should be considered if feeding will be required for longer than four weeks. In general, these tubes are less disturbing to the patient than are tubes placed via the nasal or oral route. The risks of sinusitis and nasal or pharyngeal injuries are also eliminated. Implanted tubes transverse two epithelial barriers: the skin and the mucosa of the gastrointestinal tract. Because these barriers are the primary defenses against bacterial invasion, there is a significant risk of infection at the tube site [33,34]. Also, if the patient or caregiver inadvertently removes the tube, particularly soon after it has been placed, an operative procedure of the stomach or intestine may be needed to prevent ongoing peritoneal soilage [35]. As with all surgical procedures, placement of enteral access devices entails risks of anesthetic complications and hemorrhage, in addition to infection.

Several options are available for the placement of gastrostomy tubes. Currently, the most common technique is percutaneous endoscopic gastrostomy (PEG) [36–38]. Placement of a PEG requires that an endoscope be passed into the stomach for visualization and manipulation of the insertion site. After placement, an external bolster holds the tube in position and keeps the stomach up against the abdominal wall to prevent leakage of feedings or gastric contents. This procedure can usually be performed under local anesthesia with conscious sedation and is done with either a "push" or "pull" technique [39]. Besides infection and hemorrhage, uncommon complications include inadvertent placement of the tube through the colon or another intra-abdominal viscus and erosion or extrusion of the tube, with resultant leakage of gastric contents and tube feedings into the abdominal cavity [40–43]. Within one to two weeks of placement, significant adhesions form between the stomach and the abdominal wall, and leakage of material into the peritoneal cavity is unlikely, even when the tube is removed. The general practice is to wait 24 hours after PEG tube insertion to initiate feedings; however, there is evidence that feeding can begin as soon as 4 to 6 hours after placement [44].

Fluoroscopically guided percutaneous gastrostomy is an alternative to the PEG technique, although it is done less often [45]. This technique requires the introduction of a tube into the stomach for the delivery of contrast and air for dilation of the stomach, after which the stomach is punctured percutaneously. For patients with pharyngeal or esophageal abnormalities that preclude endoscopic or fluoroscopic placement of a tube, a surgical gastrostomy may be placed. The surgical gastrostomy tube can be implanted using either an open technique (with laparotomy) or laparoscopically [46–48]. Both methods generally require general anesthesia to be administered. Because of its more invasive nature, surgical placement of a gastrostomy tube is generally associated with a higher complication rate than is endoscopic or fluoroscopic placement. However, because the stomach is secured to the abdominal wall directly, there is usually a lower risk of gastric leakage than with the other techniques [33].

The small bowel can be accessed through the abdominal wall using several different methods. A percutaneous endoscopic jejunostomy tube can be placed, using a technique similar to that for a PEG tube, except that the tube is endoscopically positioned beyond the pylorus into the jejunum. Alternatively, if the patient already has a gastrostomy tube in place or is having one inserted, a small bowel feeding tube may be inserted through the gastrostomy tube and into the duodenum or jejunum. In addition, a small bowel feeding tube can be inserted through a preexisting gastrostomy fluoroscopically [49,50]. Also available are combination tubes that have dual ports: one for drainage of the stomach and one for delivery of nutritional formulas into the small bowel. These can be inserted via an endoscopic technique or, more commonly, during an open operative procedure [51–53]. With all small bowel feeding tubes placed transgastrically, there is a risk that the distally placed small bowel tube will migrate back into the stomach; thus, the tube may have to be repositioned endoscopically or fluoroscopically in order for the patient to be fed into the small bowel [54].

A feeding jejunostomy implanted directly into the small bowel provides the most secure means of accessing the small bowel [55]. Placement of a feeding jejunostomy almost always requires an operative procedure, via either an open or a laparoscopic approach [50,56,57]. Many times, these tubes are implanted during laparotomy for another reason, such as abdominal trauma or resection of a major neoplasm. Occasionally, they are placed during a primary procedure for a patient who will require long-term enteral feeding and has contraindications to gastric feeding. There are several different types of jejunal tubes that may be placed, ranging from small-bore tubes placed via a needle catheter technique to larger tubes placed directly into the bowel through a surgically constructed serosal tunnel. The smaller-bore needle catheter jejunostomy tubes are usually used when enteral feeding will be required for shorter periods of time, because patency may be difficult to maintain and the tube cannot be replaced once it comes out [58,59].

15.4.2.1 Care of the Insertion Site

Care of the insertion site for various tube types should begin as soon as the tube is placed and continue until the tube is removed and the exit site is healed (Table 15.3). The loss of any permanent feeding tube should be considered a medical emergency. If the tube is inadvertently removed before the tract has had time to mature, the viscus into which the tube was inserted may fall away from the abdominal wall, with leakage of gastrointestinal contents into the peritoneal cavity [35]. However, the loss of a tube from a mature site requires early reinsertion if the feeding device is to be maintained. The failure to recannulate the tube tract within a few hours may result in permanent closure of the tract, with the need to perform another procedure to gain access for a new tube.

15.4.2.2 Maintaining Tube Patency

Several considerations are important in maintaining patency of all types of feeding tubes. The smaller-bore (14 French or less) polyurethane, silicone, or polyurethane–silicone combination tubes

TABLE 15.3
Care of Insertion

Type of Placement	Evaluate	Assessment	Care	Precautions
Nasal or oral	Daily	Redness, dryness, or fissures noted around nose or mouth	Lubricate nares with water-soluble lubricant. Change anchoring method.	If condition worsens, may need to change site of insertion.
Nasal or oral	Twice daily	Decreased oral hygiene	Mouth care	
Nasal	Daily	Sores or increased nasal drainage	Replace via the oral route, may require antibiotics.	May indicate sinusitis; report to MD.
Gastrostomy or jejunostomy	Daily — start 24 h post placement	Check exit site.	Clean tube site twice daily with soap and water and the area immediately around the skin opening. If site is covered by a bolster, use cotton swab for cleaning.	
	Immediately postplacement, then daily	Increased bleeding or drainage at exit site	Place additional gauze dressing around the site and the tube.	Do not place dressings directly under the external bolster — may dislodge tube. Report to MD.
	Daily	Increased tenderness, swelling, or redness	More frequent cleaning; cap feeding ports when not in use; possibly antiobiotics or tube removal	Report immediately to MD — may be sign of an infection.
	Daily	Inadvertent tube removal	Contact MD — may be able to reinsert through established tract if done quickly.	If tract is not mature, this should be considered a medical emergency.

are more prone to clogging than are larger-bore or stiffer tubes. Regular flushing with water or normal saline has been shown to be the best way to prevent clogging. The tube should be flushed with a minimum of 30 ml of water or saline solution before and after each intermittent feeding, or every 3 to 4 h during continuous feeding [60]. Medications administered via feeding tubes should be in a liquid form or crushable [61]. Tablets should be crushed finely and dissolved in water prior to administration. The tube should be flushed with 30 ml of water before and after administering medications. Medications should not be mixed with the nutritional product, because formula–medication interactions may result in coagulation of the formula and clogging of the tube or in precipitation of the medication and loss of its effectiveness. If enteral feedings are held for any reason, the tube should continue to be flushed every 3 to 4 h to maintain patency. If the feeding tube does become clogged, several maneuvers can be attempted, as outlined in Figure 15.1 [62–64].

15.5 GASTRIC VS. SMALL BOWEL ACCESS

Enteral nutritional support has become standard for many patients admitted to an intensive care unit, and the use of early enteral support has gained popularity over the past decade in many institutions [6,65–67]. There is considerable debate regarding the best site for feeding the ICU patient: prepyloric or postpyloric [68,69]. Ultimately, this decision will be based on the perceived

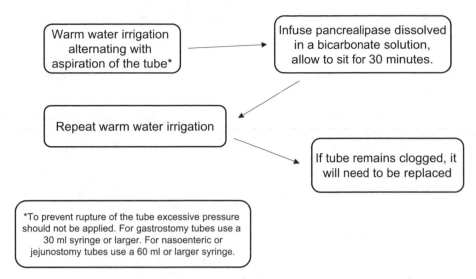

FIGURE 15.1 Steps for unclogging enteral feeding tubes.

advantages and disadvantages of either site, as well as the physician's assessment of the specific needs of the particular patient.

The advantages of gastric (prepyloric) feedings include preservation of the reservoir function of the stomach, the allowance for bolus feedings, the ease of tube placement for short-term access, the need for less equipment (such as a feeding pump), and decreased costs, because specifically trained personnel are not needed for tube placement. The disadvantages of gastric feeding relate to prolonged retention of formula in the stomach as a result of decreased gastric motility, leading to regurgitation and possible tracheobronchial aspiration, and the frequent development of high gastric residuals or feeding intolerance, which leads to a delay in achieving caloric goals [70,71].

The advantages of small bowel (postpyloric) feeding include bypassing the pylorus if gastric emptying is a problem and a theoretical decreased risk of aspiration [72–77]. It should be pointed out, however, that this latter issue remains an area of marked controversy, and a decreased risk of aspiration pneumonia with use of postpyloric feedings has not been clearly established. The disadvantages of small bowel feedings relate to the greater difficulty in placing postpyloric feeding tubes, which may necessitate transport of a critically ill patient for fluoroscopy or endoscopically guided placement, and the greater costs associated with having experienced personnel available for tube placement, the tube itself, and the use of additional equipment, particularly a pump for delivery of the formula [78–82].

Placement of small bowel feeding tubes has been reported to be highly successful with the use of endoscopic and fluoroscopic guidance [81–83]. However, the initial placement of the tube into the small bowel may give the clinician a false sense of security, because the tube may migrate out of position and back into the stomach. It this occurs, repeat endoscopy or fluoroscopy is generally required to reposition the tube, increasing costs further.

Placement of small bowel feeding tubes at the bedside obviates some of the risks and costs associated with small bowel feedings and eliminates the need for patient transport. Several methods for blind bedside placement of postpyloric feeding tubes have been described [10,25,78,84–87]. Earlier techniques required long periods for "tube migration" (4 to 72 h) prior to obtaining an abdominal radiograph to confirm correct placement [76]. Salasidis et al. [88] described a technique utilizing air insufflation and reported a 78% success rate in achieving small bowel placement; however, the authors waited two hours prior to obtaining an abdominal radiograph to allow time for tube migration. Thurlow et al. [84] utilized a corkscrew technique and reported an 87% success rate at time of placement. Zaloga et al. [85] reported a 92% success rate with this method using

TABLE 15.4
Motility Agents

	Metoclopramide	Erythromycin
Trade name	Reglan	E-Mycin
Effect on gastrointestinal (GI) tract	Increases resting esophageal sphincter tone, improves gastric tone and peristalsis, relaxes pyloric sphincter and augments duodenal peristalsis	Increases gastric emptying and improves intestinal motility (not presently FDA approved for this function)
Contraindications	Do not use in patients with seizure disorder.	Do not use in patients with preexisting liver disease or hepatic impairment.
Most common adverse reactions	Restlessness, drowsiness, diarrhea, weakness	Abdominal pain, cramping, nausea, and vomiting
Form	Available in oral or intravenous (IV)	Available in oral or IV (shortages of IV form have occurred)

trained personnel; however, when the task was given to untrained residents, the success rate dropped to 70%. Recently, the use of a magnetic device has been described; however, the success rate with this technique was lower than that reported with other techniques [89].

Promotility agents (see Table 15.4) have been used in an effort to facilitate small bowel feeding tube placements. There have been mixed reports on their efficacy in improving success rates, and the utility of these agents remains uncertain [84,90–92].

Several studies have shown that consistently higher success rates can be achieved when specifically trained personnel are designated for feeding tube placements [78,85,86]. The type of professional appears to be immaterial, with successful tube placements being achieved by physicians, nurses, and dietitians [86].

The practice at our institution is based on the technique described by Lord et al. [10], which is outlined in Table 15.5. Nasoduodenal or nasojejunal feeding tubes are placed at the bedside in most ICU patients. We have recently reported the results of blind bedside placement of small bowel feeding tubes in 1220 critically ill patients [93]. Trained professionals from the nutrition support service, including one physician, four nurses, and three dietitians, were responsible for small bowel feeding tube placements in all patients in the surgical–trauma, medical, cardiothoracic, cardiac units; neurologic ICUs; and the ICU stepdown unit. The overall success rate of this team in achieving postpyloric placement was 86% (1045/1220), with 72% of the feeding tips delivered distal to the second portion of the duodenum and 57% at or beyond the ligament of Treitz. We did note a learning curve with each newly trained practitioner. The individual with the most experience was a dietitian, who achieved a 93% success rate (401/432). Our results are consistent with the evidence indicating that designating and training specific personnel for small bowel feeding tube placement will lead to improved success with the procedure.

15.6 CONCLUSION

The clinician has a wide variety of enteral access devices and equipment from which to choose. The specific choice will be influenced by the desired site for feeding, the duration of enteral feeding needed, and the availability of trained staff for feeding tube placement. Once the enteral access device is in position, care should be taken to maintain the integrity of the site and the patency of the tube, to ensure the provision of effective enteral nutritional support.

TABLE 15.5
Sample Placement Protocol

Bedside Small Bowel Feeding Tube Placement:
A Variation of the "10-10-10" Protocol

Policy Statement: A Nutrition Support Service member or APN who has shown clinical competency with insertion will place a small bowel feeding tube (SBFT) at the bedside, with verification of placement by KUB prior to initiation of feeding.

Description: A protocol involving the insertion of all but **10** centimeters of a nonweighted 43" or 55" Corpak® feeding tube with a stylet **10** min after intravenous metoclopramide **10** mg in order to obtain small bowel placement.

Procedure:

1. Administer 10 mg intravenous metoclopramide (5 mg if patient in renal failure) over 1 to 2 min approximately 10 min prior to tube insertion.
2. Put on gloves.
3. If NGT or OGT is in place, obtain aspirate, noting color and pH, clamp NGT/OGT for SBFT insertion.
4. Set the hub of the stylet firmly into main port of feeding tube; close the medication port with cap.
5. Flush tube with approximately 10 cc tap water to check for patency or leaks, activate lubricant.
6. Elevate patient's HOB as tolerated.
7. Insert SBFT into nostril and advance to nasopharynx and into esophagus. Flexion of patient's neck or having patient swallow will facilitate passage of tube into esophagus.
8. Advance tube to 55 to 60 cm and auscultate over the epigastric area and attempt to aspirate gastric contents, comparing aspirate with previous NGT aspirate if available. Gastric aspirate is bilious in appearance. The pH may range from 1 to 7, depending on the use of gastric prophylaxis medication.
9. Continue to advance SBFT slowly with a gentle touch. Infuse approximately 60 cc air slowly, starting at 70 to 75 cm, to help open the pylorus. Never force the tube; if resistance is met, pull back and attempt to readvance. Continue to advance to the 100 cm mark. There should be a vacuum present on the syringe when the tube is in the small bowel.
10. Aspirate and check pH and color of output when tube is at 100 cm mark. Color of small bowel aspirate is generally yellow in appearance with a pH of 7+.
11. Remove stylet and check for kinks or loops, then attempt to reinsert. The stylet should be easy to insert. Upon reinsertion of stylet, if any resistance is met, pull tube back until stylet is easily inserted. After stylet is in place, readvance tube.
12. When tube is in position, remove stylet and secure tube with tape to nose. Place stylet in plastic bag to use in future if SBFT needs to be repositioned.
13. Return NGT to suction, if this was on prior to procedure.
14. Order KUB to verify placement.
15. If SBFT pulled back from original insertion cm marking, reinsert stylet and advance SBFT per preceding procedure. Obtain KUB to verify position.

15.7 CASE STUDY

K.D. is a 53-year-old male involved in a motor vehicle collision. A head and abdominal CT scan were both negative. The patient sustained a T7 vertebral body fracture, right femur fracture, left distal femur fracture, bilateral post acetabular fractures, multiple rib fractures, and a pneumothorax. A chest tube was placed. The patient was intubated and placed on mechanical ventilation. The patient has a history of atrial fibrillation and chronic pancreatitis. The patient was sent to the trauma intensive care unit.

On postadmission day 3, the patient remains intubated and the decision is made to begin enteral feeds. The plan for the next several days is for the patient to undergo several orthopedic procedures. The patient is expected to be weaned from the ventilator in approximately 7 to 10 days.

Anthropometrics: Height 5' 11", weight 86 kg, IBW 81 kg, BMI 26

Inputs/Outputs:

IVFs: D51/2NS with 20 mEq KCL @ 100 ml/h

Nasogastric tube (Salem Sump — 16 French): 2200 ml

Urine output: 2500 ml

Chest tube: 150 ml

Patient has had 2 bowel movements.

Question:

What are the possible causes of the high gastric output?

Answer:

The possible causes of the high output are decreased gastric motility, gastric outlet obstruction, and migration of the nasogastric tube tip into the duodenum. An abdominal
radiograph should be done to check for obstruction or migration of the tube.

Question:

The abdominal radiograph demonstrated the nasogastric tube to be in good position.
There was no evidence of an obstruction. It was determined the patient has decreased
gastric motility. Where should the patient be fed (stomach or small bowel), and what
is the appropriate enteral access device to use in this patient?

Answer:

To reduce the risk of aspiration, the patient should be continued on low-intermittent gastric suction. Therefore, a nasoenteric feeding tube at or beyond the ligament of Treitz
would be preferred. The patient's injuries will not affect his swallowing function. Giv-
en the short period of time (7 to 10 days) anticipated that the patient will require tube
feeds, a permanent enteral access is not warranted. Because the Salem Sump nasogastric tube is in the left nares, the nasoenteric tube is placed through the right nares.

Question:

The patient was started on IV metoclopramide 10 mg q 6 hours, and his gastric output decreased to 300 ml in 24 hours. He has developed pneumonia and is not expected to
wean from the ventilator for another 7 days. He is presently tolerating his feeds at goal
via a 10 French nasoenteric tube. The RN notes he is developing a sore on his left nares.
The patient is receiving several medications via his nasogastric tube. The patient's
weight has increased 12 kg since admission. Should any changes be made?

Answer:

The patient's poor gastric motility has resolved. Because he no longer requires gastric decompression, the stiff Salem Sump can be removed and his ulceration treated. His enteral medications should be in liquid or crushable form. Because the medications are
to be given into the small bowel, they need to be diluted with 10 to 30 ml of water; in
addition, adequate flushing between administration of medications needs to be continued.

Question:

The patient's small bowel feeding tube is pulled accidentally when the patient is being
turned. What type of tube should be placed?

Answer:

Because the patient's decreased gastric motility has resolved, a small bowel tube may no
longer be necessary. At many institutions, a specially trained professional is needed to
place the small bowel tube; the bedside nurse can place a nasogastric tube. Therefore,
a 12 French nasoenteric tube placed into the stomach would be appropriate.

REFERENCES

1. Heyland, D.K., Cook, D.J., and Guyatt, G.H., Enteral nutrition in the critically ill patient: a critical review of the evidence, *Intens. Care Med.*, 19, 435, 1993.
2. Kudsk, K.A., Croce, M.A., Fabian, T.C., et al., Enteral versus parenteral feeding: effects on septic morbidity after blunt and penetrating abdominal trauma, *Ann. Surg.*, 215, 503, 1992.
3. McMahon, M.M., Farnell, M.B., and Murray, M.J., Nutritional support of critically ill patients, *Mayo Clin. Proc.*, 68, 911, 1993.
4. Moore, E.E. and Jones, T.N., Benefits of immediate jejunostomy feeding after major abdominal trauma: a prospective, randomized study, *J. Trauma*, 26, 874, 1986.
5. Moore, F.A. and Moore, E.E., The benefits of enteric feeding, *Adv. Surg.*, 30, 141, 1996.
6. Zaloga, G.P., Bortenschlager, L., Black, K.W., et al., Immediate postoperative enteral feeding decreases weight loss and improves wound healing after abdominal surgery in rats, *Crit. Care Med.*, 20, 115, 1992.
7. Heyland, D., Cook, D.J., Winder, B., et al., Enteral nutrition in the critically ill patient: a prospective survey, *Crit. Care Med.*, 23, 1055, 1995.
8. Meyer, N.A. and Kudsk, K.A., Enteral versus parenteral nutrition: alterations in mechanisms of function in mucosal host defenses, *Nestle Nutr. Workshop Ser. Clin. Perform. Programme*, 133, 2003.
9. Ciaccia, D., Quigley, R.L., Shami, P.J., et al., A case of retrograde jejunoduodenal intussusception caused by a feeding gastrostomy tube, *Nutr. Clin. Pract.*, 9, 18, 1994.
10. Lord, L.M., Weiser-Maimone, A., Pulhamus, M., et al., Comparison of weighted vs. unweighted enteral feeding tubes for efficacy of transpyloric intubation, *J. Parenter. Enteral Nutr.*, 17, 271, 1993.
11. Levenson, R., Turner, W.W., Jr., Dyson, A., et al., Do weighted nasoenteric feeding tubes facilitate duodenal intubations?, *J. Parenter. Enteral Nutr.*, 12, 135, 1988.
12. Ugo, P.J., Mohler, P.A., and Wilson, G.L., Bedside postpyloric placement of weighted feeding tubes, *Nutr. Clin. Pract.*, 7, 284, 1992.
13. Montgomery R.C., B.-N.M., Thomas S.E., Postoperative nasogastric decompression: a prospective randomized trial, *South. Med. J.*, 89, 1063, 1996.
14. Caplan, E.S. and Hoyt, N.J., Nosocomial sinusitis, *JAMA*, 247, 639, 1982.
15. Landis, E.E., Jr., Hoffman, H.T., and Koconis, C.A., Upper airway obstruction associated with large bore nasogastric tubes, *South. Med. J.*, 81, 1333, 1988.
16. Biggart, M., McQuillan, P.J., Choudhry, A.K., et al., Dangers of placement of narrow bore nasogastric feeding tubes, *Ann. R. Coll. Surg. Engl.*, 69, 119, 1987.
17. McWey, R.E., Curry, N.S., Schabel, S.I., et al., Complications of nasoenteric feeding tubes, *Am. J. Surg.*, 155, 253, 1988.
18. Bankier, A.A., Wiesmayr, M.N., Henk, C., et al., Radiographic detection of intrabronchial malpositions of nasogastric tubes and subsequent complications in intensive care unit patients, *Intens. Care Med.*, 23, 406, 1997.
19. Rolfe, I. and Nair, B., Complications associated with the insertion of narrow-bore feeding-tubes, *Med. J. Aust.*, 152, 108, 1990.
20. Alessi, D.M. and Berci, G., Aspiration and nasogastric intubation, *Otolaryngol. Head Neck Surg.*, 94, 486, 1986.
21. Ferreras, J., Junquera, L.M., and Garcia-Consuegra, L., Intracranial placement of a nasogastric tube after severe craniofacial trauma, *Oral Surg. Oral Med. Oral Pathol. Oral Radiol. Endod.*, 90, 564, 2000.
22. Burns, S.M., Carpenter, R., and Truwit, J.D., Report on the development of a procedure to prevent placement of feeding tubes into the lungs using end-tidal CO_2 measurements, *Crit. Care Med.*, 29, 936, 2001.
23. Araujo-Preza, C.E., Melhado, M.E., Gutierrez, F.J., et al., Use of capnometry to verify feeding tube placement, *Crit. Care Med.*, 30, 2255, 2002.
24. Metheny, N., McSweeney, M., Wehrle, M.A., et al., Effectiveness of the auscultatory method in predicting feeding tube location, *Nurs. Res.*, 39, 262, 1990.
25. Stone, S.J., Pickett, J.D., and Jesurum, J.T., Bedside placement of postpyloric feeding tubes, *AACN Clin. Issues*, 11, 517, 2000.
26. Neumann, M.J., Meyer, C.T., Dutton, J.L., et al., Hold that x-ray: aspirate pH and auscultation prove enteral tube placement, *J. Clin. Gastroenterol.*, 20, 293, 1995.

27. Metheny, N., Williams, P., Wiersema, L., et al., Effectiveness of pH measurements in predicting feeding tube placement, *Nurs. Res.*, 38, 280, 1989.

28. Metheny, N., Reed, L., Wiersema, L., et al., Effectiveness of pH measurements in predicting feeding tube placement: an update, *Nurs. Res.*, 42, 324, 1993.

29. Metheny, N.A., Clouse, R.E., Clark, J.M., et al., pH testing of feeding-tube aspirates to determine placement, *Nutr. Clin. Pract.*, 9, 185, 1994.

30. Metheny, N., Reed, L., Berglund, B., et al., Visual characteristics of aspirates from feeding tubes as a method for predicting tube location, *Nurs. Res.*, 43, 282, 1994.

31. Metheny, N.A., Stewart, B.J., Smith, L., et al., pH and concentration of bilirubin in feeding tube aspirates as predictors of tube placement, *Nurs. Res.*, 48, 189, 1999.

32. Metheny, N.A., Smith, L., and Stewart, B.J., Development of a reliable and valid bedside test for bilirubin and its utility for improving prediction of feeding tube location, *Nurs. Res.*, 49, 302, 2000.

33. Shellito, P.C. and Malt, R.A., Tube gastrostomy: techniques and complications, *Ann. Surg.*, 201, 180, 1985.

34. Ephgrave, K.S., Buchmiller, C., Jones, M.P., et al., The cup is half full, *Am. J. Surg.*, 178, 406, 1999.

35. Holmes, J.H., Brundage, S.I., Yuen, P., et al., Complications of surgical feeding jejunostomy in trauma patients, *J. Trauma*, 47, 1009, 1999.

36. Gauderer, M.W., Ponsky, J.L., and Izant, R.J., Jr., Gastrostomy without laparotomy: a percutaneous endoscopic technique, *J. Pediatr. Surg.*, 15, 872, 1980.

37. Grant, J.P., Comparison of percutaneous endoscopic gastrostomy with Stamm gastrostomy, *Ann. Surg.*, 207, 598, 1988.

38. Gauderer, M.W., Percutaneous endoscopic gastrostomy and the evolution of contemporary long-term enteral access, *Clin. Nutr.*, 21, 103, 2002.

39. Hogan, R.B., DeMarco, D.C., Hamilton, J.K., et al., Percutaneous endoscopic gastrostomy: to push or pull. A prospective randomized trial, *Gastrointest. Endosc.*, 32, 253, 1986.

40. Larson, D.E., Burton, D.D., Schroeder, K.W., et al., Percutaneous endoscopic gastrostomy: indications, success, complications, and mortality in 314 consecutive patients, *Gastroenterology*, 93, 48, 1987.

41. DeLegge, M.H., Effect of external bolster tension on PEG tube tract formation, *Gastrointest. Endosc.*, 43, 349, 1996.

42. Grant, J.P., Mortality with percutaneous endoscopic gastrostomy, *Am. J. Gastroenterol.*, 95, 3, 2000.

43. Stefan, M.M., Holcomb, G.W., 3rd, and Ross, A.J., 3rd, Cologastric fistula as a complication of percutaneous endoscopic gastrostomy, *J. Parenter. Enteral Nutr.*, 13, 554, 1989.

44. Ho, C.S., Yee, A.C., and McPherson, R., Complications of surgical and percutaneous nonendoscopic gastrostomy: review of 233 patients, *Gastroenterology*, 95, 1206, 1988.

45. McLoughlin, R.F., So, B., and Gray, R.R., Fluoroscopically guided percutaneous gastrostomy: current status, *Can. Assoc. Radiol. J.*, 47, 10, 1996.

46. Peitgen, K., von Ostau, C., and Walz, M.K., Laparoscopic gastrostomy: results of 121 patients over 7 years, *Surg. Laparosc. Endosc. Percutan. Tech.*, 11, 76, 2001.

47. Murayama, K.M., Schneider, P.D., and Thompson, J.S., Laparoscopic gastrostomy: a safe method for obtaining enteral access, *J. Surg. Res.*, 58, 1, 1995.

48. Rosser, J.C., Jr., Rodas, E.B., Blancaflor, J., et al., A simplified technique for laparoscopic jejunostomy and gastrostomy tube placement, *Am. J. Surg.*, 177, 61, 1999.

49. Baskin, W. and Johanson, J.F., Trans-PEG ultra thin endoscopy for PEG/J Placement, *Gastrointest. Endosc.*, 57, 146; author reply 146, 2003.

50. Bell, S.D., Carmody, E.A., Yeung, E.Y., et al., Percutaneous gastrostomy and gastrojejunostomy: additional experience in 519 procedures, *Radiology*, 194, 817, 1995.

51. Parasher, V.K., Abramowicz, C.J., Bell, C., et al., Successful placement of percutaneous gastrojejunostomy using steerable guidewire: a modified controlled push technique, *Gastrointest. Endosc.*, 41, 52, 1995.

52. Duckworth, P.F., Jr., Kirby, D.F., McHenry, L., et al., Percutaneous endoscopic gastrojejunostomy made easy: a new over-the-wire technique, *Gastrointest. Endosc.*, 40, 350, 1994.

53. DeLegge, M.H., Patrick, P., and Gibbs, R., Percutaneous endoscopic gastrojejunostomy with a tapered tip, nonweighted jejunal feeding tube: improved placement success, *Am. J. Gastroenterol.*, 91, 1130, 1996.

54. DeLegge, M.H., Duckworth, P.F., Jr., McHenry, L., Jr., et al., Percutaneous endoscopic gastrojejunostomy: a dual center safety and efficacy trial, *J. Parenter. Enteral Nutr.*, 19, 239, 1995.

55. McGonigal, M.D., Lucas, C.E., and Ledgerwood, A.M., Feeding jejunostomy in patients who are critically ill, *Surg. Gynecol. Obstet.*, 168, 275, 1989.

56. Duh, Q.Y., Senokozlieff-Englehart, A.L., Choe, Y.S., et al., Laparoscopic gastrostomy and jejunostomy: safety and cost with local vs general anesthesia, *Arch. Surg.*, 134, 151, 1999.

57. Henderson, J.M., Strodel, W.E., and Gilinsky, N.H., Limitations of percutaneous endoscopic jejunostomy, *J. Parenter. Enteral Nutr.*, 17, 546, 1993.

58. Myers, J.G., Page, C.P., Stewart, R.M., et al., Complications of needle catheter jejunostomy in 2,022 consecutive applications, *Am. J. Surg.*, 170, 547, 1995.

59. Cogen, R., Weinryb, J., Pomerantz, C., et al., Complications of jejunostomy tube feeding in nursing facility patients, *Am. J. Gastroenterol.*, 86, 1610, 1991.

60. Massoni, M., *Gastrointestinal Care*, Springhouse Corporation, 1993.

61. Giving medication through a nasogastric tube, *Nursing*, 10, 70, 1980.

62. Tinckler, L., Nasogastric tube management, *Br. J. Surg.*, 59, 637, 1970.

63. Marcuard, S.P., Stegall, K.L., and Trogdon, S., Clearing obstructed feeding tubes, *J. Parenter. Enteral Nutr.*, 13, 81, 1989.

64. Marcuard, S.P. and Stegall, K.S., Unclogging feeding tubes with pancreatic enzyme, *J. Parenter. Enteral Nutr.*, 14, 198, 1990.

65. Inoue, S., Epstein, M.D., Alexander, J.W., et al., Prevention of yeast translocation across the gut by a single enteral feeding after burn injury, *J. Parenter. Enteral Nutr.*, 13, 565, 1989.

66. Moore, F.A., Moore, E.E., and Haenel, J.B., Clinical benefits of early post-injury enteral feeding, *Clin. Intens. Care*, 6, 21, 1995.

67. Carr, C.S., Ling, K.D., Boulous, P., and Singer M., Randomized trial of safety and efficacy of immediate postoperative enteral feeding in patients undergoing gastrointestinal resection, *BMJ*, 312, 869, 1996.

68. Hiyama, D.T. and Zinner, M.J., *Principles of Surgery*. McGraw-Hill, New York, 1994.

69. Marik, P.E. and Zaloga, G.P., Gastric versus post-pyloric feeding: a systematic review, *Crit. Care*, 7, R46, 2003.

70. Montecalvo, M.A., Steger, K.A., Farber, H.W., et al., Nutritional outcome and pneumonia in critical care patients randomized to gastric versus jejunal tube feedings. The Critical Care Research Team, *Crit. Care Med.*, 20, 1377, 1992.

71. Neumann, D.A. and DeLegge, M.H., Gastric versus small-bowel tube feeding in the intensive care unit: a prospective comparison of efficacy, *Crit. Care Med.*, 30, 1436, 2002.

72. Lazarus, B.A., Murphy, J.B., and Culpepper, L., Aspiration associated with long-term gastric versus jejunal feeding: a critical analysis of the literature, *Arch. Phys. Med. Rehabil.*, 71, 46, 1990.

73. Mullan, H., Roubenoff, R.A., and Roubenoff, R., Risk of pulmonary aspiration among patients receiving enteral nutrition support, *J. Parenter. Enteral Nutr.*, 16, 160, 1992.

74. Cataldi-Betcher, E.L., Seltzer, M.H., Slocum, B.A., et al., Complications occurring during enteral nutrition support: a prospective study, *J. Parenter. Enteral Nutr.*, 7, 546, 1983.

75. Botoman, V.A., Kirtland, S.H., and Moss, L.A., A randomized study of a pH sensor feeding tube vs a standard feeding tube in patients requiring enteral nutrition, *J. Parenter. Enteral Nutr.*, 18, 154, 1994.

76. Rees, R.G., Payne-James, J.J., King, C., and Silk, D.B.A., Spontaneous transpyloric passage and performance of "fine bore" polyurethane feeding tubes: a controlled clinical trial, *J. Parenter. Enteral Nutr.*, 12, 462, 1988.

77. Strong, R.M., Condon, S.C., Solinger, M.R., et al., Equal aspiration rates from postpylorus and intragastric-placed small-bore nasoenteric feeding tubes: a randomized, prospective study, *J. Parenter. Enteral Nutr.*, 16, 59, 1992.

78. Powers, J., Chance, R., Bortenschlager, L., et al., Bedside placement of small-bowel feeding tubes in the intensive care unit, *Crit. Care Nurse*, 23, 16, 2003.

79. Ott, D.J., Mattox, H.E., Gelfand, D.W., et al., Enteral feeding tubes: placement by using fluoroscopy and endoscopy, *Am. J. Roentgenol.*, 157, 769, 1991.

80. Hillard, A.E., Waddell, J.J., Metzler, M.H., et al., Fluoroscopically guided nasoenteric feeding tube placement versus bedside placement, *South. Med. J.*, 88, 425, 1995.

81. Patrick, P.G., Marulendra, S., Kirby, D.F., et al., Endoscopic nasogastric-jejunal feeding tube placement in critically ill patients, *Gastrointest. Endosc.*, 45, 72, 1997.
82. Prager, R., Laboy, V., Venus, B., et al., Value of fluoroscopic assistance during transpyloric intubation, *Crit. Care Med.*, 14, 151, 1986.
83. Rives, D.A., LeRoy, J.L., Hawkins, M.L., et al., Endoscopically assisted nasojejunal feeding tube placement, *Am. Surg.*, 55, 88, 1989.
84. Thurlow, P.M., Bedside enteral feeding tube placement into duodenum and jejunum, *J. Parenter. Enteral Nutr.*, 10, 104, 1986.
85. Zaloga, G.P., Bedside method for placing small bowel feeding tubes in critically ill patients: a prospective study, *Chest*, 100, 1643, 1991.
86. Taylor, B. and Schallom, L., Bedside small bowel feeding tube placement in critically ill patients using a dietitian/nurse team approach, *Nutr. Clin. Pract.*, 16, 258, 2001.
87. Lenart, S. and Polissar, N.L., Comparison of 2 methods for postpyloric placement of enteral feeding tubes, *Am. J. Crit. Care*, 12, 357, 2003.
88. Salasidis, R., Fleiszer, T., and Johnston, R., Air insufflation technique of enteral tube insertion: a randomized, controlled trial, *Crit. Care Med.*, 26, 1036, 1998.
89. Boivin, M., Levy, H., and Hayes, J., A multicenter, prospective study of the placement of transpyloric feeding tubes with assistance of a magnetic device. The Magnet-Guided Enteral Feeding Tube Study Group, *J. Parenter. Enteral Nutr.*, 24, 304, 2000.
90. Heiselman, D.E., Hofer, T., and Vidovich, R.R., Enteral feeding tube placement success with intravenous metoclopramide administration in ICU patients, *Chest*, 107, 1686, 1995.
91. Kittinger, J.W., Sandler, R.S., and Heizer, W.D., Efficacy of metoclopramide as an adjunct to duodenal placement of small-bore feeding tubes: a randomized, placebo-controlled, double-blind study, *J. Parenter. Enteral Nutr.*, 11, 33, 1987.
92. Kalliafas, S., Choban, P.S., Ziegler, D., et al., Erythromycin facilitates postpyloric placement of nasoduodenal feeding tubes in intensive care unit patients: randomized, double-blinded, placebo-controlled trial, *J. Parenter. Enteral Nutr.*, 20, 385, 1996.
93. Taylor, B., Everett, S., and Muckova, N., Bedside small bowel placement in over 1200 critically ill patients: a success story, *Crit. Care Med. (Suppl.)*, 31, A85, 2003.

16 Enteral Formulations

Ainsley M. Malone
Mount Carmel West Hospital

CONTENTS

16.1 INTRODUCTION

In the last 25 years, the availability of enteral formulas for use in hospitalized patients has increased dramatically. In the late 1970s, when enteral nutrition support was in its infancy, approximately 16 enteral formulas were available for use (1). The present-day marketplace offers well over 100 enteral formulas, many of which can be considered for use in the critically ill patient. Selecting an enteral formula can be a challenging decision. Choosing an appropriate formula is often difficult, given the multiple formula variations that exist. The clinical state of the patient, including his or her current condition and any underlying disease state, is a primary determinant of formula selection. Moreover, other factors, such as energy and protein requirements and fluid status, are important considerations when choosing an appropriate formula.

Promoting positive outcomes through the use of modified enteral formulas has become a key component in formula decision making. Does the use of an immune-enhancing formula reduce infectious complications? Does a formula for acute respiratory distress syndrome result in a reduction in the need for ventilatory support? Answering these questions and others requires a review of the available literature to assist the practitioner in selecting an enteral formula that may benefit the patient. It should be pointed out that enteral formulas are considered food supplements by the Food and Drug Association and therefore are not under regulatory control. In addition, there is a lack of prospective, randomized, controlled clinical trials supporting the proposed indications for most specialized formulas. This chapter will focus on several areas:

- Individual components of enteral formulas, their functions and characteristics
- Categories of enteral formulas, including product types within each category
- Review of the available evidence evaluating the use of specialized formulas

16.2 NUTRIENT COMPONENTS OF ENTERAL FORMULAS

16.2.1 CARBOHYDRATE

Carbohydrate represents the primary macronutrient in most enteral formulas and ranges from 28 to 82% of total calories. It is the formula component that influences overall sweetness, with the simpler form yielding a sweeter product. Table 16.1 outlines the sources of carbohydrate available in enteral formulas. Generally, the shorter the carbohydrate molecule is, the greater the osmolality and the sweeter the product requiring the least digestive capacity (2). Most enteral formulas contain either oligosaccharides containing 3 to 10 glucose units or polysaccharides, polymers containing more than 10 glucose units. Polymeric formulas provide carbohydrate primarily in the form of corn syrup solids; hydrolyzed formulas offer hydrolyzed cornstarch or maltodextrin as their source of carbohydrate. The majority of enteral formulas do not contain lactose, a disaccharide many individuals are unable to digest adequately due to insufficient quantities of the enzyme lactase (3). Many products offer variations of total carbohydrate content to assist in management of metabolic states such as hyperglycemia and hypercapnia. See the section on disease state formulations for further discussion. See Chapter 2 for a thorough review of carbohydrate metabolism in the critically ill patient.

16.2.2 PROTEIN

Proteins are the source of amino acids necessary for synthesis of structural proteins, enzymes, antibodies, and other vital functional components. In addition, amino acids, especially in the critically ill patient, are often metabolized for use as energy substrates (4). The content of protein in enteral formulas ranges from approximately 6 to 25%. A patient's protein requirements and underlying disease state are primary determinants for product selection. Both the protein quantity and the quality provided in an enteral formula are important considerations when choosing a product (3). Table 16.1 outlines various protein sources available in enteral formulas. One of the most common methods for assessing protein quality is the determination of the protein's biological value (BV). Proteins with a high BV offer a higher percentage of absorbed nitrogen required for growth and maintenance (5). The lower the protein's BV is, the greater the percentage of nonessential amino acids present in the protein, with a greater amount of total protein required to achieve nitrogen balance.

The form of protein available in enteral formulations can vary from intact proteins to hydrolyzed proteins or crystalline amino acids (see Table 16.1). In addition, some formulas offer increased doses of specific amino acids added primarily for pharmacologic function, amounts which should not be factored into a formula's total protein content. The protein form best suited for the critically

TABLE 16.1
Macronutrient Sources in Enteral Formulas

Enteral Formula Type	Carbohydrate	Protein	Fat
Polymeric formulas	Corn syrup solids	Casein	Borage oil
	Hydrolyzed cornstarch	Sodium, calcium,	Canola oil
	Maltodextrin	magnesium, and potassium	Corn oil
	Sucrose	caseinates	Fish oil
	Fructose	Soy protein isolate	High oleic sunflower oil
	Sugar alcohols	Whey protein concentrate	Medium-chain triglycerides
		Lactalbumin	Menhaden oil
		Milk protein concentrate	Monoglycerides and diglycerides
			Palm kernel oil
			Safflower oil
			Soybean oil
			Soy lecithin
Hydrolyzed formulas	Cornstarch	Hydrolyzed casein	Fatty acid esters
	Hydrolyzed cornstarch	Hydrolyzed whey protein	Fish oil
	Maltodextrin	Crystalline L-amino acids	Medium-chain triglycerides
	Fructose	Hydrolyzed lactalbumin	Safflower oil
		Soy protein isolate	Sardine oil
			Soybean oil
			Soy lecithin
			Structured lipids

ill patient has frequently been a source of controversy (3). It has often been thought that the digestive and absorptive ability of the small intestine in critical illness is impaired, a reason to support the use of more chemically defined formulas. Whether this impairment exists is not well defined (3). See Chapter 3 for an extensive review of protein metabolism.

16.2.2.1 Amino Acids

The term *elemental* formula became well accepted in the early days of enteral nutrition. The concept that free amino acids were better absorbed by the functionally impaired gut was commonly accepted, especially as it applied to the critically ill patient (6). It is well known that di- and tripeptides are absorbed from the intestinal lumen without hydrolysis (7). The use of peptide-based enteral formulas has been shown to be superior to that of free amino acids in promoting greater nitrogen absorption in both the healthy and the diseased gut (8,9). In addition, the use of intact protein may be as effective as amino acid use in promoting intestinal integrity. One study, comparing the use of amino acids vs. intact protein in patients with Crohn's disease, found that the use of intact protein was equally as effective in promoting disease remission as were free amino acids (10). The use of free amino acids in enteral formulas may be necessary in those who are intolerant of peptide-based formulas.

16.2.2.2 Peptides

Peptides are hydrolyzed proteins containing varying chain lengths, with most peptide formulas containing a mixture of di- and tripeptides. These formulas have been suggested for use in critically ill patients and in those with impaired gastrointestinal function (e.g., pancreatitis or short bowel syndrome) (2,11,12). Whether there is a benefit in using peptide-based formulas rather than intact protein formulas in the critically ill patient is unclear.

One study in critically ill patients demonstrated improvement in serum proteins in those who received a peptide-based vs. an intact protein formula (13). Whether a difference in formula tolerance or in intensive care unit length of stay occurred with the use of a peptide formula was not evaluated. Other studies have documented a reduced incidence of hypoalbuminemic-related diarrhea with the use of peptide-based formulas (11,12).

More recent data support the use of intact protein formulas in critically ill patients. In 1997, Heimburger et al. demonstrated no difference in diarrhea incidence between a peptide-based and a whole-protein formula in critically ill patients (14). Moreover, Dietscher et al., in 1998, compared a combined peptide and free amino acid formula with a whole-protein formula in ICU patients and found no difference in diarrhea incidence (15). It appears that the primary issue regarding peptide-based formula usage relates to the presence of gastrointestinal dysfunction. Clearly in those patients with malabsorption, pancreatic dysfunction, short bowel syndrome, or other evidence of gastrointestinal disease, peptide-based enteral formulas should be considered for initial use. In those with normal gastrointestinal function, however, enteral formulas with an intact protein source should be routinely utilized as the first choice in enteral product selection.

16.2.2.3   Glutamine

Glutamine, a nonessential amino acid, is a contributor to multiple metabolic functions and is considered a "conditionally essential" amino acid in periods of metabolic stress, including sepsis, trauma, burns, and critical illness. Glutamine is the most abundant amino acid in skeletal muscle and plasma and is the primary carrier of nitrogen from the skeletal muscle to the viscera due to its two amino groups. Glutamine has multiple functions, all of which are important in the critically ill patient. It assists in the regulation of acid–base balance through ammonia synthesis, is essential for the synthesis of nucleotides and nucleic acids, and is the preferred primary energy source for rapidly proliferating cells such as enterocytes, lymphocytes, and macrophages. It is known that glutamine levels in both the blood and the muscle are reduced in injury, trauma, and critical illness (21). Glutamine's function with rapidly dividing cells, especially those of the intestinal mucosa, has generated the most recent interest (22). Glutamine has been shown to increase nutrient absorption, reduce bacterial translocation, and exert trophic effects on the small bowel mucosa.

The inclusion of free glutamine in enteral products is a recent advance. (See Table 16.2 for glutamine content of selected formulas.) Previously, glutamine was available either as a component of a free amino acid formula or as a protein-bound form. With the protein-bound form, the actual glutamine content is estimated and will vary with the protein source, amount, and degree of processing. It is known that hydrolyzed formulas will have less glutamine than their constituent protein, due to losses that occur during hydrolysis (23). In addition to glutamine provided from an product's inherent protein, some enteral products contain added glutamine in the free amino acid form.

Whether providing a formula with enhanced glutamine will benefit the critically ill patient is not entirely known. Two studies have demonstrated reduced infectious complications in bone marrow transplant patients who received glutamine-supplemented parenteral nutrition compared to standard parenteral nutrition (24,25). However, in the same population, a trial evaluating enteral glutamine-supplemented formulas did not show similar results (26). Glutamine's suggested role in maintenance of gut permeability was evaluated by Velasco and colleagues (27) in 2001. They compared the effects of a standard and a glutamine-supplemented enteral formula on improvement of gut permeability in critically ill patients and found no difference. Two studies specifically evaluating glutamine in critically ill patients have yielded positive results. In 1998, Houdijk and colleagues demonstrated a significant reduction in pneumonia, bacteremia, and sepsis in critically ill multiple trauma patients receiving a glutamine-supplemented enteral formula (28). Jones et al., in 1999, evaluated a glutamine-supplemented enteral formula and found a significant reduction in

TABLE 16.2
Protein, Amino Acid, and Lipid Content of Selected Enteral Formulas

Enteral Product	% of kcals from Protein	Arginine (g/1000 kcals)	Glutamine (g/1000 kcals)	% of kcals from Fat	Linoleic Acid (g/l)	Medium-Chain Triglycerides (g/l)	ω-3 Fatty Acids (g/l) and Source
Alitraq	21.1	4.6	15.5	13.2	6.6	6.4	0
Choice DM	17.0	0	0	43.0	10.2	4.9	2.1 Canola oil
Criticare HN	14.4	1.4	1.6–2.4	4.5	3.4	0.0	0.10 Emulsifiers
Crucial	25.0	10.0	4.8	39	7.7	35	3.8 Fish oil
Deliver 2.0	15.0	0	0	45.0	37.0	29.0	5.5 Soybean oil
F.A.A.	20.0	12.0	0	10	8.4	2.8	0.0
Diabetisource AC	20.0	8.6	0	44.0	10.0	8.9	4.0 Canola oil
Fibersource HN	18.0	0	0	29.0	7.2	8.1	2.7 Canola oil
Glucerna, Glucerna Select	16.7	N/A	N/A	49.0	7.7	0.02	0.7 Canola oil
	20.0			49	9.2	0.09	1.6 Canola oil
Glytrol	18.0	N/A	N/A	42	5.4	9.4	1.8 Canola oil
Hepatic-Aid II	15.0	3.8	0	N/A	N/A	N/A	N/A
Impact, Impact 1.5, Impact with Fiber	22.0	12.5	0	25.0	2.5	7.6	1.7
				40.0	3.8	38.2	2.6
				25.0	2.5	7.6	1.7 Menhaden oil
Impact Glutamine	24.0	12.5	11.5	30.0	3.9	11.7	2.7 Menhaden oil

(continued)

TABLE 16.2 (CONTINUED)
Protein, Amino Acid, and Lipid Content of Selected Enteral Formulas

Enteral Product	% of kcals from Protein	Arginine (g/1000 kcals)	Glutamine (g/1000 kcals)	% of kcals from Fat	Linoleic Acid (g/l)	Medium-Chain Triglycerides (g/l)	ω-3 Fatty Acids (g/l) and Source
Intensical	25.0	5.5	6.9	29.0	6.6	10.3	1.9 Canola oil
Isocal HN Plus	18.0	N/A	N/A	29.0	6.1	11.5	1.3 Canola oil
Isosource HN	18.0	N/A	N/A	29.0	7.2	8.1	2.7 Canola oil
Isosource 1.5	18.0	N/A	N/A	38.0	14.7	20.1	3.6 Canola oil
Jevity 1.2	18.5	N/A	N/A	29.0	5.4	10.6	1.3 Canola oil
Jevity 1.5				29.4	6.7		1.3 Canola oil
Magnacal Renal	15.0	N/A	N/A	45.0	17.9	20.0	3.7 Canola oil
Nepro	14.0	N/A	N/A	43.0	15.5	0.01	2.9 Canola oil
Novasource Pulmonary	20.0	N/A	N/A	40.0	11.5	14.2	4.7 Canola oil
Novasource Renal	15.0	N/A	N/A	45.0	16.6	14.2	6.1 Canola oil
Novasource 2.0	18.0	N/A	N/A	39.0	14.3	11.5	6.1 Canola oil
Nutren 1.5	16.0	N/A	N/A	39.0	9.8	34.0	2.5 Canola oil
Nutren 2.0	16.0	N/A	N/A	45.0	7.8	8.0	1.5 Canola oil
NutriHep	11.0	N/A	N/A	12.0	1.6	14.8	0.4 Canola oil
NutriRenal	14.0	N/A	N/A	46.0		49.6	Canola oil
NutriVent	18.0	N/A	N/A	55.0	15.4	38.5	3.5 Canola oil

	C1	C2	C3	C4	C5	C6	C7	Oil
Optimental	20.5	5.5	4.4	25.0	3.9	4.9	4.3	Canola oil
Oxepa	16.7	N/A	N/A	55.2	14.5	23.1	10.2	Sardine and borage oils
Peptamen, Peptamen with FOS	16.0	1.2	3.0	33.0, 33.0	3.2	27.6, 27.0	.04	Soybean oil
Peptamen 1.5	18.0	1.1	3.3	33.0	6.1	41.0	0.9	Soybean oil
Peptinex, Peptinex DT	20.0	1.8, 3.0	4.9, 4.7	15.0, 15.0	7.0, 4.5	3.8, 8.4	0.9, 0.8	Soybean oil
Perative	20.5	6.2	5.4	25.0	6.8	14.8	1.2	Canola oil
Pulmocare	16.7	N/A	N/A	55.1	18.4	18.8	4.8	Canola oil
RenalCal	7.0	N/A	N/A	35.0	6.3	24.1	1.8	Canola oil
Replete and Replete with Fiber	25.0, 25.0	N/A	N/A	30.0	5.1	8.4	2.1	Canola oil
Respalor	20.0	N/A	N/A	40.0	10.3	20.0	2.2	Canola oil
Subdue, Subdue Plus	20.0	1.5	3.7	30.0, 30.0	3.1, 5.5	18.0, 24.0	0.7, 1.2	Canola oil
Tolerex	8.0	1.8	3.5	1.0	1.2	0	0	
TraumaCal	22.0	N/A	N/A	40.0	25.0	20.0	3.7	Soybean oil
TwoCal HN	16.7	N/A	N/A	40.9	10.9	17.1	1.4	Canola oil
Vivonex Plus	18.0	5.0	10.0	6.0	3.4	0	0.5	Soybean oil
Vivonex RTF	20.0	5.7	0	10.0	2.8	6.3	0.4	Soybean oil
Vivonex TEN	15.0	2.9	19	3.0	2.2	0	0	Soybean oil

Note: N/A = not available.

intensive care and hospital lengths of stay, as well as in total patient costs in those who received the glutamine-supplemented formula (29).

Two recent systematic reviews of the available data evaluating enteral glutamine in critically ill patients have concluded that the use of glutamine-supplemented formulas may be of benefit. In 2003, Garcia-de-Lorenzo et al. recommended that, due to benefits in reducing hospital length of stay and infectious complications in trauma patients, the use of enteral formulas supplemented with 15 to 25 g/d glutamine for more than five days is warranted (30). In addition, in 2003 Heyland et al. recommended that enteral glutamine should be considered in burn and trauma patients (31). Further study evaluating glutamine is necessary, not only to confirm existing benefits but also to evaluate the effects of enteral glutamine use on overall morbidity and mortality in other groups of critically ill patients (32).

16.2.2.4 Arginine

Arginine is considered an essential amino acid during periods of stress, due mainly to its increased requirements in tissue repair. Arginine serves a number of biochemical and functional roles within the body. Arginine is a precursor for the synthesis of important proteins, including proline, glutamate, and polyamine. As an intermediate in the urea cycle, arginine is important for ammonia detoxification. In addition, arginine plays a role in cell signaling and in the regulation of key cellular processes (33). It has been suggested that arginine enhances immune function through lymphocyte proliferation (34). Arginine's role in the production of nitric oxide has generated the most interest in critically ill patients. Nitric oxide is an antimicrobial agent, a neurotransmitter, and a vasodilator. Its production is regulated by nitric oxide synthase induced by increasing arginine levels (4,34). Increased nitric oxide levels have been associated with improvements in immune function in the critically ill patient (35).

The role of arginine in immune function has led to the inclusion of supplemental arginine in enteral formulas designed for the critically ill patient. Arginine content varies, because there is some arginine as a component of the primary protein source (see Table 16.2). Unfortunately, other constituents have also been included in these "immune-enhancing" formulas, so it is difficult to ascertain arginine's specific benefits. A review of recent data evaluating these types of formulas is outlined in Section 16.3.3.

16.2.3 LIPID

Lipids in enteral formulas serve as both a concentrated source of energy and a source of essential fatty acids. Due to their isotonicity, lipids exert influence on formula osmolality. Fat sources vary among formulas. Table 16.1 outlines the lipid sources included in enteral formulas. The percentage of total calories provided by fat ranges from 1 to 55%. Essential fatty acids (linoleic and linolenic acids) should comprise a minimum of 4% of total calories to meet absolute essential fatty acid requirements (3). Standard enteral formulas derive 15 to 30% of total calories from fat. Formulas with higher amounts of fat have been developed for use with specific disease states, such as pulmonary disease or diabetes (see Section 16.3 for a more thorough review).

16.2.3.1 Long-Chain Fatty Acids

Fat in enteral formulas is included as triglycerides, with constituent long-chain or medium-chain fatty acids. Recent interest has been generated in the structure of the available long-chain fat source. Initially, fatty acids in enteral formulas were predominantly of the omega-6 family. In more recent years, the omega-3 family of fatty acids has been added in combination with omega-6 fatty acids. The class of fatty acid is defined by the position of the first double bond from the terminal methyl end on the carbon chain (36). Omega-3 fats include alpha-linolenic acid, eicosapentanoic acid (EPA), and docosahexanoic acid (DHA). These fatty acids follow a differing metabolic pathway than do omega-6 fatty acids with regard to eicosanoid synthesis. Omega-3 fatty acids are precursors to the 3 series of prostaglandins and the 5 series of leukotrienes, compounds shown to have anti-inflammatory properties (37–39). Conversely, omega-6 fats are metabolized to arachidonic acid, a precursor to the 2 series of prostaglandins and 4 series of leukotrienes, known proinflammatory compounds and immunosuppressants (39). These metabolic variations form an important foundation for the alterations in fat sources utilized in enteral formulas. Table 16.2 outlines the various lipid components of selected enteral formulas.

16.2.3.2 Medium-Chain Triglycerides

Triglycerides esterified with fatty acids of medium chain length (6- to 12-carbon chains) are classified as medium-chain triglycerides (MCTs) and offer unique advantages for use in enteral formulas (36,38). MCTs do not require bile salts or pancreatic lipase for digestion and can be directly absorbed by the intestinal epithileal cell, a benefit to the patient with impaired fat digestion, as in pancreatitis or short bowel syndrome. In addition, MCTs are absorbed directly into the portal circulation and metabolized at the cellular level without the assistance of carnitine. MCTs, unlike LCTs, are not stored and are almost completely metabolized to CO_2 and H_2O (36).

Enteral formulas contain MCT amounts ranging from 0 to 85% of the total fat content. It is important to remember that MCTs do not offer a source of the essential fatty acids (linoleic and linolenic acids) and therefore must always be provided in combination with a source of long-chain fatty acids. In high quantities, MCTs are metabolized to ketones in the liver, a disadvantage to those at risk of ketosis (i.e., diabetic patients or those who are acidotic) (40). Table 16.2 specifies the lipid components of various enteral formulas.

16.2.4 FIBER

The addition of fiber in enteral formulas was introduced in the 1980s, when its beneficial role in gastrointestinal health was recognized (3). Dietary fiber is defined as structural and storage polysaccharides in plants that are not digested by human enzymes (41). Sources of fiber in enteral formulas include soy polysaccharide, hydrolyzed guar gum, oat fiber, and others (3,41). Table 16.3 provides a listing of enteral formulas and their fiber content.

A recent addition to selected formulas is fructooligosaccharides (FOS), short-chain oligosaccharides that are rapidly fermented by the colonic bacteria to short-chain fatty acids (SCFAs), which may aid in the management of diarrhea and overall gastrointestinal tract health (41). SCFAs are used as an energy source by colonic bacteria, a potential benefit in maintaining healthy gut flora (42).

Fiber can be classified by its solubility in water. Soluble fibers, such as pectin and guar, are fermented by colonic bacteria and have been shown to prevent colonic mucosal atrophy, stimulate mucosal proliferation, and provide fuel for the colonocyte (3). In addition, increased colonic sodium and water absorption has been demonstrated with soluble fiber use, a potential benefit in the treatment of diarrhea associated with tube feeding use (43). Insoluble fiber, such as soy polysaccharide, increases fecal weight, leading to increased peristalsis and decreased stool transit time (44). See Chapter 10 for a more thorough discussion of dietary fiber.

The use of fiber-fortified enteral formulas in the critically ill patient is controversial, due mainly to the paucity of data demonstrating benefit in its use (45–47). The reported incidence of diarrhea in patients receiving tube feedings ranges from 2 to 63%, with the higher incidence reported in the critically ill patient population (48). Variations in reported incidence are a result of a variety of factors, including population studied, definition of diarrhea used, and whether reports accounted for other causes of diarrhea.

Both soluble and insoluble fibers have been studied in the management of diarrhea. Insoluble fiber, such as soy polysaccharide, has not been shown conclusively to improve diarrhea, especially in the acutely ill patient (46,47). Soy polysaccharide–containing enteral formulas may be more beneficial in chronic long-term enteral feeding patients. Bass et al. demonstrated a significant

TABLE 16.3
Fiber Content of Selected Enteral Formulas

Product	Total Dietary Fiber (g/l)	% Insoluble Fiber	% Soluble Fiber
Advera	8.9	100.0	0.0
Choice DM	14.4	N/A	N/A
Compleat	4.3	74.0	26.0
Diabetisource AC	4.3	74.0	26.0
Fibersource HN	10.0	75.0	25.0
Fibersource Std	10.0	75.0	25.0
Glucerna Select	14.1	57.0	43.0
Glytrol	15.0	30.0	70.0
Isosource 1.5	8.0	48.0	52.0
Isosource VHN	10.0	48.0	52.0
Jevity 1.0	14.4	100.0	0.0
Jevity 1.2	22.0	75.0	25.0
Jevity 1.5	22.0	75.0	25.0
Novasource Pulmonary	8.0	48.0	52.0
Nutren 1.0 w/Fiber	14.0	95.0	5.0
NutriFocus	20.8	75.0	25.0
Peptamen w/FOS	4.0	100.0	0.0
Probalance	10.0	75.0	25.0
Promote w/Fiber	14.4	94.0	6.0
Protain XL	9.1	N/A	N/A
Resource Diabetic	12.8	50.0	50.0
Replete w/Fiber	14.0	95.0	5.0
Ultracal	14.4	N/A	N/A
Ultracal Plus HN	10.0	N/A	N/A

Note: N/A = not available.

reduction in diarrhea in chronically ill patients requiring tube feedings for > 25 days who received a soy polysaccharide–containing enteral formula, compared with a fiber-free formula (46). Wong reviewed the use of fiber in diarrhea management and suggested that insoluble fiber may be more effective in treating the long-term tube feeding patient, whereas soluble fiber may be beneficial in the critically ill patient (43). In a recent evaluation, Schultz et al. demonstrated a trend toward diarrhea reduction when pectin was combined with an insoluble fiber formula, compared with an insoluble fiber formula alone (49).

The use of a fiber-supplemented enteral formula in selected critically ill patients may require reevaluation. Several cases of bowel obstruction caused by the use of fiber-containing formulas have been reported in the surgical and burn population (50–51). It would be prudent to initiate a fiber-free enteral formula in patients who require motility-suppressing medications or are at risk for bowel obstruction or ischemia.

16.3 FORMULA CATEGORIES

Enteral formulas for use in the critically ill patient can be classified as standard, chemically defined, or specialized. Many formulas are available within each category; these may be significantly different from one another. For example, standard enteral formulas include formulas with varying nutrient density, inclusion or exclusion of fiber, and various macronutrient distribution, etc. The decision regarding which formula to utilize in the critically ill patient will be based on a number

---

TABLE 16.4
Factors to Consider in Enteral Formula Selection

Assessment of Patient	Assessment of Formula
Past medical history and present problems	Composition of carbohydrate, protein, and fat
Age	Calorie:nitrogen ratio
Calorie and nutrient requirements	Osmolality
Gastrointestinal function	Renal solute load
Hepatic function	pH
Renal function	Residue/fiber content
Pulmonary status	Viscosity
	Caloric density
	Convenience of administration
	Bacteriologic safety
	Cost

Source: From Gottschlich M.M., Shronts E.P., Hutchins A.M. in *Clinical Nutrition: Enteral and Tube Feeding*, 3rd edition, W.B. Saunders, Philadelphia, 1997, 207–239. With permission.

---

of factors, both patient and formula related, including, among others, gastrointestinal function, fluid status, and organ function. (Table 16.4 outlines factors to consider in enteral formula selection.) Formula selection frequently requires adjustment throughout the patient's hospital course as clinical status changes.

16.3.1 DISEASE-SPECIFIC FORMULAS

Specialized formulas encompass a wide range of formulas and are designed for a variety of clinical scenarios. Some are intended for patients with specific disease states, such as pulmonary disease, renal insufficiency, diabetes, etc. Others are recommended for use in hypermetabolic states, such as that common to the critically ill patient. A review of currently available formulas from five national manufacturers indicates there are over 35 enteral formulas designed for a particular condition or disease state.

Specialized formulas may or may not result in improved outcomes for critically ill patients, and their use is controversial (3,4,19,58–60). It is essential that clinicians evaluate specialized enteral formulas prior to their use. Manufacturers market their products for a variety of disease states or conditions that may not be supported by scientific literature. It is important to remember that nutrition is only one aspect of a critically ill patient's treatment. Therefore, it is necessary to ask, "What possible difference in outcome will this enteral formula offer to the patient?" Additionally, the concept of benefit vs. harm must be considered. Does the risk of harm outweigh the potential benefit that this type of product may offer? Table 16.5 outlines other important considerations when evaluating specialized formulas. The following formulas for specific disease states or conditions will be reviewed: diabetes mellitus, hepatic disease, critical illness or hypermetabolism (immune-enhancing), pulmonary disease (acute respiratory distress syndrome and chronic obstructive pulmonary disease), and renal insufficiency.

16.3.2 DIABETES MELLITUS

Maintenance of normal blood glucose levels in the critically ill patient is often difficult secondary to the hypermetabolic stress response (61). In the presence of counterregulatory hormones, an increased reliance on fatty acid oxidation by the skeletal muscle results in reduced glucose uptake and resultant hyperglycemia (4). Control of blood glucose levels has demonstrated both a reduced incidence of complications and improved outcomes (62–64).

TABLE 16.5
Considerations in Evaluation of Specialized Enteral Formulas

Is the nutrient profile appropriate, based on known metabolic abnormalities and nutrient requirements of the specified condition?
Has the product testing been limited to animal research only?
Have prospective, controlled, randomized clinical trials evaluating the product been conducted?
Is the research only product specific?
Can the study results be generalized to other populations or only that in which the product was studied?
Have objective criteria been developed to evaluate the specific formula?
Are recommendations for product use confined only to the population(s) studied or for use with additional population(s)?

Source: Adapted from: Malone A.M., *Support Line*, 2002, 24(1): 3–11.

TABLE 16.6
Enteral Formulas Designed for Diabetes Mellitus

Product	Manufacturer	Kcals/ml	% CHO Kcals	% PRO Kcals	% FAT kcals	Fiber (g/1000 ml)
Choice DM	Novartis Nutrition	1.06	40.0	17.0	43.0	14.4
Diabetisource AC	Novartis Nutrition	1.0	36.0	20.0	44.0	4.3
Glucerna Select	Ross Products	1.0	22.8	20.0	49.0	21.1
Glytrol	Nestlé Clinical Nutrition	1.0	40.0	18.0	42.0	15.0
Resource Diabetic	Novartis Nutrition	1.06	36.0	24.0	40.0	12.8

Several diabetic formulas are currently available (Table 16.6) with similar characteristics. Carbohydrate sources vary but generally consist of oligosaccharides, fructose, cornstarch, and fiber. The use of more complex carbohydrates, such as fructose, cornstarch, and fiber, has been shown to improve glycemic control primarily from delayed gastric emptying and reduced intestinal transit (65). Types of fiber and total fiber content vary among diabetic enteral formulas. Soluble fiber, such as guar and pectin, has been associated with improved glucose control (66). Due to the inherent viscosity of soluble fiber, most enteral diabetic formulas contain both soluble and insoluble fiber sources. Total fat content ranges from 40 to 49%, raising the concern of impaired gastric emptying with the use of a formula with increased fat content (52).

There are few randomized, controlled trials evaluating diabetic formulas. In a series of two studies, Peters et al. demonstrated that the use of a diabetic formula results in a reduced glucose response compared to standard enteral formulas (67,68). It should be noted that these studies were conducted in healthy volunteers using a study protocol that attempted to mimic continuous tube feeding administration. Results of these studies cannot be generalized to hospitalized patients. Craig et al. compared a diabetic and a standard formula in type 2 diabetics residing in a long-term care facility (69). There were no significant differences in fasting serum glucose levels at baseline, monthly, or at the study completion. Fingerstick glucose checks were not significantly different over the entire course of the study period but were significantly lower in the diabetic formula group in weeks one, five, and seven. The overall clinical significance of these results is unknown. Selected clinical outcomes, such as fever, pneumonia, and pressure ulcers were noted to be higher in the standard formula group, but these differences were not significant.

In the only evaluation of a diabetic formula in hospitalized patients, Beyers et al. compared the efficacy of blood glucose control using a standard enteral formula and a diabetic formula (70). In this small study, blood glucose levels were significantly higher when the standard enteral formula was provided. Both formulas required the use of supplemental insulin for blood glucose control. The nutrient cost of the diabetic formula was significantly higher than that of the standard formula. It is interesting to note that the amount of intravenous dextrose received when the standard formula was provided was three times that received during infusion of the diabetic formula. Although the results were not statistically significant, a larger sample size may have yielded different results. Overall, despite the small study size, the results confirm that glucose control is variable in a hospital setting and that, although the use of a diabetic formula can affect blood glucose levels, the effect may not be significant, irrespective of all other methods utilized for controlling blood glucose.

The routine use of a diabetic formula does not appear warranted (59,60). However, when blood glucose control becomes problematic, despite appropriate pharmacologic intervention and the avoidance of overfeeding, use of a diabetic formula may offer an advantage in facilitating improved glucose control. It is important, however, to consider the following questions:

- Will the use of a diabetic formula influence the intake of other nutrients?
- Will adequate protein be provided?
- Will there be an increased intake of the immunosuppressant omega-6 fatty acids?

These are important questions to take into account if a diabetic formula is considered.

16.3.3 HEPATIC DISEASE

16.3.3.1 Branched-Chain Amino Acids (See Hepatic Formulas)

In the late 1970s, research began to appear demonstrating the beneficial use of high branched-chain amino acid (BCAA — valine, leucine, and isoleucine) parenteral formulations for the patient with advanced liver disease. Patients with liver disease are often malnourished and require increased amounts of protein to maintain nitrogen equilibrium (16,17). These formulas provided increased amounts of BCAA and reduced amounts of the aromatic amino acids (AAA) phenylalanine, tyrosine, and tryptophan. These alterations have been thought to promote a reduced uptake of AAA at the blood–brain barrier, reducing the synthesis of false neurotransmitters and thereby ameliorating the neurological symptoms that occur with hepatic encephalopathy (HE) (18). Two enteral formulas with increased BCAA are available. See Table 16.7 for formula characteristics.

TABLE 16.7
Enteral Formulas Designed for Hepatic Disease

Product	Manufacturer	Kcals/ml	% CHO kcals	% Fat kcals	% Protein kcals	Comments
Hepatic-Aid II	Hormel Healthlabs	1.2	57.3	27.7	15.0	Increased levels of leucine, isoleucine, and valine Minimal phenylalanine, tryptophan, and tyrosine content Contains negligible amounts of vitamins and minerals
NutriHep	Nestlé Clinical Nutrition	1.5	77.0	11.0	12.0	Contains standard amounts of vitamins and minerals 50% BCAA and 50% AAA 66% of fat is MCT

Parenteral and enteral BCAA formulas have been studied in patients with both acute and chronic hepatic encephalopathy (HE). These studies are difficult to evaluate due to patient heterogeneity, differences in secondary therapies, and differences in nutritional regimens. Some studies evaluated BCAA without providing a nitrogen source for the control group (71).

Studies evaluating parenteral and enteral BCAA formulas in patients with acute encephalopathy have yielded conflicting results (72–76). A meta-analysis conducted by Naylor et al. reviewed nine randomized controlled trials evaluating parenteral BCAA (77). Five of the studies showed a highly significant improvement in mental recovery from acute encephalopathy and a significant reduction in mortality. The authors concluded that, due to short-term follow-up times and mortality discrepancy across the trials, recommendation of parenteral BCAA over conventional therapy is not indicated.

Several trials evaluating BCAA in chronic encephalopathy have been conducted in an attempt to determine whether BCAA improve neurological outcome or improve tolerance to dietary protein. In a multicenter trial, Horst et al. compared a BCAA-enriched and a mixed-protein enteral supplement (74). The BCAA-supplemented group achieved nitrogen balance equal to that of the control group without precipitation of HE. Additional studies, in which patients were randomized to receive either oral diets enriched with BCAA or control, failed to demonstrate clinical benefit of the BCAA-enriched diet (19). In a recent (2003) evaluation, Marchesini and colleagues compared the use of oral BCAA supplementation with standard protein or carbohydrate without protein on death, disease deterioration, and the need for hospital admission in ambulatory patients with advanced cirrhosis (78). BCAA supplementation resulted in a significant decrease in the primary occurrence events, death, and disease deterioration. The authors concluded that there are benefits to routinely supplementing BCAA in patients with advanced cirrhosis. Although this study offers a possible benefit to routine BCAA supplementation, generalizing these results to the critically ill patient with HE is not recommended.

The routine use of BCAA enriched enteral formulas does not appear to be clinically beneficial in patients with advanced liver disease, HE, or both. Standard enteral formulas can successfully be used with most patients. However, in those patients who are unable to tolerate standard protein intakes without precipitation of HE, the use of BCAA-enriched enteral formulas may be better tolerated, thus permitting achievement of desired protein intakes (19,58,60,79).

16.3.4 HYPERMETABOLISM AND CRITICAL ILLNESS

The availability of formulas with added components potentially to improve outcome began to appear in the 1990s (4). Specific nutrients, such as arginine, nucleotides, and n-3 fatty acids, were added to enteral formulas to enhance the immune system. The underlying rationale for these formula modifications was that by providing immune enhancement, the immune suppression common in critical illness and other disease states (such as trauma and surgery) could be down-regulated, resulting in improved patient outcome (80). There are multiple enteral formulas marketed for immune modulation (see Table 16.8 for a listing of available products). Table 16.2 provides additional information by offering a breakdown of the arginine, glutamine, and various lipid sources of many available enteral products.

Of all the specialized enteral products available, immune-enhancing formulas have been studied the most. A decade of research evaluating these formulas has demonstrated potential benefits in selected populations but has also raised concern regarding potential detriment (81). Early studies evaluating immune-enhancing products were harshly criticized for flaws in both study design and statistical analysis. Others included small sample sizes that failed to yield significant results (19). Recently, there have been three meta-analyses and an industry-sponsored review presenting data from studies evaluating immune-enhancing formulas in critically ill patients (81–90). Selected highlights from these findings are presented here. A more complete review can be obtained by referring to the individual publications.

TABLE 16.8
Formulas Designed for Immune Enhancement

Product	Manufacturer	Kcals/ml	% CHO Kcals	% PRO Kcals	% FAT kcals	Comments
Crucial	Nestlé Clinical Nutrition	1.5	33.7	23.5	39.0	Hydrolyzed protein, fortified with arginine (15.0 g/l), vitamins A and C, zinc, and β-carotene MCT/LCT 50/50, marine oil as source of n-3 fatty acids
Impact	Novartis	1.5	53.0	22.0	25.0	Fortified with arginine
Impact 1.5	Nutrition	1.5	38.0	22.0	40.0	(12.5 g/l, 18.7 g/l, 16.3 g/l,
Impact Glutamine		1.3	46.0	24.0	30.0	12.5 g/l, 16.3 g/l) and nucleotides
Impact with Fiber		1.0	53.0	22.0	25.0	Menhaden oil as source of n-3 fatty acids
Impact Recover		1.0	46.0	24.0	30.0	Impact Glutamine fortified with 15.0 g/l of glutamine and 10.0 g/l fiber. Impact with Fiber provides 10.0 g/l fiber.
Intensical	Ross Products	1.3	46.0	25.0	29.0	Fortified with arginine (7.2 g/l) Menhaden oil as source of n-3 fatty acids
Perative	Ross Products	1.3	54.5	20.5	25.0	Protein in peptide form Fortified with arginine (8.0 g/l)
Pivot 1.5	Ross Products	1.5	45.0	25.0	30.0	13 gm arginine/l structured lipid sardine oil as source of n-3 fatty acids

In 1999, Beale and colleagues conducted a meta-analysis of 12 studies including 1557 critically ill patients following trauma, sepsis, or major injury (82). No effect on mortality was demonstrated with immunonutrition. There were, however, significant reductions in infection rate, ventilator days, and hospital length of stay, most notably in surgical patients who received immune-enhancing formulas. The authors recommended the use of immune-enhancing formulas in the surgical population and that further study was necessary before recommendations could be made to use these formulas in all critically ill patients.

Heys et al. in 1999 conducted a meta-analysis of 11 trials evaluating immunonutrition in 1009 critically ill surgery and trauma patients (83). The use of immune-enhancing formulas was associated with a significant decrease in the incidence of wound complications and in hospital length of stay in patients undergoing gastrointestinal surgery and in those with critical illness. There were no differences, however, in death rate or in incidence of pneumonia in those who received the immune-enhancing enteral nutrition.

In 2001, Heyland et al. reviewed 22 randomized trials including 2419 patients, comparing immunonutrition with standard enteral formulas in surgical and critically ill patients (84). The overall results demonstrated no benefit of immunonutrition on mortality; however, immunonutrition was associated with a shorter hospital stay and a reduced incidence of infectious complications. In subgroup analysis, the authors found that infectious complications and hospital length of stay were significantly lower in patients receiving formulas higher in arginine content. In addition, there was a trend toward decreased mortality with the use of these formulas. Elective surgical patients, compared to critically ill patients, demonstrated a reduced incidence of infectious complications when fed an immune-enhancing formula. The authors concluded that immunonutrition may decrease rates of infectious complications; however, this effect varies with patient population. Elective surgical patients may benefit from an immune-enhancing formula. Due to the potential for harm in selected critically ill patients, the authors recommended against routine use of immune-enhancing formulas in critically ill patients.

The use of immune-enhancing formulas in critically ill patients remains controversial. Some have suggested that positive effects on outcome have been realized only in those patients "less sick" (i.e., those with lower APACHE scores) (84). These investigators have raised concern that the use of immune-enhancing formulas in sicker patients, such as those with severe sepsis, may lead to a worsening of the inflammatory process, an effect that could explain a higher mortality rate in this patient subgroup (91,92). As a result of this concern, Bertolini et al., in 2003, reported an interim analysis of a multicenter trial evaluating an immune-enhancing formula (Perative® — a low-arginine formula) and parenteral nutrition on mortality in critically ill patients (93). Subgroup analysis distinguished patients with and without severe sepsis and septic shock. Results demonstrated that those severely septic patients who received the immune-enhanced enteral nutrition had a significantly higher mortality in the intensive care unit, compared to those who received parenteral nutrition. The investigators altered their study protocol based on their results and discontinued recruiting patients with severe sepsis. They agree with recommendations by other investigators that the use of immune-enhancing formulas in severe sepsis is contraindicated.

When should immune-enhancing formulas be utilized? Several authors have evaluated the literature extensively, offering usage recommendations. In addition, an industry-sponsored symposium attempted to address this question, providing guidelines for use of these formulas. Table 16.9 outlines these recommendations. It is important to remember that the decision to use an immune-enhancing formula should be based on each patient's clinical status at the time of evaluation. As clinical condition changes, further decision making regarding product usage will be required.

16.3.5 PULMONARY DISEASE

Specialized enteral formulas have been developed for two types of pulmonary disease: chronic obstructive pulmonary disease (COPD) and acute respiratory distress syndrome (ARDS).

16.3.5.1 COPD Formulas

In the 1980s, reports began to appear in the literature describing adverse ventilatory effects when large amounts of dextrose-based parenteral nutrition solutions were provided to patients with and without COPD (95–97). It was thought that the high amount of dextrose provided in standard parenteral nutrition formulas was the primary causative factor in the reported adverse effects (95). This concept was carried over into enteral nutrition via the introduction of a modified macronutrient formula designed for the COPD patient. Replacing a portion of carbohydrate calories with those provided from fat would limit CO_2 production, resulting in improved ventilatory status (34). Several pulmonary formulas are currently available (Table 16.10).

Numerous studies exist comparing the effects of macronutrient metabolism on respiratory function and status. Most have studied ambulatory patients, making it difficult to generalize to patients in the hospital setting, but selected details can be highlighted.

In 1985, Angelillo et al. studied the effect of fat and carbohydrate content on CO_2 production in ambulatory COPD patients with hypercapnia (98). The authors found that use of a high-fat formula reduced CO_2 production and respiratory quotient, compared to those receiving a lower-fat formula. Al-Saady et al., in 1989, compared the effects of a high-fat enteral formula with a standard

TABLE 16.9
Recommendations for Use of Immune-Enhancing Enteral Formulas (IEFs)

Patients Who Should Receive Early Enteral Nutrition with an IEF
- Patients undergoing elective gastrointestinal (GI) surgery
  - Moderately or severely malnourished patients (albumin < 3.5 g/dl) undergoing major elective upper GI procedures on the esophagus, stomach, pancreas, and hepatobiliary tree
  - Severely malnourished patients (albumin < 2.8 g/dl) undergoing lower GI surgery
- Patients with blunt and penetrating torso trauma
  - Trauma patients with an injury severity score 18
  - Patients with injuries to two or more body systems
  - Patients with an abdominal trauma index 20
  - Patients with severe injuries to the colon, pancreas and duodenum, and stomach

Patients Who May Benefit from Use of IEF (Further Research Is Required)
- Elective surgery
- Patients undergoing aortic reconstruction with an anticipated prolonged need for mechanical ventilation
- Patients undergoing major head and neck surgery in whom there is preexisting malnutrition
- Severe head injury (Glasgow Coma Scale < 8 with an abnormal head CT scan)
- Burns 30% (third degree)
- Ventilator dependent, nonseptic medical and surgical patients at risk of subsequent infectious morbidity
- Intensive care unit patients with APACHE scores between 10 and 20

Patients Not Considered Candidates for an IEF
- Those with severe sepsis or septic shock
- Those expected to resume an oral diet within five days
- Those in the intensive care unit for monitoring purposes only
- Those with bowel obstruction distal to the site of access
- Those with incomplete resuscitation or splanchnic hypoperfusion
- Those with major upper GI hemorrhage

Sources: From Kudsk K.A., Schloerb P.R., DeLegge M.H., et al., *J. Parenter. Enteral Nutr.,* 2001, 25: S61–S62; Heyland D.K., *Nutr. Clin. Pract.* 2002, 17: 267–272; and McGowan K.C. and Bistrian B.R., *Am. J. Clin. Nutr.* 2003, 77: 764–770.

TABLE 16.10
Formulas Designed for Pulmonary Disease

Product	Manufacturer	Kcals/ml	% CHO Kcals	% PRO Kcals	% FAT kcals
COPD Formulas					
NovaSource Pulmonary	Novartis Nutrition	1.5	40.0	20.0	40.0
NutriVent	Nestlé Clinical Nutrition	1.5	27.0	18.0	55.0
Pulmocare	Ross Products	1.5	28.2	16.7	55.1
Respalor	Novartis Nutrition	1.5	40.0	20.0	40.0
ARDS Formula					
Oxepa	Ross Products	1.5	28.1	16.7	55.2

formula on ventilatory status in hospitalized patients (99). CO_2 levels and ventilatory time were significantly reduced in the high-fat formula group. In a more recent study (1996), Akrabawi et al. evaluated pulmonary function and gas exchange in ambulatory COPD patients (100). Patients received both a high-fat (55%) and a moderate-fat (41%) formula "meal" on two separate days. No significant differences in respiratory quotient were demonstrated between the moderate- and high-fat meals; however, CO_2 levels increased significantly during consumption of the moderate-fat formula. In addition, gastric emptying time was significantly longer following the high-fat meal. The authors concluded that because overall CO_2 levels were similar at the end of the testing period and RQ values were not different, the delayed gastric emptying observed in the high-fat meal may have influenced nutrient utilization. This may explain the lack of an observed benefit in CO_2 production with the high-fat formula.

It is important to note that in most of the early reports citing adverse respiratory effects, patients received excessive calories (1.7 to 2.25 times the measured energy expenditure) (95–97). A classic study by Talpers et al. demonstrated no significant change in CO_2 production with increasing carbohydrate intake; however, with increasing caloric intake, CO_2 production was significantly increased (101). The authors concluded that avoidance of overfeeding is of greater significance than carbohydrate intake in avoiding nutritionally related hypercapnia.

Overall results demonstrating whether "chronic" pulmonary enteral products offer a clinical advantage to the critically ill patient are inconclusive. When consideration is given to the potential disadvantages in using a pulmonary formula, delayed gastric emptying, and the potential limitation in the availability of carbohydrate (a preferred fuel source for the exercising muscle), the routine use of a pulmonary formula in hospitalized patients does not seem warranted (100,102,103).

16.3.5.2 ARDS Formula

Acute respiratory distress syndrome (ARDS) is a clinical illness characterized by hypoxemia, ultimately resulting in respiratory failure (104). The cascade of events that occurs in ARDS is thought to involve alveolar macrophages and their release of proinflammatory eicosanoids derived from the metabolism of arachidonic acid. Several of these metabolites — thromboxane A_2, leukotrienes, and prostaglandin E_2 — have been implicated in the development of acute lung injury (105,106). A specialized enteral formula (Table 16.10) has been developed that offers a modified lipid component specifically designed to potentially modulate the inflammatory cascade in ARDS. This formula contains borage and fish oils, sources of γ-linolenic and eicosapentanoic acids. These fatty acids, in conjunction with metabolic alterations known to occur in ARDS, lead to an increased production of prostaglandins of the 1 series and leukotrienes of the 5 series, metabolites associated with an anti-inflammatory and vasodilatory state. Vasoconstriction, platelet aggregation, and neutrophil accumulation are reduced when the eicosanoid balance favors anti-inflammatory rather than proinflammatory mediators (107).

The evidence supporting the use of a specialized enteral formula for ARDS is not widespread but nevertheless has merit. Preclinical animal data has demonstrated positive effects of eicosapentanoic (EPA) and γ-linolenic acids (GLA) on proinflammatory mediator production, gas exchange, and oxygen delivery (105,106). This work led to the completion of a multicenter trial evaluating the use of an ARDS formula in patients with evidence of either ARDS or acute lung injury (ALI) (108). Patients receiving the specialized formula showed a significant improvement in gas exchange, required significantly fewer days of mechanical ventilatory support, and demonstrated a decreased ICU length of stay compared to the control group. The authors concluded that the use of a specialized enteral formula would be useful in the management of those with ARDS or at risk of developing it. A recent report by Tehila has demonstrated similar results (27). Fifty-two ventilated patients with $PaO_2/F_iO_2 \leq 250$ mm Hg were randomized to receive either an ARDS or a control formula. Patients who received the ARDS formula had a significantly shorter length of ventilator time and a reduced ICU length of stay, compared to the control patients. There was no difference in either hospital length of stay or mortality between the two groups. Despite the paucity of controlled trials evaluating a specialized ARDS formula, there is a possible benefit in its use (9). Further studies are needed to validate the results demonstrated.

One potential disadvantage in the use of an ARDS formula is the negative effect of a high-fat formula on gastric emptying. Delayed gastric emptying is fairly common in the critically ill, and high-fat formulas have been associated with an increase in gastric emptying (37). Use of naso-intestinal feedings may be alternative to gastric feedings when using this type of formula or when gastric emptying is known to be impaired.

16.3.6 RENAL INSUFFICIENCY

The use of products with renal insufficiency is primarily dictated by the level of renal dysfunction and the intended treatment plan. Patients with acute renal failure are typically hypercatabolic and hypermetabolic, due to their underlying disease state. This, in addition to the type of renal replacement therapy utilized (if any), influences the patient's energy and protein requirements (109). In patients in whom dialysis is delayed or unintended, a calorically dense, reduced protein formula is indicated (3). Protein requirements for the nondialyzed patient with chronic renal failure range from 0.55 to 1.0 g/kg/d and can be achieved with reduced protein formulas (109). In addition to modified protein levels, renal formulas offer alterations in electrolyte composition, a variation that may offer the greatest benefit to patients with renal disease.

In the 1980s, the use of enteral formulas with only essential amino acids flourished in response to data demonstrating benefit with similarly designed parenteral nutrition formulas (110). Theoretically, provision of only essential amino acids would favor urea nitrogen recycling providing nitrogen for protein synthesis (111). Several enteral and parenteral nutrition products were subsequently developed with only essential amino acids to promote improved protein synthesis. Research evaluating these products failed to demonstrate efficacy in promoting metabolic or therapeutic benefit with the use of only essential amino acids (112,113). Amin-Aid® (Watson Pharma, Marina del Ray, CA), a well recognized product providing only essential amino acids, is no longer available as a tube feeding. It is available only as an oral drink.

Several calorically dense enteral products are available for the renal impaired patient (Table 16.11). Formulas vary in protein, electrolyte, vitamin, and mineral content. Formula selection is dependent on the patient's level of renal function, the renal replacement therapy in use, and the patient's overall nutrient requirements. It is important to remember that patients undergoing renal replacement therapy often have significantly increased protein requirements (109), and renal formulas may not provide levels of protein to achieve these requirements. Standard calorically dense formulas are frequently appropriate for renal failure patients. Ongoing laboratory monitoring of renal excreted electrolytes — potassium, phosphorus and magnesium — is essential when using standard enteral formulas. In patients undergoing continuous veno-venous hemodialysis (CVVHD), renal formulas may not be the most appropriate formula choice. These patients may not require significant fluid restriction and have protein requirements of 1.5 to 2.0 g/kg/d (109). A standard high-protein formula may be best suited for this type of patient.

16.4 CONCLUSION

Enteral formula selection in the critically ill patient can be a challenging process. Underlying clinical state, nutritional requirements, and gastrointestinal function are all key components in deciding which formula to utilize. Understanding the individual formula components and the specific product variations is essential in formula selection. The growth of formula availability has resulted in a large number of specialized products marketed for improving specific disease-related outcomes. It is important that the practitioner carefully evaluate these products in conjunction with supportive scientific data prior to routine use.

TABLE 16.11
Enteral Products Designed for Renal Disease

Product	Manufacturer	Kcals/ml	Protein (gm)[a]	Potassium (mEq)[a]	Phosphorus (mg)[a]	Magnesium (mg)[a]
Renal Formulas						
Magnacal Renal	Novartis Nutrition	2.0	37.5	16	400	100
Nepro	Ross Products	2.0	35.0	14	343	108
NovaSource Renal	Novartis Nutrition	2.0	37.0	14	325	100
Renalcal	Nestlé Clinical Nutrition	2.0	17.0	Negligible	Negligible	Negligible
Suplena	Ross Products	2.0	15.0	14	365	108
Standard Concentrated Formulas						
Deliver 2.0	Novartis Nutrition	2.0	37.5	21.5	555	200
NovaSource 2.0	Novartis Nutrition	2.0	45.0	19	550	210
Nutren 2.0	Nestlé Clinical Nutrition	2.0	40.0	25	670	268
Two-Cal HN	Ross Products	2.0	42.0	31	538	213

[a] Per 1000 kcals.

REFERENCES

1. Griggs B.A., Chernoff R., Hoppe M.C., and Wade J.E. *Enteral Alimentation.* American Society for Parenteral and Enteral Nutrition, Rockville, MD, 1979.
2. Fussell S.T. Enteral nutrition: a comprehensive overview. In: Matarese L.E. and Gottschlich M.M. (eds.), *Contemporary Nutrition Support Practice: A Clinical Guide,* 2nd edition. W.B. Saunders, Philadelphia, 2003, 188–200.
3. Gottschlich M.M., Shronts E.P., and Hutchins A.M. Defined formula diets. In: Rombeau J.L. and Rolandelli R.H. (eds.), *Clinical Nutrition: Enteral and Tube Feeding,* 3rd edition. W.B. Saunders, Philadelphia, 1997, 207–239.
4. Marks D.B., Marks A.D., and Smith C.M. (eds.). Intertissue relationships in the metabolism of amino acids. In: *Basic Medical Biochemistry.* Williams & Wilkins, Baltimore, 1996, 647–665.
5. Bell S.J., Bistrian B.R., Wade J.E., et al. Modular enteral diets: cost and nutritional value comparisons. *J. Am. Diet. Assoc.* 1987, 87: 1526–1530.
6. Keohane P.P. and Silk D.B. Peptides and free amino acids. In: Rombeau J.L. and Caldwell M.D. (eds.), *Clinical Nutrition: Enteral and Tube Feeding*, 1st edition. W.B. Saunders, Philadelphia, 1984, 44–59.
7. Reeds P.J. and Beckett P.R. Protein and amino acids. In: Ziegler E.E. and Filer L.J. (eds.), *Present Knowledge of Nutrition*, 7th edition. ISLI Press, Washington, DC, 1996, 67–86.
8. Silk D.B., Fairclough P.D., Clar M.L., et al. Use of peptide rather than free amino acid nitrogen source in chemically defined enteral diet. *J. Parenter. Enteral Nutr.* 1980, 4: 548–553.
9. Craft I.L, Geddes D., Hyde C.W., et al. Absorption and malabsorption of glycine and glycine peptides in man. *Gut* 1968, 9: 425–437.
10. Verma S., Brown S., Kirkwood B., and Giaffer M.H. Polymeric versus elemental diet as primary treatment in active Crohn's disease: a randomized, double-blind trial. *Am. J. Gastroenterol.* 2000, 95: 735–739.

11. Brinson R.R. and Kolts B.E. Hypoalbuminemia as an indicator of diarrheal incidence in critically ill patients. *Crit. Care Med.* 1987, 15: 506–509.

12. Brinson R.R. Enteral nutrition in the critically ill patient: role of hypoalbuminemia. *Crit. Care Med.* 1989, 17: 367–370.

13. Ziegler F., Ollivier J.M., Cynober L., et al. Efficiency of enteral nitrogen support in surgical patients: small peptides versus non-degraded proteins. *Gut* 1990, 31: 1277–1283.

14. Heimburger D.C., Geels W.J., Bilbrey J., et al. Effects of small peptide and whole protein enteral feedings on serum proteins and diarrhea in critically ill patients: a randomized trial. *J. Parenter. Enteral Nutr.* 1997, 21: 162–167.

15. Dietscher J.E., Foulks C.J., and Smith R.W. Nutritional response of patients in an intensive care unit to an elemental formula vs a standard enteral formula. *J. Am. Diet. Assoc.* 1998, 98: 335–336.

16. Raup S.M. and Kaproth P. Hepatic failure. In: Matarese L.E. and Gottschlich M.M. (eds.), *Contemporary Nutrition Support Practice: A Clinical Guide*, 2nd edition. W.B. Saunders, Philadelphia, 2003, 445–459.

17. Fischer J.E. Branched-chain enriched amino acid solutions in patients with liver failure: an early example of nutritional pharmacology. *J. Parenter. Enteral Nutr.* 1990, 14: 249S–256S.

18. Fischer J.E. The role of plasma amino acids in hepatic encephalopathy. *Surgery* 1975, 78: 276–290.

19. Matarese L.E. Rationale and efficacy of specialized enteral and parenteral formulas. In: Matarese L.E. and Gottschlich M.M. (eds.). *Contemporary Nutrition Support Practice: A Clinical Guide*, 2nd edition. W.B. Saunders, Philadelphia, 2003, 263–275.

20. Malone A.M. The clinical benefits and efficacy in using specialized enteral feeding formulas. *Support Line* 2002, 24(1): 3–11.

21. Souba W., Smith R.J., Wilmore D.W. Glutamine metabolism by the intestinal tract. *J. Parenter. Enteral Nutr.* 1985, 9:609–617.

22. Smith R.J. Glutamine metabolism and its physiological importance. *J. Parenter. Enteral Nutr.* 1990, 14(Suppl.): 40S–44S.

23. Swails W.S., Bell S.J., Borlase B.C., et al. Glutamine content of whole proteins; implications for enteral formulas. *Nutr. Clin. Pract.* 1992, 7: 77–80.

24. Ziegler T.R., Young L.S., Benfell K., et al. Clinical and metabolic efficacy of glutamine-supplemented parenteral nutrition after bone marrow transplantation: a randomized, double-blind, controlled study. *Ann. Intern. Med.* 1992, 116: 821–828.

25. Schloerb P.R. and Amare M. Total parenteral nutrition with glutamine in bone marrow transplantation and other clinical applications (a randomized, double-blind study). *J. Parenter. Enteral Nutr.* 1993, 17: 407–413.

26. Dickson T.M.C., Wong, R.M., Negrin R.S., et al. Effect of oral glutamine supplementation during bone marrow transplantation. *J. Parenter. Enteral Nutr.* 2000, 24: 61–66.

27. Velasco N., Hernandez G., Wainstain C., et al. Influence of polymeric enteral nutrition supplemented with different doses of glutamine on gut permeability in critically ill patients. *Nutrition* 2001, 17: 907–911.

28. Houdijk A.P., Rijnsburger E.R., Jansen J., et al. Randomised trial of glutamine-enriched enteral nutrition on infectious morbidity in patients with multiple trauma. *Lancet* 1998, 352: 772–776.

29. Jones C., Palmer T.E., and Griffiths R.D. Randomized clinical outcome study of critically ill patients given glutamine-supplemented enteral nutrition. *Nutrition* 1999, 15: 108–115.

30. Garcia-de-Lorenzo A., Zarazaga A., Garcia-Luna P.P., et al. Clinical evidence for enteral nutritional support with glutamine: a systematic review. *Nutrition* 2003, 19: 805–811.

31. Heyland D.K., Dhaliwal R., Drover J.W., et al. Canadian clinical practice guidelines for nutrition support in mechanically, ventilated, critically ill adult patients. *J. Parenter. Enteral Nutr.* 2003, 27: 355–373.

32. Wischmeyer P.E. Clinical applications of L-glutamine: past, present, and future. *Nutr. Clin. Pract.* 2003, 18: 377–385.

33. Basu H.N. Arginine: a clinical perspective. *Nutr. Clin. Pract.* 2002, 17: 218–225.

34. Nieves C. and Langkamp-Henken B. Arginine and immunity: a unique perspective. *Biomed. Pharmacother.* 2002, 56: 471–482.

35. Suchner U., Heyland D.K., and Peter K. Immune-modulating actions of arginine in the critically ill. *Br. J. Nutr.* 2002, 87(Suppl): S121–S132.

36. Marks D.B., Marks A.D., and Smith C.M. Digestion and transport of dietary lipids. *Basic Medical Biochemistry*. Williams & Wilkins, Baltimore, 1996, 491–500.

37. Gottschlich M.M. Selection of optimal lipid sources in enteral and parenteral nutrition. *Nutr. Clin. Pract.* 1992, 7: 152–156.

38. Mayes P.A. Lipids of physiologic significance. In: Murray R.K., Granner D.K., Mayes P.A., and Rodwell V.W. (eds.), *Harper's Biochemistry*, 24th edition. Appleton & Lange, Stamford CT, 1996, 146–157.

39. Kinsella J.E. and Lokesh B. Dietary lipids, eicosanoids and the immune system. *Crit. Care Med.* 1990, 18: S94–S113.

40. Bell S.J., Mascioli E.A., Bistrian B.R., et al. Altrnative lipid sources for enteral and parenteral nutrition: long and medium-chain triglycerides, structured triglycerides and fish oils. *J. Am. Diet. Assoc.* 1991, 91: 701–709.

41. Position of the American Dietetic Association: health implications of dietary fiber. *J. Am. Diet. Assoc.* 2002, 102: 993–1000.

42. Scheppach W. Effects of short chain fatty acids on gut morphology and function. *Gut* 1994, 35 (Suppl): S35–S38.

43. Wong K. The role of fiber in diarrhea management. *Support Line* 1998, 20(6): 16–20.

44. Compher C., Seto R.W., Lew J.I, and Rombeau J.L. Dietary fiber and its clinical applications to enteral nutrition. In: Rombeau J.L. and Rolandelli R.H. (eds.), *Clinical Nutrition: Enteral and Tube Feeding*, 3rd edition. W.B. Saunders, Philadelphia, 1997, 81–95.

45. Dobb G.J. and Towler S.C. Diarrhea during enteral feeding in the critically ill: a comparison of feeds with and without fiber. *Intens. Care Med.* 1990, 16: 252–255.

46. Bass D.J., Forman L.P., Abrams S.E., et al. The effect of dietary fiber in tube-fed elderly patients. *J. Gerontol. Nurs.* 1996, 22(10): 37–44.

47. Belknap D., Davidson L.J., and Smith C.R. The effects of psyllium hydrophilic mucilloid on diarrhea in enterally fed patients. *Heart Lung* 1997, 26: 229–237.

48. Bliss D.Z., Guenter P.A., and Settle R.G. Defining and reporting diarrhea in tube-fed patients: what a mess! *Am. J. Clin. Nutr.* 1992, 16(5): 488–489.

49. Schultz A.A., Ashby-Hughes B., Taylor R., et al. Effects of pectin on diarrhea in critically ill tube-fed patients receiving antibiotics. *Am. J. Crit. Care* 2000, 9: 403–411.

50. Scaife C.L., Saffle J.R., and Morris S.E. Intestinal obstruction secondary to enteral feedings in burn trauma patients. *J. Trauma* 1999, 47: 859–863.

51. McIvor A.C., Meguid M.M., Curtas S., and Kaplan D.S. Intestinal obstruction from cecal bezoar: a complication of fiber-containing tube feedings. *Nutrition* 1990, 6: 115–117.

52. Kollef M.H. and Schuster D.P. The acute respiratory distress syndrome. *N. Eng. J. Med.* 1995, 332: 27–37.

53. Lin H.C. and Hasler W.L. Disorders of gastric emptying. In: Yamada T. (ed.), *Textbook of Gastroenterology,* 2nd edition, vol. I. J.B. Lippincott, Philadelphia, 1995, 1318.

54. Russell M., Cromer M., and Grant J. Complications of enteral nutrition therapy. In: Gottschlich M.M. (ed.), *The Science and Practice of Nutrition Support: A Case-Based Core Curriculum*. Kendall-Hunt, Dubuque, IA, 2001, 189.

55. Malone A.M. and Brewer C.K., Monitoring for complications and efficacy. In: Rolandelli R. (ed.) *Clinical Nutrition: Enteral and Tube Feeding*, 4th edition. W.B. Saunders, Philadelphia, 2004, 276–290.

56. Harkness L. The history of enteral nutrition therapy: from raw eggs and nasal tubes to purified amino acids and early postoperative jejunal delivery. *J. Am. Diet. Assoc.* 2002, 102: 399–404.

57. Lefton J. Management of common gastrointestinal complications in tube-fed patients. *Support Line* 2002, 24(1): 19–25.

58. ASPEN Board of Directors and Clinical Guidelines Task Force. Guidelines for the use of parenteral and enteral nutrition in adult and pediatric patients. *J. Parenter. Enteral Nutr.* 2002, 26: 15A–895A.

59. Malone A.M. The clinical benefits and efficacy in using specialized enteral feeding formulas. *Support Line* 2002, 24(1): 3–11.

60. Russell M.K. and Charney P. Is there a role for specialized enteral nutrition in the intensive care unit? *Nutr. Clin. Pract.* 2002, 17: 156–168.

61. Martindale R.G., Shikora S.A., Nishikawa R., and Siepler J.K. The metabolic response to stress and alterations in nutrient metabolism. In: Shikora. S.A., Martindale R.G., and Schwaitzberg S.D. (eds.), *Nutritional Considerations in the Intensive Care Unit: Science, Rationale and Practice*. Kendall-Hunt, Dubuque, IA, 2002, 11–20.

62. Zerr K.J., Furnary A.P., Grunkemeier G.L., et al. Glucose control lowers the risk of wound infections in diabetics after open heart surgery. *Ann. Thorac. Surg.* 1997 Feb, 63(2): 356–361.

63. Trick W.E., Scheckler W.E., Tokars J.I, et al. Modifiable risk factors associated with deep sternal site infection after coronary artery bypass grafting. *J. Thorac. Cardiovasc. Surg.* 2000, 119: 108–114.

64. van den Berghe G., Wouters P., Weekers F., et al. Intensive insulin therapy in the critically ill patients. *N. Engl. J. Med.* 2001, 345(19): 1359–1367.

65. Charney P. Diabetes mellitus. In: Matarese L.E. and Gottschlich M.M. (eds.), *Contemporary Nutrition Support Practice: A Clinical Guide*, 2nd edition. W.B. Saunders, Philadelphia, 2003, 533–545.

66. Jenkins D.J.A., Leeds A.R., and Gassull M.A. Unabsorbable carbohydrate and diabetes: decreased postprandial hyperglycemia. Lancet. 1976;2:172.

67. Peters A.L. and Davidson M.B. Lack of glucose elevation after simulated tube feeding with a low-carbohydrate, high fat enteral formula in patients with type 1 diabetes. *Am. J. Med.* 1989, 87: 178–181.

68. Peters A.L. and Davidson M.B. Effects of various enteral feeding products on postprandial blood glucose response in patients with type I diabetes. *J. Parenter. Enteral Nutr.* 1992, 16: 69–74.

69. Craig L.D., Nicholson S., Silverstone F.A., and Kennedy R.D. Use of a reduced carbohydrate, modified-fat enteral formula for improving metabolic control and clinical outcomes in long-term care residents with type 2 diabetes: results of a pilot trial. *Nutrition* 1998, 14: 529–534.

70. Beyers P., Silver H., and Restler C. Hyperglycemia: is a disease specific enteral formula indicated? ASPEN 19th Clinical Congress, Miami Beach, 1996: 592 (abstract).

71. Zaloga G. and Ackerman M.H. A review of disease specific formulas. *AACN* 1994, 5: 421–435.

72. Cerra F.B., Cheung N.K., and Fischer J.F. Disease specific amino acid infusion in hepatic encephalopathy: a prospective, randomized, double-blinded controlled trial. *J. Parenter. Enteral Nutr.* 1985, 9: 288–295.

73. Michel H., Bories P., Aubin J.P., et al. Treatment of acute hepatic encephalopathy in cirrhotics with branched-chain amino acid enriched versus a conventional amino acid mixture. *Liver* 1985, 5: 282–289.

74. Horst D., Grace N.D., Conn H.O., et al. Comparison of dietary protein with an oral, branched chain enriched amino acid supplement in chronic portal-systemic encephalopathy: a randomized controlled trial. *Hepatology* 1984, 4: 279–287.

75. Cerra F.B., Cheung N.K., Fischer J.E., et al. Disease-specific amino acid infusion (F080) in hepatic encephalopathy: a prospective, randomized, double-blind, controlled trial. *J. Parenter. Enteral Nutr.* 1985, 9: 288–295.

76. Rossi-Fanelli F., Riggio O., Cangiano C., Cascino A., et al. Branched-chain amino acids vs. lactulose in the treatment of hepatic coma: a controlled study. *Dig. Dis. Sci.* 1982, 27: 929–935.

77. Naylor C.D., O'Rourke K., Detsky A.S., and Baker J.P. Parenteral nutrition with branched-chain amino acids in hepatic encephalopathy. *Gastroenterology* 1989, 97: 1033–1042.

78. Marchesini G., Bianchi G., Merli M., et al. Nutritional supplementation with branched-chain amino acids in advanced cirrhosis: a double-blind, randomized trial. *Gastroenterology* 2003, 124: 1792–1801.

79. Mizok B.A. Nutritional support in hepatic encephalopathy. *Nutrition* 1999, 15: 220–228.

80. Gottschlich M.M., Jenkins M., Warden G.D., et al. Differential effects of three dietary regimens on selected outcome variables in burn patients. *J. Parenter. Enteral Nutr.* 1990, 14: 225–236.

81. McClave S. The effects of immune-enhancing diets (IEDs) on mortality, hospital length of stay, duration of mechanical ventilation and other parameters. *J. Parenter. Enteral Nutr.* 2001, 25: S44–S50.

82. Beale R.J., Bryg D.J., and Bihari D.J. Immunonutrition in the critically ill: a systematic review of clinical outcome. *Crit. Care Med.* 1999; 27: 2799–2805.

83. Heys S.D., Walker L.G., Smith I., and Eremin O. Enteral nutritional supplementation with key nutrients in patients with critical illness and cancer. *Ann. Surg.* 1999, 329: 467–477.

84. Heyland D.K., Novak F., Drover J.W., et al. Should immunonutrition become routine in critically ill patients? A systematic review of the evidence. *JAMA* 2001, 286: 944–953.

85. Schloerb P.R. Immune-enhancing diets: products, components and their rationales. *J. Parenter. Enteral Nutr.* 2001, 25: S3–S7.

86. Jurkovich G. Outcome studies using immune-enhancing diets: blunt and penetrating torso trauma patients. *J. Parenter. Enteral Nutr.* 2001, 25: S14–S18.

87. Sax H. Effect of immune-enhancing formulas in general surgery patients. *J. Parenter. Enteral Nutr.* 2001, 25: S19–S23.

88. Oltermann M. and Rasses T. Immunonutrition in a multidisciplinary ICU population: a review of the literature. *J. Parenter. Enteral Nutr.* 2001, 25: S30–S35.

89. Moore F. Effects of immune-enhancing diets on infectious morbidity and multiple organ failure. *J. Parenter. Enteral Nutr.* 2001, 25: S36–S43.

90. Kidsk K.A., Schloerb P.R., DeLegge M.H., et al. Consensus recommendations from the U.S. summit on immune-enhancing enteral therapy. *J. Parenter. Enteral Nutr.* 2001, 25: S61–S62.

91. Heyland D.K. and Novak F. Immunonutrition in the critically ill patient: more harm than good? *J. Parenter. Enteral Nutr.* 2001, 25: S51–S55.

92. Heyland D.K. Immunonutrition in the critically ill patient: putting the cart before the horse? *Nutr. Clin. Pract.* 2002, 17: 267–272.

93. Bertolini G., Iapichino G., Radrizzani D., et al. Early enteral immunonutrition in patients with severe sepsis: results of an interim analysis of a randomized multicentre clinical trial. *Intens. Care Med.* 2003, 29: 834–840.

94. McGowan K.C. and Bistrian B.R. Immunonutrition: problematic or problem solving? *Am. J. Clin. Nutr.* 2003, 77: 764–770.

95. Askanasi J., Rosenbaum S.H., Hyman A.I., Silverberg P.A., et al. Respiratory changes induced by the large glucose loads of total parenteral nutrition. *JAMA* 1980, 243: 1444–1447.

96. Covelli H.D., Black J.W., Olsen M.S., and Beekman J.F. Respiratory failure precipitated by high carbohydrate loads. *Ann. Intern. Med.* 1981, 95: 579–581.

97. Delafosse B., Bouffard Y., Viale J.P., Annat G., et al. Respiratory changes induced by parenteral nutrition in postoperative patients undergoing inspiratory pressure support ventilation. *Anesthesiology* 1987, 66: 393–396.

98. Angelillo V.A., Sukhdarshan B., Durfee B., et al. Effects of low and high carbohydrate feedings in ambulatory patients with chronic obstructive pulmonary disease and chronic hypercapnia. *Ann. Intern. Med.* 1985, 103: 883–885.

99. Al-Saady N.M., Blackmore C.M., and Bennett E.D. High fat, low carbohydrate, enteral feeding lowers PaCO$_2$ and reduces the period of ventilation in artificially ventilated patients. *Intens. Care Med.* 1989, 15: 190–195.

100. Akrabawi S.S., Mobarhan S., Stoltz R.R. and Ferguson P.W. Gastric emptying, pulmonary function, gas exchange, and respiratory quotient after feeding a moderate versus high fat enteral formula meal in chronic obstructive pulmonary disease patients. *Nutrition* 1996, 12: 260–265.

101. Talpers S.S., Romberger D.J., Bunce S.B., et al. Nutritionally associated increased carbon dioxide production: excess total calories vs high proportion of carbohydrate calories. *Chest* 1992, 102: 551–555.

102. Malone A.M. Is a pulmonary formula warranted for patients with pulmonary dysfunction? *Nutr. Clin. Pract.* 1997, 11: 189–191.

103. McMahon M.M., Benotti P.N., and Bistrian B.R. A clinical application of exercise physiology and nutritional support for the mechanically ventilated patient. *J. Parenter. Enteral Nutr.* 1990, 14: 538–542.

104. Hudson L.D. and Steinberg K.P. Acute respiratory distress syndrome: clinical features, management and outcome. In: Fishman A.P. (ed.), *Pulmonary Diseases and Disorders*. McGraw-Hill, New York, 1998, 2549–2565.

105. Mancuso P., Whelan J., DeMichele S.J., Snider C.C., et al. Dietary fish oil and fish and borage oil suppress intrapulmonary proinflammatory eicosanoid biosynthesis and attenuate pulmonary neutrophil accumulation in endotoxic rats. *Crit. Care Med.* 1997, 25: 1198–1206.

106. Karlstad M.D., Palombo J.D., Murray M., and DeMichele S.J. The anti-inflammatory role of γ-linolenic and eicosapentanoic acids in acute lung injury. In: Haung Y.S. and Mills D.E. (eds.), *Gamma Linolenic Acid: Metabolism and Its Roles in Nutrition and Medicine*. AOCS Press, Champaign, IL, 1996, 137–167.

107. Wennberg A.K., Nelson J.L., DeMichele S.J., and Campbell A.M. *Affecting Clinical Outcome in Acute Respiratory Distress Syndrome with Enteral Nutrition.* Ross Products Division, Abbott Laboratories, Columbus, OH, 1997.
108. Gadek J., DeMichele S., Karlstad M., Murray M., et al. Effect of enteral with eicosapentanoic acid, γ-linolenic acid, and antioxidants in patients with acute respiratory distress syndrome. *Crit. Care Med.* 1999, 27: 1409–1420.
109. Goldstein D.J. and Abrahamian-Gebeshian C. Nutrition support in renal failure. In: Matarese L.E. and Gottschlich M.M. (eds.), *Contemporary Nutrition Support Practice: A Clinical Guide*, 2nd edition. W.B. Saunders, Philadelphia, 1998, 447–471.
110. Mirtallo J.M., Kudsk K.A., and Ebbert M.L. Nutritional support of patients with renal disease. *Clin. Pharm.* 1984, 3: 253–263.
111. Giovanetti S. and Maggiore Q. A low nitrogen diet with protein of high biological value for severe chronic uremia. *Lancet* 1964, 1: 1000–1003.
112. Mirtallo J.M., Schneider P.J., Mavko K., Ruberg R.L., and Fabri P.J. A comparison of essential and general amino acid infusions in the nutritional support of patients with compromised renal function. *J. Parenter. Enteral Nutr.* 1982, 6: 109–113.
113. Kopple J.D. and Swendseid M.E. Nitrogen balance and plasma amino acid levels in uremic patients fed an essential amino acid diet. *Am. J. Clin. Nutr.* 1974, 27: 806–812.

17 Parenteral Formulations

Michael L. Christensen
University of Tennessee Health Science Center, LeBonheur Children's
Medical Center

CONTENTS

17.1 INTRODUCTION

Parenteral nutrition has been a lifesaving procedure for patients with short gut syndrome, very low birthweight infants, and certain other patients with gut failure. The modern era of parenteral nutrition began in the 1960s, with the development of a technique to catheterize the central venous circulation and the demonstration that normal growth and development could be achieved in immature dogs fed exclusively with parenteral nutrition (1,2). The placement of a central venous catheter allowed the provision of hypertonic parenteral nutrition formulas that were rapidly diluted in the high-flow central vein. Prior to this time, the provision of parenteral nutrition was limited to isotonic formulas that could be infused through a peripheral vein. The principal limitations were the large fluid volumes necessary to meet the nutritional needs of the patients, leading to fluid overload and the loss of peripheral venous access in patients who required prolonged support with parenteral nutrition.

TABLE 17.1
Normal Fluid Requirements

< 2.5 kg	150 ml/Kg
2.5–10 kg	100 ml/kg
10–20 kg	1000 ml + 50 ml/kg (for each kg > 10 kg)
≥ 20 kg	1500 ml ± 20 ml/kg (for each kg ≥ 20 kg)

Considerable knowledge about the provision of parenteral nutrition has evolved over the past 40 years. There is now a multitude of commercial products — amino acids, carbohydrates, fat emulsions, electrolytes, minerals, vitamins, and trace elements — available for inclusion in parenteral nutrition formulations. Parenteral nutrition is indicated when the enteral route is inadequate, the enteral route should be avoided, or when the enteral route may be harmful. A number of meta-analyses of the use of parenteral nutrition in different patient populations, including intensive care, oncology, and surgery, have not shown a benefit and have generally reported increased complications; therefore, careful selection of patients for parenteral nutrition is necessary (3–7). The American Society for Parenteral and Enteral Nutrition (ASPEN) has recently published revised guidelines for the use of parenteral nutrition in adult and pediatric patients (8).

17.2 WATER

Water is the most abundant constituent of the human body, accounting for approximately 60% of total body weight in the adult and 70 to 75% in the infant. Water balance depends on fluid intake, urine and stool output, metabolic and respiratory rates, evaporative losses from skin, and body temperature. Fluid requirements vary, depending on the age of the patient and concurrent disease. Normal fluid requirements, summarized in Table 17.1, range from 150 ml/kg in preterm neonates to 30 ml/kg in normal adults (9). Factors that increase fluid requirement included elevated body temperature, burn injury, fistula drainage, nasogastric losses, and diarrhea. In infants, radiant warmers and phototherapy increase evaporative losses. Factors that decrease fluid requirements include renal failure, congenital or congestive heart failure, and respiratory disorders. In evaluating fluid amounts in parenteral nutrition, it is important to consider fluids administered with parenteral drug administration, other intravenous fluids, and enteral feedings or oral intake.

17.3 ENERGY SOURCES

Intravenous sources of energy include carbohydrates, protein, and fat. The dietary reference intake in the adult diet is 45 to 65% carbohydrate, 25 to 35% fat, and 10 to 35% protein (10). The provision of optimal nutrition support to hospitalized patients is necessary to improve nutritional status while preventing complications associated with overfeeding or underfeeding. Measurement of energy expenditure using direct or indirect calorimetry or the double-labeled water method provides the most accurate method for determining energy requirements. These methods are expensive and time consuming, and require trained personnel. A number of predictive equations have been developed as more practical means for estimating energy requirements. The accuracy and applicability of these equations have been questioned (11–13). Clinicians must carefully choose the method for estimating energy requirement, understanding the degree of accuracy that is acceptable and the limitations in its application. (See Chapter 6.)

17.3.1 DEXTROSE

Dextrose is the most common energy source used in parenteral nutrition. Intravenous dextrose monohydrate provides 3.4 kcal/g. Anhydrous dextrose provides 4 kcal/g, whereas dextrose in aqueous solution is hydrated, lowering the caloric content to 3.4 kcal/g. Commercial dextrose solution concentrations are available from 2.5 to 70%. Most institutions have the availability of an automated compounding system and predominantly use 70% dextrose that can be admixed with sterile water to create a wide range of lower final dextrose concentrations. Dextrose solutions have an acidic pH of 3.5 to 5.5.

Parenteral nutrition solutions with final dextrose concentrations less than 12.5% usually can be infused into a peripheral vein. The use of peripheral parenteral nutrition depends on having suitable veins that can tolerate high volume rates. In general, peripheral parenteral nutrition should be limited to a short period of time, usually less than 1 week. The osmolality of peripheral parenteral nutrition solutions can reach 800 to 900 mOsm/l, making these solutions relatively hypertonic. Coadministration of fat emulsion with the peripheral parenteral nutrition solution or the addition of heparin to the peripheral parenteral nutrition solution may increase the duration of the peripheral catheter (14–18). Dextrose concentration exceeding 12.5% or a total osmolality exceeding 900 mOsm/l should be infused into a central vein.

17.3.2 LIPIDS

Intravenous fat emulsions are used widely in parenteral nutrition as an energy source and to provide essential fatty acids (19). The first fat emulsion introduced in the United States in the 1960s contained cottonseed oil. Severe adverse reactions led to its withdrawal from the market soon after its introduction. The next fat emulsion introduced was derived from soybean oil, which is high in long-chain triglycerides (LCTs), notably linolenic acid. A safflower oil fat emulsion followed the soybean oil fat emulsion. Safflower oil is low in linolenic acid, and concern over the possible development of linolenic acid deficiency led to its replacement with a combination soybean oil–safflower oil fat emulsion. Fat emulsions are available in 10% (1.1 kcal/ml), 20% (2.0 kcal/ml), and 30% (3.0 kcal/ml). These products contain egg phospholipid as an emulsifying agent and glycerol to make the product approximately isotonic. Outside the U.S., there is a greater variety of fat sources included in the fat emulsion with soybean oil, including olive oil (monounsaturated fatty acids), fish oil (n-3 polyunsaturated fatty acids [PUFAs]), and coconut oil (medium-chain triglycerides [MCTs]), as well as structured lipids. Representative fat emulsions are listed in Table 17.2. Structured lipid emulsions are manufactured triglycerides where medium-chain and long-chain fatty acids are esterified on the same glycerol backbone.

Fat emulsions are generally given continuously to infants and may be given intermittently to older children and adults or included in a total nutrient admixture. To meet essential fatty acid requirements, only 2 to 4% of the nonprotein calories need to be provided as essential fatty acid, or about 10% as total fat. Adults usually receive 0.5 to 1.0 g/kg, up to a maximum dose of 2.5 g/kg. Infants usually receive 2 to 3 g/kg, up to a maximum dose of 4 g/kg (20). In infants, lipids are usually started at 0.5 to 1.0 g/kg and advanced 0.5 to 1 g/kg as tolerated. Slower titration schedules in preterm infants are often required because of the immaturity in clearance and metabolism pathways.

The currently available fat emulsions have a very different composition from lipids normally found in regular diet, infant formulas, or human milk (21). The 10% fat emulsion product provides twice the amount of phospholipid as the 20%, when given on a gram-equivalent amount. The excessive amount of phospholipid administered with the 10% fat emulsion has been associated with abnormal plasma lipid profile in infants (22,23).

TABLE 17.2
Fatty Acid Composition of Intravenous Fat Emulsions

Fatty Acid Content (%) Manufacturer	Intralipid® 10%, 20%, 30% (Kabi-Vitrum)	Liposyn II® 10%, 20% (Abbott)	Liposyn III® 10%, 20%, 30% (Abbott)	Lipofundin® 10, 20% (B. Braun)	ClinOleic® 20% (Baxter)	Omegaven® 10% (Fresenius Kabi)
Oil source	Soybean	Soybean, safflower	Soybean	Soybean, coconut	Soybean, olive	Soybean, fish
Caprylic (C8:0)	—	—	—	27	—	—
Capric (C10:0)	—	—	—	18	—	—
Lauric (C12:0)	—	—	—	1	—	—
Myristic (C14:0)	—	—	—	—	—	4.9
Palmitic (C16:0)	10	5	10	16	13	10.7
Palmitoleic (C16:1n-7)	—	—	—	—	1	8.2
Stearic (C18:0)	4	2	4	3	3	2.4
Oleic (C18:1n-9)	21	15	21	12.5	60	12.3
Linoleic (C18:2n-6)	56	66	55	27	18	3.7
Linolenic (C18:3n-3)	8	4.2	8	3.5	2	1.3
Arachidonic (C20:4n-6)	1	—	—	0.5	0.3	2.6
Eicosapentaneoic (C20:5n-3)	—	—	—	—	—	18.8
Docosapentaenoic (C22:5n-3)	—	—	—	—	—	2.8
Docosahexaenoic (C22:6n-3)	—	—	—	—	—	16.5

Fat emulsions are prone to the formation of hydroperoxides on exposure to light, and photo-therapy may enhance the formation of hydroperoxides (24–26). Preterm infants have limited antioxidant reserves and may be at increased risk for oxidative damage. Protecting the fat emulsion from light has been advocated as a method to limit hydroperoxide formation (27).

The other major concerns with the administration of fat emulsion are the infection risk and the effect on immune function. Infection risk with a fungal organism *Malazzeia furfur* and *Staphylo-coccus epidemitus* has been reported with the use of fat emulsion (28,29). The effect of the administration of fat emulsion on immune function is controversial and has been the subject of several reviews (30–34). No difference in the incidence of infection was observed in bone marrow transplant patients receiving a standard dose (25 to 30% of energy intake) or a low dose (6 to 8%) of a soybean fat emulsion (35). The high content of PUFAs, primarily of the n-6 series, in soybean oil–based fat emulsion may adversely affect the immune system, inflammation, and oxidant stress levels (36). PUFAs are precursors to different eicosanoids (leukotrienes, prostaglandins, and throm-boxanes). The metabolism of n-6 PUFAs leads to eicosanoids that are proinflammatory and suppress the immune function, whereas n-3 PUFAs decrease the production of inflammatory eicosanoids and enhance immune function. MCTs have a higher utilization rate and lower the amount of n-6 PUFAs when incorporated into the intravenous fat emulsion.

17.3.3 GLYCEROL

Glycerol, a sugar alcohol that provides 4.3 cal/g, is a nonprotein caloric source in the parenteral nutrition product ProcalAmine® (B. Braun, Irvine, CA). ProcalAmine contains 3% amino acids and 3% glycerol premixed in 1 l containers (Table 17.3). This product is intended for the short-term administration to postsurgical patients. ProcalAmine contains standard electrolytes that may not be appropriate for all patients. The potential benefits of short-term administration of ProcalAmine must be weighed against the infusion of standard intravenous fluids. Glycerol as a nonprotein caloric source does offer an advantage over dextrose in that it does not require insulin for uptake into the cell. Postsurgical insulin-dependent patients had lower insulin requirements when given parenteral nutrition with glycerol, as compared to glucose, as the nonprotein caloric source (37–39).

17.3.4 ENERGY UTILIZATION OF PARENTERAL CARBOHYDRATE SOURCES

The maximum infusion of dextrose in patients receiving parenteral nutrition depends on the age of the patient and the underlying clinical condition. Net fat synthesis occurred when parenteral glucose intake exceeded 12.5 mg/kg/min in postsurgical newborns and 12.6 mg/kg/min in stable infants (40,41). In critically ill children, maximal glucose oxidation occurred at glucose intakes of 5 mg/kg/min (42,43). The fraction of exogenous glucose that was oxidized decreased as glucose infusion rates increased, up to an infusion rate of 8 mg/kg/min. Children with lipogenesis had an average glucose intake of 8.5 mg/kg/min (42).

These results in critically ill children are similar to the glucose oxidation rates reported in critically ill adults. In adults, increasing glucose infusion rates from 4 to 8 mg/kg/min is associated with increased glucose oxidation rates, although efficiency of oxidation decreases (44,45). When glucose infusion rates exceeded 9 mg/kg/min, there was no significant increase in glucose oxidation (45). Glucose infusion rates in excess of the oxidative capacity will enter nonoxidative metabolic pathways, including glycolysis, glycogenesis, and lipogenesis. Alternately, excessive glucose infu-sion rates can lead to hyperglycemia and glycosuria, which has been associated with higher morbidity and mortality rates in critically ill adults (46–48).

TABLE 17.3
Glycerol-Containing Amino Acid Solution

Preparation Manufacturer	ProcalAmine® 3% (3% Amino Acid and 3% Glycerin with Electrolytes) B. Braun
Nitrogen g/100 ml	0.46
Essential amino acids (mg/100 ml)	
Histidine	85
Isoleucine	210
Leucine	270
Lysine	220
Methionine	160
Phenylalanine	170
Threonine	120
Tryptophan	46
Valine	200
Nonessential amino acids (mg/100 ml)	
Alanine	210
Arginine	290
Proline	340
Serine	180
Taurine	—
Tyrosine	—
N-acetyl-l-tyrosine	—
Glycine	420
Cysteine	< 20
Glutamic acid	—
Aspartic acid	—
Electrolytes (mEq/l)	
Calcium	3
Sodium	35
Potassium	24
Magnesium	5
Chloride	41
Acetate	47
Phosphate (mmol/l)	3.5
mOsm/l	735
pH	6.5–7

17.3.5 PROTEIN SOURCES

Parenteral protein products have undergone considerable change during the past 40 years. The initial protein sources were hydrolysates of casein and fibrin. They could be produced in large quantities at reasonable cost and met most of the essential amino acid requirements of adults. Deficiencies of hydrolysates included the uncertain metabolic fate of peptides, the uncontrollable batch-to-batch variation in the hydrolysate composition, the production of hyperammonemia (especially in infants, likely due to low arginine rather than preformed ammonia), and the occasional severe allergic-type reaction. Early crystalline amino acid formulations resulted in a profound hyperchloremic metabolic acidosis in infants that was less severe in older children and adults. The discussion of standard and modified disease-specific amino acids will focus on those products available in the U.S. Similar products by different manufacturers are available outside the U.S.

17.3.5.1 Standard

The amino acid composition of standard amino acid solutions has been based on high-quality dietary proteins such as egg white, but modified to replace glutamine and asparagine with glycine (Table 17.4). Standard amino acid solutions are intended to meet the protein needs of stable adults. Standard amino acid solutions are available in concentrations ranging from 3.5 to 15%, with or without added electrolytes. More highly concentrated amino acid solutions are often used in pharmacies that have automated formulators and may be used in fluid-restricted patients. Amino acid solutions that contain electrolytes are best used in stable patients who do not have unusual electrolyte requirements. The standard amino acid solutions may be inadequate in certain disease states and during infancy. This has led to the development of modified disease-specific amino acid solutions and amino acid solutions for use in infants.

17.3.5.2 Kidney Disease

There are currently four commercially available modified amino acid solutions that have been formulated for patients with renal failure (Table 17.5). These products contain predominantly essential amino acids and histidine. One product also contains arginine, which is important in the urea cycle, and another contains lower amounts of nonessential amino acids. The essential amino acid solutions for renal failure were based on the principles established for treating patients with chronic renal failure with a low-protein diet and an essential amino acid supplement. Because of underlying differences in the metabolic response between chronic and acute renal failure, essential-only amino acid solution may not meet protein needs.

The benefits of modified amino acid solutions for renal failure over standard amino acids in acute renal failure remain controversial (49–52). Patients with acute renal failure are highly variable in terms of hypermetabolism and hypercatabolism, as well as renal function. Protein and energy requirements will depend on their underlying disease state rather than their renal failure. Nutrition therapy must be individualized, given the degree of critical illness, use of renal replacement therapy, and nutritional status.

17.3.5.3 Liver Disease

There is only one modified amino acid solution approved for use in patients with hepatic failure (Table 17.5). HepatAmine® (B. Braun, Irvine, CA) contains high amounts of branched-chain amino acids and low amounts of aromatic amino acid solutions.

The basis for the formulation of the hepatic failure amino solution emerges from the false neurotransmitter and unified theories of hepatic encephalopathy (53,54). Patients with hepatic encephalopathy have elevated plasma aromatic amino acids (AAA), because of decreased liver metabolism, and decreased plasma branched-chain amino acids (BCAA), because of peripheral metabolism (55–58). The reduction in the BCAA–AAA ratio favors brain uptake of AAA which compete with BCAA to cross the blood–brain barrier. The aromatic amino acid derived neuroamines (phenylethylamine, tyramine, phenylehtanolamine, octopamine, serotonin, and tryptamine) are elevated in the blood and in the CNS. These substances have been associated with hepatic encephalopathy.

Patients with hepatic encephalopathy often have protein-calorie malnutrition. The traditional approach to nutritional intervention in patients with hepatic encephalopathy was protein restriction. When the diet is restrictive, undernutrition and its associated complications further compromise patients with liver failure. Most patients can be supported with standard amino acid formulation with careful attention to protein intake. For patients who decompensate while receiving modest doses of standard amino acids, use of the hepatic failure amino acid solution should be considered. Clinical studies support the hepatic-failure amino acid formulation to be beneficial in liver failure (59–65). Because the hepatic-failure amino acid solution is more costly than standard amino acid solutions, strict criteria should be implemented to prevent the inappropriate use of this product.

TABLE 17.4
Standard Amino Acid Solutions

Preparation Manufacturer	Aminosyn® 8.5% Abbott	Aminosyn® 10% Abbott	Aminosyn II® 8.5% Abbott	Aminosyn II® 10% Abbott	Aminosyn II® 15% Abbott
Nitrogen g/100 ml	1.34	1.57	1.30	1.53	2.3
Essential Amino Acids (mg/100 ml)					
Histidine	260	300	255	300	450
Isoleucine	620	720	561	660	990
Leucine	810	940	700	1000	1500
Lysine	624	720	735	1050	1575
Methionine	340	400	120	172	258
Phenylalanine	380	440	209	298	447
Threonine	460	520	280	400	600
Tryptophan	150	160	140	200	300
Valine	680	800	350	500	750
Nonessential Amino Acids (mg/100 ml)					
Alanine	1100	1280	695	993	1490
Arginine	5850	980	713	1018	1527
Proline	750	860	505	722	1083
Serine	370	420	371	530	795
Taurine	—	—	—	—	—
Tyrosine	44	44	189	—	—
N-acetyl-l-tyrosine	—	—	—	270	405
Glycine	1100	1280	350	500	750
Cysteine	—	—	—	—	—
Glutamic acid	—	—	517	738	1107
Aspartic acid	—	—	490	700	1050

Electrolytes mEq/l

	FreAmine III® 8.5% B. Braun	FreAmine III® 10% B. Braun	Travasol® 8.5% Baxter	Travasol® 10% Baxter	Novamine® 15% Baxter
Calcium	—	—	—	—	—
Sodium	—	—	31.3	44.4	62.7
Potassium	5.4	5.4	—	—	—
Magnesium	—	—	—	—	—
Chloride	35	—	—	—	—
Acetate	90	148	50.3	71.8	107.6
Phosphate (mmol/l)	—	—	—	—	—
mOsm/l	850	1000	612	870	1300
pH	5.3	5.3	5—6.5	5.8	5.8

Preparation	FreAmine III® 8.5%	FreAmine III® 10%	Travasol® 8.5%	Travasol® 10%	Novamine® 15%
Manufacturer	B. Braun	B. Braun	Baxter	Baxter	Baxter
Nitrogen g/100 ml	1.3	1.53	1.43	1.65	2.37

Essential Amino Acids (mg/100 ml)

Histidine	240	280	372	480	894
Isoleucine	590	690	406	600	749
Leucine	770	910	526	730	1040
Lysine	620	730	492	580	1180
Methionine	450	530	492	400	749
Phenylalanine	480	560	526	560	1040
Threonine	340	400	356	420	749
Tryptophan	130	150	152	180	250
Valine	560	660	390	580	960

(continued)

TABLE 17.4 (CONTINUED)
Standard Amino Acid Solutions

Preparation Manufacturer	FreAmine III® 8.5% B. Braun	FreAmine III® 10% B. Braun	Travasol® 8.5% Baxter	Travasol® 10% Baxter	Novamine® 15% Baxter
Nonessential Amino Acids (mg/100 ml)					
Alanine	600	710	1760	2070	2170
Arginine	810	950	880	1150	1470
Proline	950	1120	356	680	894
Serine	500	590	—	500	592
Taurine	—	—	—	—	—
Tyrosine	—	—	34	40	39
N-acetyl-1-tyrosine	—	—	—	—	—
Glycine	1190	1400	1760	1030	1040
Cysteine	< 20	<20	—	—	—
Glutamic acid	—	—	—	—	749
Aspartic acid	—	—	—	—	434
Electrolytes (mEq/l)					
Calcium	—	—	—	—	—
Sodium	10	10	—	—	—
Potassium	—	—	—	—	—
Magnesium	—	—	—	—	—
Chloride	≤3	<3	34	40	—
Acetate	72	89	73	87	151
Phosphate (mmol/l)	10	10	—	—	—
mOsm/l	810	950	890	1000	1388
pH	6–7	6–7	6	6	5.6

TABLE 17.5
Modified Amino Acid Solutions

Preparation	FreAmine HBC® 6.9%	BranchAmin® 4%	HepatAmine® 8%	Aminees® 5.2%	Aminosyn RF® 5.2%	NephrAmine® 5.4%	RenAmin® 6.5%
Manufacturer	B. Braun	Baxter	B. Braun	Baxter	Abbott	B. Braun	Baxter
Nitrogen g/100 ml	0.97	0.44	1.2	0.66	0.79	0.64	1
Essential Amino Acids (mg/100 ml)							
Histidine	160	—	240	412	429	250	420
Isoleucine	760	1380	900	525	462	560	500
Leucine	1370	1380	1100	825	726	880	600
Lysine	410	—	610	600	535	640	450
Methionine	250	—	100	825	726	880	500
Phenylalanine	320	—	100	825	726	880	490
Threonine	200	—	450	375	330	400	380
Tryptophan	90	—	66	188	165	200	160
Valine	880	1240	840	600	528	640	820
Nonessential Amino Acids (mg/100 ml)							
Alanine	400	—	770	—	—	—	560
Arginine	580	—	600	—	600	—	630
Proline	630	—	800	—	—	—	350
Serine	330	—	500	—	—	—	300
Taurine	—	—	—	—	—	—	—
Tyrosine	—	—	—	—	—	—	40
N-acetyl-l-tyrosine	—	—	—	—	—	—	—
Glycine	330	—	900	—	—	—	300
Cysteine	<20	—	<20	—	—	<20	—
Glutamic acid	—	—	—	—	—	—	—
Aspartic acid	—	—	—	—	—	—	—
Electrolytes mEq/l							
Calcium	—	—	—	—	—	—	—
Sodium	10	—	10	—	—	5	—
Potassium	—	—	—	—	5.4	—	—
Magnesium	—	—	—	—	—	—	—
Chloride	≤3	—	<3	—	—	<3	31
Acetate	57	—	62	50	105	44	60
Phosphate (mmol/l)	—	—	10	—	—	—	—
mOsm/l	620	316	785	416	475	435	600
pH	6–7	6	6–6.8	6.4	5.2	6–7	6

17.3.5.4 Trauma/Stress

Trauma, sepsis, or major surgery results in profound hypercatabolism. During the catabolic state, there is significant breakdown of skeletal muscle, resulting in increased release to meet the increased demand for hepatic protein synthesis and increased metabolism of BCAAs as a preferred local energy source. It has also been observed that providing BCAAs, notably leucine, reduced skeletal muscle catabolism and increased skeletal muscle and hepatic protein synthesis (66). Two modified amino acid products have been formulated with a high content of BCAAs (Table 17.5). A third product contains BCAAs and is added to standard amino acid solution. Studies of BCAA-enriched parenteral nutrition solutions have not demonstrated a decreased catabolic rate or a reduction in morbidity or mortality. (67–70). Although there are theoretical reasons for the use of BCAA-enriched solutions, they have not been shown to be superior to standard amino acid solution.

17.3.5.5 Pediatric

Infants have a number of immature enzymatic metabolic pathways, rendering certain amino acids considered nonessential for adults essential in infants. The most notable inactive amino acid metabolic pathways are the conversion of phenylalanine to tyrosine and the transulfuration pathway. When standard amino acid solutions are administered to infants, aberrant plasma amino acids have been observed, including elevated plasma concentrations of methionine and phenylalanine and low concentrations of tyrosine, cysteine, and taurine (71). Three pediatric amino acid solutions are available in the United States (Table 17.6). One pediatric amino acid solution (TrophAmine®, B. Braun, Irvine, CA) was designed to normalize plasma amino acids to a postprandial reference range developed in healthy one-month-old breastfed infants (71–74). This product, compared to a standard amino acid solution, was associated with higher weight gain and nitrogen balance in postsurgical infants (75). Recently, a generic version (Premasol®, Baxter, Deerfield, IL) has been introduced. Another pediatric amino acid solution (Aminosyn PF®, Abbott, Abbott Park, IL) is a modification of the company's standard amino acid solution, incorporating additional amino acids thought to be essential in the infants, including glutamic acid, aspartic acid, and taurine; reducing alanine, glycine, methionine, and valine; and increasing leucine and arginine.

17.3.5.6 Cysteine

Preterm and newborn infants have a functional immaturity in the transulfuration pathway, leading to impairment in the metabolism of sulfur-containing amino acids. Low cysteine concentrations have been reported in infants receiving parenteral nutrition containing minimal amounts of cysteine. The initial pediatric amino acid solution released in the U.S. was designed to have cysteine added to the parenteral nutrition solution at the time of preparation. Cysteine addition to a pediatric amino acid solution resulted in higher taurine levels, and at 40 mg/g of amino acids, plasma taurine concentrations were within the normal reference range for infants (76,77). Cysteine is not included in the pediatric amino acid solution because it is not stable in solution for prolonged periods of time. When cysteine is included in the amino acid solution, it forms the dimer cystine, which has limited solubility in solution and precipitates out of solution. Cysteine HCl is available as a 50 mg/ml solution and is added to the parenteral nutrition solution at a dose of 40 mg per gram of amino acids.

17.3.5.7 Glutamine

Glutamine is a nonessential amino acid but may be essential in certain clinical settings (e.g., critical illness), because the body is unable to synthesize sufficient amounts. Glutamine is not included in parenteral amino acid solutions because of limited solubility (3.5 g/dl) and stability (degradation with heat sterilization and prolonged storage). These problems have been overcome by the synthesis

TABLE 17.6
Pediatric Amino Acid Solutions

Preparation Manufacturer	Aminosyn-PF® 7% Abbott	Aminosyn-PF® 10% Abbott	TrophAmine® 6% B. Braun	TrophAmine® 10% B. Braun	Premasol® 6% Baxter	Premasol® 10% Baxter
Nitrogen g/100 ml	1.07	1.52	0.93	1.55	0.93	1.55
Essential Amino Acids (mg/100 ml)						
Histidine	220	312	290	480	0.29	0.48
Isoleucine	534	760	490	820	0.49	0.82
Leucine	831	1200	840	1400	0.84	1.40
Lysine	475	677	490	820	0.49	0.82
Methionine	125	180	200	340	0.20	0.34
Phenylalanine	300	427	290	480	0.29	0.48
Threonine	360	512	250	420	0.25	0.42
Tryptophan	125	180	120	200	0.12	0.20
Valine	452	673	470	780	0.47	0.78
Nonessential Amino Acids (mg/100 ml)						
Alanine	490	698	320	540	0.32	0.54
Arginine	861	1227	730	1200	0.73	1.20
Proline	570	812	410	680	0.41	0.68
Serine	347	495	230	380	0.23	0.38
Taurine	50	70	15	25	0.015	0.025
Tyrosine	44	44	140e	240e		
N-acetyl-l-tyrosine						
Glycine	270	385	220	360	0.22	0.36
Cysteine			<14e	< 16e	< 0.014	< 0.016
Glutamic acid	576	820	300	500	0.30	0.50
Aspartic acid	370	527	190	320	0.19	0.32
Electrolytes (mEq/l)						
Calcium						
Sodium	3.4	3.4	5	5	0	0
Potassium						
Magnesium						
Chloride			< 3	< 3	< 3*	< 3*
Acetate	32.5	46	56	97	57	94
Phosphate (mmol/l)						
mOsm/l	586	829	52	875	520	865
pH	5.4	5.4	5–6	5–6	5.5 (5.0–6.0)	5.5 (5.0–6.0)

TABLE 17.7
Normal Daily Electrolyte and Mineral Requirements

	Adults	Infants and Children
Sodium	50–250 mEq	2–4 mEq/kg
Potassium	30–200 mEq	2–3 mEq/kg
Chloride	50–250 mEq	2–3 mEq/kg
Phosphate	10–40 mmol	0.5–2 mmol/kg
Calcium	10–20 mEq	1–3 mEq/kg
Magnesium	10–30 mEq	0.25–0.5 mEq/kg

of glutamine-containing dipeptides, alanyl-glutamine and glycyl-glutamine, which are available outside the U.S. The dose of parenteral glutamine has ranged from 0.26 to 0.57 g/kg/d. The addition of glutamine to parenteral nutrition solutions and the patient population that would most benefit from this addition remain controversial (78–81). Continued study of glutamine supplementation of parenteral nutrition is needed to define which patients will benefit.

17.4 ELECTROLYTES AND MINERALS

Management of electrolyte and mineral status in acutely ill patients receiving parenteral nutrition remains the most challenging aspect of providing parenteral nutrition. Once a patient's estimated caloric and protein needs have been met through the titration of the parenteral nutrition solution, most of the clinician's effort is focused on maintaining electrolyte and mineral status. Electrolytes may be added to parenteral nutrition solution using single or multiple electrolyte formulations. Multiple electrolyte formulations are most appropriately used in patients who have normal organ function and normal serum electrolytes. The usual requirements of electrolytes and minerals are listed in Table 17.7. Sodium and potassium are available as chloride, acetate, and phosphate salts, and magnesium is available as the sulfate salt. Calcium gluconate is the preferred salt for parenteral nutrition but is also available as calcium chloride. The concern for calcium phosphate precipitation limits the amount of calcium and phosphate that can be added to parenteral nutrition solutions. Therefore, preterm neonates, who have the highest requirements for both calcium and phosphate, have the greatest risk of calcium phosphate precipitation in parenteral nutrition solutions. Outside the U.S., organic phosphates are available that have much greater compatibility with calcium.

17.5 VITAMINS

Parenteral multivitamin products (Table 17.7) have been formulated according to the recommendations of the American Medical Association National Advisory Group (AMA-NAG) in adult and pediatric patients (82,83). The Food and Drug Administration (FDA) Division of Metabolic and Endocrine Drug Products and the AMA's Division of Personal and Public Health Policy sponsored a workshop in 1985 that led to recommended changes to adult multivitamin products. These included an increase in the dosage of vitamins B1, B6, C, and folic acid, as well as the addition of vitamin K (Table 17.8) (84).

Two vitamin shortages due to manufacturing issues have delayed implementation of these recommended changes. The importance of parenteral vitamins' addition to parenteral nutrition solutions has been highlighted by a number of national shortages of parenteral adult and pediatric multivitamins. The most serious consequence of the shortage was the development of refractory lactic acidosis due to thiamine deficiency, resulting in significant morbidity and mortality (85). Notably, there continues to be a lack of a parenteral multivitamin product formulated to meet the unique needs of preterm neonates.

TABLE 17.8
Multivitamin Preparations

	Current Adult Formulation	Proposed Adult Formulation	Pediatric Formulation
Fat-Soluble Vitamins			
Vitamin A	3300 IU	3300 IU	2300 IU
Vitamin D	200 IU	200 IU	400 IU
Vitamin E	10 IU	10 IU	7 IU
Vitamin K	—	150 mcg	200 mcg
Water-Soluble Vitamins			
Thiamine (B1)	3 mg	6 mg	1.2 mg
Riboflavin (B2)	3.6 mg	3.6 mg	1.4 mg
Pyridoxine (B6)	4 mg	6 mg	1 mg
Cyanocobalamin	5 mcg	5 mcg	1 mcg
Ascorbic acid (C)	100 mg	200 mg	80 mg
Niacin	40 mg	40 mg	17 mg
Biotin	60 mg	60 mg	20 mg
Folic acid	400 mcg	600 mcg	140 mcg
Pantothenic acid	15 mg	15 mg	5 mg

TABLE 17.9
Guidelines for Daily Trace Elements

	Adults	Children	Neonates
Zinc	2.5–4.0 mg	100 mcg/kg	300 mcg/kg
Copper	0.5–1.5 mg	20 mcg/kg	20 mcg/kg
Manganese	0.15–0.8 mg	2–10 mcg/kg	2–10 mcg/kg
Chromium	10–15 mcg	0.14–0.2 mcg/kg	0.14–0.2 mcg/kg
Selenium	40–80 mcg	2–3 mcg/kg	2–3 mcg/kg

17.6 TRACE ELEMENTS

Trace elements are essential micronutrients that are necessary cofactors for the function of a number of enzymatic systems. Trace elements are available as single-entity and multiple–trace element products. The AMA-NAG has published guidelines for four trace elements known to be important to human nutrition (83,86). The recommended amounts for zinc, copper, manganese, and chromium are listed in Table 17.9. Selenium may also be an important trace element that should be considered for addition to parenteral nutrition solutions (87,88). Guidelines for the supplementation of molybdenum and iodine have not been established. Iron is an important element that is not routinely added to parenteral nutrition solutions but should be considered in patients who are receiving long-term parenteral nutrition and unable to take oral iron supplementation.

Zinc requirements are increased in metabolic stress, secondary to increased urinary excretion, and in gastrointestinal diseases, secondary to increased ostomy, fistula, or diarrheal losses. Manganese and copper are excreted via the biliary tract and should be restricted or withheld in patients with cholestatic liver disease. Zinc, chromium, and selenium are renally excreted, and restriction or elimination may be needed with impaired renal function. Evidence is accumulating that there is adequate chromium contamination in parenteral nutrition solutions, so chromium addition to parenteral nutrition may not be necessary (89,90).

17.6.1 ALUMINUM

Aluminum is the most abundant metal in the earth's crust and is ubiquitous in its distribution but has no known biological function. The accumulation of aluminum in human tissue has now been recognized for more than a quarter-century. Aluminum contamination is associated with osteomalacia, encephalopathy, and microcytic anemia, and may contribute to cholestasis in infants. Patients with impaired renal function and neonates are at the greatest risk for exposure to unsafe amounts of aluminum. Aluminum toxicity was first reported as an encephalopathy in adult patients on dialysis and subsequently in children with renal disease not on dialysis but receiving aluminum-containing phosphate binders (91–94). High concentrations of aluminum were found in the gray matter of dialysis patients (95). Subsequently, severe osteomalacia was reported in patients undergoing dialysis with tap water contaminated with high concentrations of aluminum (96). High concentrations of aluminum have been found in the bone, urine, and plasma of infants receiving parenteral nutrition (97,98). Accumulation of aluminum has been observed in patients with normal renal function who received long-term parenteral nutrition (99).

The FDA published new labeling requirements mandating that manufacturers include information regarding aluminum content present in large- and small-volume parenterals. The aluminum content of all large- and small-volume parenterals used in the preparation of parenteral nutrition will be required to have an aluminum concentration that does not exceed 25 mcg/l, which must be stated on the product label (100–102). This requirement applies to all large-volume parenterals used in parenteral nutrition including, but not limited to, amino acid solution, concentrated dextrose solution, sterile water, and lipid emulsion. The new packaging requirement for these products will include a statement in the precautions section of the labeling that the product contains no more 25 mcg/ml of aluminum. Small-volume parenterals will require the immediate container label to state the aluminum content as "Contains no more than ____ mcg/l of aluminum." For products that are lyophilized powders used in the preparation of parenteral nutrition solutions, the label will contain a statement "When reconstituted in accordance with the package insert instructions, the concentration of aluminum will be no more than ___ mcg/ml." The warning section of the label will contain a statement indicating that the product contains aluminum, which may be toxic. Prolonged parenteral administration may lead to toxic aluminum concentrations in patients with impaired kidney function and neonates. Aluminum intakes that exceed 4 to 5 mcg/kg/d accumulate aluminum at levels associated with CNS and bone toxicity. The implementation date continues to be pushed back by the FDA, but the latest implementation date was July 2004.

The American Society for Clinical Nutrition and the American Society for Parenteral Nutrition committee have stated that a safe intake of aluminum is 2 mcg/kg/d and an unsafe intake is 15 to 30 mcg/kg/d (103). All parenteral products have some aluminum contamination. Calcium and phosphate salts are the chief source of aluminum contamination associated with parenteral nutrition. Pharmacists who prepare and deliver parenteral nutrition solutions are responsible for choosing products with the lowest aluminum content for the preparation of parenteral nutrition solutions, calculating the aluminum content for the compounded parenteral nutrition solution, and informing the recipient's physician whether the aluminum content is safe, unsafe, or toxic. *Safe* is defined as the amount of aluminum intake per patient per day that did not result in aluminum accumulation in tissue or fluids and was associated with no toxic effect. *Unsafe* is defined as the amount of aluminum intake per patient per day that resulted in tissue loading but not documented toxicity. *Toxic* is defined as the amount of aluminum taken in per patient per day that resulted in tissue loading and symptoms of toxicity.

17.7 ORDERING PARENTERAL NUTRITION SOLUTIONS

Parenteral nutrition is one of the most complicated pharmaceutical products administered to patients. The complexity of this solution makes it prone to errors, both in the prescribing and in the preparation. Standardized order forms for parenteral nutrition are commonly used to reduce potential errors. The order form is designed to meet the unique needs of the practitioners and patient population of the institution. The order form can be fairly rigid, allowing the prescribing of a few standardized parenteral nutrition solutions with only minimal additions allowed, or a flexible order form that identifies the major components of the parenteral nutrition solution with the daily amounts written in by the practitioner. An example of an adult and a pediatric flexible order form is provided (Table 17.10 and Table 17.11), listing the major components (the amount of which must be written in for a 24-hour basis) and space for ordering other additives to the parenteral nutrition solution. A number of institutions use the back of the parenteral nutrition order form to provide specific instructions and general guidelines for writing parenteral nutrition orders. Institutions must have written policies and procedures for the ordering and preparing parenteral nutrition solutions and monitoring patients requiring parenteral nutrition. Prior to initiating parenteral nutrition, it is important to confirm the location of the venous access device. The order form must indicate whether the parenteral nutrition solution is to be administered via a central or a peripheral catheter. Parenteral nutrition solutions orders must be written or reviewed on a daily basis.

17.8 PREPARATION OF PARENTERAL NUTRITION SOLUTIONS

Typically, parenteral nutrition solutions contain 2.5 to 5% amino acids and 20 to 25% dextrose, plus electrolytes, minerals, vitamins, and trace elements sufficient to meet the patient's estimated daily requirements. Intravenous fat emulsions offer a concentrated source of calories and can be used as a source of essential fatty acids. In some medical centers and in home parenteral nutrition programs, the fat emulsion is added directly to the parenteral nutrition solution (104). Manual or automated methods of parenteral nutrition preparation are available. The manual method allows the pharmacist to decide the order of mixing and must be undertaken carefully to avoid potential incompatibilities. Manufacturers of automated compounders need to provide the compounding sequence to ensure safety and compatibility.

Parenteral nutrition solutions should be prepared in the pharmacy by appropriately trained staff using strict aseptic procedures and a laminar airflow hood. Although the hypertonicity of the solutions is not ideal for growth of many bacterial organisms, some pathogens, such as *Candida albicans*, can readily proliferate in these solutions at room temperature (105,106). The total 24-hour requirements for fluids and nutrients are generally prepared in a single container or, occasionally, in multiple containers, depending on the volume of infusate. Parenteral nutrition solutions should be refrigerated immediately if not administered to a patient soon after preparation.

The complex nature of parenteral nutrition solution, including the amino acid–dextrose solutions (2 in 1) and total nutrient admixtures containing the intravenous fat emulsion, requires careful attention to stability and compatibility issues. Total nutrient admixtures add another level of complexity. Acid pH, di- and trivalent cations, and trace elements can be disruptive to the fat emulsion. Only total nutrition admixture formulations that have been well documented should be used, exactly as described. Proper preparation instructions should be obtained directly from the manufacturer of the amino acids and fat emulsion.

Both the American Society for Health-Systems Pharmacists (ASHP) and ASPEN have published quality assurance guidelines on the preparation of sterile products and safe practices related to parenteral nutrition (107,108). These guidelines emphasize policies and procedures for all personnel involved in the preparation of parenteral nutrition, appropriate training and education, facilities and equipment requirements, process validation, expiration dating, and labeling requirements. Observ-

TABLE 17.10
Adult General Parenteral Nutrition Order Form

Adult Parenteral Nutrition Order Form

TPN orders must be written by 1400.

Date:_____   Time:_____   ☐ Central Use Only

Weight:_____   PN Day #: _____   ☐ Peripheral Use Only

ORDER TOTAL AMOUNT PER 24 HOURS

Amino Acids (Source _____)   _____ g

Dextrose   _____ g

Sodium, Total (_____ mEq)	Sodium Chloride	_____ mEq
_____ mEq/l	Sodium Acetate	_____ mEq
	Sodium Phosphate	_____ mEq
Potassium, Total (_____mEq)	Potassium Chloride	_____ mEq
_____ mEq/l	Potassium Acetate	_____ mEq
	Potassium Phosphate	_____ mEq
Calcium Gluconate (_____mEq/l)		_____ mEq
Magnesium Sulfate (_____mEq/l)		_____ mEq
Multivitamins _____		_____ ml
Zinc		_____ mg

_____

_____   _____

_____   _____

_____   _____

         _____

Total Final Volume: _____ ml   to infuse at _____ ml/h

Fat Emulsion 20% _____ ml   to infuse at _____ ml/h

Signature:_____   Print Name:_____

Beeper: _____

TABLE 17.11
Pediatric General Parenteral Nutrition Order Form

Pediatric Parenteral Nutrition Order Form

TPN orders must be written by 1400.

Date:_____   Time:_____   ☐ Central Use Only

Weight:_____   PN Day #: _____   ☐ Peripheral Use Only

ORDER TOTAL AMOUNT PER 24 HOURS

Amino Acids (Source _____)	_____ g
Dextrose _____ g	

Sodium, Total (_____ mEq)	Sodium Chloride	_____ mEq
_____ mEq/l	Sodium Acetate	_____ mEq
	Sodium Phosphate	_____ mEq

Potassium, Total (_____ mEq)	Potassium Chloride	_____ mEq
_____ mEq/l	Potassium Acetate	_____ mEq
	Potassium Phosphate	_____ mEq

Calcium Gluconate (_____mEq/l)	_____ mEq
Magnesium Sulfate (_____mEq/l)	_____ mEq
Multivitamins _____	_____ ml
Zinc	_____ mg

_____   _____

_____   _____

_____   _____

_____   _____

Total Final Volume: _____ ml	to infuse at _____ ml/h
Fat Emulsion 20% _____ ml	to infuse at _____ ml/h

Signature:_____   Print Name:_____

Beeper: _____

ing the physical appearance of the final admixture for gross particulate contamination is one of the most fundamental quality assurance measures that pharmacists routinely apply. For total nutrient admixtures, the products should be inspected for any visual signs of phase separation. When possible, quantitative end-product testing of the accuracy of all additives to the parenteral nutrition solution should be done on a routine basis.

REFERENCES

1. Dudrick, S.J. et al., Long-term TPN with growth, development, and positive nitrogen balance, *Surgery*, 64, 134, 1968.
2. Wilmore, D.W. and Dudrick, S.J., Growth and development of an infant receiving all nutrients exclusively by vein, *JAMA*, 203, 140, 1968.
3. Heyland, D.K. et al., TPN in the critically ill patient: meta analysis, *JAMA*, 280, 2013, 1998.
4. Heyland, D.K. et al., Total parenteral nutrition in the surgical patient: a meta-analysis, *Can. J. Surg.*, 44, 102, 2001.
5. Torosian, M.H., Perioperative nutrition support for patients undergoing gastrointestinal surgery: critical analysis and recommendations, *World J. Surg.*, 23, 565, 1999.
6. McGeer, A.J., Detsky, A.S., and O'Rourke, K., Parenteral nutrition in cancer patients undergoing chemotherapy: a meta analysis, *Nutrition*, 6, 233, 1990.
7. Koretz, R.L., Lipman, T.O., and Klein, S., AGA technical review on parenteral nutrition, *Gastroenterology*, 212, 770, 2001.
8. Guideline for the use of parenteral and enteral nutrition in adult and pediatric patients, *JPEN*, 26, 1SA, 2002.
9. Holliday, M.A. and Segar, W.E., The maintenance need for water in parenteral fluid therapy, *Pediatrics*, 19, 823, 1957.
10. Food and Nutrition Board, Institute of Medicine, Dietary reference intakes for energy, carbohydrate, fiber, fat, fatty acids, cholesterol, protein, and amino acids, National Academy Press, Washington, DC, 2002.
11. Flancbaum, L. et al., Comparison of indirect calorimetry, the Fick method, and prediction equations in estimating the energy requirements of critically ill patients, *Am. J. Clin. Nutr.*, 69, 461, 1999.
12. Reeves, M.M. and Capra, S., Predicting energy requirements in the clinical settings: are methods evidence based? *Nutr. Rev.*, 61, 143, 2003.
13. MacDonald, A. and Hildebrandt, L., Comparison of formulaic equations to determine energy expenditure in the critically ill patient, *Nutrition*, 19, 233, 2003.
14. Phelps, S.P. and Cochran, E.B., Effect of the continuous administration of fat emulsion on the infiltration of intravenous lines in infants receiving peripheral parenteral nutrition solutions, *JPEN*, 13, 628, 1989.
15. Randolph, A.G. et al., Benefit of heparin in peripheral venous and arterial catheters, *BMJ*, 316, 969, 1998.
16. Shah, P. and Shah, V., Continuous heparin infusion to prevent thrombosis and catheter occlusion in neonates with peripherally placed percutaneous central venous catheters, *Cochrane Database Syst. Rev.*, 3, CD002772, 2001.
17. Barrington, K.J., Umbilical artery catheters in the newborn: effects of heparin, *Cochrane Database Syst. Rev.*, 2, CD000507, 2000.
18. Kamala F. et al., Randomized controlled trial of heparin for prevention of blockage of peripherally inserted central catheters in neonates, *Acta. Paediatr.*, 91,1350, 2002.
19. Dupont, I.E. and Carpentier, Y.A., Clinical use of lipid emulsions, *Curr. Opin. Clin. Nutr. Metab. Care*, 2, 139, 1999.
20. American Academy of Pediatrics Committee on Nutrition, Recommendations for use of intravenous fat emulsions in children, *Pediatrics*, 68, 738, 1981.
21. Uauy, R. and Castillo, C., Lipid requirements of infants: Implications for nutrient composition of fortified complementary foods, *J. Nutr.*, 133, 2962S, 2003.
22. Haumont, D. et al., Plasma lipid and plasma lipoprotein concentrations in low birth weight infants given parenteral nutrition with twenty or ten percent lipid emulsion, *J. Pediatr.*, 115, 787, 1989.

23. Haumont, D. et al., Effect of liposomal content of lipid emulsions on plasma lipid concentration in low birth weight infants receiving parenteral nutrition, *J. Pediatr.*, 121, 759, 1992.
24. Silvers, K.M., Darlow, B.A., and Winterbourn, C.C., Lipid peroside and hydrogen peroxide formation in parenteral nutrition solutions containing multivitamins, *JPEN*, 25, 14, 2001.
25. Neuzil, J. et al., Oxidation of parenteral lipid emulsion by ambient and phototherapy lights: potential toxicity of routine parenteral feeding, *J. Pediatr.*, 126, 785, 1995.
26. Helbock, H.J., Motchnik, P.A., and Ames, B.N., Toxic hydroperoxides in intravenous lipid emulsions used in preterm infants, *Pediatrics*, 91, 83, 1993.
27. Baird, L.L., Protecting TPN and lipid infusions from light: reducing hydroperoxides in NICU patients, *Neonatal Netw.*, 20, 17, 2001.
28. Freeman, J. et al., Association of intravenous lipid emulsion and coagulase negative staphylococcal bacteremia in neonatal intensive care units, *N. Eng. J. Med.*, 323, 301, 1990.
29. Avila-Figueroa, C. et al., Intravenous lipid emulsions are major determinant of coagulase negative staphylococcal bacteremia in very low birth weight newborns, *Pediatr. Infect. Dis. J.*, 17, 10, 1988.
30. Guillou, P.J., The effects of lipids on some aspects of the cellular immune response, *Proc. Nutr. Soc.*, 52, 91, 1993.
31. Pomposelli, J.J. and Bistrian, B.R., Is total parenteral nutrition immunosuppressive? *New Horiz.*, 2, 224, 1994.
32. Suchner, U. and Senftleben, U., Immune modulation by polyunsaturated fatty acids during nutrition therapy: interactions with synthesis and effects of eicosanoids, *Infusionsther. Transusionsmed.*, 21, 167, 1994.
33. Garnacho Montero, J. et al., Lipids and immune function, *Nutr. Hosp.*, 11, 230, 1996.
34. Yaqoob, P., Lipids and the immune response, *Curr. Opin. Clin. Nutr. Metab. Care*, 1, 163, 1998.
35. Lennsen, P. et al., Intravenous lipid dose and incidence of bacteremia and fungemia in patients undergoing bone marrow transplantation, *Am. J. Clin. Nutr.*, 67, 927, 1998.
36. Carpentier, Y.A. and Dupont, I.E., Advances in intravenous lipid emulsions, *World J. Surg.*, 24, 1493, 2000.
37. Freeman, J.B. et al., Safety and efficacy of a new peripheral intravenously administered amino acid solution containing glycerol and electrolytes, *Surg. Gynecol. Obstet.*, 156, 625, 1983.
38. Lev-Ran, A. et al., Double-blind study of glycerol vs. glucose in parenteral nutrition of postsurgical insulin-treated diabetic patients, *JPEN,* 11, 271, 1987.
39. Waxman, K. et al., Safety and efficacy of glycerol and amino acids in combination with lipid emulsion for peripheral parenteral nutrition support, *JPEN*, 16, 374, 1992.
40. Bresson, J.L. et al., Energy substrate utilization in infants receiving total parenteral nutrition with different glucose to fat ratios, *Pediatr. Res.*, 25, 645, 1989.
41. Jones, M.O. et al., Glucose utilization in the surgical newborn infant receiving total parenteral nutrition, *J. Pediatr. Surg.*, 28, 1121, 1993.
42. Coss-Bu, J.A. et al., Energy metabolism, nitrogen balance, and substrate utilization in critically ill children, *Am. J. Clin. Nutr.*, 74, 644, 2001.
43. Sheridan, R.L. et al., Maximal parenteral glucose oxidation in hypermetabolic young children: a stable isotope study, *JPEN*, 22, 212, 1998.
44. Burke, J.J. et al., Glucose requirements following burn injury. Parameters of optimal glucose infusion and possible hepatic and respiratory abnormalities following excessive glucose intake, *Ann. Surg.*, 190, 274, 1979.
45. Wolfe, R.R. et al., Investigation of factors determining the optimal glucose infusion rate in total parenteral nutrition, *Metabolism*, 29, 892, 1980.
46. Van den Berghe, G. et al., Intensive insulin therapy in critically ill patients. *N. Engl. J. Med.*, 345, 1359, 2001.
47. Van den Berghe, G. et al., Outcome benefit of intensive insulin therapy in the critically ill: insulin dose versus glycemic control, *Crit. Care Med.*, 31, 359, 2003.
48. Finney, S.J. et al., Glucose control and mortality in the critically ill patients. *JAMA*, 290, 2041, 2003.
49. Abel, R.M. et al., Improved survival from acute renal failure after treatment with intravenous essential L-amino acids, *N. Engl. J. Med.*, 228, 695, 1973.

50. Freund, H.R., Atamian, S., and Fischer, J.E., Comparative study of parenteral nutrition in renal failure using essential and nonessential amino acid containing solutions, *Surg. Gynecol. Obstet.*, 151, 652, 1980.

51. Mirallo, J.M. et al., A comparison of essential and general amino acid infusion in the nutritional support of patients with compromised renal function, *JPEN*, 6, 109, 1982.

52. Feinstein, E.L. et al., Clinical and metabolic responses to parenteral nutrition in acute renal failure: a controlled double-blind study, *Medicine*, 60, 124, 1981.

53. Fsicher, J.E. and Baldessarini, J.R., False neurotransmitters and hepatic failure, *Lancet*, 2, 75, 1971.

54. James, J.H. et al., Hyperammonaemia, plasma amino acid imbalance, and blood–brain amino acid transport: a unified therapy of portal-systemic encephalopathy, *Lancet* 2, 772, 1979.

55. Ferenci, P. and Wewalka, F., Plasma amino acids in hepatic encephalopathy, *J. Neural. Transm. Suppl.*, 14, 87, 1978.

56. Cacino, A. et al., Plasma amino acids imbalance in patients with liver disease, *Am. J. Dig. Dis.*, 23, 591, 1978.

57. Watanabe, A. et al., Characteristics changes in serum amino acid levels in different types of hepatic encephalopathy, *Gastroenterol. Jpn.*, 17, 218, 1982.

58. Campollo, O., Sprengers, D., and McIntyre, N., The BCAA/AAA ratio of plasma amino acids in three different groups of cirrhotics, *Rev. Invest. Clin.*, 44, 513, 1992.

59. Cerra, F.B. et al., Disease specific amino acid infusion (F080) in hepatic encephalopathy. A prospective, randomized, double-blind controlled trial, *JPEN*, 9, 288, 1985.

60. Rocchi, E. et al., Standard or branched-chain amino acid infusions as short-term nutritional support in liver cirrhosis?, *JPEN*, 9, 447, 1985.

61. Naylor, C.D. et al., Parenteral nutrition with branched-chain amino acids in hepatic encephalopathy: a meta-analysis, *Gastroenterology*, 97, 1033, 1989.

62. Egberts, E.H. et al., Branched-chain amino acids in the treatment of latent portosystemic encephalopathy: a double-blind placebo-controlled crossover study, *Gastroenterology*, 88, 887, 1985.

63. Marchesini, G. et al., Nutritional supplementation with branched-chain amino acids in advanced cirrhosis: a double-blind randomized trial, *Gastroenterology*, 127, 1792, 2003.

64. Vilstrup, H. et al., Branched-chain enriched amino acid versus glucose treatment of hepatic encephalopathy: a double-blind study of 65 patients with cirrhosis, *J. Hepatol.*, 10, 291, 1990.

65. Michel, H. et al., Treatment of acute hepatic encephalopathy in cirrhotics with a branched-chain amino acids enriched versus a conventional amino acids mixture: a controlled study of 70 patients, *Liver*, 5, 282, 1985.

66. Buse, M.G. and Reid, S.S., Leucine: a possible regulator of protein turnover in muscle, *J. Clin. Invest.*, 56, 1250, 1975.

67. Cerra, F. et al., The effect of stress level, amino acid formula, and nitrogen dose on nitrogen retention in traumatic and septic stress, *Ann. Surg.*, 205, 282, 1987.

68. Von Meyenfeldt, M.F. et al., Effect of branched-chain amino acid enrichment of total parenteral nutrition sparing and clinical outcome of sepsis and trauma: a prospective randomized double-blind trial, *Br. J. Surg.*, 77, 924, 1990.

69. Kuhl, D.A. et al., Use of selected visceral protein measurements in the comparison of branched-chain amino acids with standard amino acids in parenteral nutrition support of injured patients, *Surgery*, 107, 503, 1990.

70. Bower, R.H. et al., Branched chain amino acid enriched solution in the septic patient: a randomized prospective trial, *Ann. Surg.*, 203, 13, 1986.

71. Winters, R.W. et al., Plasma amino acids in infants receiving parenteral nutrition, in *Clinical Nutrition Update: Amino Acids*, Greene, H.L., Holliday, M.A., and Munro, H.N., Eds., American Medical Association, Chicago, 1977, 147.

72. Wu, P.Y.K., Edwards, N.B., and Storm, M.C., The plasma amino acid pattern of normal term breast-fed infants, *J. Pediatr.*, 109, 347, 1986.

73. Heird, W.C. et al., Pediatric parenteral amino acid mixture in low birth weight infants, *J. Pediatr.*, 81, 41, 1988.

74. Heird, W.C. et al., Evaluation of an amino acid mixture designed to maintain normal plasma amino acid patterns in infants and children receiving parenteral nutrition, *Pediatrics*, 80, 401, 1987.

75. Helms, R.A. et al., Comparison of a pediatric versus standard amino acid formulation in preterm neonates requiring parenteral nutrition, *J. Pediatr.*, 110, 466, 1987.

76. Helms, R.A. et al., Cysteine supplementation results in normalization of plasma taurine concentrations in children receiving home parenteral nutrition, *J. Pediatr.,* 134, 358, 1999.

77. Storm, M.C. and Helms, R.A., Cysteine supplementation normalizes plasma taurine concentrations in low birth weight premature infants requiring parenteral nutrition support, *JPEN,* 27, S4, 2003.

78. Novak, F. et al., Glutamine supplementation in serious illness: a systematic review of the evidence, *Crit. Care Med.*, 30, 2022, 2002.

79. Boelens, P.G. et al., Glutamine alimentation in catabolic state, *J. Nutr.*, 131, 2569S, 2001.

80. Heyland, D.K., In search of the magic nutraceutical: problems with current approaches, *J. Nutr.,* 131, 2591S, 2001.

81. Buchman AL., Glutamine: commercially essential or conditionally essential? A critical appraisal of the human data., *Am. J. Clin. Nutr.,* 74, 25, 2001.

82. American Medical Association Department of Foods and Nutrition, Multivitamin preparations for parenteral use: a statement by the Nutrition Advisory Group, *JPEN,* 3, 258, 1979.

83. Green, H.L. et al., Guidelines for the use of vitamins, trace elements, calcium magnesium, and phosphorous in infants and children receiving total parenteral nutrition: report of the Subcommittee on Pediatric Parenteral Nutrient Requirements from the Committee on Clinical Practice issues of the American Society for Clinical Nutrition, *Am. J. Clin. Nutr.*, 48, 1324, 1988.

84. Parenteral multivitamins products, drugs for human use: drug efficacy study implementation: amendment (21 CFR 5.70), *Federal Register*, April 20, 2000, 65, 21200.

85. Lactic acidosis traced thiamine deficiency related to nationwide shortage of multivitamins for total parenteral nutrition, *Morb. Mortal. Wkly. Rep.*, 46, 523, 1997.

86. American Medical Association Department of Foods and Nutrition, Guideline for essential trace element preparations for parenteral use: a statement by an expert panel, *JAMA*, 241, 2051. 1979.

87. Baptista, R.J. et al., Utilizing selenious acid to reverse selenium deficiency in total parenteral nutrition patients, *Am. J. Clin. Nutr.*, 39, 816, 1984.

88. Hunt, D.R. et al., Selenium depletion in burn patients, *JPEN,* 8, 865, 1984.

89. Moukarzel, A.A. et al., Excessive chromium intake in children receiving total parenteral nutrition, *Lancet*, 339, 385, 1992.

90. Mouser, J.F. et al., Chromium and zinc concentrations in pediatric patients receiving long-term parenteral nutrition, *Am. J. Health Syst. Pharm.*, 56, 1950, 1999.

91. Polinsky, M.S. and Gruskin, A.B., Aluminum toxicity in children with chronic renal failure, *J. Pediatr.*, 105, 758, 1984.

92. Baluarte, H.J. et al., Encephalopathy in children with chronic renal failure, *Proc. Dial. Transplant. Forum*, 7, 95, 1977.

93. Foley, C.M. et al., Encephalopathy in infants and children with chronic renal disease, *Arch. Neurol.*, 38, 656, 1981.

94. Sedman, A.B. et al., Encephalopathy in childhood secondary to aluminum toxicity, *J. Pediatr.*, 105, 836, 1984.

95. Alfrey, A.C., LeGendre, G.R., and Kaehny, W.D., The dialysis encephalopathy syndrome: possible aluminum intoxication, *N. Engl. J. Med.*, 294, 184, 1976.

96. Ward, M.K. et al., Osteomalacic dialysis osteodystrophy: evidence for a water-borne aetiological agent, probably aluminum, *Lancet*, 1, 841, 1978.

97. Sedman, A.B. et al., Response to aluminum in parenteral nutrition during infancy, *J. Pediatr.*, 109, 877, 1986.

98. Koo, W.W.K. et al., Aluminum in parenteral solutions: sources and possible alternative, *JPEN,* 10, 591, 1986.

99. Ott, S.M. et al., Aluminum is associated with low bone formation in patients receiving chronic parenteral nutrition, *Ann. Intern. Med.*, 98, 910, 1983.

100. Department of Health and Human Services, Food and Drug Administration, Aluminum in large and small volume parenteral used in total parenteral nutrition. Proposed rule, *Fed. Regist.*, 63, 176, 1998.

101. Department of Health and Human Services, Food and Drug Administration, Aluminum in large and small volume parenteral used in total parenteral nutrition. Final rule, *Fed. Regist.*, 65, 4103, 2000.

102. Department of Health and Human Services, Food and Drug Administration, Aluminum in large and small volume parenteral used in total parenteral nutrition. Final rule; delay of effective date, *Fed. Regist.*, 68, 32979, 2003.

103. ASCN/ASPEN Working Group on Standards for Aluminum Content of Parenteral Solutions, Klein, G.L., Alfrey, A.C., Shike, M., Sherrard, D.J., Parenteral drug products containing aluminum as an ingredient or a contaminant: response to FDA notice of intent, *Am. J. Clin. Nutr.*, 53, 399, 1991.

104. Brown, R., Quercia, R.Q., and Sigman, T., Total nutrient admixture; a review, *JPEN*, 10, 650, 1986.

105. Goldman, D.A., Martin, W.R., and Worthington, J.W., Growth of bacteria and fungi in total parenteral nutrition solutions, *Am. J. Surg.*, 126, 314, 1973.

106. Brennan, M.F. et al., The growth of *Candida albicans* in nutritive solutions given parenterally, *Arch. Surg.*, 103, 705, 1971.

107. ASHP guidelines on quality assurance of pharmacy-prepared sterile products. American Society of Health System Pharmacists, *Am. J. Health Syst. Pharm.*, 57, 1150, 2000.

108. Safe practices for parenteral nutrition formulations: national advisory group on standards and practice guidelines for parenteral nutrition, *JPEN*, 22, 1, 1998.

18 Complications of Parenteral Feeding

Elaina E. Szeszycki
CVS Pharmacy and Coram Healthcare

Suzanne Benjamin
Indiana University Hospital

CONTENTS

18.1 INTRODUCTION

Research and reporting in nutrition support has escalated in the past century, and with updated information, parenteral nutrition (PN) requirements have been refined. The constant fine-tuning of PN solutions and individualizing requirements for certain patient populations should be based on sound evidence and appropriate clinical judgment. The goal is to meet the patient's individual needs while providing the safest solution possible. Although meeting the patient's requirements is not always possible, especially in the critically ill patient, PN should always be provided in the safest manner by those writing for, compounding, and administering these solutions.

Unfortunately, PN is not without risk, but there is some guidance for minimizing complications related to parenteral nutrition. Monitoring nutrition support in critically ill patients is complicated by comorbid disease states and altered hemodynamic status. These confounding factors always need to be appreciated when prescribing and monitoring PN. This chapter is dedicated to identifying complications related to parenteral nutrition and how best to prevent or minimize these complications. Complications are generally separated into three categories: technical, infectious, and metabolic.

18.2 TECHNICAL COMPLICATIONS

Most technical complications are related to the insertion of intravenous catheters and can be very serious or potentially fatal. The most common are listed in Table 18.1. Catheter placement should only be performed by experienced personnel who are familiar with their institution's policies and procedures for catheter placement.

18.2.1 PERIPHERAL

Peripheral lines are for parenteral solutions containing 900 mOsm/l or less, whereas central venous lines are for solutions greater than 900 mOsm/l. Incidence of phlebitis, pain, inflammation, and scarring increase dramatically when solution osmolality exceeds 900 mOsm/l via a peripheral line.[1] Besides osmolality, other factors that can contribute to phlebitis include insertion site, vein size, duration of insertion, cannular size, material, and colonization. Peripheral lines should be rotated every 48 to 72 hours to prevent thrombosis and phlebitis.[2] Heparin 1 unit/ml and hydrocortisone 10 mg/l have been added to peripheral parenteral nutrition in hopes of decreasing phlebitis.[3]

There is limited use for peripheral lines in the intensive care patient, but these may be the only alternative if central venous access cannot be obtained due to catheter-related sepsis, high risk of bleeding, or poor venous access (e.g., long-term PN for short bowel patients).

18.2.2 PERIPHERALLY INSERTED CENTRAL CATHETER (PICC)

PICC lines may be an option for central parenteral nutrition if a central venous line cannot be placed and PN is required for longer than two weeks. This is still not ideal for critically ill patients, with the availability of only single- or double-lumen PICCs. Double-lumen PICCs are known for increased mechanical problems.[4] Most patients will still require additional venous access for intravenous fluids, medications, blood products, and blood sampling. Infectious complications tend to be fewer in PICC lines than in percutaneous central venous catheters, but mechanical complications and limited access are significant disadvantages of PICC lines in the intensive care patient.[5]

18.2.3 CENTRAL

Central venous access is the preferred route in critically ill patients when parenteral nutrition is indicated, as discussed in Chapter 5 and Chapter 12. Central access allows for maximizing nutrient delivery while minimizing volume. Again, these devices and their placement are not without risk, and the diagnosis and treatment of mechanical complications are reviewed in detail in Chapter 14 and elsewhere.[5,6]

Catheter occlusion can be divided into thrombotic or nonthrombotic, with ~95% of occlusions being thrombotic.[5] Catheter occlusion is not seen routinely in critically ill patients but is still worth discussing, because patients on long-term PN may become acutely ill and require intensive care. Central venous thrombosis can be a significant problem if it develops into pulmonary embolism, an infected clot, or loss of central venous access at the involved site.[6] Factors contributing to venous thrombosis have been well described as the Triad of Virchow and include damage to the vessel wall, changes in blood flow, and alterations in the composition of the blood.[7] Fibrin sheaths made up of fibrin and platelets form at the tip of the catheter as a result of foreign body response. The sheath will eventually clot a catheter, and a thrombolytic agent, such as urokinase, heparin, TPA, or reteplase, will be required to open the catheter. Thrombolytic therapy is contraindicated in several patient populations (Table 18.2).[8]

TABLE 18.1
Catheter-Related Complications Associated with Parenteral Nutrition (PN)

Complication	Possible Etiology	Symptoms	Treatment	Prevention
Pneumothorax	Catheter placement by inexperienced personnel	Tachycardia, dyspnea, persistent cough, diaphoresis	A small pneumothorax may resolve untreated; a larger pneumothorax may require chest tube placement	Catheter placement by experienced personnel
Air embolism	Occurs when line is interrupted and air is inspired while the line is uncapped	Cyanosis, tachypnea, hypotension, churning heart murmur (classic sign)	Immediately place patient on the left side and lower the head of the bed; this may keep the air within the apex of the right ventricle until it is reabsorbed	Line placement by appropriately trained personnel
Catheter embolization	Pulling the catheter back through the needle used for insertion	Cardiac arrhythmias	Surgically remove the catheter tip	Avoid withdrawing the catheter through the insertion needle
Venous thrombosis	Mechanical trauma to vein, hypotension, solution osmolality, hypercoagulopathy, sepsis	Swelling or pain in neck or one or both arms or shoulders	Anticoagulation therapy with urokinase or streptokinase; remove catheter	Use of silicone catheter; addition of heparin to PN; low-dose warfarin therapy
Catheter occlusion	Hypotension; failure to maintain line patency; formation of fibrin sheath outside the catheter; solution precipitates	Increasing need for greater pressure to maintain a continuous infusion rate	Anticoagulation therapy with urokinase or streptokinase	Use of a large-diameter catheter as appropriate; routine flushes of catheter; monitor for solution precipitation
Improper tip location	Venous vasculature anomalies; catheter placement by inexperienced personnel	Phlebitis; severe cardiorespiratory distress; possible thrombosis	Remove catheter	Proper catheter placement by properly trained personnel
Phlebitis	Peripheral administration of hypertonic solution (osmolarity ≥ 900 mOsm/kg); line infiltration	Redness, swelling, pain at peripheral site	Change peripheral line site, start central PN if appropriate	Minimize osmolarity of peripheral solution by using lipids as primary source of calories; reduce addition of electrolytes and other PN additives as possible
Catheter-related sepsis	Inappropriate technique in line placement; poor catheter care; contaminated solution	Unexplained fever, chills; red, indurated area around catheter site; possible catheter tip	Remove catheter and replace at another site	Development of strict protocols for line placement and catheter care

Source: From Skipper, A. and Marian, M.J., *Nutrition Support Dietetics Core Curriculum*, 2nd ed., ASPEN, Silver Spring, MD, 1993. With permission

TABLE 18.2
Contraindications to Thrombolytic Therapy

1. Active internal bleeding
2. Recent cerebral vascular accident (CVA)
3. Intracranial or intraspinal surgery within 2 months
4. Recent trauma
5. Intracranial neoplasm
6. Arteriovenous (AV) malformation
7. Aneurysm
8. Known bleeding diatheses
9. Severe uncontrolled arterial hypertension

Nonthrombotic occlusion can occur due to lipid sludge, calcium–phosphate precipitates, or precipitate from incompatible medications. These occlusions can be treated, respectively, with ethanol,[9] hydrochloric acid,[10] and sodium bicarbonate.[5] Parenteral solutions should be monitored closely for any precipitate or destabilized emulsion of a total nutrient admixture. The human eye can only detect ≥ 50 microns but a precipitate or globule 5 microns in size can occlude a pulmonary capillary.[11] For this very reason, professionals responsible for ordering and compounding PN solutions should adhere to their institution's specific compatibility guidelines for electrolytes, vitamins, minerals, and medications. Exceeding the guidelines may result in precipitate or globule occlusion and even fatality, as seen with erroneous compounding of a PN formula.[12] Pharmacists involved with nutrition support or the compounding of parenteral nutrient solutions should be consulted whenever a compatibility question arises.

18.3 INFECTIOUS COMPLICATIONS

Infectious complications are the greatest cause of morbidity and mortality in patients receiving specialized intravenous nutrition support. Many infections are related to the central venous catheter (CVC), with the incidence ranging from 3 to 20% in hospitalized patients. Rates are 2 to 5 times higher in the critically ill patient. Bacterial systemic infections related to the catheter occur in 3 to 7% of CVCs.[2] Risk factors influencing sepsis include patient characteristics, therapy, catheter properties, and maintenance procedures.[13] Refer to Table 18.3 for guidelines regarding prevention of catheter-related infections.[14] Because the glucose content in central PN is a good medium for bacterial growth, it is recommended that PN be administered through a dedicated port of a central line that has not been used for any other therapy.[2] Refer to Section 18.4.2 for specific lipid administration guidelines.

PN is associated with an increase in non–catheter-related infections, which may be related to overfeeding, hyperglycemia, immunosuppression by intravenous (IV) lipid, missing nutrients (e.g., taurine, choline, vitamins, minerals), and nonluminal delivery of nutrients.[15] Great strides have been made in the past 10 to 20 years to improve the constituents of PN and how PN is delivered. Recommended calorie intake is less, more aggressive blood glucose control is becoming a standard of therapy, enteral nutrition is encouraged when possible, new lipid products are being evaluated, and a variety of missing nutrients are being studied for their usefulness in specialized nutrition support. (See Chapter 11.)

18.4 METABOLIC COMPLICATIONS

Metabolic complications related to macronutrient and micronutrient composition of PN can be minimized by following published guidelines and fastidious monitoring.

TABLE 18.3
Guidelines for Prevention of Catheter-Related Infections in Parenteral Nutrition Patients

1. Insertion and maintenance of intravascular catheters by experienced staff or specialized IV teams
2. Adequate nursing staff
3. Continuous quality assurance and education
4. Routine infection-control surveillance
5. Maximal barrier precautions
6. Observe hand hygiene and aseptic technique during care of catheters.
7. Chlorhexidine for skin antiseptic
8. Designate one port exclusively for PN when multilumen catheter in place.
9. Antimicrobial/antiseptic-impregnated catheters and cuffs in high risk patients when standard procedures fail
10. Systemic antibiotic and antibiotic lock prophylaxis is not recommended for routine use, due to possible resistance.
11. Antibiotic ointments are not recommended routinely due to possible resistance and catheter incompatibility.
12. Monitor catheter sites visually or by palpation through intact dressing on a regular basis.
13. Change dressings at least weekly and more frequently if site of dressing becomes damp, loosened, or soiled.
14. Prophylactic heparin is used routinely to prevent central venous thrombosis.
15. Routine parenteral fluids should be admixed in the pharmacy in a laminar-flow hood using aseptic technique.
16. Replacement of administration sets every 24 h is recommended for total nutrient admixtures and separate lipids.
17. Complete separate lipid infusions within 12 h if possible and total nutrient admixtures within 24 h of hang time.
18. Replace catheter if catheter-related infection or mechanical problem is suspected, no routine change recommended.
19. Discontinue catheter when medically possible.

Individual substrates will be discussed in detail as to the possible ensuing complications and how best to prevent these complications. Table 18.4 summarizes most metabolic complications that can occur while patients are receiving PN. Hypervolemia is more common in critically ill patients than hypovolemia, due to fluid overload from increased vascular permeability associated with the systemic inflammatory response syndrome (SIRS).[16] Because of this, fluid restriction to as low as 1 l/d is sometimes necessary. Compounding with concentrated dextrose 70%, amino acid 15%, and lipid 30% solutions are useful in these situations to maximize the PN formula. It is difficult to provide adequate nutrition support in this small volume, but limiting the dangers of fluid overload on lung function and gas exchange is a priority. Once the fluid balance improves, PN volume can be increased to meet the nutritional needs of the patient more adequately.

18.4.1 Dextrose

Carbohydrate, provided as dextrose, administered in excess can cause hyperglycemia, increased carbon dioxide production leading to respiratory compromise, and hepatic complications. In addition to hyperglycemia, critically ill patients are hyperinsulinemic and exhibit peripheral insulin resistance. Prolonged hyperglycemia may cause mobilization of fatty acids and therefore elevated triglyceride levels.

Hyperglycemia can also occur if the rate of initiation of the parenteral nutrition is not gradually increased, especially in the critically ill patient. Parenteral dextrose may aggravate existing hyperglycemia caused by the stress response that occurs due to the release of counterregulatory hormones.[17] This results in increased hepatic glucose production and decreased peripheral glucose uptake. Cytokines and interleukins, also released during an inflammatory response, may negatively affect carbohydrate metabolism and glucose levels. Fingerstick or arterial blood glucose should be monitored every two to six hours, depending on insulin requirements and overall clinical status of the patient, with a goal of maintaining blood glucose at 100 to 200 mg/dl.[18] If blood glucose continues to be elevated, patients may require subcutaneous insulin via a sliding scale. Likewise, if the rate of administration and the concentration of glucose in the PN solution remain stable, two-thirds of the 24-hour quantity of supplemental insulin can be added to the next bag of PN.

TABLE 18.4
Metabolic Complications Associated with Parenteral Nutrition (PN)

Complication	Possible Etiology	Symptoms	Treatment	Prevention
Hypervolemia	Excess fluid administration; renal dysfunction; congestive heart failure; hepatic failure	Dyspnea, bounding pulse, moist rales, edema, weight gain	Restrict fluid; use diuretics; dialysis in extreme cases	Initiate PN once fluid balance stable; monitor input and output; monitor serum and urine osmolality
Hypovolemia	Inadequate fluid administration; overdiuresis	Dehydration, thirst, dry mucous membranes, decreased urine output, decreased weight	Increase fluid intake	Monitor daily intake and output; monitor serum and urine osmolality
Hyperkalemia	Renal dysfunction; excessive potassium administration; metabolic acidosis; use of potassium-sparing medication	Diarrhea, tachycardia, cardiac arrest, oliguria, paresthesias	Decrease potassium intake; use potassium binders	Monitor serum levels for trends; assess for drug–nutrient interactions, especially potassium-sparing diuretics
Hypokalemia	Inadequate potassium provision; increased potassium losses (diarrhea, diuretics, intestinal fistulas)	Nausea, vomiting, confusion, arrhythmias, cardiac arrest, respiratory depression	Increase PN potassium or provide intravenously	Give 40 mEq of potassium daily unless contraindicated, 3 mEq of potassium per gram of nitrogen needed with anabolism
Hypernatremia	Inadequate free water administration; excessive sodium intake; excessive water losses; fever, burns, hyperventilation	Thirst; decreased skin turgor; mild irritability in some cases; elevated serum sodium, BUN, and hematocrit	Decrease sodium intake; replenish fluids	Avoid excess sodium intake; monitor fluid status; monitor urine sodium
Hyponatremia	Excessive fluid administration; nephritis and/or adrenal insufficiency; dilutional states (congestive heart failure, SIADH,[a] cirrhosis with ascites)	Confusion, hypotension, irritability, lethargy, seizures	Restrict fluid intake; increase sodium intake as dictated by clinical status	Avoid overhydration; provide 60 to 100 mEq/d unless contraindicated by cardiac, renal, or fluid status; monitor urine sodium
Hyperglycemia	Rapid infusion of concentrated dextrose solution, sepsis, pancreatitis, postoperative stress, chromium deficiency, use of steroids, advanced age, multiple sources of dextrose from both oral and IV routes	Blood glucose > 200 mg/dl; metabolic acidosis; polyuria, polydipsia	Use insulin; reduce dextrose concentration in PN	Slow initiation and advancement of PN; use mixed substrate solution

Complication	Cause	Signs/Symptoms	Treatment	Prevention/Monitoring
Hypoglycemia	Abrupt discontinuation of PN; insulin overdose	Weakness, sweating, palpitations, lethargy, shallow respirations	Administer dextrose	Taper PN solution; with abrupt discontinuation of TPN, hang 10% dextrose at the same rate as the TPN to prevent rebound hypoglycemia; monitor serum glucose levels with use of insulin
Hypertriglyceridemia	Lipid provision exceeds ability to clear lipids from bloodstream (>4 mg/kg per minute); sepsis, multisystem organ failure, pathologic hyperlipidemia, lipoid nephrosis; medication usage alters fat metabolism (i.e., cyclosporin)	Serum triglyceride level 300–350 mg/dl 6 h past lipid initiation; elevated levels in previously stable patients (i.e., sepsis)	Decrease lipid volume administered; lengthen infusion time; simultaneously infuse glucose	Assess for preexisting history of hyperlipidemia before initiation of PN; avoid lipid administration > 2.5 g/kg per day or >60% of total calories
Hypercalcemia	Renal failure, tumor lysis syndrome; bone cancer; excess vitamin D intake; prolonged immobilization and stress; hyperparathyroidism	Confusion, dehydration, muscle weakness, nausea, vomiting, coma	Administer isotonic saline; inorganic phosphate supplementation; administer corticosteroids, mithramycin	Encourage weight-bearing activity; evaluate vitamin D intake
Hypocalcemia	Decreased vitamin D intake; hypoparathyroidism; citrate binding of calcium due to excessive blood transfusions; hypoalbuminemia	Paresthesias, tetany, irritability, ventricular arrhythmias	Calcium supplementation if truly hypocalcemic, [correction factor = (normal albumin − observed albumin) × 0.8][b]	Provide 15 mEq of calcium daily
Hypermagnesemia	Excessive magnesium administration; renal insufficiency	Respiratory paralysis, hypotension, premature ventricular contractions, lethargy, cardiac arrest, coma, liver dysfunction	Decrease magnesium provision	Monitor serum levels for trends
Hypomagnesemia	Refeeding syndrome; alcoholism; diuretic usage; increased losses (e.g., diarrhea); medications (cyclosporin); diabetic ketoacidosis; chemotherapy	Cardiac arrhythmias, tetany, convulsions, muscular weakness	Magnesium supplementation	Monitor serum levels for trends
Hyperphosphatemia	Excess phosphate administration; renal dysfunction	Paresthesias, flaccid paralysis, mental confusion, hypertension, cardiac arrhythmias, tissue calcification long term	Decrease phosphate administration; phosphate binders	Monitor serum levels for trends

(continued)

TABLE 18.4 (CONTINUED)
Metabolic Complications Associated with Parenteral Nutrition (PN)

Complication	Possible Etiology	Symptoms	Treatment	Prevention
Hypophosphatemia	Refeeding syndrome, alkalosis, insulin therapy, Gram-negative sepsis, persistent vomiting or malabsorption, phosphate binders, hypercalcemia, hyperthyroidism	Muscle weakness, altered speech, "thickened tongue," coma, anemia, peripheral paresthesias	Supplement with potassium phosphate or sodium phosphate, being sure calcium supplementation is adequate	Monitor serum levels for trends; add adequate phosphate to PN: 7–10 mmol/1000 kcals
Prerenal azotemia	Dehydration; excess protein provision; inadequate nonprotein calorie provision with mobilization of own protein stores	Elevated serum BUN	Increase fluid intake; decrease protein load; increase nonprotein calories	Monitor serum BUN for trends; perform nitrogen balance study
Overfeeding	Excess carbohydrate and/or protein administration	Excess carbohydrate: CO_2 retention, cardiac tamponade, liver dysfunction; Excess protein: elevated BUN, excess nitrogen excretion, elevated BUN/Cr ratio	Decrease carbohydrate/protein provision as needed	Avoid excess carbohydrate/protein administration
Essential fatty acid deficiency (EFAD)	Inadequate fat intake	Dermatitis; alopecia; alterations in pulmonary, neurologic, and red cell membranes	Lipid administration	Provide 2–4% of calories as linoleic acid, or 8–10% of calories from fat, especially in patients severely malnourished or expected not to take food by mouth for more than 3 weeks

[a] SIADH: syndrome of inappropriate secretion of antidiuretic hormone.
[b] Correction factor should be added to the observed calcium level.

Source: Adapted from Skipper, A. and Marian, M.J., *Nutrition Support Dietetics Core Curriculum*, 2nd ed., ASPEN, Silver Spring, MD, 1993.

Commonly, critically ill patients are hyperglycemic prior to the initiation of PN, so it is suggested that 0.05 to 0.1 units of regular insulin per gram of dextrose be added to the PN solution. Regular insulin can be advanced by 0.05 units/g up to 0.2 units/g of dextrose. If adequate glucose control is still not obtained, it is suggested to discontinue insulin in the PN and subcutaneous sliding scale and begin a separate, continuous intravenous insulin infusion.[18,19]

Van den Berghe and associates performed a prospective, randomized, controlled study over 12 months in 1548 patients admitted to a surgical intensive care unit. They compared intensive insulin therapy (maintenance of blood glucose between 80 and 110 mg/dl) to conventional insulin therapy (maintenance of blood glucose between 180 and 200 mg/dl) and found reduced mortality and morbidity in the intensive insulin group. The greatest reduction occurred in patients requiring intensive care for more than 5 days.[20] These results and future studies may encourage tighter blood glucose control in critically ill patients than has been previously established.

Strict monitoring is required due to sudden changes in clinical course related to infection, treatment of infection, and other medical therapy; all of which can affect glycemic control. Hypoglycemia may occur if a patient's central PN is abruptly discontinued. If abrupt cessation of PN is necessary, dextrose 10% should be infused until PN can be restarted. Peripheral PN can be abruptly discontinued without complications of hypoglycemia. Although hypoglycemia is uncommon in discontinuation of PN without insulin, it is still recommended to taper the rate over 1 to 2 hours to avoid hypoglycemia.[18]

In order to avoid such complications, it is recommended to initiate PN with 100 to 150 g dextrose per day.[19] It is imperative to take all dextrose-containing solutions into account when calculating daily carbohydrate intake. Most patients in an ICU are fluid restricted but may be receiving multiple medications diluted in dextrose, or renal replacement therapy. Renal replacement therapy may provide an additional 500 to 1000 calories per day, depending on percent dianeal used and amount of fluid replaced. The dialysate solutions used for peritoneal dialysis vary in dextrose concentration from 1.5 to 4.25% and could provide up to 1000 calories, depending on dwell time and frequency of infusions.[21] Identifying all calorie sources is very important, because overfeeding has been associated with hyperglycemia, lipogenesis, hypercapnia, electrolyte abnormalities, increased metabolic rate, and impaired phagocytosis.[5] One study suggests that underfeeding due to inability to reach target needs was associated with better outcomes than higher levels of calorie intake in medical intensive care patients.[22]

Hepatic complications can occur if the patient is being overfed or receiving more carbohydrate than the liver can oxidize. The maximum oxidation rate of carbohydrate is 4 to 7 mg/kg/min in the stressed patient to prevent fat synthesis and deposition of nonoxidized glucose in the liver.[19,23] Alterations in hepatic enzymes may not be seen for two to three weeks, but liver enzymes should be monitored on a weekly basis. Elevation of the serum transaminases and alkaline phosphatase can be seen within one week, whereas an increase in bilirubin usually occurs later. The order in which the preceding levels rise is variable.[24,25] If elevations do occur, all etiologies of hepatic inflammation and dysfunction should be investigated before assuming PN is the culprit. PN administration has been associated with cholestasis, fatty changes, portal inflammation or triaditis, bile duct proliferation, and fibrosis. A retrospective descriptive review by Wolfe and associates, however, concludes otherwise.[26] The authors found a positive correlation between abnormal histologic features in preexisting liver disease, abdominal sepsis, renal failure, and blood transfusions, but not administration of parenteral nutrition. If PN has been determined to be the cause of elevated liver enzymes or cholestasis, total calories can be reduced if the patient is being overfed. If the total calorie intake is appropriate, it may be reasonable to replace some of the carbohydrate calories with lipid. Table 18.5 lists a stepwise approach for minimizing hepatic alterations related to PN.

Patients with chronic obstructive pulmonary disease, bronchitis, or emphysema have a tendency to retain carbon dioxide. Because glucose has a higher (1.0) respiratory quotient, glucose in PN can induce excessive carbon dioxide production and negatively impact respiratory parameters. Also, excessive carbohydrate can increase difficulty in weaning patients from the ventilator. A percentage

TABLE 18.5
Stepwise Approach for Minimizing Hepatic Complications

1. Reevaluate calorie and protein needs and adjust if necessary.
2. Adjust dextrose–lipid ratio up to 40% lipid as nonprotein calories if lipid clearance adequate.
3. Decrease calorie-to-nitrogen ratio closer to 100:1.
4. Review current medications and disease state for hepatotoxic effect.
5. Initiate enteral nutrition when possible.
6. Consider glutamine for maintenance of gastrointestinal tract integrity.

of glucose calories can be replaced with lipid calories to reduce potential respiratory problems, because lipids have a lower respiratory quotient (0.7). Usually, in these patients, 60 to 70% of the calories are provided by carbohydrate, and 30 to 40% of the calories are provided as lipid.[27]

18.4.2 LIPID

Intravenous (IV) lipid emulsions are used routinely in PN as a nonglucose source and for prevention of essential fatty acid deficiency (EFAD). Their advantage as a calorie source is due to the lower respiratory quotient, increased caloric density (~9 kcal/g), and isotonicity, which is beneficial for peripheral PN.[28,29] Contraindications to the use of IV fat include hypertriglyceridemia, hypercholesterolemia, hyperlipidemia and fat metabolism disturbances, and allergy to egg phospholipids.[30] Serum triglyceride levels should be drawn before lipids are infused and then monitored weekly thereafter when lipids are infused daily.

Infusion of fat can saturate the metabolic pathways that generate energy from fats and cause an increase in serum triglycerides. Therefore, IV fat administration should be monitored by following fasting serum triglyceride levels with bolus infusion and steady-state levels. *Fasting levels* are levels that are drawn while the patient is nil per os (NPO). If the patient is receiving continuous IV fat infusion, the triglyceride level can be drawn at any time (if patient is NPO) and assumed at steady-state level. If fat is infused intermittently over 10 to 12 hours, the triglyceride level should be drawn at least 4 hours after the infusion is completed. An acceptable range for the serum triglyceride level is patient specific, but a level of ≤ 400 mg/dl is preferred in the critically ill patient.[31] If postinfusion triglyceride levels equal baseline levels, it is assumed that the IV fat has appropriately cleared.

The maximum hang time for IV fat emulsions recommended by the Centers for Disease Control is 12 hours. This recommendation was subsequent to reports of increased microbial growth in contaminated IV fat emulsions hung for greater than 12 hours, as well as reports of Gram-negative sepsis associated with the administration of IV fat emulsion.[32] Infusion of lipids over 4 to 8 hours in patients with adult respiratory distress syndrome (ARDS) has resulted in pulmonary hypertension, increased lung microvascular pressure, and arterial hypoxemia.[33,34] Although there are reports that contradict these results,[35] the current recommendation is to infuse lipids that are given separately from PN at a slower rate over 10 to 12 hours in critically ill patients to avoid any effect on pulmonary gas exchange. The advantages of adding lipid to PN to make a total nutrient admixture (TNA) are that it allows for slower infusion over 24 hours and further decreases the risk of bacterial growth, because the pH in a TNA prohibits bacterial growth.[36]

Current recommendations for IV fat or lipid administration is 25 to 30% of total calories and no more than 1 g/kg/d in critically ill patients.[5,37] Percent of total calories may be decreased further in septic patients or even eliminated in those patients demonstrating impaired clearance with elevated triglyceride levels (> 400 mg/dl). On the other hand, EFAD can develop after prolonged administration of fat-free PN, so infusion of EFA as 4% of total calories or lipids (not 100% EFA) as 10% of total calories is necessary to prevent EFAD.[38] This can be accomplished by infusing Intralipid® 20% (Kabi Pharmacia Inc., Clayton, NC) 250 ml twice weekly, thereby providing the required EFA intake in less volume over 10 to 12 hours. Potential clinical signs of EFAD include dermatitis, abnormal eye and neurological function, hyperlipidemia, hypercoagulation, and abnormal eicosanoid metabolism.[39] Finally, propofol, a sedative commonly used in the ICU, is contained in a 10% fat emulsion (1.1 kcal/ml) and, depending on the rate of infusion, could provide significant calories and grams of IV fat. These calories and grams of fat need to be taken into consideration when determining lipid intake.

Available commercial lipid preparations in the United States consist exclusively of long-chain triglycerides (LCTs). Earlier studies have demonstrated adequate tolerance, maintenance of nitrogen balance, and prevention or reversal of EFAD,[40–44] but their conclusions cannot be extrapolated to critically ill patients, especially those in a septic state. Additional studies evaluated the effect of lipid emulsion on various immunologic and hematolgoic parameters. Tumor necrosis factor and IL-1 are elevated as part of the stress response to injury and are known to inhibit the activity of lipoprotein lipase that decreases fat clearance. This has prompted a plethora of *in vitro* and *in vivo* animal and human studies. Also, LCTs may not be readily oxidized due to their slow clearance from systemic circulation.[45]

Phagocytotic activity in septic rats was not different between the glucose group and the lipid group.[46] Injured rats had improved function of the reticuloendothelial system (RES) on a medium-chain triglyceride (MCT)–LCT mixture vs. nonprotein calories provided as glucose alone or as glucose plus LCT. Nonprotein calories were equal for all groups.[45] Results of a study done in humans evaluating the effect of LCT emulsion on RES function suggested impaired function after 3 days of daily 10-hour infusions.[47] In contrast, neonates receiving low-dose lipid infusion did not experience any changes in their polymorphonuclear leukocytes or platelet activity after the 16-hour infusion.[48] This was only a one-day study, and results cannot be extrapolated to prolonged IV fat administration.

Monson et al. performed a small, prospective, crossover study in postoperative surgical patients and found improvement of immunological parameters in the PN containing lipid group vs. the PN without lipid group.[49] Battistella and associates found opposite results in their prospective, randomized trial of IV fat emulsion in trauma patients. In this study, one group received a portion of nonprotein calories as lipid and the other group did not, and calories were not replaced with dextrose. The researchers found a higher number of infectious complications and depressed T-cell function in the lipid group and so concluded that these critically injured patients had an increased susceptibility to infection, prolonged pulmonary failure, and delayed recovery. The study groups did not receive isocaloric regimens, and the volume intake may have been less in the glucose only group, so it is unclear whether it was the hypocaloric regimen in less volume or the absence of lipids that affected the results.[50]

A meta-analysis of total parenteral nutrition (TPN) in the critically ill patient was performed using pertinent studies from 1980 to 1998.[51] The results were influenced by patient population, use of lipid, methodological quality, and year of publication. Lower complications, but no difference in mortality, were seen in malnourished patients in earlier studies with lower method scores. No effect on treatment or mortality was seen in studies published since 1989 with higher method scores. Complication rates were lower in studies that did not use lipid, but there was no effect on mortality between studies that did or did not use lipids. Studies evaluating critically ill patients tended to have higher complications and mortality rates than studies with surgical patients.[51]

Canadian clinical practice guidelines for nutrition support in mechanically ventilated, critically ill adult patients were recently published.[52] These guidelines were developed by an expert panel that reviewed randomized clinical trials or meta-analyses of randomized, controlled trials published between 1980 and 2002. These guidelines recommend hypocaloric regimens or withholding lipids in critically ill patients who are not malnourished or are tolerating some enteral feeds, or when PN is indicated for the short term (< 10 days). This particular guideline was based on two studies aiming for ~20 to 25 kcal/kg/d, but patients actually received 65 to 70% of the goal.[22,53] This is only a guideline, and individual patient needs should be addressed. There are insufficient data to make recommendations in patients requiring long-term PN (> 10 days).[52]

More recent data tend to suggest less or no lipid usage in critically ill patients requiring short-term PN, at least until more conclusive evidence is available regarding lipid emulsions containing a mixture of MCT–LCT or MCT—LCT–fish oil. MCTs provide an alternative fat source and have the advantage of being hydrolyzed more rapidly and completely. Formulations with large quantities of MCT do not contain significant quantities of precursors for prostaglandin production and therefore may not exacerbate the stress response in severe illness.[45] Fish oil or omega-3 fatty acids have been found to reduce inflammatory and thrombotic responses, which could be very useful in critically ill patients. The omega-3 fatty acids appear to be incorporated into cell membranes fairly quickly.[54]

The search continues for an ideal lipid emulsion that can be utilized in intensive care patients. The Department of Surgery in Bochum, Germany, studied the impact of omega-3 fatty acid–enriched TPN on leukotriene synthesis by leukocytes after major surgery. This was a prospective, double-blind, randomized study of two parallel groups. Group 1 received Lipoplus® (B. Braun Melsungen AG, Melsungen, Germany) (MCT:LCT:fish oil = 5:4:1), an omega-3 fatty acid (FA)–enriched 20% lipid emulsion. Group 2 received Intralipid®, a standard 20% lipid emulsion. Daily lipid infusion for both groups was 0.7 g/kg body weight (BW) for the first 2 days and 1.4 g/kg BW thereafter. After 5 days of postoperative TPN, the omega-3 FA group had a significant increase in the leukotriene B 5 series (LTB_5). This series exerts considerably less biological activity than the proinflammatory lipid mediator leukotriene B 4 series (LTB_4). There was some increase in the generation of the leukotriene C series that are potent constrictors of vascular and bronchial smooth muscle, but the level came back to baseline by day 5 and there was no difference between groups.[55] Lipoplus is not currently available in the United States, but once an appropriate ratio of omega-6 and omega-3 fatty acids is determined for hyperinflammatory situations, manufacturers of PN solutions should utilize this information to develop a commercially available product.

18.4.3 PROTEIN

Current recommendations for critically ill patients range from 0.6 to 2.0 g/kg/d, depending on liver function, renal clearance, type of renal replacement therapy, and other potential sources of nitrogen loss.[31,16] Earlier studies recommended intakes of up to 3.0 g/kg/d,[56] but later studies showed that increasing protein intake up to 2.2 g/kg/d increased catabolism.[16] The hemodynamic effects of exogenous protein include raising the metabolic rate, body temperature, and carbon dioxide production.[16] Excessive protein can also contribute to prerenal azotemia, which is aggravated by underlying dehydration.[38] Monitoring of blood urea nitrogen, body weight, and fluid balance can help to prevent this complication. These negative effects, plus the fact that it is very difficult to reverse the loss of lean body mass in severe stress and injury, have encouraged more conservative protein guidelines for the critically ill.[16,17] In reality, it may be difficult to meet your protein goal due to volume constraints, unless renal replacement therapy is continuous and effective.

The nonprotein calorie to nitrogen (NPC:N) ratio represents the amount of calories required to incorporate 1 g of nitrogen into tissue and not be used as an energy source. This does not always mean that each gram of nitrogen is used for tissue accretion, but providing an appropriate ratio of nonprotein calories to nitrogen may aid in attenuating the loss of lean body tissue. The ratio may range from 150:1 to 200:1 for stable hospitalized patients but decrease to 100:1 in critically ill patients, because these patients tend to require more protein in an increasingly catabolic state. They may also require fewer nonprotein calories, due to an inefficient utilization of carbohydrate and lipid calories, as mentioned earlier.[57] Conversely, the NPC:N ratio may increase to 300:1 in patients with renal and hepatic insufficiency, due to the intolerance of large amounts of protein. The NPC:N ratio is to be used as a general guideline in formulating parenteral and enteral nutrition regimens, in conjunction with clinical status of the patient and other available nutrition parameters.

18.4.4 ELECTROLYTES AND MINERALS

Table 18.4 lists the possible etiology, symptoms, treatment, and prevention of metabolic complications associated with PN. Usual daily requirements are discussed in Chapter 9 but may be altered due to disease process, impaired renal clearance, excessive losses from urine or gastrointestinal fluid, medication effect, or redistribution intracellularly due to refeeding. The refeeding phenomenon is a frequent occurrence in malnourished patients or those without nutrient intake for a number of days, which is common in critically ill patients. The administration of nutrients, specifically dextrose, results in secretion of insulin for intracellular transfer of phosphate and glucose for glucose metabolism and protein synthesis.[58] Approximately 7 to 10 mmol of phosphorus/1000 kcal of dextrose are required to prevent hypophosphatemia from refeeding; this could be more, depending on other factors promoting phosphorus excretion.[5] Also, keep in mind that lipid emulsions provide 7.5 mmol of phosphorus per 500 ml.[30] This may not be clinically significant unless hyperphosphatemia due to renal failure is an issue. Hypokalemia and hypomagnesemia are also commonly associated with refeeding due to intracellular shifts,[59] so it is imperative to monitor all electrolyte and mineral levels daily during PN, or more frequently if levels are outside the normal range and require treatment. Calcium is highly protein bound, so it is common to see low serum calcium levels with hypoalbuminemia. Ionized calcium is the most accurate determination of calcium status in critical illness but may be difficult to obtain. Calculating a corrected calcium level, as listed in Table 18.4, is a practical method of assessing calcium status in hypoalbuminemic patients.[59] Calcium supplementation may be harmful during critical illness, as demonstrated in models of shock.[60] A conservative approach to calcium administration in critically ill patients may be warranted until more information is available. Refer to Chapter 20 regarding drug–nutrient interactions for a list of medications affecting electrolyte and mineral levels.

18.4.5 VITAMINS AND TRACE MINERALS

There are no conclusive results yet available regarding altered vitamin and mineral requirements in the critically ill, so most patients receive standard intravenous multivitamin and trace mineral doses, as dictated in Chapter 8. The FDA recently revised the parenteral vitamin requirements for adults, which included adding 150 mcg of vitamin K to multivitamin preparations.[61] In most cases, this would not cause a problem, but for patients who are warfarin resistant or at risk for developing thromboses, this may become an issue.

The additional vitamin K content in lipid emulsions further complicates the issue. Vitamin K content varies from ~6 to 72 mcg/100ml in commonly used lipid emulsions.[62] Clinicians need to be aware of this information so that the frequency of monitoring can be adjusted accordingly.

Additional thiamine at 100 mg/d for at least 3 days may be beneficial in malnourished patients to avoid wet and dry beriberi disease, especially during aggressive refeeding with carbohydrate.[63] Wernicke–Korsakoff syndrome involves confusion, ataxia, opthalmoplegia, and nystagmus, which may develop in chronic alcoholics due to thiamine deficiency and warrants IV supplementation.[63]

Oxidative stress in disease and the role of antioxidants, such as vitamin E, vitamin C, carotenoids, glutathione, flavenoids, selenium, and zinc, are of particular interest in the critically ill, where increased oxidative activity and oxidative tissue injury have been identified. There is a role for oxidants and free radicals in normal physiologic processes, but various endogenous and exogenous factors may negatively affect their role and lead to cellular injury and death.[64] Antioxidant nutrient levels are decreased in a variety of conditions, so it is hypothesized that supplementation with antioxidants may prevent or limit oxidative injury. Some early clinical trials are promising;[65,66] however, conflicting evidence exists.[67] Further research is warranted before any guidelines can be developed for clinical practice.

Trace mineral levels fluctuate during the acute-phase response due to altered protein binding and transfer into other body compartments, and patients do not necessarily require additional supplementation when low levels are detected.[68] There are situations in which trace mineral additives need to be adjusted, but all levels need to be scrutinized during inflammation. Refer to Chapter 8 for trace mineral requirements.

Caution should be exercised when providing increased amounts of vitamins and minerals in PN, due to compatibility concerns. With respect to the addition of vitamin C to PN, formation of calcium oxalate is possible, depending on the amount of vitamin C, the concentration of calcium, pH, and amino acid profile of the solution.[69] Current compatibility data supports the addition of vitamin C to PN — but with caution and close monitoring of solution stability.[70] Even though increased supplementation of thiamine occurs in PN, there is a concern for the effect of bisulfite content and differences in pH among the amino acid solutions on thiamine stability and bioavailability.[71] Studies are needed to determine the maximum amount of thiamine stable in various PN solutions that are used in current practice. Supplemental copper sulfate and zinc sulfate need to be added cautiously to total nutrient admixtures, due to their di- and trivalent nature, which can disrupt the emulsion.[72]

It is imperative to understand the importance of individualizing therapy for each patient, depending on age, nutritional status, disease, comorbid states, and stress level, so that the least harmful and most effective PN solution can be administered to the patient. Incorporating results from prospective, randomized, controlled trials into clinical practice ensures that patients are receiving the most appropriate care.

18.5 CASE STUDY

M.A. is a 63-year-old African American female with a 14-year history of short bowel syndrome secondary to multiple bowel resections, requiring chronic PN therapy. At home, she consumes a regular diet in addition to TPN. This has resulted in significant fluid requirements to compensate for the large ileostomy output (i.e., the total volume of her TPN is 4500 ml, which is cycled over 12 hours). As a result of poor maintenance of central line and ports, she has had multiple episodes of bacteremia and fungemia, requiring hospitalization. She recently presented to the ER department due to feeling poorly, with nausea, vomiting, and fever. She reports her baseline chronic abdominal pain has increased as well.

18.5.1 PMH

- Short bowel syndrome secondary to multiple abdominal surgeries, on home TPN
- History of multiple related line infections including *Enterococcus fecalis* bacteriemia, Torulopsis, *Klebsiella* bacteriemia, *Candida albicans*
- Status post cholecystectomy
- Status post perforated appendix
- Status post panniculitis
- Status post TAH, BSO
- Status post left cataract surgery
- History of hypercoagulable state with DVT on chronic anticoagulation
- Status post ileostomy

18.5.2 HOSPITAL COURSE

Upon admission, the patient had a temperature of 39°C. Blood cultures were obtained, which eventually grew out coagulase negative staph, as well as *Candida albicans*. The patient was also in acute renal failure secondary to dehydration from her high ostomy output. Her BUN/Cr at that time were 53 mg/dl and 3.5 mg/dl, respectively. She was also hyperglycemic, with a BG of

357 mg/dl. Her home TPN was providing 1.6 grams of protein/kg/d and 39 total calories/kg/d, with 100 units of insulin in the bag. Again, the total volume of her TPN was 4500 ml.

Shortly after arrival on the ward, the patient became hypotensive and was transferred to the ICU. She was then placed on dopamine and levophed. She continued to receive her "usual" TPN, and after several days of input significantly exceeding output, she was started on renal replacement therapy (i.e., CVVH) due to total volume overload and uremia. She also became hyponatremic at that time, with a serum sodium of 128 mmol/l. The decision was then made to decrease the total volume of her TPN because her ileostomy output had significantly decreased (in large part due to her NPO status) and to decrease her nonprotein calories (NPCs) to provide 28 total kcal/kg/d.

Over the next few days, her clinical status improved. The dopamine and levophed were discontinued, she became afebrile, and her serum sodium and BG normalized, as did her serum creatinine. Her BUN remains slightly elevated 22 mg/dl, reflecting her now-chronic renal insufficiency; however, her urine output continues to be adequate. The patient was subsequently discharged with a designated home care company to provide antibiotics and TPN. They will also monitor her ileostomy output and adjust the TPN volume accordingly. Additional discharge plans include reviewing catheter care with patient and caregivers, evaluating the need for a new catheter if catheter-related infections continue, and instituting a short-bowel diet in hopes of decreasing ileostomy output and therefore intravenous volume and calorie requirements.

REFERENCES

1. ASPEN Board of Directors Guidelines for the use of parenteral and enteral nutrition in adult and pediatric patients, *JPEN*, 26, 1SA, 2002.
2. Vanek, V.W., The ins and outs of venous access: part 1, *Nutr. Clin. Prac.*, 17, 85, 2002.
3. Krzywda, E.A. et al., Parenteral access devices, in *The Science and Practice of Nutrition Support: A Case-Based Core Curriculum*, Gottschlich, M.M., Ed., Kendall/Hunt, Dubuque, IA, 2001, chap.11.
4. James, L., Bledsoe, L., and Hadaway, L.C., A retrospective look at tip location and complications of peripherally inserted central catheter lines, *J. Intr. Nurs.*, 16, 104, 1993.
5. Fuhrman, M.P., Complication management in parenteral nutrition, in *Contemporary Nutrition Support Practice*, Gottschlich, M.M., Ed., W.B. Saunders, St. Louis, MO, 242, 2003.
6. Dempsey, D.T., Complications of parenteral and enteral nutritional support, in *Nutrition for the Hospitalized Patient Basic Science and Principles of Practice*, Torosian, M.H., Ed., Marcel Dekker, New York, 1995, chap. 18.
7. McDonough, J. and Altemeier, W., Subclavian venous thrombosis secondary to indwelling catheters, *Surg. Gynecol. Obstet.*, 133, 397, 1971.
8. Hematological agents, in *Facts and Comparisons*, Cada, D.J., Ed., Wolters Kluwer, St. Louis, 2003 (updated monthly), chap. 2.
9. Pennington, C.R. and Pithie A.D., Ethanol lock in the management of catheter occlusion, *JPEN*, 11, 507, 1987.
10. Shulman, R.J. et al., Use of hydrochloric acid to clear obstructed central venous catheters, *JPEN*, 12, 509, 1988.
11. Driscoll, D.F., Compounding of TPN admixtures: then and now, *JPEN*, 27, 433, 2003.
12. Food and Drug Administration: FDA safety alert: Hazards of precipitation associated with parenteral nutrition, *Am. J. Hosp. Pharm.*, 51, 2834, 1994.
13. Johnson, A. and Oppenheim, B.A., Vascular catheter-related sepsis: diagnosis and prevention, *J. Hosp. Inf.*, 20, 67, 1992.
14. CDC. Guidelines for prevention of intravascular catheter-related infections: recommendations and reports, *MMWR* 2002, 51 (RR-10).
15. Gastroenterology Teaching Project Committee, Slide 48, TPN trial results: proposed reasons for poor outcomes, *Unit #15: Clinical Nutrition I: Specialized Nutritional Support*, AGA, 2001.
16. Campbell, I.T., Limitations of nutrient intake. The effect of stressors: trauma, sepsis and multiple organ failure, *Eur. J. Clin. Nutr.*, 53, S143, 1999.

17. Chiolero, R., Revelly, J., and Tappy, L., Energy metabolism in sepsis and injury, *Nutrition*, 13, 45S, 1997.

18. Hurley, D.L., Neven, A.K., and McMahon, M.M., Diabetes mellitus, in *The Science and Practice of Nutrition Support: A Case-Based Core Curriculum*, Gottschlich, M.M., Ed., Kendall/Hunt, Dubuque, IA, 2001, chap.32.

19. McMahon, M. et al., Parenteral nutrition in patients with diabetes mellitus: theoretical and practical considerations, *JPEN*, 13, 545, 1989.

20. Van den Berghe, G. et al., Intensive insulin therapy in critically ill patients, *N. Engl. J. Med.*, 345, 1359, 2001.

21. Monson, P. and Mehta, R.L., Nutritional considerations in continuous renal replacement therapies, *Seminars in Dialysis*, 9, 152, 1996.

22. Krishnan, J.A. et al., Caloric intake in medical ICU patients: consistency of care with guidelines and relationship to clinical outcomes, *Chest*, 124, 297, 2003.

23. Phelps, S.J. et al., Toxicities of parenteral nutrition in the critically ill patient, *Crit. Care. Clinics*, 7, 725, 1991.

24. Bower, R.H., Hepatic complications of parenteral nutrition, *Seminars in Liver Disease*, 3, 216, 1983.

25. Robertson, J.F.R., Garden, D.J., and Shenkin, A., Intravenous nutrition and hepatic dysfunction, *JPEN*, 10, 172, 1986.

26. Wolfe, B.M. et al., Effect of total parenteral nutrition on hepatic histology, *Arch. Surg.*, 123, 1084, 1988.

27. Ireton-Jones, C.S., Borman, K.R., and Turner, W.W., Nutrition considerations in the management of ventilator-dependent patients, *NCP*, 8, 60, 1993.

28. Louie, N. and Niemiec, P.W., Parenteral nutrition solutions, in *Parenteral Nutrition*, 2nd vol. of Rombeau, J.L. and Caldwell, M.D., Eds., *Clinical Nutrition*, W.B. Saunders, Philadelphia, 1986, chap.14.

29. Phelps, S.J. and Cochran E.B., Effect of continuous administration of fat emulsion on the infiltration of intravenous lines in infants receiving peripheral parenteral nutrition solutions, *JPEN*, 13, 628, 1989.

30. Intralipid® 20% A 20% I.V. Fat Emulsion, *Package Insert*, Kabi Pharmacia, Clayton, NC, 1991.

31. ASPEN Board of Directors and the Clinical Guidelines Task Force, Guidelines for the use of parenteral and enteral nutrition in adult and pediatric patients, *JPEN*, 1SA, 2002.

32. Brown, D.H. and Simkover, R.A., Maximum hang times for i.v. fat emulsions, *Am. J. Hosp. Pharm.*, 44, 282, 1987.

33. Venus, B. et al., Hemodynamic and gas exchange alterations during intralipid infusion in patients with adult respiratory distress syndrome, *Chest*, 95, 1278, 1989.

34. Mowatt-Larssen, C.A. and Brown, R.O., Specialized nutrition support in respiratory disease, *Clin. Pharm.*, 12, 276, 1993.

35. Zakinthinos, S., Baltopoulos, G., and Roussos, C.H., Fat emulsions and ARDS, *Chest*, 98, 509, 1990.

36. Gilbert, M. et al., Microbial growth patterns in a total parenteral nutrition formulation containing lipid emulsion, *JPEN*, 10, 494, 1986.

37. Cresci, G.A. and Martindale, R.G., Parenteral nutrition, in *Handbook of Nutrition and Food*, Berdanier, C., Ed., CRC Press, Boca Raton, FL, 2002, chap. 43.

38. Matarese, L.E., Metabolic complications of parenteral nutrition therapy, in *The Science and Practice of Nutrition Support: A Case-Based Core Curriculum*, Gottschlich, M.M., Ed., Kendall/Hunt, Dubuque, IA, 2001, chap.13.

39. Siguel, E.N., Nutrient chart no. 13, Nutrient: essential fatty acids (EFA), *Nutr. Supp. Serv.*, 8, 24, 1988.

40. Meng, H.C., Fat emulsion in parenteral nutrition, in *Total Parenteral Nutrition*, Fischer, J.E., Ed., Little, Brown, Boston, 1976, 305.

41. Holman, R.T., Johnson, S.B., and Hatch, T.F., A case of human linolenic acid deficiency involving neurological abnormalities, *Am. J. Clin. Nutr.*, 35, 617, 1982.

42. Kaminski, Jr., M.V. et al., Comparative study of clearance of 10% and 20% fat emulsion, *JPEN*, 7, 126, 1983.

43. Baker, J.P. et al., Randomized trial of total parenteral nutrition in critically ill patients: metabolic effects of varying glucose–lipid ratios as the energy source, *Gastroenterology*, 87, 53, 1984.

44. Nagayama, M. et al., Fat emulsion in surgical patients with liver disease, *J. Surg. Research*, 47, 59, 1989.

45. Hamaway, K.J. et al., The effect of lipid emulsions on reticuloendothelial system function in the injured animal, *JPEN*, 9, 559, 1985.

46. Nishiwaki, H. et al., Influences of an infusion of lipid emulsion on phagocytotic activity of cultured Kupffer's cells in septic rats, *JPEN*, 10, 614, 1986.

47. Seidner, D.L. et al., Effects of long-chain triglyceride emulsions on reticuloendothelial system function in humans, *JPEN*, 13, 614, 1989.

48. Herson, V.C. et al., Effects of intravenous fat infusion on neonatal neutrophil and platelet function, *JPEN*, 13, 620, 1989.

49. Monson, J.R.T. et al., Immunorestorative effect of lipid emulsions during total parenteral nutrition, *Br. J. Surg.*, 73, 843, 1986.

50. Battistella, F.D. et al., A prospective, randomized trial of intravenous fat emulsion administration in trauma victims requiring total parenteral nutrition, *J. Trauma*, 43, 52, 1997.

51. Heyland, D.K. et al., Total parenteral nutrition in the critically ill patient: a meta-analysis, *JAMA*, 280, 2013, 1998.

52. Heyland, D.K. et al., and the Canadian Critical Care Clinical Practice Guidelines Committee, Canadian clinical practice guidelines for nutrition support in mechanically ventilated, critically ill adult patients, *JPEN*, 27, 355, 2003.

53. McCowen, K.C. et al., Hypocaloric total parenteral nutrition: effectiveness in prevention of hyperglycemia and infectious complications: a randomized clinical trial, *Crit. Care Med.*, 28, 3606, 2000.

54. Carpentier, Y.A. et al., Recent developments in lipid emulsions: relevance to intensive care, *Nutrition*, 13, 73S, 1997.

55. Koller, M. et al., Impact of omega-3 fatty acid enriched TPN on leukotriene synthesis by leukocytes after major surgery, *Clin. Nutr.*, 22, 59, 2003.

56. Cochran, E.B. et al., Parenteral nutrition in the critically ill patient, *Clin. Pharm.*, 8, 783, 1989.

57. Stein, T.P., Protein metabolism and parenteral nutrition, in *Parenteral Nutrition*, 2nd vol. of Rombeau, J.L. and Caldwell, M.D., Eds., *Clinical Nutrition*, W.B. Saunders, Philadelphia, 1986, chap. 5.

58. Dwyer, K., Barone, J.E., and Rogers, J.F., Severe hypophosphatemia in postoperative patients, *Nutr. Clin. Pract.*, 7, 279, 1992.

59. Zaloga, G.P. and Chernow, B., Life-threatening electrolyte and metabolic abnormalities, in *Current Therapy in Critical Care Medicine*, Parillo, J.E., Ed., Decker, Toronto, 1987, 245.

60. Trump, B.F. and Berezesky, I.K., Calcium-mediated cell injury and cell death, *Crit. Care Med.*, 4, 139, 1996.

61. Fed. Reg. 65: 64607–64619, 2000.

62. Singh, H. and Duerksen, D.R., Vitamin K and nutrition support, *Nutr. Clin. Pract.*, 18, 359, 2003.

63. Mascarenhas, M.R., Vitamins, in *Nutrition for the Hospitalized Patient: Basic Science and Principles of Practice*, Torosian, M.H., Ed., Marcel Dekker, New York, 1995, chap. 8.

64. Jones, C.R. et al., Plasma antioxidant status after high-dose chemotherapy: a randomized trial of parenteral nutrition in bone marrow transplantation patients, *Am. J. Clin. Nutr.*, 72, 181, 2000.

65. Tanaka, H. et al., Reduction of resuscitation fluid volumes in severely burned patients using ascorbic acid administration: a randomized, prospective study, *Arch. Surg.*, 135, 326, 2000.

66. Berger, M.M. and Cavadini, C., Unrecognised intake of trace elements in polytraumatized and burnt patients, *Ann. Fr. Anesth. Reanim.* (France), 13, 289, 1994.

67. Clemens, M.R. et al., Supplementation with antioxidants prior to bone marrow transplantation, *Wein. Klin. Wochenschr.* (Austria), 109, 771, 1997.

68. Galloway, P., McMillan, D.C., and Sattar, N., Effect of the inflammatory response on trace element and vitamin status, *Ann. Clin. Biochem.*, 37, 289, 2000.

69. Louie, N., Stability of vitamins in total parenteral nutrient solutions, *Am. J. Hosp. Pharm.*, 43, 2138, 1986.

70. Mirtallo, J.M., Parenteral formulas, in *Parenteral Nutrition*, Rombeau, J.L. and Rolandelli, R.H., Eds., *Clinical Nutrition*, 3rd ed., W.B. Saunders, Philadelphia, 2001, chap. 7.

71. Niemiec, Jr., P.W. and Vanderveen, T.W., Compatibility considerations in parenteral nutrient solutions, *Am. J. Hosp. Pharm.*, 41, 893, 1984.

72. Clintec Nutrition Company in cooperation with Wagner, D.P. and Atkins, J., *Total Nutrient Admixtures: Clinical and Practical Guidelines*, Clintec Nutrition Company, Deerfield, IL, 1992, 47.

19 Enteral Feeding Challenges

*Carol Rees Parrish, Joseph Krenitsky,
and Carolyn Kusenda*
University of Virginia Health System

CONTENTS

19.1 INTRODUCTION

Nutrition support of the critically ill patient remains an area of controversy. Randomized controlled trials have yielded enlightening results on a number of aspects of critical care. These findings have prompted inquiry into the most basic questions of providing nutrition to the critically ill population. Questions such as the timing of nutrition, nutrient needs, and specific nutrients that would best affect outcomes remain active topics. The best available evidence is that enteral nutrition (EN) provides improved outcomes in the critically ill patient, compared to parenteral nutrition (PN).[1]

Many barriers may be encountered in the hospital setting that prevent adequate infusion of EN into patients. The literature reports that "gastrointestinal intolerance" is responsible for the majority of lost feeding time.[2–9] See Table 19.1 for a list of barriers that alter effective infusion of EN in a typical ICU.

The real barrier, however, may be the perceptions and misinformation regarding gastrointestinal (GI) intolerance, due to a lack of evidence-based and uniform practice in assessing GI function during initiation and progression of EN. How do we effectively provide enteral feeding to a patient population with inherent "endogenous ICU barriers" that thwart our efforts at feeding? This chapter provides a review of GI function to better assess "EN tolerance" in these patients. The most common GI intolerance issues facing clinicians will be addressed:

- Aspiration
- Bowel sounds
- Residual volumes
- Nausea and vomiting
- Diarrhea
- Osmolality and dilution of EN
- Constipation
- Initiation and progression of EN
- Clogged feeding tubes

In addition, suggestions to surmount EN intolerance will be provided.

TABLE 19.1
Barriers to EN Delivery in the Hospital Setting

Diagnostic procedures
Diprivan (propofol)
Enteral access problems (clogged or pulled tubes or obtaining postpyloric access)
Feedings held due to drug–nutrient interactions
Hemodialysis
Hypotensive episodes
Inadvertent hypocaloric TEN orders
NPO at midnight for tests, surgery, or procedures
Physical or occupational therapy
Transportation off the unit
GI intolerance or dysfunction

Source: From The University of Virginia Health System Nutrition Support Traineeship Syllabus. With permission.

19.2 ASPIRATION

Aspiration is defined as the passage of materials into the airway below the level of the true vocal cords.[11] The aspirated substance may be saliva, nasopharyngeal secretions, bacteria, food, beverage, or gastric contents. Studies that investigate the risk or management of aspiration related to enteral feeding are unable to differentiate the source of the aspirated material unless the feeding is radioactively labeled.[12,13] However, few studies are so designed. The incidence of aspiration pneumonia in patients who receive enteral tube feeding is difficult to determine due to varying definitions of aspiration, pneumonia, and varying ability to recognize aspiration events. Studies that have investigated methods to decrease aspiration pneumonia in tube-fed patients have described aspiration pneumonia rates between 5 and 36%.[14–16]

19.2.1 DETECTION OF ASPIRATION

Several methods of monitoring patients for aspiration risk have been popularized through conventional wisdom, including:

- The routine monitoring of gastric residual volumes (see Section 19.4)
- Checking tracheal secretions for the presence of glucose
- The addition of blue food color to feeding formulas

The presence of glucose in tracheal secretions is not a specific or sensitive method of detecting aspiration of enteral feedings. Tracheal glucose can be positive in patients who are not receiving feeding, and in one study tracheal glucose correlated with serum glucose but not aspiration.[17,18] Some tube-feeding formulas will not trigger a positive result even when aspirated, due to low glucose content of the formula.[18]

Several studies have provided data that the use of blue dye in feeding formulas had a very low sensitivity.[17,19,20] In addition, some food dyes are absorbed by critically ill patients and are mitochondrial toxins when absorbed.[21,22] The use of food color or methylene blue to detect aspiration is not recommended, due to low sensitivity and concern for toxicity in critically ill patients. On September 29, 2003, the Food and Drug Administration released a Public Health Advisory regarding reports of toxicity associated with the use of FD&C Blue No. 1 (Blue 1) in enteral feeding solutions.[23]

19.2.2 REDUCING ASPIRATION RISK

19.2.2.1 Body Position

There is evidence that the position of the patient is one of the primary factors that can influence aspiration risk. Several studies have demonstrated that aspiration and pneumonia are significantly more likely when patients are supine.[24,25] Semirecumbent position cannot guarantee absolute protection against all aspiration or pneumonia events, but it is a method that is neither expensive nor time consuming, and it is a variable that can be controlled. Strict use of semirecumbent position (head of bed elevated approximately 45 degrees) is the most consistent and potent means to reduce the likelihood of aspiration.

19.2.2.2 Tube Size and Placement Issues

The best available data suggest that the size of the nasal or oral placed feeding tube does not influence the incidence of aspiration or pneumonia.[26] It *is* critical that the placement of the feeding tube be properly confirmed via radiograph before feedings begin.[26]

TABLE 19.2
Conditions in Which Jejunal Feeding Tubes
Should Be Considered

Neuromuscular disease involving aerodigestive tract
Structural abnormalities of aerodigestive tract
Gastroparesis or severely delayed gastric emptying
Persistently high gastric residuals
Patients who require supine positioning

Although a tube crossing the gastro-esophageal junction might appear to increase the risk of aspiration, the evidence would suggest otherwise. Several studies have demonstrated that the incidence of aspiration does not differ between gastrostomy and nasogastric feedings.[28,29] It is not uncommon for clinicians to place the tip of a feeding tube beyond the pylorus, in the hope of decreasing aspiration events. However, placement of feeding tubes into the small bowel does not appear to reduce aspiration risk, compared to gastric feeding.[14,30] More than ten studies have attempted to investigate the relationship of small bowel feeding and the incidence of aspiration and pneumonia.[9,12–16,30–34] No single study has shown a significant association, due to low incidence and small sample sizes. In addition, not all of the studies positioned the tip of the feeding tube beyond the ligament of Treitz, and most did not regularly reconfirm feeding tube position during the study period.[9,30,31] If the feeding tube location is not monitored throughout the study, the question remains whether a properly positioned tube would reduce aspiration events. Meta-analysis of these studies has been reported in an attempt to compensate for the small sample size of each individual study.[14,30] However, despite the increased numbers of patients available for analysis, it remains unclear whether a properly positioned jejunal tube can reduce aspiration; therefore, from a purely evidence-based perspective, the question of jejunal placement of feeding tubes and aspiration risk remains unanswered.

One practical observation that can be gleaned from these studies is that, taken together, a large number of critically ill patients appear to have received gastric tube feedings in a safe and effective manner. In studies in which protocols for aspiration precautions were established, patients received full tube feedings with very low rates of aspiration pneumonia.[15,16] Considering the time and expense that can be associated with jejunal placement of feeding tubes, it would appear reasonable to feed routinely via the gastric route unless patients demonstrate intolerance to gastric feedings. Patients suspected to be at increased risk for aspiration of gastric contents due to altered anatomy or motility should be considered for jejunal-placed tubes (see Table 19.2).

19.2.2.3   Feeding Delivery Methods

The delivery rate of the feeding formula may also influence aspiration and pneumonia. Bolus administration of 350 ml of EN has been demonstrated to reduce lower esophageal sphincter pressure, which can precipitate reflux of feeding.[35] Continuous EN has been associated with improved feeding tolerance and reduced aspiration events.[36,37] One group has reported reduced aspiration events in patients fed with cyclic drip feedings, compared to a continuous feeding.[38] The authors postulated that cyclic EN might allow a reduction in gastric pH with reduced colonization of gastric contents. However, randomized trials have failed to find a difference in gastric pH or in gastric colonization or pneumonia incidence between patients fed with cyclic vs. continuous feedings.[39,40] The increased use of continuous insulin drips in many intensive care units also raises the concern that cyclic feeding schedules may increase the chance of hypoglycemic episodes.

TABLE 19.3
Risk Reduction for Aspiration Pneumonia

- Maintain a semirecumbent position with the head (shoulders) elevated > 30 to 45 degrees or place the patient patient in reverse Trendelenberg at 30 to 45 degrees if there is no contraindication to that position. Patients with femoral lines can be at 30 degrees.
- Good oral care.
- Minimize use of narcotics.
- Verify appropriate placement of feeding tube.
- Clinically assess GI tolerance:
  - Abdominal distention
  - Fullness/discomfort
  - Vomiting
  - Excessive residual volumes
- Remove nasoenteric or oroenteric feeding tubes as soon as possible.

Source: From The University of Virginia Health System Nutrition Support Traineeship Syllabus. With permission.

19.2.2.4 Pharmacological Interventions

Several prokinetic medications have been investigated for efficacy in improving enteral feeding tolerance. In critically ill patients, metoclopramide and erythromycin improve gastric emptying, compared to a placebo.[41–45] Erythromycin has been documented to have a practical impact on improving the delivery of nutrition to the patient.[44,46] There are limited data on the use of promotility agents in reducing the incidence of aspiration pneumonia. One prospective study in 305 ICU patients receiving nasogastric feedings investigated the use of metoclopramide on pneumonia incidence. No significant difference was noted in the incidence of pneumonia or mortality between the group receiving a placebo and those receiving metoclopramide.[47]

A recent study in mechanically ventilated patients receiving opioid analgesia reported that enteral use of the narcotic antagonist naloxone decreased gastric residual and the incidence of pneumonia.[48] The median volume of gastric residual (54 vs. 129 ml, $p = 0.03$) and frequency of pneumonia (34 vs. 56%, p = 0.04) were significantly lower in the naloxone group. The use of enteral naloxone did not change the requirement for opioid administration in this study.[48] See Table 19.3 for guidelines to help prevent aspiration pneumonia during enteral feedings.

19.3 BOWEL SOUNDS — TO HAVE OR HAVE NOT

Listening for bowel sounds (BS) is a tool that has been in practice for many years as an aid to the clinician in determining readiness to initiate oral or enteral feedings. It is based on the assumption that BS are an indication of peristalsis and lack of BS would indicate aperistalsis. Without peristalsis, a functional ileus would exist. If gastric stasis should occur above the pylorus due to lack of peristalsis, then the 3 to 4 liters of secretions produced per day would build up, causing distension and ultimately emesis, unless nasogastric decompression is instituted.

BS are a function of the air–fluid interface moving through the bowel. Without air in the bowel, there will be no bowel sounds. BS are nonspecific markers and can reflect the presence of air in either the small bowel or the colon. In the presence of an ileus, BS can be nonexistent or hypoactive vs. louder, higher pitched, or hyperactive with an obstruction.[49] As a result, bowel sounds are not an accurate indicator of peristalsis, due to their nonspecific nature.

Despite the universal use of BS, there are no prospective, randomized, clinical trials comparing patients fed with or without BS and clinical outcomes. Peristalsis is propagated by two distinct waves of contractile patterns: fed and fasting.[50] Feeding activates several neural and humoral systems, elicits powerful propulsive contractions along the GI tract, and provides a stimulus for

TABLE 19.4
Suggested Guidelines in the Assessment of GI Function when Bowel Sounds Are Absent

- Does patient require gastric decompression? If so, is it meaningful based on the clinical exam (i.e., is the volume similar to normal secretions above the pylorus, or is it a small volume every shift)? Distinguish severity by differentiating those patients requiring:
  - Low constant suction vs.
  - Gravity drainage vs.
  - An occasional gastric residual check every 4 to 6 hours (small bowel aspirates should not be checked)
- Abdominal exam — firm, distended, tympanic?
- Is the patient nauseated, bloated, feeling full, vomiting?
- Is the patient passing gas or stool?
- What is the differential diagnosis? Are abdominal issues high on the list? If the preceding clinical parameters are benign, consider a trial of TEN at low rate of 10 to 20 ml/h and observe for the symptoms listed previously.

Source: From The University of Virginia Health System Nutrition Support Traineeship Syllabus. With permission.

---

secretion of GI hormones that have promotility effects. The second pattern, the migrating motor complex (or "intestinal housekeeper") is responsible for moving luminal contents along the GI tract between meals. In the postoperative setting, this is the only mechanism of importance if patients are not fed. In the postop literature, there are reports of bowel sounds being associated with the initiation of enteral feeding.[51,52] Enteral feeding may stimulate a reflex that results in coordinated propulsive activity and elicit gastrointestinal hormone secretion enhancing bowel motility — "if you feed them, bowel sounds will follow," so to speak. One small study also demonstrated earlier time to flatus and stooling after EN initiation.[53] There are many practitioners who *believe* BS are not necessary before enteral feedings begin.[6,54–57] Until further evidence is available, a common-sense approach is provided in Table 19.4.

19.4 RESIDUAL VOLUME: THE STOMACH AS A RESERVOIR — A BRIEF REVIEW OF GASTRIC FUNCTION

In order to discuss residual volume (RV), one must appreciate the various factors that contribute to RV. In addition, a reminder, one of the main functions of the stomach is to act as a reservoir. Approximately 3 to 4 l enter the GI tract above the pylorus; this does not include *any* exogenous intake. Table 19.5 lists the contributions of endogenous GI secretions, and Table 19.6 demonstrates typical gastric volumes produced and infused in the clinical setting.

Clearly, if 200 ml (or even 500 ml) are obtained after 4 hours, then significant emptying has occurred during that time period, especially if medications and water were also given.

19.4.1 OTHER FACTORS TO CONSIDER WHEN CHECKING RESIDUAL VOLUMES

19.4.1.1 Normal Gastric Emptying

Normal gastric emptying is estimated to be approximately 188 ml/h of endogenous secretions alone (gastric juice and saliva).[59] Nutrient density will alter gastric emptying; for example, 500 ml of normal saline empties at a rate of 70% per hour; 500 ml of 10% glucose at a rate of 35%/h, and enteral formulas range between 20 and 50%/h.[59] Theoretically, then, if 125 ml/h of EN were to be infused in addition to the 188 ml/h of secretions/h made, a total of ~313 ml/h would be crossing the pylorus *per hour*. If there were no gastric emptying after 4 hours, then 1250 ml would remain.

19.4.1.2 Cascade Effect

The cascade effect mimics a waterfall. The spine of a patient in the supine position protrudes upward, effectively cutting the stomach into two halves. Hence, a functional barrier is created, and

TABLE 19.5
Absorption and Secretion of Fluid in the GI Tract

Gastrointestinal Fluid Movement	
	ml
Additions	
Diet	2000
Saliva	1500
Stomach	2500
Pancreas/bile	2000
Intestine	1000
Subtractions	
Colointestinal	8900
Net stool loss	100

Source: From Harig, J.M., *American Gastroenterological Association Postgraduate Course Syllabus*, American Gastroenterological Association, Boston, 1993, 199.

TABLE 19.6
Typical Patient Receiving Enteral Nutrition

Consider the following scenario:

Saliva and gastric secretions/24 h (conservative estimate) = 3 l; hence, approximately 125 ml/h

EN infusing at 75 ml/h (typical flow rate in an ICU)

125 ml + 75 ml = 200 ml/h × 4 h (standard time frame between RV checks) = 800 ml RV

(Medications and water flushes are excluded for simplicity.)

Source: From The University of Virginia Health System Nutrition Support Traineeship Syllabus. With permission.

gravity keeps secretions from leaving the fundus, or proximal section, until enough volume is collected to "cascade over" the spine like a waterfall into the antrum, allowing secretions to leave the stomach. If the feeding port happens to sit in the fundus during infusion, then an artificial residual will accumulate until it is high enough to cascade over to the pyloric end and out the stomach.[60]

The mere words *residual volume* conjure up the idea that having one is not acceptable. Assumptions are often made that any type of residual in the stomach is abnormal or that undesirable clinical consequences may follow, such as fullness, nausea, vomiting, and aspiration followed by pneumonia. Table 19.7 lists other factors clouding the issue of RV.

Throughout the literature, one of the primary reasons EN is held in critically ill patients is the result of a predetermined, arbitrary RV.[2–9,59] This arbitrary volume frequently results in inadequate delivery of nutrients. However, the volume for which EN is often held is much lower than the *combined* volume of EN, medications, normal endogenous GI secretions, and the water given as flushes over the measured period. This suggests, in actuality, that *significant net emptying* has occurred (refer to Table 19.6). Furthermore, there is no agreement among practitioners regarding the RV at which EN needs to be held; to date, it is an arbitrary number, based on practitioner experience and training. The maximum allowed RV cited in the literature ranges from 60 to 500 ml.[61] Another frequently quoted RV cutoff used is 1.5 to 2 times the EN flow rate. The most frequently

---

TABLE 19.7
Factors Clouding the Issue of Residual Volume Efficacy

1. Does checking RV correlate with a decrease in aspiration events?
2. Furthermore, how does one check an RV? Consider:
   - Type of tube (feeding tube vs. Salem Sump type)
   - Location of tube tip in stomach (fundus, antrum, or G-tube)
   - Position of patient (supine vs. right or left side vs. prone)
   - Method of aspirating (20 to 60 ml syringe vs. gravity drainage vs. low constant suction)
   - The volume withdrawn from the stomach may depend on any or all of the preceding. Therefore, do the RVs obtained mean something different depending on the setting? If so, is validation and a different cutoff needed for each?
3. What volume is too much?
4. What effect does the use of histamine-2 receptor blockers and proton pump inhibitors play in the assessment of RV?
5. What is done with the contents once they have been removed — reinfuse or discard?

Source: From The University of Virginia Health System Nutrition Support Traineeship Syllabus. With permission.

---

accepted RV threshold was 100 to 150 ml, based on a telephone survey of hospitals in the United States;[62] however, the origin of this range is uncertain. Due to decades of use, 100 to 150 ml has become standard practice by default. Several in-depth critiques of the use of RV are available in the literature.[63–65]

19.4.1.3 Clinical Relevance of Residual Volume

The practice of checking RV has existed for decades; however, the first study attempting to evaluate its utility as a reliable tool in the clinical setting was McClave in 1992.[66] McClave compared RV with physical exam and radiographic findings in enterally fed patients and healthy volunteers. Vital HN was infused continuously via 10 Fr nasogastric tubes (NGT) to volunteers (N = 20), critically ill patients (N = 10), and floor patients with percutaneous endoscopic gastrostomies (PEG) (N = 8). The important findings of this study included the following:

- RV did not correlate with physical exam or radiographic evidence.
- Physical exam and radiographic findings correlated significantly.
- Forty percent of volunteers had an RV of > 100 ml during the study vs. 39% of subjects.
- Because of the short duration of the study (8 hours total), no conclusions could be made as to the safety or value of RV > 100 to 200 ml, but the question remains, what is the validity of checking RV?

In another study, Pinella et al. compared two continuous feeding protocols in 80 naso- or orogastric-fed medical, surgical, and trauma patients:[59]

- Group 1 (RV threshold of 150 ml)
- Group 2 (RV threshold of 250 ml)

Formula selection was based on the discretion of the intensivist, and calorie level was based on the Harris–Benedict formula multiplied by a stress factor. Prokinetic agents were used at the discretion of the intensivist in group 1, but mandatory use was required in group 2. The outcome measures were GI intolerance, time to reach a goal flow of TEN, and the percentage of the required EN delivered. The treatment group experienced fewer episodes of elevated RV; however, time to goal flow and total percentage of nutritional requirements received were similar to controls. This study supports the use of a higher RV threshold of 250 ml, with mandatory use of a prokinetic; however, it does not address the benefit (or lack thereof) of using RV in the first place.

Powell et al. hypothesized that checking gastric RV leads to the occlusion of small-bore feeding tubes.[67] General medicine patients were continuously fed a polymeric formula through an 8 Fr NGT. Group A (N = 15) had RV checked every 4 hours; group B's (N = 13) RV was not checked. Occlusion rates were significantly higher in group A than in group B (p = 0.02). Unfortunately, actual RV was not reported, and the study was neither designed nor powered to demonstrate sensitivity of RV as a marker for aspiration.

A recent consensus statement, which arose from a summit meeting composed of respected nutrition support practitioners, suggested 500 ml is probably an acceptable cutoff for RV.[68] The basis for this recommendation came primarily from two studies and an abstract.[59,61,69] The first, a simulated module of gastric emptying, surmised that in a normal gut, gastric emptying is significant such that 500 ml should not pose a risk.[59] Although the article is an excellent review of gastric physiology, it is a simulated model. Therefore, it does not account for all the factors that affect patients, such as the influence of medications, anesthesia and surgery, illness severity or injury, individual organs that may not be working, mechanical ventilation, and a combination of comorbid states with which our patients present.

In the second study, Mentec et al. conducted a prospective, descriptive study of critically ill patients (N = 153) to determine the frequency, risk factors, and complications of upper digestive intolerance (vomiting and increased gastric aspirate volumes [GAV] defined as 150 to 500 ml).[61] Patients were fed 25 kcal/kg at goal flow from day 1 by 14 Fr NGT. Forty-nine patients (32%) had an increased GAV; 40 patients (26%) experienced vomiting. Of the 40 patients that vomited, 52% did not have increased GAV vs. 47% who did have increased GAV. The authors concluded that GAV *by itself* was not significantly associated with pneumonia, but vomiting was (p = 0.05).

Lukan et al. added yellow microspheres and blue food coloring (BFC) directly to tube feeding and obtained RV and specimens from oropharynx and trachea from critically ill, ventilated patients fed via NGT (N = 13), PEG (N = 13), or NGT then PEG (N = 2).[69] Aspiration and regurgitation events were defined by detection of yellow color on fluorometry. Although RV reached > 400 ml in 0.7% of samples, RV did not correlate with aspiration or regurgitation events. The authors concluded that a RV < 400 ml is an insensitive marker for risk of aspiration. Of note, aspiration pneumonia does not necessarily follow regurgitation and aspiration events.

Mounting evidence is available to suggest that the standard practice of 150 to 200 ml RV cutoff is over conservative and results in unnecessary withholding of EN. The evidence behind the recent consensus statement that a RV up to 500 ml is probably safe during enteral feeding in critically ill patients has yet to be validated.[33,61,68,69] What is becoming more apparent, however, is that RV itself is not a validated tool to assess tube feeding tolerance or aspiration risk. A very large, prospective, controlled trial with adequate power will be necessary to put this controversy to rest. For now, the healthcare team must be vigilant in good clinical judgment to ensure safe enteral feeding. For suggested strategies until further evidence is available, see Table 19.8.

19.5 NAUSEA AND VOMITING

The idea of initiating EN in a patient experiencing nausea and vomiting (N/V) may appear somewhat counterintuitive. Nausea and vomiting are often the result of medication side effects, a procedure, surgery, or an underlying disease process; this is especially true in the critical care setting. Critically ill patients with persistent nausea and vomiting are at a high risk for malnutrition (if this is not already present). After careful assessment, the underlying cause can often be identified and treated. While efforts at curtailing N/V are initiated, EN can be started. Due to the subjective nature of nausea and intermittent bouts of vomiting, antiemetics are often ordered on a prn basis. If nausea or vomiting is significant enough to prevent EN, consider standing orders for medications aimed at providing symptomatic relief. See Table 19.9 for suggestions for the treatment of N/V. Additionally, an excellent review of the management of nausea and vomiting is available elsewhere.[70,71]

TABLE 19.8

Suggested Guidelines to Evaluate Residual Volume

1. Is it a residual? (For example, is it less than the flow rate?)
2. What does the residual look like? (Formula or gastric secretions?)
3. *Clinically* assess the patient for nausea, vomiting, abdominal distension, fullness, bloating, discomfort.
4. Place the patient on his or her right side for 15 to 20 minutes before checking an RV to avoid *the cascade effect.*
5. Review *all* enterally given fluids, including medications and water for flushes and medication delivery.
6. Try a prokinetic agent or antiemetic, then review orders for prn vs. standing vs. elixir vs. tablets. Typical doses for available prokinetics:
   • Metoclopramide: 5–20 mg qid (may need to give IV initially)
   • Erythromycin: 50–200 mg qid
   • Domperidone: 10–30 mg qid
7. Seek transpyloric access of feeding tube.
8. Switch to a more calorically dense product to decrease the total volume infused.
9. Tighten glucose control to less than 200 mg% to avoid gastroparesis from hyperglycemia.
10. Consider analgesic alternatives to opiates.
11. Consider a proton pump inhibitor (PPI) in order to decrease sheer volume of endogenous gastric secretions (e.g., omeprazole, lansoprazole, esomeprazole, pantoprazole, rabeprazole). In patients whose increased gastric secretions are an issue, use of PPIs can decrease dependency on or use of IV hydration. This option is typically used for those patients who will be going home on TEN. PPIs can decrease the sheer volume of gastric secretions and often allows discharge without IV hydration in addition to TEN or can decrease it enough that reinfusion of gastric secretions through the j-port is manageable.
12. Raise the threshold for what constitutes a residual volume up to 400–500 ml.
13. Consider stopping the RV checks if the patient is clinically stable, has no abdominal complaints, or the RV checks have been "acceptable" for 48 hours.

Source: From The University of Virginia Health System Nutrition Support Traineeship Syllabus. With permission.

TABLE 19.9

Suggestions to Overcome Nausea and Vomiting in TEN-Fed Patients

1. Review medications — any contributing? Can they be changed to an alternative?
2. Try a prokinetic agent or antiemetic, then review orders for prn vs. standing vs. elixir vs. tablets.
3. Switch to a more calorically dense product to decrease the total volume infused.
4. Seek transpyloric access of feeding tube.
5. Tighten glucose control to less than 200 mg% to avoid gastroparesis from hyperglycemia.
6. Consider analgesic alternatives to opiates.
7. Consider a proton pump inhibitor in order to decrease sheer volume of endogenous gastric secretions (e.g., omeprazole, lansoprazole, esomeprazole, pantoprazole, rabeprazole).
8. If bacterial overgrowth is a possibility, treat with enteral antibiotics.

Source: From The University of Virginia Health System Nutrition Support Traineeship Syllabus. With permission.

19.6 DIARRHEA

The diagnosis and management of diarrhea in critically ill, enterally fed patients can be a challenge. Historically, the use of EN has been implicated as a primary cause of diarrhea in this population. Available evidence does not support these implications.[72–75] Successful management of diarrhea in the critically ill patient depends on accurate identification and treatment of the source. Manipulation of EN has often been a primary means of attempting to prevent or treat diarrhea. However, the vast majority of diarrhea in enterally fed patients has been associated with the use of medications or with infectious agents.[73–77] Therapies to treat diarrhea have included using low fat or elemental feeds, slowing the feeding rate, using less-concentrated solutions, or stopping EN altogether. These interventions are often implemented without an investigation of the primary etiology of the diarrhea. Not only are these treatments often unnecessary; they also may prevent the patient from receiving optimal nutrition support.[75]

19.6.1 INCIDENCE OF DIARRHEA IN EN

The reported incidence of diarrhea among tube-fed patients ranges from 2 to 68%.[78,79] Subjective measures, such as stool frequency, consistency, and volume, may not be clinically relevant. More objective, quantifiable measures are difficult to obtain and include stool weight (> 300 g/d)[80] or volume (> 500 ml/d).[76] In one tube-fed population, a 46% incidence of diarrhea was reported using subjective data, and a 0% incidence was reported using objective data.[81] In the clinical setting, recording stool characteristics (volume, consistency, and frequency) while concomitantly looking for clinical signs and symptoms of diarrhea (dehydration, electrolyte imbalance, sacral and perianal skin irritation) can assist with evaluation of need for treatment.

19.6.2 FLOW RATE

EN has been customarily initiated at lower flow rates in an attempt to avoid abdominal distress and diarrhea. The need to use starter-type regimes (initiation of EN at a lower rate or osmolality or both) in order to give the GI tract a chance to adapt has been refuted.[75,82] The functional GI tract has been shown to tolerate up to 150 cc/h gastrically and 267 cc/h transpylorically.[82,83] Adjustment of flow rate has not been determined to be associated with increased incidence of abdominal discomfort, diarrhea, or malabsorption.

19.6.3 FORMULA COMPOSITION

The use of elemental diets is not routinely indicated for use in patients with diarrhea.[84] Patients with functional GI tracts tolerate polymeric formulas as well as elemental formulas.[77] In a prospective, randomized clinical trial, Heimburger et al. compared use of peptide-containing formulas with intact protein formulas in 50 critically ill patients. Both formulas were well tolerated, and the incidence of diarrhea was attributed to medications.[76]

Although the GI tract may be affected in many ways by critical illness, its overall absorptive capacity is significant. For malabsorption to occur, 90% of organ function must be impaired.[84] The use of elemental formulas should be limited to those patients with severely impaired gastrointestinal function.[75]

19.6.4 OSMOLALITY

See Section 19.7.

19.6.5 MEDICATIONS

The most common cause of diarrhea in tube-fed patients has consistently been found to be the use of hyperosmotic medications.[76,85] Edes et al. reported a 26% incidence of diarrhea in a population of tube-fed patients. Medications were directly responsible in 61% of the cases.[76] Antibiotic use, with its association with *C. difficile*, has been cited as a primary cause of diarrhea.[73–75,86] Examples of medications commonly associated with diarrhea and their osmolalities are listed in Table 19.10. Possible options for resolving medication-related diarrhea include changing the medication itself, diluting the medication to make it more isotonic prior to administration, and changing the route of administration from enteral to IV.

TABLE 19.10
Osmolality of Selected Liquids and Medications

Typical Liquids	(mOsm/kg)	Drug	(mOsm/kg)
TEN formulas	250–710	Acetaminophen elixir	5400
Milk/eggnog	275/695	Diphenoxylate susp.	8800
Gelatin	535	KCl elixir (sugar-free)	3000
Broth	445	Chloral hydrate syrup	4400
Sodas	695	Furosemide (oral)	3938
Popsicles	720	Metoclopramide	8350
Juices	~990	Multivitamin liquid	5700
Ice cream	1150	Sodium Phosphate	7250
Sherbet	1225	Cimetidine liquid	4035

Source: From The University of Virginia Health System Nutrition Support Traineeship Syllabus. With permission.

19.6.6 GASTROINTESTINAL

Diarrhea can be caused by malabsorption; however, diarrhea does not *cause* malabsorption. In a patient with persistent diarrhea, once the obvious culprits have been investigated, a review of anatomy, underlying disease states, concomitant problems, and secondary effects of treatments or medications is in order. If malabsorption is suspected, it should be tested, diagnosed, and treated. Manipulation of feeding regimes has not been proved to treat such GI dysfunctions, and commercial claims of such should be highly scrutinized.

19.6.7 TREATMENT OF DIARRHEA

After etiology has been determined, appropriate medical management can be initiated. See Table 19.11 for suggested strategies for treatment.

TABLE 19.11
Systematic Approach when Addressing Diarrhea in EN-Fed Patients

1. Quantify stool volume — is it really diarrhea?
2. Review medication list. (Did medications switch from the IV to enteral route when enteral access was achieved?)
   - Common offenders include:
   - Acetaminophen and theophylline elixir
   - NeutraPhos
   - Lactulose
   - Standing orders for stool softeners or laxatives
3. Check for *C. difficile* or other infectious cause (lactoferrin, leukocytes).
4. Try fiber:
   - Few clinical studies
   - Supports the health of colonocytes
5. Once infectious causes are ruled out:
   - Try an anti-diarrheal agent (may need standing order vs. prn).
6. Continue to feed.

Source: From The University of Virginia Health System Nutrition Support Traineeship Syllabus. With permission.

19.6.8 DIARRHEA AND PROBIOTICS

The use of probiotic cultures to prevent or treat diarrhea remains an area of investigation. Lactobacillus GG has been shown to reduce the duration of diarrhea associated with rotovirus in children and to reduce the incidence of antibiotic-associated diarrhea from 16% in the placebo group to 5% in the Lactobacillus group.[87,88] Lactobacillus supplements have not been adequately tested in adults receiving tube feedings to assess whether there are beneficial effects in terms of diarrhea or acquisition of *Clostridium difficile*. A probiotic yeast, *Saccharomyces boulardii*, has been studied in a prospective, multicenter, double-blind trial in critically ill patients receiving EN. The use of 500 mg *S. boulardii* four times a day reduced the mean percentage of days with diarrhea from 18.9 to 14.2% (p = 0.0069).[89] However, *S. boulardii* has been reported to be a potential pathological agent in the critically ill population.[90] Severely ill, mechanically ventilated patients were pretreated with *S. boulardii* in a 12-bed ICU. Seven cases of fungemia with *S. boulardii* were reported over a two-year period. Investigators confirmed the genomic identity between isolates of blood culture and yeasts from the packets administered to the patients.[90]

Routine use of probiotic supplements is not recommended until additional data are available regarding efficacy and risks in a critically ill population (see Chapter 10).

19.7 OSMOLALITY AND DILUTION OF TUBE FEEDINGS

Osmolality is often blamed for GI intolerance of TEN. Hypertonic formulas (> 300 mOsm) are sometimes diluted to make them "isotonic." However, there are no data to support the practice of diluting TEN. Two studies have demonstrated that hypertonic formulas (ranging from 503 to 620 mOsm/kg), infused either gastrically or at the ligament of Treitz, achieve isotonicity or near-isotonicity very rapidly within the jejunum.[91,92] In fact, the osmolality of TEN formulas should not cause a clinical problem for several reasons. The osmolality of liquids that are routinely taken orally by hospitalized patients is far greater than that of TEN, but most clinicians would never recommend a half- or quarter-strength clear liquid diet. Consider also the osmolality of common medications delivered via the enteral route (see Table 19.10). The osmolality of medications is far greater than that of TEN, yet most focus on the TEN formula as problematic.

At times, patients have increased hydration needs that justify diluted tube feedings. Using diluted feedings (at increased rates) allows the delivery of both adequate nutrition and increased hydration without the need for the nurse or caregiver to give frequent water boluses.

19.8 CONSTIPATION

Although bowel movement frequency is highly individual, ≤ 2 stools weekly have been included as one of the Rome consensus criteria for the symptom.[93] When evaluating constipation in the critical care setting, several factors need to be considered, including patient's normal stool history, time since last bowel movement, and comprehensive assessment of the abdomen by an experienced practitioner. Factors contributing to the incidence of constipation in the critically ill patient include use of anticholinergics, narcotics, and sedatives; inadequate provision of fluid; immobilization; and neuromuscular or GI motility disorders.

Daily monitoring of GI function is important to help avoid more serious cases of constipation. Left untreated, stool can accumulate, filling the entire large bowel. Patients with signs and symptoms of constipation should be evaluated for impaction, bowel obstruction, and ileus. Treatment options include slow increase in fluid and fiber in the diet, followed by inclusion of a saline agent such as milk of magnesia. If these interventions fail, inclusion of a stimulant agent should be considered.[93]

TABLE 19.12
Examples of EN Initiation

Continuous — Standard Textbook
Standard: 20–50 cc/h
    Note: (30 ml = 2 Tb)
Progression: By 10–25 cc/h every 6–24 h
University of Virginia Health System:
    Initiation: Full strength (all products except 2 cal/ml) at 50 ml/h and increase by 25 ml every 4 h to goal rate. A 2.0 cal/ml product is started at 25 ml/h (few patients need ≥ 50 ml/h to meet needs). The final goal rate is dependent on the patient's caloric requirements and GI comfort.

Intermittent/Bolus — Standard Textbook
Typical: 120 ml q 4 hrs, then
Progression: 60 ml q 8–12 hrs as tolerated
University of Virginia Health System:
    Initiation: 125 ml, full strength (regardless of product) every 3 h for two feedings; increase by 125 ml every 2 feedings to final goal volume per feeding during waking hours.

Source: From The University of Virginia Health System Nutrition Support Traineeship Syllabus. With permission.

19.9 INITIATION AND PROGRESSION OF TUBE FEEDINGS

The starting rate and advancement of enteral feedings have been dictated more by tradition than by objective evidence. Nutrition support texts generally recommend starting continuous EN at 20 to 50 ml/h and advancing by 10 to 25 ml every 4 to 24 hours.[56,94,95] Intermittent feeding recommendations are generally to start with 60 to 120 ml of EN every 4 hours and advance by 30 to 60 ml every 8 to 12 hours. However, no references are given for these recommendations. Few investigators have attempted to study the question of the ideal startup and advancement rate for enteral feeding.

Healthy volunteers can tolerate infusion rates of 30 to 60 ml/*minute*. Only at rates of 85 ml/min (5100 ml/h) did subjects show intolerance.[96] Rees continuously infused 87 ml/h into 14 patients with impaired GI function and achieved 100% of prescribed volume in nine patients.[97] In a later study of patients with moderately impaired GI function, Rees did not use a starter regimen in his EN-fed patients.[98] These patients were set to receive 2.25 l of either an intact or a predigested EN product; patients averaged 1985 kcal/d, suggesting they tolerated EN well.

These studies were not designed to establish the limits of tolerance or the ideal tube-feeding progression. Nevertheless, it is clear that many patients, even those with impaired GI function, will tolerate initiation and progression of feedings much faster than has traditionally been recommended. See Table 19.12 and Table 19.13 for sample tube-feeding protocols for initiation, progression, and run times of EN. When discussing flow rates, it is important to keep the actual delivery volume in perspective. For example, 30 ml/h is only 2 tablespoons, and 60 ml/h is one-quarter cup delivered over an entire hour.

19.10 OBSTRUCTED FEEDING TUBES

Feeding tube obstruction occurs in 6 to 10% of tube-fed patients. Factors that increase the incidence of clogging include pump malfunction, tubes, improper administration of medications, failure to adequately flush tube with water, and precipitation of tube feeding proteins. Precipitation of tube

TABLE 19.13
Sample Run-Time Orders of EN at the University of Virginia Health System

- ICU setting: 22 hours
- Floor beds: 16–20 hours (if protocol is to hold for phenytoin suspension BID-TID)
- Stable medical ICU patients: The run time is changed to 1500–0900 to allow for planned trips off the unit for procedures unless on an insulin drip
- If TEN delivery still falls short of 100% of estimated needs, the following alternatives are tried (cyclic TEN defined as less than 24-hour infusion):
  - Run TEN at 75 ml/h from 1900–0700 for total of 900 ml
  - Start TEN at 1900 and run at 75 ml/h until 5 cans infused
  - Adjust pump setting to provide a "dose delivery" of TEN (e.g., start TEN at 1900 and run at 100 ml/h until 1250 ml infused)

Source: From The University of Virginia Health System Nutrition Support Traineeship Syllabus. With permission.

TABLE 19.14
Preventing Feeding Tube Occlusion and Declogging Techniques Once Occluded

Prevention of Clogging

Use liquid medications whenever possible.

Adequately crush pills to powder form prior to administration.

Irrigate feeding tube with water before and after administration of medications.

Flush tube before and after aspirating for gastric residuals to eliminate acid precipitation of formula in the feeding tube.

Avoid mixing tube feedings with liquid medications having a pH value of 5.0 or less.

Suggested Technique for Unclogging Feeding Tubes

Attempt to unclog tube with lukewarm water.

If unsuccessful, mix viokase and sodium bicarbonate mixture:

   (1 crushed viokase tablet [or 1 teaspoon viokase powder], 1 nonenteric-coated 325 mg $NaHCO_3$ [or 1/8 teaspoon baking powder]; dissolve in 5 cc lukewarm water)

Gently aspirate the tube contents proximal to the clog to allow solution direct contact with clog.

Inject the pancreatic enzyme solution into the feeding tube, clamp it, and allow mixture to remain in tube for 30 minutes.

Unclamp feeding tube and gently flush tube with warm tap water to restore patency.

feeding occurs with gastric feedings more frequently than with small bowel feedings, due to the acidic environment of the stomach.[99] Small-bore feeding tubes require more care than larger-bore tubes because they are more likely to clog.

Carbonated beverages and various fruit juices have historically been misused in an attempt to unclog feeding tubes. It has been shown that use of sugar-containing, hyperosmotic liquids can actually aggravate tube clogging. These liquids stick to feeding tubes and promote precipitation of formula, due to their sugar content and acidic nature. For these reasons, such beverages should not be utilized as potential unclogging agents.

Prevention of clogging is important because placement of small-bore feeding tubes can be timely and costly. Giving lavage flushes of warm water may be enough to remove a clog and should be attempted first. If this method fails, the use of a pancreatic enzyme solution has been shown to be highly effective.[99] Different strategies for preventing tube clogging and declogging feeding tubes are listed in Table 19.14. In addition, commercially available decloggers can be found in Table 19.15.

TABLE 19.15
Commercially Available Tube Decloggers

DeCloggers™
Bionix
	Soft, flexible, screw-threaded device to
	   be inserted down the tube to clear
	   build-up or clog
	Available in various lengths and sizes
		www.bionix.com
		800-551-7096

Clog Zapper™
CORPAK
Viasys MedSystems
	Combines a "multienzyme cocktail,"
	   acids, buffers, and antibacterial
	   agents in its formulation. Will break
	   up formula clogs but may not work
	   with clogs from medications.
	Kit contains chemical powder, syringe,
	   and applicator. Unopened kit has a
	   shelf life of 12 months. Once
	   reconstituted, should be used within
	   24 hours.
		www.viasyshealthcare.com
		800-323-6305

PEG Cleaning Brush BARD	Flexible catheter with feather-cut brush at distal end	www.crbard.com 800-826-BARD (2273)

Source: From Barnadas, G., *EN Module*, 2003. With permission.

19.11 CONCLUSION

For now, enteral nutrition is the accepted standard of care for nourishing critically ill patients who are unable to eat on their own. Until evidence becomes available to change this practice, efforts at improving the delivery of EN to this patient population will continue. This chapter has reviewed the evidence for many of the issues that impede effective EN delivery and attempted to make suggestions to overcome these barriers, based on the evidence and on the clinical experience of the authors.

REFERENCES

1. Braunschweig, C.L., et al., Enteral compared with parenteral nutrition: a meta analysis. *Am. J. Clin. Nutr.,* 2001, 74, 534.
2. De Beaux, I., et al., Enteral nutrition in the critically ill: a prospective survey in an Australian intensive care unit, *Anaesth. Intens. Care,* 29, 619, 2001.
3. De Jonghe, B., Appere-De-Vechi, C., Fournier, M., et al., A prospective survey of nutritional support practices in intensive care unit patients: what is prescribed? What is delivered? *Crit. Care Med.,* 29, 8, 2001.
4. McClave, S.A., et al., Enteral tube feeding in the intensive care unit: factors impeding adequate delivery, *Crit. Care Med.,* 27, 1252, 1999.
5. Heyland, D., et al., Enteral nutrition in the critically ill patient: a prospective survey, *Crit. Care Med.,* 23, 1055, 1995.
6. Heyland, D.K., et al., How well do critically ill patients tolerate early, intragastric enteral feeding? Results of a prospective, multicenter trial, *Nutr. Clin. Pract.,* 14, 23, 1999.
7. Adam, S. and Batson, S., A study of problems associated with the delivery of enteral feed in critically ill patients in five ICUs in the U.K., *Intens. Care Med.,* 23, 261, 1997.
8. Montejo, J.C., Enteral nutrition-related gastrointestinal complications in critically ill patients: a multicenter study, *Crit. Care Med.,* 27, 1447, 1999.

9. Montejo, J.C., et al., Multicenter, prospective, randomized, single-blind study comparing the efficacy and gastrointestinal complications of early jejunal feeding with early gastric feeding in critically ill patients. *Crit. Care Med.*, 30, 796, 2002.

10. Parrish, C.R., Krenitsky, J., and McCray, S., *University of Virginia Health System Nutrition Support Traineeship Syllabus*, University of Virginia Medical Center Nutrition Services Department, Charlottesville, VA, 2003.

11. Teasell, R.W., Bach, D., and McRae, M., Prevalence and recovery of aspiration poststroke: a retrospective analysis, *Dysphagia*, 9, 35, 1994.

12. Heyland, D.K. et al., Effect of postpyloric feeding on gastroesophageal regurgitation and pulmonary microaspiration: results of a randomized controlled trial, *Crit. Care Med.*, 29, 1495, 2001.

13. Esparza, J., et al., Equal aspiration rates in gastrically and transpylorically fed critically ill patients, *Intens. Care Med.*, 27, 660, 2001.

14. Heyland, D.K., Drover, J.W., Dhaliwal, R., and Greenwood, J., Optimizing the benefits and minimizing the risks of enteral nutrition in the critically ill: role of small bowel feeding. *J. Parenter. Enteral Nutr.*, 26(6): S51–5, 2002.

15. Kearns, P.J. et al., The incidence of ventilator-associated pneumonia and success in nutrient delivery with gastric versus small intestinal feeding: a randomized clinical trial, *Crit. Care Med.*, 28, 1742, 2000.

16. Neumann, D.A. and DeLegge, M.H., Gastric versus small-bowel tube feeding in the intensive care unit: a prospective comparison of efficacy, *Crit. Care. Med.*, 30, 1436, 2002.

17. Metheny, N.A. and Clouse, R.E., Bedside methods for detecting aspiration in tube fed patients. *Chest*, 103, 724, 1997.

18. Kinsey, G.C. et al., Glucose content of tracheal aspirates: implications for the detection of tube feeding aspiration, *Crit. Care Med.*, 10, 1557, 1994.

19. Potts, R.G. et al., Comparison of blue dye visualization and glucose oxidase test strip methods for detecting pulmonary aspiration of enteral feedings in intubated adults, *Chest*, 103, 117, 1993.

20. Montejo-Gonzalez, J.C. et al., Detecting pulmonary aspiration of enteral feeding in intubated patients. *Chest*, 106, 1632, 1994.

21. Czop, M. and Herr, D.L., Green skin discoloration associated with multiple organ failure. *Crit. Care Med.*, 30, 598, 2002.

22. Reyes, F.G., Valim, M.F., and Vercesi, A.E., Effect of organic synthetic food colours on mitochondrial respiration, *Food Addit. Contam.*, 13, 5, 1996.

23. Reports of blue discoloration and death in patients receiving enteral feedings tinted with the dye, FD&C Blue No. 1. FDA Public Health Advisory FDA/Center for Food Safety & Applied Nutrition. September 29, 2003, http://www.cfsan.fda.gov/~dms/col-ltr2.html, accessed November 1, 2004.

24. Drakulovic, M.B. et al., Supine body position as a risk factor for nosocomial pneumonia in mechanically ventilated patients: a randomized trial, *Lancet*, 354, 1851, 1999.

25. Torres, A. et al., Pulmonary aspiration of gastric contents in patients receiving mechanical ventilation: the effect of body position. *Ann. Intern. Med.*, 116, 540, 1992.

26. Dotson, R.G., Robinson, R.G., and Pingleton S.K., Gastroesophageal reflux with nasogastric tubes: effect of nasogastric tube size, *Am. J. Respir. Crit. Care Med.*, 149, 1659, 1994.

27. Pratt, J.C. and Tolbert, C.G., Tube feeding aspiration. *Am. J. Nurs.*, 96, 37, 1996.

28. Baeten, C. and Hoefnagels, J., Feeding via nasogastric tube or percutaneous endoscopic gastrostomy: a comparison, *Scand. J. Gastroenterol. Suppl.*, 194, 95, 1992.

29. Cole, M.J. et al., Aspiration after percutaneous gastrostomy: assessment by Tc-99m labeling of the enteral feed, *J. Clin. Gastroenterol.*, 9, 90, 1987.

30. Marik, P.E. and Zaloga, G.P., Gastric versus post-pyloric feeding: a systematic review, *Crit. Care*, 7, R46, 2003.

31. Montecalvo, M.A. et al., Nutritional outcome and pneumonia in critical care patients randomized to gastric versus jejunal tube feedings, *Crit. Care Med.*, 20, 1377, 1992.

32. Davies, A.R. et al., Randomized comparison of nasojejunal and nasogastric feeding in critically ill patients, *Crit. Care Med.*, 30, 586, 2002.

33. Strong, R.M. et al., Equal aspiration rates from postpylorus and intragastric-placed small-bore nasoenteric feeding tubes: a randomized, prospective study, *J. Parenter. Enteral Nutr.*, 16, 59, 1992.

34. Kortbeek, J.B., Haigh, P.I., and Doig, C., Duodenal versus gastric feeding in ventilated blunt trauma patients: a randomized controlled trial, *J. Trauma*, 46, 992, 1999.

35. Coben, R.M. et al., Gastroesophageal reflux during gastrostomy feeding, *Gastroenterology*, 106, 13, 1994.

36. Kocan, M.J. and Hickisch, S.M., A comparison of continuous and intermittent enteral nutrition in NICU patients, *J. Neurosci. Nurs.*, 18, 333, 1986.

37. Ciocon, J.O. et al., Continuous compared with intermittent tube feeding in the elderly, *J. Parenter. Enteral Nutr.*, 16, 525, 1992.

38. Jacobs, S. et al., Continuous enteral feeding: a major cause of pneumonia among ventilated intensive care unit patients, *J. Parenter. Enteral Nutr.*, 14, 353, 1990.

39. Spilker, C.A., Hinthorn, D.R., and Pingleton, S.K., Intermittent enteral feeding in mechanically ventilated patients: the effect on gastric pH and gastric cultures, *Chest*, 110, 243, 1996.

40. Bonten, M.J. et al., Intermittent enteral feeding: the influence on respiratory and digestive tract colonization in mechanically ventilated intensive-care-unit patients, *Am. J. Respir. Crit. Care Med.*, 15, 394, 1996.

41. Booth, C.M., Heyland, D.K., and Paterson, W.G., Gastrointestinal promotility drugs in the critical care setting: a systematic review of the evidence, *Crit. Care Med.*, 30, 1429, 2002.

42. Jooste, C.A., Mustoe, J., and Collee, G., Metoclopramide improves gastric motility in critically ill patients, *Intens. Care Med.*, 25, 464, 1999.

43. MacLaren, R. et al., Sequential single doses of cisapride, erythromycin, and metoclopramide in critically ill patients intolerant to enteral nutrition: a randomized, placebo-controlled, crossover study, *Crit. Care Med.*, 28, 1237, 2000.

44. Boivin, M.A. and Levy, H., Gastric feeding with erythromycin is equivalent to transpyloric feeding in the critically ill, *Crit. Care Med.*, 29, 1916, 2001.

45. Berne, J.D. et al., Erythromycin reduces delayed gastric emptying in critically ill trauma patients: a randomized, controlled trial, *J. Trauma*, 53, 422, 2002.

46. Reignier, J. et al., Erythromycin and early enteral nutrition in mechanically ventilated patients, *Crit. Care Med.*, 30, 1237, 2002.

47. Yavagal, D.R., Karnad, D.R., and Oak, J.L., Metoclopramide for preventing pneumonia in critically ill patients receiving enteral tube feeding: a randomized controlled trial, *Crit. Care Med.*, 28, 1408, 2000.

48. Meissner, W., Dohrn, B., and Reinhart, K., Enteral naloxone reduces gastric tube reflux and frequency of pneumonia in critical care patients during opioid analgesia, *Crit. Care Med.*, 31, 776, 2003.

49. Waxman, K., The acute abdomen, in *Textbook of Critical Care*, 4th ed., Grenvik A, ed., W.B. Saunders, Philadelphia, 2000, 1603.

50. Livingston, E.H., Passaro E.P., et al., Postoperative ileus, *Dig. Dis. Sci.*, 35, 121, 1990.

51. Luckey, A., et al., Mechanisms and treatment of postoperative ileus, *Arch. Surg.*, 138, 206, 2003.

52. Holte, K. and Kehlet, H., Postoperative ileus: a preventable event, *Brit. J. Surg.*, 87, 1480, 2000.

53. Beier-Holgersen, R. and Boesby, S., Influence of postoperative enteral nutrition on postsurgical infections, *Gut*, 39, 833, 1996.

54. Zaloga, G.P., Enteral nutrition in hospitalized patients: a consensus summary, in *Enteral Nutrition Support for the 1990s: Innovations in Nutrition, Technology, and Techniques; Report of the Twelfth Ross Roundtable on Medical Issues*, Campbell, S.M. and McCamish, M.A., eds., Ross Laboratories, Columbus, OH, 1992, 47.

55. Booth, F.V., Practical issues in tube feeding, *J. Crit. Care Nutr.*, 1, 33, 1993.

56. Charney, P., Enteral nutrition: indications, options, and formulations, in *The Science and Practice of Nutrition Support*, Gottschlich, M.M., ed., Kendall/Hunt, Dubuque, IA, 2001, 141.

57. MacLaren, R., Intolerance to intragastric enteral nutrition in critically ill patients: complications and management, *Pharmacother.*, 20, 1486, 2000.

58. Harig, J.M., Pathophysiology of small bowel diarrhea, in *American Gastroenterological Association Postgraduate Course Syllabus*, Kahrilas, P.J., Vanagunas, A. eds., American Gastroenterological Association, Boston, 1993, 199.

59. Lin, H.C. and Van Citters, G.W., Stopping enteral feeding for arbitrary gastric residual volume may not be physiologically sound: results of a computer simulation model, *J. Parenter. Enteral Nutr.*, 21, 286, 1997.

60. Pinilla, J.C., et al., Comparison of gastrointestinal tolerance to two enteral feeding protocols in critically ill patients: a prospective, randomized controlled trial, *J. Parenter. Enteral Nutr.*, 25, 81, 2001.

61. Mentec, H., et al., Upper digestive intolerance during enteral nutrition in critically ill patients: frequency, risk factors, and complications, *Crit. Care Med.*, 29, 1955, 2001.

62. Payne, C., Krenitsky, K., and Morse, J., The use of gastric residual volumes as a determinant of tube feeding tolerance: a survey of clinical practice, (Abstract), *American Society for Parenteral and Enteral Nutrition 20th Clinical Congress Syllabus*, Washington, DC, 396, 1996.

63. Parrish, C.R., Enteral feeding: the art and the science, *Nutr. Clin. Pract.*, 18, 76, 2003.

64. McClave, S.A. and Snider, H.L., Clinical use of gastric residual volumes as a monitor for patients on enteral feeding, *J. Parenter. Enteral Nutr.*, 26, S43, 2002.

65. Edwards, S.J. and Metheny, N.A., Measurement of gastric residual volume: state of the science, *Medsurg Nurs.*, 9, 125, 2000.

66. McClave, S.A., et al., Use of residual volume as a marker for enteral feeding intolerance: retrospective blinded comparison with physical examination and radiographic findings, *J. Parenter. Enteral Nutr.*, 16, 99, 1992.

67. Powell, K.S., et al., Aspirating gastric residuals causes occlusion of small-bore feeding tubes, *J. Parenter. Enteral Nutr.*, 17, 243, 1993.

68. McClave, S.A., et al., North American Summit on Aspiration in the Critically Ill Patient: consensus statement, *J. Parenter. Enteral Nutr.*, 26, S80, 2002.

69. Lukan, J., et al., Poor validity of residual volume as a marker for risk of aspiration, *Am. J. Clin. Nutr.*, 75, 417S, 2002.

70. Quigley, E.M.M., Hasler, W.L., and Parkman, H.P., AGA technical review on nausea and vomiting, *Gastroenterology*, 120, 263, 2001.

71. Garrett, K., et al., Managing nausea and vomiting, *Crit Care Nurse*, 23, 31, 2003.

72. Levinson, M. and Bryce, A., Enteral feeding, gastric colonization and diarrhoea in the critically ill patient: is there a relationship? *Anaesth. Intens. Care*, 21, 85, 1993.

73. Bliss, D.Z. et al., Acquisition of *Clostridium difficile* and *Clostridium difficile*–associated diarrhea in hospitalized patients receiving tube feeding, *Ann. Intern. Med.*, 129, 1012, 1998.

74. Heimburger, D., Sockwell, D.G., and Geels, W.J., Diarrhea with enteral feeding: prospective reappraisal of putative causes, *Nutrition*, 10, 392, 1994.

75. Keohane, P., et al., Relation between osmolality of diet and gastrointestinal side effects in enteral nutrition, *Br. Med. J.*, 288, 678, 1984.

76. Edes, T.E., Walk, B.E., and Austin, J.L., Diarrhea in tube-fed patients: feeding formula not necessarily the cause, *Am. J. Med.*, 88, 91, 1990.

77. Jones, B.J.M., et al., Comparison of an elemental and polymeric enteral diet in patients with normal gastrointestinal function, *Gut*, 24, 78, 1983.

78. Cataldi-Betcher, E.L. et al., Complications occurring during enteral nutrition support: a prospective study, *J. Parenter. Enteral Nutr.*, 7, 546, 1983.

79. Kelly, T.W.J., Patrick, M.R., and Hillman, K.M., Study of diarrhea in critically ill patients, *Crit. Care Med.*, 11, 7, 1983.

80. Hwang, T.L., et al., The incidence of diarrhea in patients with hypoalbuminemia due to acute or chronic malnutrition during enteral feeding, *Am. J. Gastroenterol.*, 89, 376, 1994.

81. Benya, R., Layden, T.J., and Mobarhan, S., Diarrhea associated with tube feedings: the importance of using objective criteria, *J. Clin. Gastroenterol.*, 13, 167, 1991.

82. Zarling, E.J. et al., Effect of enteral formula infusion rate, osmolality, and chemical composition upon clinical tolerance and carbohydrate absorption in normal subjects, *J. Parenter. Enteral Nutr.*, 10, 588, 1986.

83. Kandil, H.E., et al., Marked resistance of normal subjects to tube-feeding-induced diarrhea: the role of magnesium, *Am. J. Clin. Nutr.*, 57, 73, 1993.

84. Silk, D.A. and Grimble, G.K., Relevance of physiology of nutrient absorption to formulation of enteral diets, *Nutrition*, 8, 1, 1992.

85. Guenter, P.A., Settle, R.G., and Perlmutter, S., Tube feeding related diarrhea in acutely ill patients, *J. Parenter. Enteral Nutr.*, 15, 277, 1991.

86. Bliss, D, Guenter, P.A., and Settle, R.G., Defining and reporting diarrhea in tube-fed patients—what a mess! *Am. J. Clin. Nutr.*, 55, 753, 1992.

87. Szajewska, H. and Mrukowicz, J.Z., Probiotics in the treatment and prevention of acute infectious diarrhea in infants and children: a systematic review of published randomized, double-blind, placebo-controlled trials, *J. Pediatr. Gastroenterol. Nutr.*, 33, S17, 2001.

88. Arvola, T. et al., Prophylactic Lactobacillus GG reduces antibiotic-associated diarrhea in children with respiratory infections: a randomized study, *Pediatrics*, 104, e64, 1999.

89. Bleichner, G. et al., *Saccharomyces boulardii* prevents diarrhea in critically ill tube-fed patients: a multicenter, randomized, double-blind placebo-controlled trial, *Intens. Care Med.,* 23, 517, 1997.

90. Lherm, T. et al., Seven cases of fungemia with *Saccharomyces boulardii* in critically ill patients, *Intens. Care Med.*, 28, 797, 2002.

91. Miller, L.J., Malagelada, J.R., and Go, V.L.W., Postprandial duodenal function in man, *Gut*, 19, 699, 1978.

92. Hecketsweiler, P. et al., Absorption of elemental and complex nutritional solutions during a continuous jejunal perfusion in man, *Digestion*, 19, 213, 1979.

93. American Gastroenterological Association medical position statement: guidelines on constipation, *Gastroenterology*, 119, 1761, 2000.

94. Guenter, P. et al., Delivery systems and administration of enteral nutrition, in *Enteral and Tube Feeding*, 3rd ed., Rombeau J.L. and Rolandelli R.H., eds., W.B. Saunders, Philadelphia, 1997, 255.

95. Ideno K.T., Enteral nutrition, in *Nutrition Support Dietetics Core Curriculum*, 2nd ed., Gottschlich M.M., Matarese L.E., and Shronts E.P., eds., American Society for Parenteral and Enteral Nutrition, Silver Spring, MD, 1993, 89.

96. Heitkemper M, Hanson R, Hansen B., Effects of rate and volume of tube feeding in normal subjects, *Commun. Nurs. Res.*, 10, 71, 1977.

97. Rees, R.P.G. et al., Do patients with moderately impaired gastrointestinal function requiring enteral nutrition need a predigested nitrogen source? A prospective crossover controlled trial, *Gut*, 33, 877, 1992.

98. Rees, R.P.G. et al., Tolerance of elemental diet administered without starter regimen, *Br. Med. J.*, 290, 1869, 1985.

99. Marcuard, S.P., Stegall, K.L., and Trogdon, S., Clearing obstructed feeding tubes, *J. Parenter. Enteral Nutr.*, 13, 81, 1989.

100. Barnadas, G., Nutrition in homecare, *EN Module,* 2003.

20 Drug–Nutrient Interactions

Rex O. Brown
University of Tennessee Health Science Center

CONTENTS

20.1 INTRODUCTION

The interaction of drugs and nutrition is an extremely important component of clinical monitoring of patients [1]. The number of drugs used in the critical care setting has increased exponentially over the last ten years, and early use of nutrition support is being advocated for the critically ill patient. This creates an environment for many possible clinically significant drug–nutrient interactions. This chapter addresses the clinically significant drug–nutrient interactions that may occur in the critical care setting. There are several clinically significant drug–nutrient interactions (e.g., grapefruit juice and many drugs metabolized by the CYP 3A4 enzyme) that would likely not occur in the critical care setting, so they will not be addressed in this chapter.

Chan has suggested that drug–nutrient interactions be placed in four distinct categories [2]:

- Biopharmaceutical inactivations
- Absorption
- Systemic or physiologic dispositions
- Alteration of elimination or clearance

Although this categorization has not been universally accepted, it allows for a systematic clinical evaluation of the different drug–nutrient interactions and possibly identifies areas for concentrated clinical research. Drug-related problems in patients receiving nutrition support in an acute care setting were studied by Cerulli et al. [3]. They reported 220 clinically important interventions in 440 patients. Another patient population at high risk of drug–nutrient interactions, because of the number of medications needed, are solid-organ transplant patients [4]. This chapter addresses clinically important drug–nutrient interactions using two major categories:

- Drugs affecting nutrition
- Nutrition affecting drugs

20.2 DRUG EFFECTS ON NUTRITION THERAPY

20.2.1 GASTROINTESTINAL EFFECTS

Because enteral nutrition (EN) is advocated in critically ill patients, assessment of gastrointestinal tolerance is an important component of clinical monitoring. Drugs that cause gastrointestinal disorders need to be recognized, especially when one is trying to separate EN intolerance from a drug-induced gastrointestinal disorder (Table 20.1).

Nonsteroidal anti-inflammatory drugs often cause gastropathies that include gastric or small bowel ulceration. These drugs are primarily used for mild to moderate pain and fever in the critical care setting. These types of ulcers would interfere with the administration of EN, because frank bleeding can occur as well as nausea and vomiting. Drug vehicles have been under close scrutiny as etiologies of diarrhea because they are often hyperosmolar. Edes et al. reported that approximately 80% of diarrhea in acute care patients was caused by concomitant drug therapy [5]. The major etiologies in this study were sorbitol used as a drug vehicle (48%), diarrhea from *Clostridia difficile* (17%), magnesium-containing antacids (10%), and quinidine (3%).

Liquid drug preparations would be logical choices for critical care patients who have small-bore feeding tubes or permanent ostomies. Many of these liquid products have a substantial sorbitol content and osmolalities than exceed 1000 mOsm/l [6,7]. Preparations like acetaminophen elixir can have an osmolality > 5000 mOsm/l. See Table 20.2 for examples of osmolality for some liquid drug products. When products like this are bolused into tubes, especially jejunostomy tubes, the osmotic load may cause diarrhea. In the case of acetaminophen, switching to crushed tablets followed by 15 to 30 ml water flushes will alleviate this problem. Other interventions include diluting the hyperosmotic liquid preparation with water potentially to improve gastrointestinal tolerance. Prokinetic drugs like metoclopramide are used for improving gastrointestinal emptying during EN in critically ill patients; however, they also act on the small bowel. These drugs can potentially cause gastrointestinal intolerance in some patients. When gastric emptying is improved with the administration of metoclopramide, the drug should then be discontinued or the dose should be reduced as appropriate to prevent diarrhea in the patient receiving EN.

20.2.2 FLUID AND ELECTROLYTES

A major part of clinical monitoring of the critical care patient who is receiving EN or parenteral nutrition (PN) is treating fluid and electrolyte imbalances. These problems occur quite often in this patient care setting and may be even more common in patients receiving nutrition support [8]. There are many drugs that induce electrolyte imbalances, and an appreciation of these can markedly improve clinical monitoring. Some electrolyte imbalances may be inherited by the nutrition support service (NSS). Because most of the electrolyte components are in the PN or EN formulations, there is an expectation that the nutrient formulations will help treat these disorders.

TABLE 20.1
Gastrointestinal Disorders Caused by Drug Therapy

Drug	Result
NSAIDS, aspirin	Gastrointestinal ulceration
Hyperosmolar liquids	Diarrhea
Sorbitol-containing preparations	Diarrhea
Metoclopramide	Diarrhea

Note: NSAIDS = Nonsteroidal anti-inflammatory drugs.

TABLE 20.2
Osmolality of Selected Liquid Drug Products Used in Critical Care

Drug	Osmolality (mOsm/kg)
Acetaminophen elixir (650 mg/10 ml)	5400
Acetaminophen with codeine elixir	4700
Amoxacillin suspension (250 mg/5ml)	2250
Cimetidine elixir (300 mg/5 ml)	5550
Trimethoprim–sulfamethoxazole suspension	2200
Dexamthasone elixir (1 mg/10 ml)	3350
Dextromethorphan syrup (10 mg/5 ml)	5950
Docusate sodium syrup (100 mg/30 ml)	4700
Erythromycin ethylsuccinate suspension (200 mg/5 ml)	1750
Ferrous sulfate liquid (300 mg/5 ml)	4700
Furosemide solution (40 mg/4 ml)	2050
Lactulose syrup (20 g/30 ml)	3600
Metoclopramide syrup (10 mg/10 ml)	8350
Multivitamin liquid	5700
Phenytoin suspension (125 mg/5 ml)	1500
Potassium chloride liquid 10%	3550

Source: Adapted from Dickerson, R.N. and Melnik G., *Am. J. Hosp. Pharm.*, 45, 832, 1988; and Lutomski, D.M. et al., *Ann. Pharmocother.*, 27, 269, 1993.

TABLE 20.3
Hyponatremia and Nutrition Support

Type of Hyponatremia	Treatment
Hypotonic hypovolemic	Continue PN or EN
	Replace volume deficits with NS or LR
Hypotonic euvolemic	Concentrate PN to decrease free water
	Concentrate EN to decrease free water
	Decrease other water intake (IVF)
Hypotonic hypervolemic	Eliminate sodium and concentrate PN
	Concentrate EN by using 2 kcal/ml formulation
	Discontinue IVF/water boluses

Note: NS = normal saline; LR = lactated Ringer's; IVF = intravenous fluid.

Sodium imbalances are the most difficult to diagnose and treat. Patients with hyponatremia need to be evaluated for extracellular volume status concurrently (Table 20.3). Hypovolemic hyponatremia requires replacement of salt and water, usually as normal saline or lactated Ringer's in the critical care setting. Euvolemic hyponatremia usually requires water restriction in the critical care setting, and hypervolemic hyponatremia would require salt and, especially, water restriction. Some drugs like loop diuretics have an intended effect to increase the renal excretion of sodium, usually for an overhydrated state. Other drugs like trimethoprim–sulfamethoxazole and cisplatin cause renal wasting of sodium, but they are often overlooked as etiologies [9,10]. In critical care patients, there are many causes of the syndrome of inappropriate secretion of antidiuretic hormone (SIADH), with drugs being a major contributor to this problem [11]. Carbamazepine, thiazide diuretics, and amiodarone have all been implicated to cause SIADH [12–14]. Patients with hyponatremia from these drugs will need free water restricted by concentrating the nutrient formulation, especially if the drug cannot be changed. This would require higher concentrations of dextrose, amino acids, and lipid in the PN formulation so the infusion rate could be decreased and still meet the patient's nutritional needs. With EN, administration of a 1.5 or 2 kcal/ml formulation would be used to minimize water and still meet nutritional needs. Hypernatremia usually implies a deficit in water; however, extracellular volume status must be assessed so that proper treatment can be prescribed. Excessive administration of lactulose has resulted in hypovolemic hypernatremia, presumably from excessive stool losses of water [15]. Replacement with salt and water initially to perfuse vital organs should be followed by the administration of hypotonic fluid like water, one-quarter normal saline, one-half normal saline, or D5W. Obviously, the dose of the drug should be reduced to reduce stool losses to an acceptable volume (e.g., 1 to 2 soft stools per day).

Potassium balance in the critical care patient can be particularly challenging because multiple factors (e.g., urine output, pH) can change and influence the concentration of this cation. Potassium is particularly important in nutrition support patients because it is the major intracellular cation; as new cells are synthesized, potassium will be incorporated into them. Many drugs affect potassium balance. Loop and thiazide diuretics, antipseudomonal penicillins, corticosteroids, and amphotericin B can all cause increased urinary excretion of potassium, resulting in hypokalemia. Drugs like piperacillin have been shown to decrease not only potassium, but also serum concentrations of magnesium and calcium [16]. Amphotericin B has been reported to increase urinary excretion of both potassium and magnesium. Other drugs, like insulin and beta-2 agonists, promote the movement of potassium into the intracellular space and can result in hypokalemia. Dickens et al. demonstrated a mean decrease of 0.8 mEq/l in serum potassium concentration following a single nebulized 2.5 mg dose of albuterol [17].

It is common to have patients in the critical care setting receiving nutrition support and several of the preceding drugs at one time. Standard amounts of potassium in PN or EN formulations will not maintain potassium balance in these patients when they are receiving these drugs. They will need frequent bolus doses of potassium and to have the concentration increased in PN. See Table 20.4 for general guidelines for administering electrolytes for hypokalemia, hypophosphatemia, hypomagnesemia, and hypocalcemia. Parenteral potassium products should be used when potassium is admixed with EN formulations to increase the dose of this electrolyte. Oral liquid preparations of potassium are generally incompatible with enteral feeding formulations.

Several drugs are known to induce hyperkalemia. Hyperkalemia secondary to potassium-sparing diuretics, angiotensin-converting enzyme inhibitors, and angiotensin-receptor blocking agents is well appreciated in all settings. Heparin is now known to be a cause of hyperkalemia, especially with therapeutic doses in patients with diabetes or renal failure [18]. Heparin is known to inhibit aldosterone, which normally causes sodium retention and potassium excretion. Antagonism of aldosterone results in sodium excretion and potassium retention. Trimethoprim, which is a component with sulfamethoxazole in an antibiotic product, is also a weak potassium-sparing diuretic [19]. Two clinical studies have reported mean increases in the serum potassium concentration > 1 mEq/l in patients receiving the sulfamethoxazole–trimethoprim combination [20,21].

Calcium imbalances in the critical care setting are fairly common. One recent study of 100 critically ill patients reported a 21% incidence and a 6% incidence of hypocalemia and hypercalcemia, respectively, using ionized calcium concentrations [22]. It should be noted that it is very difficult to separate true hypocalcemia from hypocalcemia secondary to hypoalbuminemia using total calcium concentrations, because the common conversion equations are inaccurate in the ICU setting [22]. In the critical care setting, ionized calcium concentrations, if available, should be used exclusively to assess calcium status.

Foscarnet, a drug used for cytomegalovirus in patients with HIV infection, has a profound effect on ionized calcium concentrations by inducing hypocalcemia. Four of six patients receiving a 90 mg/kg dose developed hypocalcemia, whereas all 11 patients receiving a 120 mg/kg dose

TABLE 20.4
Treatment of Common Electrolyte Disorders Requiring
Replacement in Critically Ill Patients[a]

Hypokalemia[b]

Lab Value (mEq/l)	Intravenous Replacement Dose (mEq)
3.5–3.9	40
3–3.4	40×2
< 3	40×3

Hypophosphatemia[c]

Lab Value (mg/dl)	Intravenous Replacement Dose (mmol/kg)
2.3–3	0.16
1.6–2.2	0.32
≤ 1.5	0.64

Hypomagnesemia[d]

Lab Value (mg/dl)	Intravenous Replacement Dose (g/kg)
1.6–1.8	0.05
1–1.5	0.10
< 1	0.15

Hypocalcemia[e]

Lab Value (mmol/l)	Intravenous Replacement Dose (g)
1–1.12	1
0.9–0.99	2
< 0.9	3

[a] These guidelines are only for patients with normal renal function. Intravenous replacement doses are usually required in critically ill patients secondary to the acuity of the patient and potential for serum concentrations to decrease further. Oral replacement may be appropriate for patients who are hemodynamically stable and have a functional and accessible gastrointestinal tract.

[b] Do not administer faster than 20 mEq/h.

[c] Do not administer faster than 7.5 mmol/h.

[d] Do not administer faster than 1 g/h.

[e] May give 3 g over 1 h.

developed this electrolyte disorder [23]. Patients receiving intravenous foscarnet should be monitored frequently and vigorously supplemented with calcium during and after administration of this drug.

A nutrient (calcium carbonate) and a drug (levothyroxine) that are often given to geriatric patients may potentially interact [24]. When these are administered concurrently, it has been shown *in vitro* that levothyroxine may adsorb to calcium carbonate. This could lead to increases in the dosing of the thryroid product. When patients are receiving both drugs, it would be prudent to space the administration times so that the levothyroxine is given 2 to 4 hours apart from the calcium administration.

Calcium gluconate and calcium chloride are products used commonly for parenteral treatment or replacement of hypocalcemia in the critically ill. It should be appreciated that 1 g of calcium chloride provides three times as much calcium per gram as calcium gluconate (13.5 mEq/g vs. 4.5 mEq/g). Most clinicians use calcium gluconate for parenteral replacement of calcium in the critical care setting. Oral calcium is used most frequently for bone health; however, these products could theoretically be used to treat hypocalcemia in patients who are hemodynamically stable with functional and accessible gastrointestinal tracts. The two products used most frequently are calcium carbonate (20 mEq of elemental calcium/g) and calcium acetate (12.7 mEq of elemental calcium/g).

Similar to potassium, the need for phosphorus will be markedly enhanced as new cells are synthesized during administration of nutrition support, because phosphate is the major intracellular anion. It has been demonstrated that patients with hypophosphatemia also have a deficit of phosphorus skeletal muscle [25]. This issue is particularly important in patients with underlying pulmonary disease (e.g., COPD) or in patients receiving mechanical ventilation in the critical care setting.

Drugs that contribute or cause hypophosphatemia include antacids or sucralfate through gastrointestinal tract binding of the anion and beta-2 adrenergic agonists that may enhance the intracellular uptake of phosphorus [26,27]. When administration of these drugs is added to administration of nutrition support in the critical care setting, the potential to develop hypophosphatemia is greatly enhanced.

Many clinicians begin the replacement of phosphorus when patients have serum concentrations of phosphorus in the low-normal range [28]. This could theoretically prevent moderate to severe hypophosphatemia and the accompanying sequellae. With PN, the phosphorus concentration can be increased to 30 mmol/l safely in most formulations. With EN, phosphorus can be added directly to the formulation using sodium phosphate (Fleet Phosphosoda) or injectable potassium phosphate. Many patients will need intravenous replacement as well as having the phosphate concentration increased in the PN or EN formulations. Oral replacement of phosphorus is an option for patients with mild hypophosphatemia; however, the gastrointestinal tract is limited to what can be tolerated because phosphate is an osmotic laxative and can cause diarrhea.

Hyperphosphatemia is rare outside of acute or chronic renal failure; however, a few cases of this disorder secondary to administration of oral phosphorus in patients with compromised renal function have been reported [29]. It should also be noted that colonic absorption of phosphorus can occur following administration of phosphate-containing enemas. Severe hyperphosphatemia (serum phosphorus concentration > 6 mg/dl) invariably requires removal of all phosphorus from the PN formulation. Metastatic calcification of calcium phosphate in soft tissues can occur with severe hyperphosphatemia. This is particularly important in the patient who has any degree of renal compromise. With EN, formulations with lower concentrations of phosphorus can be used or phosphate binders (e.g., calcium acetate) may be added.

Hypomagnesemia is another electrolyte disorder that occurs fairly frequently in the critical care setting. Although lower gastrointestinal losses and alcohol abuse are contributing causes of magnesium depletion, drugs are major factors in critical care patients. Several drugs have been identified to cause or contribute to hypomagnesemia through renal wasting of this electrolyte. Cisplatin, cyclosporine, aminoglycosides, loop or thiazide diuretics, and amphotericin B have all been shown to increase urinary excretion of magnesium [30–33]. Elliott et al. demonstrated a significant increase in magnesium fractional excretion rate from 3.4 ± 0.8 to $11.8 \pm 6.4\%$ following the administration of gentamicin [34]. Foscarnet has been reported to cause hypomagnesemia in addition to its effects on calcium status [35]. Considering that several of these drugs can be given to critical care patients concurrently, hypomagnesemia can become a major problem when serum electrolyte monitoring and appropriate supplementation are not implemented.

Hypomagnesemia can also cause hypokalemia because it is important in maintaining proper functioning of the sodium–potassium ATPase pump. Also, magnesium is critically important in the function of parathyroid hormone, which maintains calcium balance. Therefore, moderate to severe hypomagnesemia can also cause hypocalcemia. With PN, the concentration of magnesium sulfate can be increased to 32 mEq/l in many formulations. A standard concentration range used by many

---

TABLE 20.5
Drugs that Can Potentially Alter Glucose
Homeostasis in the Critical Care Setting

Generic Name	Trade Name
Hyperglycemia	
Hydrochlorothiazide	Hydrodiuril and others
Cyclosporine	Sandimmune/Neoral
Hydrocortisone	Solu-Cortef
Methylprednisolone	Solu-Medrol
Diltiazem	Cardizem
Hypoglycemia	
Gatifloxacin	Tequin
Pentamidine	Pentam 300
Regular insulin	Multiple
Glyburide	Diabeta/Micronase
Glipizide	Glucotrol

---

institutions is from 8 to 12 mEq/l. Intravenous replacement of magnesium sulfate is often needed in addition to increasing the concentration in the PN formulation. With EN, it is difficult to replace a large magnesium deficit via the gastrointestinal tract because of its cathartic properties. In the critical care setting, intravenous replacement is the most reliable method of treatment, especially for those patients with moderate to severe hypomagnesemia. Magnesium oxide or magnesium gluconate are oral forms of magnesium that can be administered PO or via tube in patients receiving EN with mild hypomagnesemia. Gastrointestinal tolerance must be monitored closely during administration of the previously mentioned salts because they can be cathartic laxatives in some patients.

Glucose homeostasis in the critically ill has recently received a great amount of attention. Van den Berghe et al. demonstrated improved mortality when critical care patients' glucose concentrations were kept in the normal range using continuous regular insulin infusions [36]. Drugs that cause hyperglycemia or hypoglycemia need to be appreciated (Table 20.5). This will also help the nutrition support clinician determine how aggressive glucose control must be. It is well recognized now that protease inhibitors can cause hyperglycemia [37,38]. In fact, Tsiodras et al. demonstrated a relative risk factor of 5 for patients developing hyperglycemia when taking a protease inhibitor, compared to a control group [37]. Cyclosporine is another drug associated with the development of hyerglycemia [39]. Both decreased synthesis and increased clearance of insulin have been shown to occur with the administration of cyclosporine [39]. Corticosteroid administration will promote hepatic gluconeogenesis and resultant hypergycermia.

Patients who receive PN and drugs that induce hyperglycemia must be monitored and treated carefully. Most clinicians will add regular insulin to the PN formulation to assist in glucose control. Many institutions have "tightened" sliding scales with regular insulin (e.g., > 120 mg/dl) and now have a lower threshold for initiating regular insulin infusions because of the benefits of controlling hyperglycemia in the critical care population. Patients receiving EN can be changed to a high-fat, low-carbohydrate formulation and have a more aggressive regimen with regular insulin to scale for short-term control of hyerglycemia in patients in the critical care setting [40,41].

Hypoglycemia has been associated with the administration of gatifloxacin, a fluroquinolone recently introduced in the U.S. [42,43]. Most cases have involved type 2 diabetic patients who were also taking oral hypoglycemic agents. Although the mechanism is unknown, patients receiving nutrition support and gatifloxacin should be monitored very closely for hypoglycemia.

20.2.3 VITAMINS

There are a number of clinically important drug–nutrient interactions involving vitamins; however, the majority of these will be encountered in chronic care and will not be covered in this chapter. Two independent studies have identified the risk of developing thiamine deficiency following the administration of the loop diuretic furosemide [44,45]. It is thought that the loop diuretic enhances the urinary excretion of thiamine, leading to a deficient state. This is likely to occur when furosemide is prescribed in multiple doses for several days or as a continuous intravenous infusion. Because therapeutic doses of thiamine (100 mg BID) are relatively benign, supplementation of this vitamin when loop diuretics are used over several days appears to be prudent.

It is appreciated that the absorption of vitamin B-12 (cyanocobolamin) is markedly decreased when patients are treated with proton pump inhibitors [46]. Although the development of a macrocytic anemia would take a few years to develop with chronic therapy, many patients are placed on proton pump inhibitors for acid suppression while in intensive care units, especially if they had been receiving the drug before admission. This is an excellent time to monitor the patient for anemia as part of routine clinical care. Some clinicians will monitor for macrocytic anemia using enzymes that are dependent on folic acid and cyanocobalamin. For instance, elevated serum concentrations of homocysteine and methylmalonic acid are consistent with cyanocobalamin deficiency in a patient with a macrocytic anemia. Intramuscular treatment of cyanocobalamin is the treatment of choice for this type of patients, especially if they must continue to receive proton pump inhibitors.

Drug vehicles can have important implications to the nutrition support clinician when a substantial dose of nutrition is delivered to the critically ill patient. Propofol, an intravenous anesthetic and sedative, is frequently used for several days in selected patients in the critical care setting [47]. This product is particularly useful in severe head trauma when frequent neurological evaluations are desired. The short half-life of propofol allows periodic stopping and evaluation of mental status. It is contained in a 10% lipid emulsion vehicle, so patients receive a continuous infusion of fat emulsion when this drug is given for sedation (Table 20.6). Several authors have identified the importance of including lipid calories from propofol when prescribing nutrition support [48,49]. If the dose of lipid (e.g., 9 to 10 kcal/kg/d) from propofol approaches the desired lipid dose with PN, lipid can be omitted from the PN formulation until the propofol is weaned or discontinued. EN patients who are receiving a substantial number of calories from propofol can be treated with a low-calorie, high-protein EN formulation so the fat calories from the drug vehicle will be

TABLE 20.6
Lipid Calories Delivered from Different Doses
of Propofol Infusion

Rate (ml/h)	Propofol Dose (mg/h)	Calories/24 h
10	100	264
15	150	396
20	200	528
25	250	660
30	300	792

accounted for. Even though one group has suggested that propofol infusions do not increase serum triglyceride concentrations [50], this has not been the experience of many clinicians [48,49]. Therefore, serum triglyceride concentrations should be monitored frequently (e.g., two to three times per week) when patients are receiving higher doses of propofol (e.g., > 5 mg/kg/h). If patients develop serum triglyceride concentrations > 500 mg/dl during propofol infusions, an alternative sedative agent like lorazepam or midazolam should be considered. There are now several lipid preparations of amphotericin B marketed in the U.S.; however, their caloric contribution is negligible [51].

20.2.4 METABOLIC ALTERATIONS

Several drugs are known to affect resting energy expenditure of patients, especially some of the agents that are used in the critical care setting. The barbiturate nembutal is used in patients with traumatic brain injury who are refractory to standard interventions to reduce intracranial pressure. This drug will clearly reduce energy expenditure. Dempsey et al. demonstrated that patients with traumatic brain injury not receiving nembutal had a mean resting energy expenditure of 126% above basal energy expenditure [52]. Conversely, those patients with traumatic brain injury who received nembutal demonstrated a resting energy expenditure of 86% of basal energy expenditure. This highly significant difference equated to a change of 600 kcal/d. Therefore, appreciation of what a barbiturate coma will do to resting energy expenditure is important when prescribing nutrition support in this critically ill population. Beta-adrenergic blockers have also been reported to reduce resting energy expenditure significantly (approximately 8%) [53].

20.3 NUTRITIONAL EFFECTS ON DRUG THERAPY

Substantial data involve the effect of nutrition on the metabolism of drugs [54]; however, many of the clinically significant issues do not involve critical care patients like the grapefruit juice–drug interactions. Also, several of these interactions that are statistically significant are not really clinically important. It is known, however, that volume of distribution for many drugs is increased in severe starvation due to an expanded extracellular volume compartment. Also, conjugation of many drugs may be impaired in patients with malnutrition [54]. It is very clear that the clearance of aminoglycoside antibiotics like gentamicin is enhanced with the administration of dietary protein [55]. Because these types of drugs have a narrow therapeutic index (i.e., small difference between drug failure, drug efficacy, and drug toxicity), appreciation of this drug–nutrient interaction is critical. Patients who are receiving aminoglycosides and have PN or EN started should have a marked increase in renal clearance of these drugs. This is especially true of critical care patients, where high-protein formulations are the standard of practice provided patients have normal renal function. Clinicians managing this type of patient should expect to increase the dose of aminoglycosides to maintain or attain therapeutic drug concentrations.

The effect of EN on drug therapy has become an important issue in the critical care setting. EN is being promoted as the feeding method of choice, so many patients now have enteral access via small-bore feeding tubes who would not have had this in the past. Therefore, drug therapy via tube becomes a reality in many different scenarios [56]. Several oral dosage forms are prepared as sustained-release preparations. Generally, these should not be crushed and administered via a feeding tube (Table 20.7) [57]. In many cases, the sustained-release capsule can be opened and the intact pellets may be poured down the feeding tube, followed by a water flush. This maintains the integrity of the sustained-release product but allows it to be administered via a tube if the patient cannot or will not swallow. Proton pump inhibitors (lansoprazole, pantoprazole) generally should be given with an acidic juice when administered via a gastric feeding tube; they can be given with a sodium bicarbonate capsule and water when given via a jejunostomy feeding tube [56].

TABLE 20.7
Selected Drugs Used in Critical Care that Should Not Be Crushed

Trade Name(s)	Generic Name	Reason
Adalat CC	Nifedipine	Slow release
Artane Sequels	Trihexyphenidyl	Slow release
ASA Enseals	Aspirin	Enteric coated
Dulcolax	Bisacodyl	Enteric coated
Calan SR	Verapamil	Slow release
Cardizem CD or SR	Diltiazem	Slow release
Cellcept	Mycophenolate	Teratogenic potential
Cipro	Ciprofloxacin	Taste
Colace	Docusate	Taste
Creon-10 or 20	Pancreatic enzymes	Enteric coated
Depakote	Valproic acid	Enteric coated
EES 400, E-mycin	Erythromycin	Enteric coated
Feosol spansule	Iron sulfate	Slow release
Glucotrol XL	Glipizide	Slow release
Humibid LA	Guiafenesin	Slow release
Inderal LA	Propranolol	Slow release
Isordil sublingual	Isosorbide	Sublingual preparation
K-Dur	Potassium chloride	Slow release
MS Contin	Morphine sulfate	Slow release
Nitrostat	Nitroglycerin	Sublingual preparation
Norpace CR	Disopyramide	Slow release in capsule
Prevacid	Lansoprazole	Slow release
Prilosec	Omeprazole	Slow release
Slow-K	Potassium chloride	Slow release
Slow-Mg	Magnesium sulfate	Slow release
Trental	Pentoxifylline	Slow release

Source: Adapted in part from Mitchell, J.E., *Hosp. Pharm.*, 35, 553, 2000.

One of the most appreciated drug–nutrient interactions is between phenytoin and EN formulations. Despite being recognized for over 20 years [58], there is still debate about the cause and the clinical significance of the interaction [59,60]. Bauer demonstrated a significant decrease in phenytoin serum concentrations in neurosurgical patients who received both the drug and EN concurrently, compared to patients receiving only the drug [58]. He suggested holding EN two hours before and after the phenytoin dose to improved absorption [58]. Other authors have suggested to increase the phenytoin dose when given with EN until a therapeutic serum concentration and adequate seizure control or prophylaxis is attained [61]. Others have supported the recommendations of Bauer and suggest holding EN around the phenytoin dose or doses [60]. *In vitro* data suggest that phenytoin suspension adheres to caseinate salts, which are often used as the protein component of EN formulations [62]. A study in healthy volunteers demonstrated that phenytoin suspension given via tube during EN administration showed delayed absorption, compared to injectable phenytoin given the same way (i.e., via the enteral route) [63]. This is consistent with earlier reports that the interaction is quite profound in patients but less so in normal volunteers [58]. The data available certainly suggest that there is an interaction between phenytoin and EN. Holding the EN infusion around phenytoin doses appears to be successful in having the patient achieve therapeutic drug concentrations and seizure control. From a nutritional standpoint, it is important to realize that the desired EN dose would need to be infused over 20 hours if a daily dose of phenytoin is given while

EN is held two hours before and after the administration. For patients receiving phenytoin suspension three times per day, the EN administration should be held at least one hour before and after each dose. This would require that the desired EN dose be infused over 18 hours each day. Because phenytoin is another drug with a narrow therapeutic index, regular measurements of serum concentrations should be done as well as close monitoring for seizures, especially in those patients following traumatic brain injury in whom the drug is used primarily for prophylaxis.

Another potentially major drug–nutrient interaction occurs between warfarin and EN or PN formulations. Some clinical data suggest that this interaction occurs and that the drug may actually bind to the protein component of EN [64]. *In vitro* data from Kuhn et al. support this mechanism [65]. Some clinicians hold the EN one hour before and after the daily dose, but this practice has not been supported by clinical studies to date. Several reports exist of warfarin resistance during the administration of lipid-containing PN [66,67]. It is interesting to note that 500 ml of 10% intravenous fat emulsion contains 154 mcg of vitamin K from the plant oils of the soybean used to make these products. Other formulations, using a combination of soybean and safflower plant oils, may provide < 100 mcg of vitamin K. Some clinicians believe that the vitamin K from these products will make anticoagulation very difficult. This becomes even more important as many institutions make the transition to new daily parenteral vitamin products that contain 150 mcg of vitamin K. Prothrombin time and INR monitoring during warfarin administration are imperative in the patient receiving concomitant PN, especially with intravenous fat emulsion and vitamins containing vitamin K.

Another group of drugs that have been extensively studied during the administration of EN formulations is the fluoroquinolones. Because the absorption of these drugs is significantly reduced when they are coadministered with ferrous sulfate or antacids, it would be natural to question the bioavailability of these agents during coadministration with EN. Unfortunately, the literature to date addressing this potential drug–nutrient interaction is conflicting. Some *in vitro* work, where the drug was mixed with several different EN formulations, demonstrated an 83% loss of ciprofloxacin, a 61% loss of levofloxacin, and a 46% loss of oflaxacin [68]. A single-dose, randomized crossover study using ciprofloxacin 750 mg orally taken with either water or an enteral supplement demonstrated a 25% decrease in absorption of the drug when taken with the supplement [69]. Yuk et al. conducted a study in healthy volunteers, who received three separate 750 mg doses of ciprofloxacin with appropriate washout periods between each dose [70]. The doses where given orally, via a nasogastric tube, and via a nasogastric tube with continuous-infusion EN. The investigators did not find a significant difference in area under the curve or bioavailability during the three methods of administration. Other investigators have found the availability of ciprofloxacin to be adequate when the drug was given concurrently with continuously infused EN in critically ill patients [71,72]. It also appears that gatifloxacin has adequate bioavailability when co administered with continuous EN in critically ill patients [73]. Therefore, the current data suggest that the fluoroquinolones may be given during continuous infusion of EN, even though some institutions hold the feeding one hour before and after each dose. The location of the feeding tube, however, may be very important because it relates to the administration of the fluoroquinolones. The major site of absorption is the duodenum, so administration of this drug via a jejunostomy feeding tube cannot be recommended at this time.

20.4 SUMMARY

Screening drug therapy for potential drug–nutrient interactions will always be an important part of clinical monitoring during delivery of PN or EN to critically ill patients. The clinically significant drug–nutrient interactions must be recognized so that clinicians can make rational decisions in caring for this patient population. The introduction of new drugs and nutritional products will undoubtedly increase the number of these interactions, which will continually change the way clinicians practice during the provision of nutrition support.

20.5 CASE STUDY

L.L. is a 70-year-old male who was involved in a motor vehicle crash. He sustained a broken femur, severe head injury, and pulmonary contusions. After undergoing a craniotomy and pinning of the femur, he requires mechanical ventilation and sedation with propofol. The patient is 6 feet tall and weights 80 kg. He has a past medical history for congestive heart failure and hypertension. Current medications in the critical care setting are:

- Phenytoin 100 mg IV Q8H
- Furosemide 40 mg IV BID
- Pantoprazole 40 mg IV daily
- Albuterol treatments Q6H
- Heparin 5000 units SQ BID
- Propofol 20 ml/h

On hospital day 3, he has bowel sounds, so EN is started at 40 ml/h (1 kcal/ml, 63 g protein/l formula). On day 4, EN is advanced to 60 ml/h, and on day 5, it is advanced to 85 ml/h. The following laboratory values are available on day 5:

- Sodium = 150 mEq/l
- Potassium = 3.2 mEq/l
- Chloride = 118 mEq/l
- Bicarbonate = 22 mEq/l
- Blood urea nitrogen = 10 mg/dl
- Serum creatinine = 1 mg/dl
- Ionized calcium = 1.05 mmol/l
- Phosphorus = 1.5 mg/dl
- Magnesium = 1.2 mg/dl
- Triglycerides = 180 mg/dl
- Arterial blood gas: pH = 7.5 pCO2 = 30 pO2 = 95 HCO3 = 23

Questions:

1. What drugs or clinical conditions contributed to LL's hypokalemia?
2. What drug contributed to LL's hypocalcemia?
3. What drug contributed to LL's hypomagnesemia?
4. Design a regimen of electrolyte boluses for LL.
5. What drug likely contributed to LL's hypertriglyceridemia?
6. How many calories are being given via drug vehicles? How many calories/kg/d are being given via drug vehicles?
7. The patient had a seizure shortly after injury, so phenytoin will be continued beyond 1 week. It is changed to 300 mg daily as capsules. What intervention would allow absorption of the drug and deliver the desired nutrition support?

Answers:

1. Furosemide by renal wasting of potassium, albuterol by promoting intracellular movement, and respiratory alkalosis.
2. Furosemide by renal wasting of calcium.
3. Furosemide by renal wasting of magnesium.
4. K phosphate 50 mmol IV over 7 h.

Magnesium SO4 8 g IV over 8 h.

Ca gluconate 1 g IV over 15 to 30 min.

5. Propofol.
6. 528 calories or 6.6 kcal/kg/d.
7. Hold the EN 2 hours before and after the daily phenytoin dose. Increase EN to run 100 ml/h × 20 h to deliver the desired nutrition support.

REFERENCES

1. Sacks, G.S. and Brown, R.O., Drug–nutrient interactions in patients receiving nutritional support, *Drug Ther.*, 24, 35, 1994.
2. Chan, L.N., Redefining drug–nutrient interactions, *Nutr. Clin. Prac.*, 15, 249, 2000.
3. Cerulli, J. and Malone, M., Assessment of drug-related problems in clinical nutrition patients, *J. Parenter. Enteral Nutr.*, 23, 218, 1999.
4. Chan, L.N., Drug–nutrient interactions in transplant recipients, *J. Parenter. Enteral Nutr.*, 25, 132, 2001.
5. Edes, T.E., Walk, B.E., and Austin, J.L., Diarrhea in tube-fed patients: feeding formula not necessarily the cause, *Am. J. Med.*, 88, 98, 1990.
6. Dickerson, R.N. and Melnik G., Osmolality of oral drug solutions and suspensions, *Am. J. Hosp. Pharm.*, 45, 832, 1988.
7. Lutomski, D.M. et al., Sorbitol content of selected oral liquids, *Ann. Pharmocother.*, 27, 269, 1993.
8. Driscoll, D.F., Drug-induced metabolic disorders and parenteral nutrition in the intensive care unit: a pharmaceutical and metabolic perspective, *DICP, Ann. Pharmacother.*, 23, 363, 1989.
9. Kaufman, A.M., Hellman, G., and Abramson, R.G., Renal salt wasting and metabolic acidosis with trimethoprim-sulfamethoxazole therapy, *Mount Sinai J. Med.*, 50, 238, 1983.
10. Hutchison, F.N., et al., Renal salt wasting in patients treated with cisplatin, *Ann. Intern. Med.*, 108, 21, 1988.
11. Belton, K. and Thomas, S.H., Drug-induced syndrome of inappropriate antidiuretic hormone secretion, *Postgrad. Med. J.*, 75, 509, 1999.
12. Lahr, M.B., Hyponatremia during carbamazepine therapy, *Clin. Pharmacol. Ther.*, 37, 693, 1985.
13. Sonnenblick, M., Friedlander, Y., and Rosin, A.J., Diuretic-induced severe hyponatremia: review and analysis of 129 reported patients, *Chest*, 103, 601, 1993.
14. Patel, G.P. and Kasiar, J.B., Syndrome of inappropriate antidiuretic hormone-induced hyponatremia associated with amiodarone, *Pharmacotherapy*, 22, 649, 2002.
15. Nelson, D.C., McGrew, W.R., and Hoyumpa, A.M., Hypernatremia and lactulose therapy, *JAMA*, 249, 1295, 1983.
16. Polderman, K.H. and Girbes, A.R., Piperacillin-induced magnesium and potassium loss in intensive care unit patients, *Intens. Care Med.*, 28, 520, 2002.
17. Dickens, G.R., et al., Effect of nebulized albuterol on serum potassium and cardiac rhythm in patients with asthma or chronic obstructive pulmonary disease, *Pharmacotherapy*, 14, 729, 1994.
18. Oster, J.R., Singer, I., and Fishman, L.M., Heparin-induced aldosterone suppression and hyperkalemia, *Am. J. Med.*, 98, 575, 1995.
19. Velazquez, H. et al., Renal mechanism of trimethoprim-induced hyperkalemia, *Ann. Intern. Med.*, 119, 296, 1993.
20. Greenberg, S. et al., Trimethoprim-sulfamethoxazole induces reversible hyperkalemia, *Ann. Intern. Med.*, 119, 291, 1993.
21. Alappan, R., Perazella, M.A., and Buller, G.K., Hyperkalemia in hospitalized patients treated with trimethoprim-sulfamethoxazole, *Ann. Intern. Med.*, 124, 316, 1996.
22. Dickerson, R.N. et al., Accuracy of methods to estimate ionized and corrected serum calcium concentrations in critically ill multiple trauma patients receiving specialized nutrition support, *J. Parenter. Enteral Nutr.*, 27, S5, 2003 (abstract).
23. Jacobson, M.A. et al., Foscarnet-induced hypocalcemia and effects of foscarnet on calcium metabolism, *J. Clin. Endocrinol. Metab.*, 72, 1130, 1991.

24. Singh, N., Singh, P.N., and Hershman, J.M., Effect of calcium carbonate on the absorption of levothyroxine, *JAMA*, 283, 2822, 2000.

25. Fiaccadori, E. et al., Hypophosphatemia in course of chronic obstructive pulmonary disease, *Chest*, 97, 857, 1990.

26. Brown, G.R. and Greenwood, J.K., Drug- and nutrition-induced hypophosphatemia: mechanisms and relevance in the critically ill, *Ann. Pharmacother.*, 28, 626, 1994.

27. Miller, S.J. and Simpson, J., Medication-nutrient interactions: hypophosphatemia associated with sucralfate in the intensive care unit, *Nutr. Clin. Prac.*, 6, 199, 1991.

28. Clark, C.L. et al., Treatment of hypophosphatemia in patients receiving specialized nutrition support using a graduated dosing scheme: results from a prospective clinical trial, *Crit. Care Med.*, 23, 1504, 1995.

29. Sutters, M., Gaboury, C.L., and Bennett, W.M., Severe hyperphosphatemia and hypocalcemia: a dilemma in patient management, *J. Am. Soc. Nephrol.*, 7, 2056, 1996.

30. Schilsky, R.L. and Anderson, T., Hypomagnesemia and renal magnesium wasting in patients receiving cisplatin, *Ann. Intern. Med.*, 90, 929, 1979.

31. Nozue, T. et al., Pathogenesis of cyclosporine-induced hypomagnesemia, *J. Pediatr.*, 120, 638, 1992.

32. Zaloga, G.P. et al., Hypomagnesemia is a common complication of aminoglycoside therapy, *Surg. Gynecol. Obstet.*, 158, 561, 1984.

33. Sheehan, J. and White, A., Diuretic-associated hypomagnesemia, *Br. Med. J.*, 285, 1157, 1982.

34. Elliott, C., Newman, N., and Madan, A., gentamicin effects on urinary electrolyte excretion in healthy subjects, *Clin. Pharmacol. Ther.*, 67, 16, 2000.

35. Gearhart, M.O. and Sorg, T.B., Foscarnet-induced severe hypomagnesemia and other electrolyte disorders, *Ann. Pharmacother.*, 27, 285, 1993.

36. Van den Berghe, G. et al., Intensive insulin therapy in critically ill patients, *N. Engl. J. Med.*, 354, 1359, 2001.

37. Tsiodras, S. et al., Effects of protease inhibitors on hyperglycemia, hyperlipidemia, and lipodystrophy: a 5-year cohort study, *Arch. Intern. Med.*, 160, 2050, 2000.

38. Kaufman, M.B. and Simionatto, C., A review of protease inhibitor-induced hyperglycemia, *Pharmacotherapy*, 19, 114, 1999.

39. Dresner, L.S. et al., Effects of cyclosporine on glucose metabolism, *Surgery*, 106, 163, 1989.

40. Coulston A.M., Clinical experience with modified enteral formulas for patients with diabetes, *Clin. Nutr.*, 17, 46, 1998 (supplement 2).

41. Sanz-Paris A. et al., High-fat versus high-carbohydrate enteral formulae: effect on blood glucose, c-peptide, and ketones in patients with type 2 diabetes treated with insulin or sulfonylurea. *Nutrition*, 14, 840, 1998.

42. Menzies, D.J. et al., Severe and persistent hypoglycemia due to gatifloxacin interaction with oral hypoglycemic agents, *Am. J. Med.*, 113, 232, 2002.

43. Baker, S.E. and Hangii, M.C., Possible gatifloxacin-induced hypoglycemia, *Ann. Pharmacother.*, 36, 1722, 2002.

44. Seligman, H. et al., Thiamine deficiency in patients with congestive heart failure receiving long-term furosemide therapy: a pilot study, *Am. J. Med.*, 91, 151, 1991.

45. Brady, J.A., Rock, C.L., and Horneffer, M.R., Thiamin status, diuretic medications, and the management of congestive heart failure, *J. Am. Diet. Assoc.*, 95, 541, 1995.

46. Marcuard, S.P., Albernaz, L., and Khazanie, P.G., Omeprazole therapy causes malabsorption of cyanocobalamin (vitamin B12), *Ann. Intern. Med.*, 120, 211, 1994.

47. Kang, T.M., Propofol infusion syndrome in critically ill patients, *Ann. Pharmacother.*, 36, 1543, 2002.

48. Lowrey, T.S. et al., Pharmacologic influence on nutrition support therapy: use of propofol in a patient receiving combined enteral and parenteral nutrition support, *Nutr. Clin. Prac.*, 11, 147, 1996.

49. Roth, M.S., Martin, A.B., and Katz, J.A., Nutritional implications of prolonged propofol use, *Am. J. Health-Syst. Pharm.*, 54, 694, 1997.

50. McLeod, G. et al., Propofol 2% in critically ill patients: effects on lipids, *Crit. Care Med.*, 25, 1976, 1997.

51. Graybill, J.R., Lipid formulations for amphotericin B: does the emperor need new clothes? *Ann. Intern. Med.*, 124, 921, 1996.

52. Dempsey, D.T. et al., Energy expenditure in acute trauma to the head with and without barbiturate therapy, *Surg. Gynecol. Obstet.*, 160, 128, 1985.

53. Welle, S., Schwartz, R.G., and Statt, M., Reduced metabolic rate during beta-adrenergic blockade in humans, *Metabolism*, 40, 691, 1991.

54. Walter-Sack, I. and Klotz, U., Influence of diet and nutritional status on drug metabolism, *Clin. Pharmacokinet.*, 31, 47, 1996.

55. Dickson, C.J., Schwartzman, M.S., and Bertino, J.S., Factors affecting aminoglycoside disposition: effects of circadian rhythm and dietary protein intake on gentamicin pharmacokinetics, *Clin. Pharmacol. Ther.*, 39, 325, 1986.

56. Beckwith, M.C., Barton, R.G., and Graves, C., A guide to drug therapy in patients with enteral feeding tubes: dosage form selection and administration methods, *Hosp. Pharm.*, 32, 57, 1997.

57. Mitchell, J.E., Oral dosage forms that should not be crushed: 2000 update, *Hosp. Pharm.*, 35, 553, 2000.

58. Bauer, L.A., Interference of oral phenytoin absorption by continuous nasogastric feedings, *Neurology*, 32, 570, 1982.

59. Au Yeung, S.C. and Ensom, M.H., Phenytoin and enteral feedings: does evidence support an interaction? *Ann. Pharmacother.*, 34, 896, 2000.

60. Gilbert, S., How to minimize interaction between phenytoin and enteral feedings: two approaches — a strategic approach, *Nutr. Clin. Prac.*, 11, 28, 1996.

61. Hatton, J. and Magnuson, B., How to minimize interaction between phenytoin and enteral feedings: two approaches — therapeutic options, *Nutr. Clin. Prac.*, 11, 30, 1996.

62. Smith, O.B., et al., Recovery of phenytoin from solutions of caseinate salts and calcium chloride, *Am. J. Hosp. Pharm.*, 45, 365, 1988.

63. Doak, K.K. et al., Bioavailability of phenytoin acid and phenytoin sodium with enteral feedings, *Pharmacotherapy*, 18, 637, 1998.

64. Penrod, L.E., Allen, J.B., and Cabacungan, L.R., Warfarin resistance and enteral feedings: 2 case reports and a supporting *in vitro* study, *Arch. Phys. Med. Rehab.*, 82, 1270, 2001.

65. Kuhn, T.A. et al., Recovery of warfarin from an enteral nutrient formula, *Am. J. Hosp. Pharm.*, 46, 1395, 1989.

66. Lutomski, D.M., Palascak, J.E., and Bower, R.H., Warfarin resistance associated with intravenous lipid administration, *J. Parenter. Enteral Nutr.*, 11, 316, 1987.

67. MacLaren, R. et al., Warfarin resistance associated with intravenous lipid administration: discussion of propofol and review of the literature, *Pharmacotherapy*, 17, 1331, 1997.

68. Wright, D.H. et al., Decreased *in vitro* fluoroquinolone concentrations after admixture with an enteral feeding formulation, *J. Parenter. Enteral Nutr.*, 24, 42, 2000.

69. Piccolo, M.L., Toossi, Z., and Goldman, M., Effect of coadministration of a nutritional supplement on ciprofloxacin absorption, *Am. J. Hosp. Pharm.*, 51, 2697, 1994.

70. Yuk, J.H. et al., Relative bioavailability in healthy volunteers of ciproloxacin administered through a nasogastric tube with and without enteral feeding, *Antimicrob. Agents Chemother.*, 33, 1118, 1989.

71. de Marie, S. et al., Bioavailability of ciprofloxacin after multiple enteral and intravenous doses in ICU patients with severe gram-negative intra-abdominal infections, *Intens. Care Med.*, 24, 343, 1998.

72. Mimoz, O. et al., Pharmacokinetics and absolute bioavailability of ciprofloxacin administered through a nasogastric tube with continuous enteral feeding to critically ill patients, *Intens. Care Med.*, 24, 1047, 1998.

73. Kanji, S. et al., Bioavailability of gatifloxacin by gastric tube administration with and without concomitant enteral feeding in critically ill patients, *Crit. Care Med.*, 31, 1347, 2003.

Section IV

Nutrition throughout the Lifecycle in the Critically Ill

21 Pregnancy

Patricia J. Bishop
Ursuline College, Breen School of Nursing

Elizabeth B. Sedlak
Bedford Medical Center

CONTENTS

21.1   INTRODUCTION

The critically ill pregnant patient provides a unique challenge to the health care team with a combination of altered maternal physiology, the presence of a fetus, increased nutritional demands, and the occurrence of disease processes. The nutritional requirements during pregnancy are dependent on the nutritional status of the woman prior to pregnancy. The nutrient demand varies as pregnancy advances through each trimester.[1] Maternal nutrition and body stores are protected during starvation at the expense of the fetus. Malnutrition may result in intrauterine growth retardation (IUGR) or fetal death. Prolonged periods longer than 13 hours without food can elevate maternal corticotropin-releasing hormone concentrations. This has been associated with premature delivery.[2]

21.2   PHYSIOLOGICAL ALTERATIONS IN PREGNANCY

Pregnancy alters the physiology in many maternal organs, systems, and metabolic pathways.[3] See Table 21.1. The expansion in circulating blood volume increases renal blood flow and glomerular filtration rate, promoting urinary excretion of glucose, uric acid, and protein. Aldosterone and renin are secreted to combat the increased renal sodium excretion. Restriction in sodium may cause a potential reduction in plasma volume and cardiac output.[5]

TABLE 21.1
Physiologic Changes during Pregnancy

	Changes during Pregnancy
Blood volume	Increased 30–50%[3]
Cardiac output	Increased 30–40% by 25–32 weeks gestation[4]
Plasma volume	Increased 40–50%[5]
Hematocrit	Decreased[6]
Oxygen consumption	Increased 20–30%[4]
Minute ventilation	Increased 48%[4]
Glomerular filtration rate	Increased 50%[3]
Creatinine	Decreased[3]
Gastrointestinal motility	Decreased[3]
Blood pressure	Decreased initially, followed by slight increase[6]

Although the slowing of the gastrointestinal tract from increased levels of plasma progesterone promotes absorption of iron and calcium, it causes increased heartburn, constipation, and delayed gastric emptying, with a risk for aspiration of stomach contents regardless of when the patient last ate. Labor or administration of narcotic analgesics also delays gastric emptying and increases the risk of aspiration.[6] In addition, the effectiveness of the esophageal sphincter is decreased from the displacement of the position of the stomach as pregnancy advances.[3]

21.3 PHYSIOLOGICAL CHANGES FOR FETAL SUPPORT

Complex interplay of maternal and fetal circulatory, endocrine, and metabolic systems maintains fetal growth.[7] The increased tissue needs for oxygen increase the basal metabolic rate 15 to 20%.[6] The metabolic demands of the pregnancy are affected by the gestational age and the total fetal mass.[8] The glucose-dependent fetus siphons fuel for energy from the maternal system, regardless of the state of maternal feeding or fasting. Placental metabolism or maternal circulation provides the 30 g of glucose daily that the fetus at term requires. The glucose reaches the fetus by facilitated diffusion, with a gradient from higher levels in the mother to lower levels in the fetus through the placenta.[9] The placenta functions as an active metabolic organ to buffer and provide the additional alteration to the nutrient stream, making what enters the fetal circulation different from what was delivered to the uterus.[6] Studies have reported a relationship between maternal hypoglycemia and impaired placental perfusion resulting in a decrease in maternal–fetal glucose transfer and fetal hypoglycemia.[7] Ketone bodies diffuse freely to the fetus during maternal fasting and can be a less effective precursor for brain protein synthesis. Impaired placental perfusion of glucose has been associated with IUGR.[9] Growth restriction prior to 26 weeks gestation may lead to neurological impairment.[6,8,9]

Transfer of free fatty acids from the maternal to the fetal circulation are needed for the developing fetal brain and central nervous system. Essential fatty acids are generally transferred more efficiently than nonessential fatty acids. Lipoprotein receptors and lipase activity within the placenta make maternal free fatty acids and triglycerides available for transfer to the fetus. The process is supported in the third trimester by the maternal hypertriglyceridemia.[7] The essential fatty acids arachidonic acid (AA) and docosahexaenoic acid (DHA) are important to the fetal brain and blood vessels. Placental development and size are associated with transfer of AA and DHA to the fetus. Some infants are born at a nutritional disadvantage due to a decreased transfer of AA and DHA *in utero*. During the period of rapid brain development, an inadequate supply of AA and DHA could lead to cell membrane breakdown from fragility and leakage. The fetus could suffer severe consequences, such as cerebral palsy from cell death in the brain.[10]

TABLE 21.2
Recommended Weight Gain during Pregnancy

	Weight Gain
Normal BMI	25–35 pounds
BMI less than 20	28–40 pounds
BMI greater than 26	15–25 pounds
Twin gestation	35–45 pounds
Decreased plasma volume and increased risk of intrauterine growth restriction	Less than 15 pounds

Sources: From Hamaoui E. and Hamaoui, M., *Gastroenterol. Clin. North Am.*, 32, 59, 2003; Johnson, T.R.B. and Niebyl, J.R., in *Obstetrics: Normal and Problem Pregnancies*, 4th ed., Gabbe, S.G., Niebyl, J.R., and Simpson, J.L., Eds., Churchill Livingstone, Nashville, TN, 2002, chap. 6; and Johnson, J.W.C. and Yancey, M.K., *Am. J. Obstet. Gynecol.*, 174, 254, 1996.

New nutritional goals set the foundations for a future healthy adult while the fetus is still developing *in utero*. Epidemiological studies have associated certain adult chronic diseases with fetal nutrition and birth weight. The infant diagnosed at birth as small for gestational age (SGA), IUGR, or low birth weight (LBW) is a deviation from the predicted weight at a given gestation. The LBW 4-pound infant at term is differentiated from the 4-pound preterm newborn delivered at 34 weeks gestation. Epidemiological studies have reported an inverse relationship between birth weight (excluding preterm) and risk of adult depression, type 2 diabetes, obesity, and coronary heart disease. Studies have reported poorer adult health outcomes in normal-birthweight individuals with impaired fetal growth, as in IUGR.[1,11] Birth weights < 2.6 kg have been associated with less-than-optimum outcomes, including elevated LDL cholesterol in adolescent males.[11,12]

21.4 RELATIONSHIP OF MATERNAL WEIGHT AND FETAL GROWTH

Weight gain during pregnancy is related to preconception nutritional status.[3] Increases in maternal body fat, protein stores, and blood volume provide the majority of the weight gain. The maternal nutrient stores provide a reserve for the fetus to draw upon for growth.[6] Inadequate maternal weight gain has been associated with an increased risk of a low-birthweight newborn, but the greatest effect on the fetus appears to be with the woman who is of low or normal prepregnant weight.[13]

The recommendations for weight gain during pregnancy are based on body mass index (BMI) to produce a normal-weight newborn. See Table 21.2. The weight gain should be distributed throughout the trimesters related to fetal growth and physiological processes. Total weight gain during the first trimester should be 3 to 6 pounds. During the second and third trimesters, the rate of weight gain should be 0.5 to 1 pound each week.[13] The fetus may gain 30 g weight per day during the third trimester of pregnancy. To achieve these goals, the pregnant woman should receive an additional intake of approximately 300 calories per day during the second and third trimesters. A twin pregnancy requires an additional intake of 150 calories per day more than a singleton pregnancy. The pregnant adolescent, as defined by the five-year period after onset of menarche, should gain a total of 30 to 33 pounds due to her own growth needs.[11]

21.5 MICRONUTRIENT DEFICIENCIES

Some populations begin pregnancy at a nutritional risk. Adolescents may be at the highest nutritional risk during pregnancy due to consumption of diets low in micronutrients, including zinc, iron, calcium, folate, and vitamins A, B_6, and C.[15] The pregnant patient who has had bariatric surgery for obesity may have a developing fetus susceptible to the micronutrient deficiencies that result from malabsorption.[11] The patient with the human immunodeficiency virus may have malnutrition and electrolyte imbalances related to dysphagia, changes in the oral cavity, and diarrhea.[16]

Attention to appropriate nutrient supplementation is important. Diets supplemented with calcium have been associated with decreased blood pressure levels and a lower rate of preterm deliveries. Vitamin A deficiency is rare in the U.S. due to dietary intake, but hypervitaminosis of A has been associated with teratogenicity in pregnancy.[15] Zinc deficiency has been associated with increased risk of premature rupture of membranes, placental abruption, and prolonged labor.[17] It is recommended that a 30 mg iron supplement be given to prevent anemia from the expansion of blood volume and deposition of iron stores in fetal tissues.[11,18] The United States Centers for Disease Control (CDC) recommend that women of childbearing years increase their intake of folic acid to 0.4 mg/d to prevent maternal megablastic anemia, neural tube defects, spontaneous abortions, and low birth weight. The pregnant woman who has previously had a child with a neural tube defect should take 4 mg of folic acid daily under medical supervision. The consumption should begin one month before trying to get pregnant and continue through the first three months of pregnancy. In addition, women who are on anticonvulsant medications are at higher risk for drug-induced folate deficiency.[11,19] Magnesium supplementation has been recommended for protection from sudden infant death syndrome.[20]

21.6 THE CRITICALLY ILL PREGNANT PATIENT

The overall prevalence of obstetric patients who may require critical care may range from 0.1 to 0.9%.[3] Pregnant patients can be critically ill without the need to occupy an intensive care unit (ICU) bed. Factors influencing placement of the patient may include level of ICU, geographical region, Interqual criteria, hospital protocols, and level of obstetrical unit. Caring for the critical patient requires communication among the intensivists, the maternal–fetal medicine consultants, and the team of healthcare providers.[21,22] The nutritional assessment includes the diagnosis, pertinent laboratory values, maternal weight gain history, prepregnancy weight, and BMI.

21.7 INDICATIONS FOR ICU ADMISSION

Conditions or diseases specific to pregnancy, or not related to pregnancy, can cause the pregnant patient to become critically ill.[3] Fetal well-being must be considered in terms of its own physiological requirements and susceptibility to maternal physiological, pharmacological, and nutritional hazards.[6] Adolescents under the age of 15 are at higher risk for medical complications, including anemia, lung or renal disease, and pregnancy-induced hypertension (PIH).[15]

The major indications for pregnant patients in the ICU are hemodynamic instability and respiratory failure.[6] Pregnant patients with the following conditions may warrant invasive monitoring and critical care:[23,24]

- Hypovolemic shock unresponsive to volume resuscitation
- Vasopressor therapy for septic shock
- Oliguria in PIH
- Need for intensive antihypertensive therapy
- Intubation for adult respiratory distress syndrome
- Class 3 or 4 cardiac disease or pulmonary hypertension in labor or postoperative
- Amniotic fluid embolism
- Pulmonary edema unresponsive to initial therapy

Stabilization of systems affected by a disease process (i.e., diabetic ketoacidosis due to illness or serum glucose levels greater than 200 mg/dl) may be required.[25] Obstetric comanagement with fetal monitoring of a viable fetus is often necessary when maternal hypoxemia, hypovolemia, preterm labor, postanesthesia states, or hypertensive crises are present.[26] For most pregnant patients in the ICU, the average obstetric length of stay (LOS) may range from 1 to 2 days.[27]

Balancing risks to the fetus remaining *in utero* with the risks of its extrauterine life against the risks associated with the health of the mother determine interventions and plan of care. In most critical care pregnant patients, delivery after immediate maternal stabilization is the goal.[4] An exception is the pregnant patient with a myocardial infarction near term. Risk of maternal death increases due to accelerated demands of late pregnancy and labor on an ischemic cardiovascular system. Conservative treatment to the cardiac condition without immediate delivery may be needed.[28] Thromboembolism, obstetric hemorrhage, hypertensive disease, amniotic fluid embolism, and anesthetic complications present increased maternal mortality rates.[6,28]

21.8 FETAL CONSIDERATIONS

Fetal survival and outcome are dependent on fetal weight, lung maturity, and condition at delivery.[4] Studies of fetal and neonatal deaths delivered at 22 to 25 weeks gestation report survival rates increasing with each additional week of pregnancy.[29,30] Studies in the 1990s of preterm deliveries reported survival rates from 34% at 23 weeks gestation increasing to 50 to 70% at 25 to 26 weeks gestation, to 90+% at 28 weeks and 100% at 30 weeks. The administration of antenatal steroids has been associated with decreased mortality on the first day of neonatal life. The incidence of moderate or severe neurodevelopmental disability was reported to be approximately 30 to 50% but continues to decrease as survival rates increase.[4,31]

21.9 TREATMENT CONSIDERATIONS

Treatment considerations during pregnancy must be approached with greater flexibility to consider the maternal–fetal unit.[3] The altered maternal physiology and the presence of a fetus present unique challenges to the plan of care. Uteroplacental blood flow is dependent on maternal cardiac output, hydration, and positioning. Maternal venous pO2 is optimal when the patient is afebrile with normal ventilation and blood pressure. Supine hypotension syndrome, with decreased cardiac output, uterine blood flow, and blood pressure, is prevented with left uterine displacement of the uterus.[6] Any reduction in blood return to the heart results in hypoperfusion of pulmonary vasculature with hypoxemia, which can lead to maternal and fetal death. Interventions are needed to correct maternal anemia and hemodynamic, blood gas, or glucose values to significantly increase maternal arterial and fetal cerebral oxygenation.[28] Bolus infusions of dextrose can cause maternal hyperglycemia that results in fetal hyperglycemia with insulin secretion, hypoxia, and acidosis secondary to the need for increased fetal oxygen consumption.[4]

Respiratory impairment may be caused by pathology that limits the expansion of lung tissue or interferes with ventilation. Diagnoses such as pneumonia, pulmonary edema, asthma, and acute respiratory distress syndrome (ARDS) require careful intravenous fluid support and ventilation for systemic perfusion of oxygen and nutrients to the maternal–fetal unit.[4] The decreased colloid osmotic pressure from PIH or after delivery has been associated with higher risk for pulmonary edema and need for ventilatory support.[24]

Maternal hypovolemia may require hemodynamic monitoring in the ICU. The pregnant patient may show signs of shock with a 10 to 20% blood loss or a gradual loss of 35% of circulating blood volume before it is clinically obvious due to the 50% increase in plasma blood volume during pregnancy. The secretion of catecholamines from the blood loss causes vasoconstriction and a reduction in uterine perfusion of up to 20% before an alteration in maternal blood pressure is observed. Maternal blood pressure, pulse, and oxygen saturation are unreliable signs of hypovolemia, whereas acidosis, lactate, and bicarbonate levels are useful indicators of maternal under-resuscitation and hypoperfusion.[6]

Fluid resuscitation to correct intravascular depletion can be achieved with lactated Ringer's solution. Large quantities of normal saline should be avoided to prevent hyperchloremic acidosis. Blood transfusions may be indicated if hypovolemia is not corrected with 2 l of crystalloid fluid replacement. To reduce the 50% mortality rate associated with amniotic fluid embolus, crystalloid fluids, vasopressor therapy, and oxygenation for the pulmonary vasospasm and right ventricular failure with a predominant left heart failure may be ordered.[6,28]

Antibiotic prophylaxis during labor or surgery has decreased the incidence of sepsis in pregnancy, although this still constitutes a major source of death.[28] The pregnant patient in septic shock with vascular collapse needs immediate attention to airway, due to possible ARDS. The risks of disseminated intravascular coagulation (DIC) and alterations in cardiac output and systemic vascular resistance result in a mortality rate of 0 to 28% for obstetrics, compared to 10 to 81% in nonobstetrics.[28,32]

The management of the pregnant patient with a severe burn differs little from treatment of the nonpregnant patient.[33] Stability of maternal systems is needed until a plan for delivery is made, dependent on assessment of fetal well-being and gestational age.[34]

Hyperemesis gravidarum (HG) may not warrant care in the ICU, but the care requires intensive nutritional support and team management to achieve a term pregnancy. Severe HG restricts nutrient intake, threatening metabolic and electrolyte balance in the most vulnerable period of fetal development.[35]

The pregnant patient with traumatic injuries needs assessment and stabilization via advanced trauma life support protocols followed by early fetal assessment. Liberal use of radiographic, obstetric diagnostic, surgical, and therapeutic modalities is employed to evaluate and maximize pregnancy outcomes.[36] Fluid and blood replacement, left uterine displacement with a wedge under the right hip, laboratory studies to assess for DIC, and fetal monitoring to assess for risks with hypovolemia, hypotension, or placental injury are included in the multidisciplinary plan of care. Cardiopulmonary resuscitation (CPR) can only generate up to 30% of the normal cardiac output due to positioning of the pregnant uterus and reduced venous return. Perimortem operative delivery of a viable fetus within 4 minutes after cardiac arrest with unsuccessful CPR may improve both maternal and fetal outcomes.[28]

Brain death or persistent vegetative state caused by irreversible brain damage in pregnancy is uncommon and poses ethical challenges.[37] Decisions are made whether to deliver the fetus immediately, provide supportive care including nutrition until fetal maturation, or allow them both to die as a unit.[38] Case reports describe prolongation of pregnancy from the period of brain death to delivery of a viable fetus to be 24 to 107 days and 1 to 189 days.[28,37]

The etiology of the brain death dictates the initial therapy. Etiologies that markedly reduce maternal and fetal oxygenation, such as drowning, drug overdose, smoke inhalation, or delayed CPR, are associated with poor maternal and fetal outcomes.[39] Brain death may frequently precipitate diabetes insipidus with polyuria, electrolyte, and acid–base changes. Serum hyperosmolality, hypernatremia, dehydration, and hypovolemia require monitoring of laboratory values, with adjustments in fluid and electrolyte replacement. Nutritional support, with enteral tube feedings alone or in combination with parenteral nutrition (PN), is initiated early for the pregnant patient with brain death to prevent a state of starvation.[37]

21.10   DECISION FOR NUTRITIONAL SUPPORT

After hemodynamic stability is achieved, micronutrient and macronutrient needs of the pregnant patient are addressed.[11] To determine whether nutritional intervention is indicated or discontinued, the question is asked, "Is current intake meeting nutritional needs?". The primary indication for

TABLE 21.3
Changes in Basal Energy Requirements

Basal Energy Requirement Change

Fever	13% increase for each Celsius degree of fever
Sepsis and trauma	20–30% increase
Burns	Up to 100%

Source: From Whittaker, J.S. et al., in *First Principles of Gastroenterology: The Basis of Disease and an Approach to Management*, Thomson, A.B.R. and Shaffer, E.A., Eds., retrieved at http://gastroresource.com/GITextbook/en/chapter2/default.htm.

nutritional intervention is that the intake of one or more nutrients is not matching the needs of the pregnancy and a deficit occurs. The risks of nutritional support are weighed against the risks of unnecessary intervention.[5] The aim of any intervention is to maintain maternal blood glucose levels between 90 and 120 mg/dl and treat any evidence of maternal hyperglycemia with insulin to prevent increased fetal insulin production.[38,40]

The Harris–Benedict formula is used to estimate basal energy expenditure (BEE). The formula is adjusted for pregnancy as follows:[5]

$$BEE = 655 + (9.6 \times weight\ (kg) + [1.8 \times height\ (cm) - 4.7\ age\ (yr)]),\ then$$

$$BEE \times 1.25 + 300\ kcal\ (single\ fetus)\ or\ 500\ kcal\ (twins)$$

where 1.25 is the stress factor for pregnancy and weight is the actual body weight if the mother is < 130% ideal body weight.[38]

When enteral or parenteral nutrition is ordered for the pregnant patient, the nutritional prescription is adjusted empirically to achieve the desired weight gain. Adjustments in the caloric intake depend on the diagnosis. An additional 300 kcal/d above baseline needs are recommended for a singleton pregnancy. Other conditions that increase the caloric requirement to 3000 to 4000 kcal/d include the presence of sepsis, catabolism, or head injury. See Table 21.3.

Decerebrate patients may require 4500 kcal/24-h period.[42] In the pregnant patient with brain death, the resting energy expenditure may be lower than predicted by the Harris–Benedict equation due to loss of spontaneous muscle activity, hypothermia, or absent brain energy consumption.[5,38] Continuous indirect calorimetry to measure metabolic parameters is considered to be the gold standard for nutritional assessment, due to the complexity in calculating the individualized metabolic response to illness and stress.[38,43]

21.11 ROUTES OF NUTRITIONAL SUPPORT

The route of nutritional repletion is determined by the severity of nutritional depletion, the degree and expected duration of gastrointestinal (GI) compromise, and the acceptance by the patient. Invasive intervention is justified when maternal and fetal nutritional risks are high. If the GI tract is functional, enteral nutrition (EN) is considered before initiating PN, because of decreased cost and reduced risks of sepsis, thrombophlebitis, and technical complications of catheter insertion.[44] EN provides less risk of nosocomial infection, organ failure, and hospitalization in the patient with sepsis, burns, or trauma, although it is associated with a risk of aspiration, nausea, and vomiting. Investigators have advocated postpyloric placement of feeding tubes, percutaneous endoscopic gastrojejunostomy, or endoscopically placed nasoenteral tubes. Self-propelling tubes entered into the stomach pass with peristalsis with a low rate of complication, are well tolerated, and are cost effective as an alternative to total parenteral nutrition (TPN).[45] Percutaneous endoscopic gastrostomy (PEG) tubes are generally not placed in pregnancy, due to risk of uterine or fetal damage, infection, or premature labor. Two successful placements of PEGs in gravid patients have been reported when enteral support was desired and nasogastric or nasoduodenal tubes were not tolerated. It has been suggested that additional experience is necessary to ascertain the safety of the procedure in this patient population.[46]

Pancreatitis, small bowel obstruction, trauma, short bowel syndrome, Crohn's disease, ulcerative colitis, and inflammatory bowel disease are conditions that lead to malnutrition and fetal growth restriction from impaired GI absorption and intolerance to EN.[40] Until adequate oral or EN intake is reestablished, the fatty acids in PN provide for growth of the fetal brain and lung tissues.[47]

Establishing and maintaining intravenous access for long-term use in the pregnant patient has brought challenges to the patient and the health care team. The percutaneously placed central catheter inserted in the subclavian, femoral, or internal jugular vein by a physician is the usual technique for extended use; however, it is associated with a risk of hemorrhage, infection, or pneumothorax. The peripherally inserted central catheter (PICC) placed in the superior vena cava by access of the basilic or cephalic vein has a reported complication rate of 20 to 26%, including phlebitis and mechanical problems.[48–50] A five-year retrospective chart review of PICC lines used in pregnancy reported complications from the 52 cases, including the following:[51]

- 17% culture-proved line infections
- 12% presumed line infections
- 8% cellulites
- 8% mechanical line failure
- 4% pain requiring line discontinuation
- 2% superficial thrombophlebitis

Preterm labor was associated with the increased risk of PICC line complications (P = 0.012). The 37% infection rate was higher than in the nonpregnant population (20 to 26%). There are reports of increased risk of infection due to the immunologic suppression in pregnancy or associated with the patient's preexisting condition of infection in the genital tract or amniotic fluid. The hypercoagulable state of pregnancy may increase the risk of thrombosis.[52]

TPN solution via central venous access administered to the pregnant patient carries additional risks specific to pregnancy.[53] In a study by Russo-Stieglitz et al. (1999), 10 of the 26 women receiving PN for HG had hyperglycemia and central venous catheter complications.[52] In addition, a reported case of a woman with a 28-week pregnancy admitted for intractable vomiting received standard TPN solution containing the commercial combination of vitamins B_1, B_2, B_6, A, C, and E. The fetus appeared stable for three weeks, until an ultrasound revealed a fetal subdural hematoma. After delivery, the neonate had an elevated plasma PKVKA-II concentration as a sign of vitamin K deficiency. This rare case stresses the need for the pregnant patient to receive TPN with vitamins A, B, C, E, and K. Prophylactic vitamin K supplementation or a weekly subcutaneous injection is administered to prevent possible fetal hemorrhagic complications, such as subdural hematoma.[54]

21.12 NUTRIENT SUPPLEMENTATION

Protein intake should be augmented by 10 to 14 g/d during the second and third trimesters, in addition to baseline needs of 60 g/d or an increase of 20%.[6,40] Amino acid oxidation varies widely during pregnancy and among individuals. The metabolic differences in synthesis, conservation of nitrogen, and use of protein resources may account for birthweight outcome differences despite adequate supply.[55] It is unknown whether mobilized proteins from flaccid paralysis become available nutrients for the fetus. Nitrogen losses from inactive musculature may produce a noncatabolic increase in urinary urea nitrogen, which yields a false estimate of nitrogen needs.[38]

It is recommended that 20 to 25% of nonprotein calories be supplied as fat for humans to avoid essential fatty acid deficiency.[38,40] Studies of lipid formulations no longer available in the U.S. reported a proposed mechanism of synthesis of AA as the precursor of prostaglandin correlated with premature labor.[52,56] The use of current soybean and soybean–safflower lipid emulsions has not been associated with premature labor.[40] Fat emulsions have been found to be safe when supplying < 50% of the calculated nonprotein calories.

In addition to protein and lipid supplementation, continued vitamin, folic acid, and trace element support is essential to the fetus. Commercially available supplements for parenteral admixture and enteral formulas may not meet the recommended daily allowances during pregnancy.[38] Critical attention to daily weights, intake and output, and laboratory studies including liver function, serum electrolyte, and hematology values is needed. Levels of iron, ferritin, vitamin B_{12}, and folate need to be monitored.[53]

If a pregnant patient is receiving nutritional support via TPN or EN after a period of weight loss, she is monitored for refeeding syndrome complications, including hypophosphatemia, hypokalemia, and hypomagnesemia. Refeeding syndrome results from the rapid uptake of these ions from the expanding fetal and maternal cells, causing muscle weakness, arrhythmias, seizures, respiratory failure, and death.[5] Serum albumin levels should be monitored during nutritional support. A low serum albumin may reflect inadequate protein intake, hepatic insufficiency, or redirection of hepatic protein synthesis. When evaluating triglyceride and cholesterol levels, it is important to note that there is a 40% increase due to the gestational hormone-induced fat mobilization.[11]

21.13 CASE STUDY

A 20-year-old female at 25 weeks pregnant was admitted with a known cardiomyopathy exacerbated by pregnancy. She was subsequently intubated secondary to a diagnosis of pulmonary edema with metabolic and respiratory acidosis. After stabilization with fluid and drug therapy using hemodynamic monitoring, attempts at weaning from the ventilator were unsuccessful. TPN and lipids were initiated through the central venous catheter. Enteral feedings were not used at that time, because the patient was receiving vasopressors to improve her cardiac output. Her intensivist did not want to risk worsening gut ischemia during the period of compromised gut blood flow. Blood glucose levels were maintained at 90 to 120 mg/dl without need for insulin. Fetal status was deemed stable by intermittent fetal monitoring performed by obstetric staff. The patient remained in semi-Fowler's position with left tilt for uterine displacement to maximize venous return.

After 6 days, her cardiac status improved and pulmonary edema resolved. Management of maternal cardiac and fetal well-being continued until she had a cesarean birth at 32 weeks. Mother's hemodynamic status after delivery was closely monitored until she was discharged on postpartum day 4. The 1640 g female infant was admitted to the neonatal intensive care unit for initial stabilization and monitoring. She was discharged to home at day of life 25 with no adverse outcome.

Administration of TPN was based on caloric requirements utilizing the basal energy expenditure (BEE) formula adjusted for pregnancy.

$$BEE \text{ of pregnant female} = 655 + (9.6 \times 55 \text{ kg}) + (1.8 \times 162 \text{ cm}) - 4.7 \text{ (20 yrs)}$$

$$655 + 528 + 291.6 - 94 = BEE \text{ of } 1380.6$$

$$1380.6 \times 1.25 \text{ kcal stress factor} = 1725.75 \text{ or } 1725$$

$$1725 + 300 = 2025 \text{ kcal/d needed}$$

Using a standard 10% amino acid solution:

$$2000 \text{ ml} = 200 \text{ g of protein}$$

$$200 \text{ g} + 10 \text{ g protein (pregnancy)} \times 4 \text{ kcal/g} = 840 \text{ kcal protein}$$

The nonprotein caloric requirement for this patient is:

$$2025 \text{ kcal} - 840 \text{ kcal} = 1185 \text{ kcal of nonprotein calories to be given}$$

No more than 30 to 35% of the 1185 should be fat, therefore:

$$1185 \text{ kcal} \times 0.35 = 415 \text{ kcal fat to be given}$$

Using a standard 20% Intralipid solution of 2 kcal/ml, approximately 208 ml of Intralipids are administered over a 24-hour period. The balance of the total caloric intake is supplied by carbohydrates.

$$2025 - (840 \text{ kcal protein} + 415 \text{ kcal fat}) = 745 \text{ kcal carbohydrates to be given}$$

$$745 \text{ kcal/3.4 kcal/g} = 219 \text{ g of carbohydrate}$$

To administer approximately 200 g of carbohydrates in a 2000 ml solution, a 10% dextrose solution can be used:

$$2000 \text{ ml} \times 0.10 = 200 \text{ g}$$

Therefore, the TPN solution to be administered will include D_{10}, 10% amino acid solution to infuse at 83 ml/h with 208 ml of 20% Intralipid to infuse over 24 hours. The patient's total fluid intake will be monitored to prevent overload. The balance of her intravenous fluid intake will be used to administer medications.

REFERENCES

1. Jackson, A.A. and Robinson, S.M., Dietary guidelines for pregnancy: a review of current evidence, *Public Health Nutr.*, 4, 625, 2001.
2. Hermann, T.S., Prolonged periods without food intake during pregnancy increase risk for elevated maternal corticotropin-releasing hormone concentrations, *Am. J. Obstet. Gynecol.*, 185, 403, 2001.
3. Naylor, D.F. and Olson, M.M., Critical care obstetrics and gynecology, *Crit. Care Clin.*, 19, 127, 2003.
4. Catanzarite, V. and Cousins, L., Respiratory failure in pregnancy, *Immunol. Allergy Clin. North Am.*, 20, 775, 2000.
5. Hamaoui, E. and Hamaoui, M., Nutritional assessment and support during pregnancy, *Gastroenterol. Clin. North Am.*, 27, 89, 1998.
6. Lapinsky, S.E., Kruczynski, K., and Slutsky, A.S., Critical care in the pregnant patient, *Am. J. Respir. Crit. Care Med.*, 152, 427, 1995.
7. McClellan, R. and Novak, D., Fetal nutrition: how we become what we are, *J. Pediatr. Gastroenterol. Nutr.*, 33, 233, 2001.
8. Battaglia, F.C., The comparative physiology of fetal nutrition, *Am. J. Obstet. Gynecol*, 148, 850, 1984.
9. Gabbe, S. and Quilligan, E.J., Fetal carbohydrate metabolism: its clinical importance, *Am. J. Obstet. Gynecol.*, 127, 92, 1977.

10. Crawford, M.A., Placental delivery of arachidonic and docosahexaenoic acids: implications for the lipid nutrition of preterm infants, *Am. J. Clin. Nutr.*, 71, 275, 2000.
11. Hamaoui E. and Hamaoui, M., Nutritional assessment and support during pregnancy, *Gastroenterol. Clin. North Am.*, 32, 59, 2003.
12. Kuzawa, C.W. and Adair, L.S., Lipid profiles in adolescent Filipinos: relation to birth weight and maternal energy status during pregnancy, *Am. J. Clin. Nutr.*, 77, 960, 2003.
13. Johnson, T.R.B. and Niebyl, J.R., Preconception and prenatal care: part of the continuum, in *Obstetrics: Normal and Problem Pregnancies*, 4th ed., Gabbe, S.G., Niebyl, J.R., and Simpson, J.L., Eds., Churchill Livingstone, Nashville, TN, 2002, chap. 6.
14. Johnson, J.W.C. and Yancey, M.K., A critique of the new recommendations for weight gain in pregnancy, *Am. J. Obstet. Gynecol.*, 174, 254, 1996.
15. Lenders, C.M., McElrath, T.F., and Scholl, T.O., Nutrition in adolescent pregnancy, *Curr. Opin. Pediatr.*, 12, 291, 2000.
16. Kuczkowski, K.M., Human immunodeficiency virus in the parturient, *J. Clin. Anesth.*, 15, 224, 2003.
17. Christian, P., Maternal nutrition, health, and survival, *Nutr. Rev.*, 60, S59, 2002.
18. Reifsnider, E. and Gill, S.L., Nutrition for the childbearing years, *JOGNN*, 29, 43, 2000.
19. Centers for Disease Control, Recommendations for the use of folic acid to reduce the number of cases of spina bifida and neural tube defects, *MMWR*, 41, 1, 1992.
20. Caddell, J.L., The apparent impact of gestational magnesium deficiency on the sudden infant death syndrome, *Magnes. Res.*, 14, 291, 2001.
21. Velez, L.L., Toal, K., and Goodwin, S.A., Two lives on the line: a case study in obstetrical critical care, *Crit. Care Nurs.*, 22, 20, 2002.
22. Zeeman, G.G., Wendel, G.D., and Cunningham, F.G., A blueprint for obstetric critical care, *Am. J. Obstet. Gynecol.*, 188, 532, 2003.
23. Poole, J.H., Aggressive management of HELLP syndrome and eclampsia, in *AACN Clin. Issues,* 8, 524, 1997.
24. Bridges, E.J. et al., Hemodynamic monitoring in high-risk obstetrics patients. II: Pregnancy-induced hypertension and preeclampsia, *Crit. Care Nurs.*, 23, 52, 2003.
25. Jovanovic, L., Medical emergencies in the patient with diabetes during pregnancy, *Endocrinol. Metab. Clin. North Am.*, 29, 771, 2000.
26. Parry, S. and Morgan, M.A., Care of the maternal–fetal unit, in *The Intensive Care Unit Manual*, Lanken, P.N., Ed., W.B. Saunders, Philadelphia, 2001, chap. 21.
27. Panchal, S., Arria, A.M., and Harris, A.P., Intensive care utilization during hospital admission for delivery, *Anesthesiology*, 92, 1537, 2000.
28. Gonik, B., Intensive care monitoring of the critically ill pregnant patient, in *Maternal–Fetal Medicine,* 4th ed., Creasy, R. and Resnik, R., Eds., W.B. Saunders Co., Philadelphia, 1999, chap. 50.
29. Lemons, J.A. et al., Very low birth weight outcomes of the National Institute of Child Health and Human Developmental Neonatal Research Network January 1995 through December, 1996, *Pediatrics*, 2000.
30. Wood, N.S. et al., Neurologic and developmental disability after extremely preterm birth, *N. Engl. J. Med.,* 343, 378, 2002.
31. MacDonald, H., Perinatal care at the threshold of viability, *Pediatrics*, 110, 1024, 2002.
32. Mabie, W.C. and Sibai, B.M., Septic shock in pregnancy, *Obstet. Gynecol.*, 90, 553, 1997.
33. Monafo, W.W., Initial management of burns, *N. Engl. J. Med.*, 335, 1581, 1996.
34. Nguyen, T.T. et al., Current treatment of severely burned patients, *Ann. Surg.*, 223, 14, 1996.
35. Coad, J., Al-Rasasi, B., and Morgan, J., Nutrient insult in early pregnancy, *Proc. Nutr. Soc.,* 61, 51, 2002.
36. Kauff, N.D. and Tejani, N., Trauma in the obstetric patient: evaluation and management, *Prim. Care Update OB/GYNS,* 5, 16, 1998.
37. Feldman, D.M. et al., Irreversible maternal brain injury during pregnancy: a case report and review of the literature, *Obstet. Gynecol. Survey*, 55, 708, 2000.
38. Powner, D. and Bernstein, I., Extended somatic support for pregnant women after brain death, *Crit. Care Med.*, 31, 1241, 2003.
39. Dillon, W.P. et al., Life support and maternal brain death during pregnancy, *JAMA*, 24B, 1089, 1982.

40. ASPEN Board of Directors and the Clinical Guidelines Task Force, Guidelines for the use of parenteral and enteral nutrition in adult and pediatric patients, *J. Parenter. Enteral Nutr.,* 26, 45S, 2002.

41. Whittaker, J.S. et al., Nutrition in gastrointestinal disease, in *First Principles of Gastroenterology: The Basis of Disease and an Approach to Management,* Thomson, A.B.R. and Shaffer, E.A., Eds., retrieved at http://gastroresource.com/GITextbook/En/chapter2/default.html.

42. Nuutinen, L.S., Alahuhta, S.M., and Heikkinen, J.E., Nutrition during ten-week life support with successful fetal outcomes in a case with fatal maternal brain damage, *J. Parenter. Enteral Nutr.,* 13, 432, 1989.

43. Headley, J.M., Indirect calorimetry, *AACN Clin. Issues,* 14, 155, 2003.

44. Viall, C.D., Enteral nutrition, in *American Critical Care Nurses Procedure Manual for Critical Care,* 3rd ed., Boggs, R.L. and Wooldridge-King, M., Eds., W.B. Saunders, Philadelphia, 1993, chap. 32.

45. Pearce, C.B. et al., Enteral nutrition by nasojejunal tube in hyperemesis gravidarum, *Clin. Nutr.,* 20, 461, 2001.

46. Shaheen, N.J. et al., The use of percutaneous endoscopic gastrostomy in pregnancy, *Gastroint. Endosc.,* 46, 564, 1997.

47. Ishijima, N. et al., Delivery of a normal newborn after intensive medical treatment for an acute exacerbation of ulcerative colitis during pregnancy: a case report, *Jpn. J. Surg.,* 29, 1257, 1999.

48. Ng, P.K. et al., Peripherally inserted central catheters in general medicine, *Mayo Clin. Proc.,* 72, 225, 1997.

49. Loughran, S.C. and Borzatta, M., Peripherally inserted central catheters: a report of 2506 catheter days, *J. Parenter. Enteral Nutr.,* 19, 133, 1995.

50. Merrell, S. et al., Peripherally inserted central venous catheters: low-risk alternatives for ongoing venous access, *West. J. Med.,* 160, 25, 1994.

51. Ogura, J.M. et al., Complications associated with peripherally inserted central catheter use during pregnancy, *Am. J. Obstet. Gynecol.,* 188, 1223, 2003.

52. Russo-Stieglitz, K.E. et al., Pregnancy outcome in patients requiring parenteral nutrition, *J. Matern. Fetal Med.,* 8, 164, 1999.

53. Viall, C.D., Total parenteral nutrition, in *American Critical Care Nurses Procedure Manual for Critical Care,* 3rd ed., Boggs, R.L. and Wooldridge-King, M., Eds., W.B. Saunders, Philadelphia, 1993, chap. 31.

54. Sakai, M. et al., Maternal total parenteral nutrition and fetal subdural hematoma, *Obstet. Gynecol.,* 101, 1142, 2003.

55. Duggleby, S.L. and Jackson, A.A., Higher weight at birth is related to decreased maternal amino acid oxidation during pregnancy, *Am. J. Clin. Nutr.,* 76, 852, 2002.

56. Iams, J., Preterm birth, in *Obstetrics: Normal and Problem Pregnancies,* 4th ed., Gabbe, S.J., Ed., Churchill Livingstone, Philadelphia, 2002, 764.

22 Nutrition Support for the Critically Ill Neonate

Sandor Nagy and Jatinder Bhatia
Medical College of Georgia

CONTENTS

22.1 INTRODUCTION

Over the past several decades, advances in neonatal care have increased the survival of more and more premature infants at lower and lower gestational ages. These changes create new challenges for the clinician, not only in terms of technological support but also in terms of nutritional support.

The traditional goal in nutrition for the term infant is to assist in the transition from *in utero* nutrition to *ex utero* nutrition. Growth and biochemical responses in a healthy term breast-fed infant remain the gold standard. In the premature infant, however, the optimal nutritional requirements are not completely defined. Present recommendations are designed to approximate the rate of growth and composition of gain of a fetus of the same postmenstrual age [1]. The premature infant, depending on the extent of prematurity, will dictate different approaches to initiate, advance, and maintain appropriate nutrient delivery and growth. We need to provide the appropriate mixture of nutrients to assist in reaching maturity (i.e., term postconceptional age and beyond) but at the same time to maintain appropriate growth. Determining the ideal growth pattern for the preterm infants

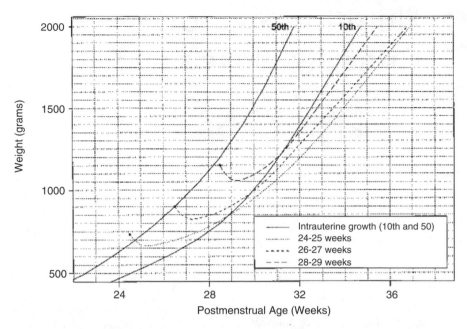

FIGURE 22.1 Postnatal growth in preterm infants in relation to intrauterine growth curves. (From Ehrenkranz RA, Younes NA, and Lemons JA, *Pediatrics*, 1999, 104:280-9.)

remains problematic. The "reference fetus" term created by Ziegler et al. serves as a model for estimating nutrient requirements for extrauterine growth [2]. Existing growth curves generated from measurements of infants born prematurely can help us at least to approximate their weight gain, linear growth, and head growth [3,4]. Based on these curves, a preterm infant should gain 12 to 15 g/kg of body weight a day, 0.75 to 1.0 cm length per week, and 0.75 to 1.0 cm head circumference per week. More recently, extrauterine growth has been described for a large cohort of premature infants from 24 to 29 weeks and compared to intrauterine growth curves using the data of Alexander et al. (Figure 22.1) [5,6]. This may be a better representation of current neonatal growth data, because the previously published curves mainly represented certain regions only [4].

22.2 ENERGY REQUIREMENT OF THE NEONATE

Energy provided by nutrition is distributed according to the classical energy balance equation:

$$E_{intake} = E_{expended} + E_{stored} + E_{excreted}$$

Energy expenditure includes the energy used for resting (or basal) metabolism, activity, thermoregulation, and energy utilized for new tissue synthesis. The basal metabolic rate (BMR) is the minimal energy needed to maintain life in the resting state. This is the largest portion of the total energy expenditure. Ideally, BMR should be measured in a thermoneutral environment and in a fasting state for 12 to 18 hours. The latter would not be feasible for preterm infants; current estimates are based on measurements during sleep for 2 to 3 hours. The estimated BMR for preterm infants is 50 kcal/kg/d [7]. This BMR is somewhat lower initially, when compared to term infants, but it gradually rises in both term and preterm babies, and eventually preterm infants demonstrate a higher BMR [8]. The energy expenditure during muscle activity is more important in the larger preterm and term infant, because the smaller and sick preterm infant is usually less active. Cold stress and energy used for thermoregulation are major factors in preterm infants; these infants show an

TABLE 22.1
Estimated Caloric Requirement of the Preterm Infant

Energy Expenditure	kcal/kg/d
Resting metabolic rate	50
Activity	15
Thermoregulation	10
Synthesis	8
Energy stored	25
Energy excreted	12
TOTAL	120

Source: From American Academy of Pediatrics, Committee on Nutrition, *Pediatric Nutrition Handbook*, 5th edition, 2003, 23–54.

increased energy need for thermoregulation, compared to term infants, because of a higher rate of heat loss from their relatively larger body surface area (see Table 22.1) [9]. The advent of better technology to maintain a thermo-neutral environment with incubators has minimized heat loss. The energy utilized during tissue synthesis is different from the stored energy, because energy is not being retained in the tissue but "burned up" during growth. To achieve the 15g/kg/d weight gain, about 20 to 30 kcal/kg energy will be stored in the tissue [10]. Energy excretion is mainly stool losses (and some minimal loss in urine), due to the fat and carbohydrate content that passes unabsorbed. As absorption improves, one can expect an 85 to 95% retention rate by 2 to 3 weeks of life, even in the low-birthweight (LBW) infants [11].

Most infants show steady weight gain when provided this energy intake enterally. In certain conditions (e.g., chronic lung disease), the energy intake must be increased to compensate for energy needed for the ongoing tissue remodeling and work of breathing [12]. Similarly, small-for-gestational-age and very small premature infants may require higher energy intakes to maintain appropriate growth.

Term infants show appropriate growth with an energy intake around 90 to 110 kcal/kg/d, with formula-fed babies requiring a slightly higher intake [13,14].

22.3 FLUID–ELECTROLYTE BALANCE OF THE NEONATE

After birth, there is a contraction of the extracellular fluid compartment that is followed by natriuresis, diuresis, and weight loss [15]. The typical weight loss is in the range of 7 to 10% of body weight. This does not happen in the first 24 to 48 hours, so most infants are oliguric initially. This initial sodium loss appears to be obligatory [16]; therefore, initial fluids should not contain any sodium, because this would put an extra burden on the kidneys. Restricting sodium intake in the first few days of life actually shows some other benefits, such as decreased oxygen requirement and lower incidence of bronchopulmonary dysplasia (BPD), without compromising growth [17,18].

After this initial fluid shift, infants require sodium to maintain growth. The preterm kidney shows a higher fractional excretion of sodium (FeNa) because of the immaturity of the tubular system. The FeNa appears to be correlated with the prematurity, where lower gestational age translates to higher FeNa. These infants are at risk for late hyponatremia [19] and may require higher sodium intake to maintain adequate growth. Extremely premature infants may need 4 to 8 mEq/kg/d of sodium intake during their growing phase [20]; older infants grow well with 2 to 3 mEq/kg/d of sodium.

TABLE 22.2
Factors Influencing Insensible Water Loss

Factors that Increase IWL
Prematurity
Radiant warmer heat
Phototherapy
Skin defects — omphalocele, gastroschisis
Tachypnea
Nonhumidified oxygen/environment

Factors that Decrease IWL
Mature skin
Heat shields
Topical skin agents — paraffin, Aquaphor
Covering skin defects
Humidified oxygen/environment

Source: From Parish, A and Bhatia, J, *Nutritional Considerations in the Intensive Care Unit: Science, Rationale and Practice*, 2002.

TABLE 22.3
Maintenance Fluid Requirement by Birth Weight for the First Month of Life

Birth Weight (g)	Insensible Losses (ml/kg/d)	Water Requirement		
		Day 1–2 (ml/kg/d)	Day 3–7 (ml/kg/d)	Day 8–30 (ml/kg/d)
< 750	100–200	100–200	150–200	120–180
750–1000	60–70	80–150	100–150	120–180
1001–1500	30–65	60–100	100–150	120–180
> 1500	15–30	60–80	100–150	120–180

Source: Adapted from Fanaroff AA (Ed), *Neonatal-Perinatal Medicine: Diseases of the Fetus and Infant*, 7th ed., Mosby, St. Louis, MO, 2002.

Potassium is the main intracellular cation. Its daily requirement is 2 to 3 mEq/kg/d and does not show much variation between term and preterm infants. Preterm infants are susceptible to hyperkalemia during the first few days of life, even in the absence of overt renal failure [21].

Insensible water loss takes up a major part in the fluid requirements for preterm infants. LBW infants have a disproportionately larger loss because of their relatively larger body surface and the immaturity of their skin to prevent evaporation [22]. Although most term infants can be started on 60 to 80 ml/kg/d of fluid maintenance, some extremely premature infants may require 200 ml/kg/d (or even more) to prevent hypernatremia. Factors that affect insensible water loss (IWL) are listed in Table 22.2. Table 22.3 provides fluid maintenance requirements for the first month of life.

For the infant less than 1000 g, a suggested fluid and nutrition regimen adapted from Parish and Bhatia is provided in Table 22.4 [23].

TABLE 22.4
Suggested Nutrition Regimen for Infants < 1000 g

	600–800 g	801–1000 g
Radiant warmer		
IVF, ml/kg/d	100–120	80–100
Dextrose%	5[a]	10[b]
AA, g/kg/d	1.0[b]	1.0[c]
Lipids,[a] g/kg/d	0.5	0.5
Incubator		
IVF, ml/kg/d	80–100	80
Dextrose%	7.5–10[b]	10[b]
AA, g/kg/d	1.5[c]	1.5[c]
Lipids,[a] g/kg/d	0.5	0.5

Note: AA = Amino acid (pediatric formulation).

[a] Start on DOL 2, 0.5 g/kg/d; increase in 0.5 g/kg/d increments to a max of 2–3 g/kg/d. Monitor triglycerides at every increase and maximum.
[b] Infants less than 1000 g may be intolerant to higher concentrations of glucose and may need adjustment based on serum glucose. Advancing glucose delivery is also dictated by tolerance.
[c] Beginning on DOL 1, increase by 0.5 g/kg/d to maximum of 2.5–3.0g/kg/d.

22.4 MACRONUTRIENTS

22.4.1 CARBOHYDRATE

For intensive care patients, the initial source of carbohydrate is glucose, because they are on intravenous fluids, at least at the beginning of their course. The normal glucose requirement is about 6 to 8 mg/kg/min to maintain euglycemia. The glucose should be increased in increments to maintain normal serum concentrations. The typical dextrose concentration used is D10W, with D5W being used in smaller infants; the use of the latter is due to glucose intolerance exhibited by very small premature infants. Moreover, if higher fluid intakes are required, adjustments in glucose concentration to maintain appropriate glucose delivery should be made. It is not unusual for the extremely premature infant to require only 2 to 3mg/kg/min of glucose to maintain serum glucose in the appropriate range. Hypoglycemia (blood glucose < 40 mg/dl) and hyperglycemia (blood glucose > 175 mg/dl) are not infrequent findings in sick newborns.

The major source of carbohydrate in breast milk and in most term formulas is lactose. Lactase activity is deficient in preterm infants compared to term babies. On the other hand, glycosidase enzymes are fully functional even in very premature infants [24,25]. Therefore, commercial formulas prepared for preterm infants contain 50 to 60% of their carbohydrate in other forms, such as glucose polymers, which are easily digested by the premature gut.

22.4.2 PROTEIN

Mature human breast milk contains 0.9 to 1.0g/dl of protein. The protein content of the colostrum (< 5 days) is much higher, 2.6 g/dl, and decreases to 1.6 g/dl in transitional milk (6 to 10 days). The whey-to-casein ratio is approximately 70:30, which helps digestion and absorption. Therefore, a typical term infant taking about 180 ml/kg of breast milk daily would receive around 2.2 g/kg/d of protein. Breast milk contains lactalbumin as the main nitrogen source. Commercially available preparations contain slightly more protein (1.4 to 1.6 g/dl), and the whey-to-casein ratio is 60:40.

TABLE 22.5
Nutritional Components of Preterm (PT) and Term (T) Breast Milk

Nutrient	\multicolumn{10}{c}{Days Postpartum}

	\multicolumn{2}{c}{3}	\multicolumn{2}{c}{7}	\multicolumn{2}{c}{14}	\multicolumn{2}{c}{21}	\multicolumn{2}{c}{28}
Nutrient	**PT**	**T**	**PT**	**T**	**PT**	**T**	**PT**	**T**	**PT**	**T**
Energy (kcal/dl)	51.4	48.7	67.4	60.6	72.3	64.2	65.6	68.6	70.1	69.7
Protein (g/dl) §	3.24	2.29	2.44	1.87	2.17	1.57	1.82	1.52	1.81	1.42
Fat (g/dl)	1.63	1.71	3.81	3.06	4.40	3.48	3.68	3.89	4.00	4.01
Lactose (g/dl) §	5.96	6.16	6.05	6.52	6.21	6.78	6.49	7.12	6.95	7.26
Sodium (mEq/l) §	26.6	22.3	21.8	16.9	19.7	11.0	13.4	10.8	12.6	8.5
Potassium (mEq/l)	17.4	18.5	17.6	16.5	16.2	15.4	16.3	15.8	15.5	15.0
Chloride (mEq/l) §	31.6	26.9	25.3	21.3	22.8	14.5	17.0	15.2	16.8	13.1
Calcium (mg/dl)	208	214	247	254	219	258	204	266	216	249
Phosphorous (mg/dl)	95	110	142	151	144	168	149	153	143	158
Magnesium (mg/dl)	28	25	31	29	30	26	24	29	25	25

Note: Numbers are expressed as mean; § denotes significant difference ($P < 0.05$).

Source: Adapted from Gross SJ, Geller J, and Tomarelli RM, *Pediatrics*, 1981, 68(4): 490–493.

The predominant whey protein in cow milk is alpha-lactoglobulin. Compared to human milk–fed infants, infants fed whey-predominant formulas have higher serum concentrations of threonine, phenylalanine, valine, and methionine. There are differences in composition of human milk based on delivery of a term or preterm infant (Table 22.5).

The optimal daily protein requirement for the preterm infant is somewhat more problematic and probably is best determined in relation to intrauterine growth rate and protein accretion rate. Another important factor in assessing dietary requirements for preterm infants is the protein-to-energy ratio. If energy intake is limited, the protein will go to the oxidative route to provide energy; on the other hand, providing too much protein might place a burden on the nitrogen-clearing capacity of the liver and kidneys without providing any benefit in terms of retention of more muscle body mass.

Kashyap et al. followed the growth of LBW infants divided into three groups [26]. Groups 1 and 2 received similar energy intakes (119 and 120 kcal/kg/d, respectively) while receiving different amounts of protein (2.8 g/kg and 3.8 g/kg, respectively). Group 3 was placed on high-calorie formula and received 142 kcal/kg and the higher amount of protein intake (3.8 g/kg). The growth rate and the protein retention rate in group 1 were slightly higher than the intrauterine accretion rate, suggesting that this amount of intake is sufficient to maintain *in utero* growth rate. On the other hand, groups 2 and 3 both showed better growth than the lower-protein group, showing the efficacy of higher protein intake to promote better growth. However, blood urea nitrogen and amino acid concentrations were also higher in both these groups, reflecting lower protein utilization with the higher intake. Moreover, the higher energy intake in group 3 did not increase the weight gain significantly compared to group 2.

Schulze et al. monitored the growth of three groups of LBW infants with only a slightly different regimen [27]:

- Group A had 2.24 g/kg/d protein with 113 kcal/kg/d
- Group B had 3.6 g/kg/d protein and 115 kcal/kg/d
- Group C had 3.5 g/kg/d protein and 149 kcal/kg/d

Although group A was still able to maintain *in utero* growth rate, groups B and C both showed better weight gain. Although group C had significantly better weight gain than group B, the nitrogen retention rates were similar. This shows that the extra energy provided to group C was not associated with greater protein synthesis but with storage of nonprotein energy, such as lipids or glycogen. In summary, to provide the balance between adequate growth and optimal protein-to-energy ratio, the current recommendation for preterm infants is in the range of 3.0 to 3.5 g/kg/d or 2.3 to 2.9 g/100 kcal of protein [8,11].

In short-term studies, Bhatia et al. demonstrated similar growth but improved cognitive function in infants fed 3.2 g protein/100 kcal, compared to 2.7 or 2.2 g/100 kcal [28]. Infants on total parenteral nutrition (TPN) need at least 2.5 g/kg/d of protein and 70 kcal/kg/d of nonprotein energy to maintain positive nitrogen balance. To achieve intrauterine growth rate (15 g/kg weight gain per day), infants need 3.0 g/kg of protein and 80 kcal/kg nonprotein energy intake daily [29].

22.4.3 LIPID

Lipids are the major energy source in both enteral and parenteral nutrition. A human milk lipid system provides approximately 50% of the energy, whereas fats in cow milk–based formulas make up 40 to 50% of the energy content. Various fat blends are used to provide the short-, medium-, and long-chain and essential fatty acids. Recently, docosahexanoic and arachadonic acids have been added to most formulas in the United States. The AAP Committee on Nutrition recommends that at least 3% of total calories should be in the form of linoleic acid and linolenic acids to meet the newborn's essential fatty acid requirement.

Long-chain polyunsaturated fatty acids (LCPUFAs) have attracted considerable interest in recent years. The most important are arachidonic acid (ARA) and docosahexaenoic acid (DHA). These are important components of membrane phospholipids and several biologically important mediators. Human milk contains both of them, but commercial formulas have been supplemented only recently.

Several studies have demonstrated that term infants receiving LCPUFA-supplemented formula have more mature retinal function and cortical processing as measured by visual evoked potential, electoretinography, and visual acuity by behavioral methods [30–32]. A meta-analysis of 12 published trials supports the benefit of LCPUFAs on visual acuity [33]. Improved cognitive function with LCPUFA supplementation has been reported by some [34–36], but not by others [37–40]. The differences in the results may be due to many factors, including variations in fatty acid supplementation and levels, testing age, and procedures and experimental design. None of the studies, however, demonstrated adverse effects. Preterm infants delivered in the third trimester of pregnancy do not have the advantage of the placental transfer of these LCPUFAs and should benefit more from LCPUFA supplementation. O'Connor et al. followed preterm infants fed with supplemented formula and demonstrated improved visual acuity and better scores on the Fagan test of novelty preference at six months of age [41]. Vocabulary comprehension was also greater at 14 months in supplemented infants, after infants of Spanish-speaking families and twins were excluded from the analysis. There were no demonstrable growth benefits or disadvantages. In contrast, Innis et al. demonstrated significantly faster weight gain with supplemented preterm formula feeding and weight-to-length ratios similar to those of term breast-fed infants at 48 and 57 weeks PMA [42]. In a similar study, preterm infants who were fed supplemented formulas for 92 weeks PMA were evaluated at 118 weeks; developmental scores using the BSID II were significantly better in the infants supplemented with a single-cell source of DHA and ARA [43]. In contrast, Fewtrell et al., in a short-term study, could not demonstrate differences in developmental scores in supplemented or control infants at 18 months of age; of concern is the shorter length of the supplemented infants at 18 months [44]. The reasons for the latter findings are not clear.

In a systematic review, Simmer found that supplementation of formula provides some increase in the early rate of visual development for preterm infants but not for term infants [45,46]. No long-term benefit has been shown so far in either group. Also, no adverse effects on growth have been demonstrated.

22.5 MINERALS, VITAMINS, AND MINOR NUTRIENTS

The *in utero* accretion rate is about 120 to 140 mg/kg/d for calcium and 60 to 75 mg/kg/d for phosphorus [8]. This intake cannot be provided in parenteral solutions because of limited solubility. Hypocalcemia is a frequent finding in premature infants, so calcium supplementation is routinely started in infants < 1800 g and adjusted based on serum levels.

One of the biggest challenges in nutrition for the preterm infant is to provide enough calcium and phosphorus for bone development. The recommended daily oral intake for preterm infants is 200 mg/kg/d for Ca and 100 mg/kg/d for P, taking into consideration the limited gut absorption of these nutrients [8]. Although prolonged parenteral nutrition and the use of unfortified human milk can lead to metabolic bone disease, especially in the small preterm infant, currently available preterm formulas provide adequate amounts of calcium and phosphorus. Human milk fortifiers also enhance the amounts of calcium and phosphorus when used appropriately. The risk of metabolic bone disease is inversely related to gestational age and birth weight and is higher in the sicker infants [47].

The bulk of the iron stores in neonates is acquired transplacentally during the third trimester. Term infants have sufficient reserve for 4 to 6 months [48]. SGA and preterm infants have a limited supply and may require supplementation in the first few weeks. Term infants require 1 mg/kg/d of iron, whereas healthy preterm infants need 2 to 4 mg/kg/d to prevent anemia of prematurity. Infants who receive erythropoetin (Epo) therapy may need > 6 mg/kg iron daily to optimize the benefit of Epo supplementation [49,50]. A recent multicenter, randomized, controlled trial conducted in infants less than 1250 g birth weight did not show a difference in transfusion requirement in the Epo-treated group [51]. The trial did not recommend routine use of early Epo in this group of infants.

Vitamin K is given to all newborns to prevent hemorrhagic disease. After that, the intestinal flora usually produces this vitamin, and deficiency is rare. Vitamin D deficiency can be seen in certain high-risk groups, such as totally breast-fed infants with limited sun exposure. The recently released AAP guideline on vitamin D intake recommends a minimum of 200 IU/d intake, starting during the first two months of life. Vitamin A deficiency has been associated with BPD [52], and vitamin E deficiency has been reported to cause hemolytic anemia [53]. However, with the change in vitamin E-to-PUFA ratio in infant formulas, the incidence of vitamin E deficiency anemia is extremely low. Typical nutritional management (both enteral and parenteral) provides enough supplements to maintain normal levels of these vitamins.

Recent data have raised concerns regarding zinc sufficiency in preterm infants. The estimated fetal accretion of zinc is approximately 850 μg/d. Clinical zinc deficiency has been reported in human milk–fed preterm infants, and the concentration of zinc in human milk declines postpartum [54]. Current recommendation of 600 μg to 1 mg/kg/d can be met with the use of preterm and term formulas and fortified human milk. Trace elements are usually sufficiently supplied by breast milk or formulas. For parenteral nutrition, suggested intakes are depicted in Table 22.6 [55].

22.6 TOTAL PARENTERAL NUTRITION

In the NICU, most admissions involve some kind of intravenous nutrition for a period of time. It is more prolonged in the very immature infants and most of the surgical patients, because of the inability to use enteral feeding. In certain cases, TPN can supplement enteral feeding until about 75 to 80% of energy and protein requirements are reached by the enteral route. TPN has been used in neonates for the past three decades. It evolved from experiences in adults, with appropriate adjustments to consider the requirements of neonates.

TABLE 22.6
Trace Minerals and Vitamins in Parenteral Nutrition

Nutrient [Amount/kg/d]	< 14 d	>14 d
Manganese (µg)	0.0–0.75	1.0
Chromium (µg)	0.0–0.05	0.2
Selenium (µg)	0.0–1.3	2.0
Molybdenum (µg)	0	0.25
Iodine (µg)	0.0–1.0	1.0
Vitamin C (mg)	80	
Vitamin A (mg)	0.7	
Vitamin D (µg)	10 (= 400 IU)	
Vitamin B1 (mg)	1.2	
Vitamin B2 (mg)	1.4	
Vitamin B6 (mg)	1	
Niacin (mg)	17	

Note: Provided as MVI-Pediatric; each 5 ml provides amounts shown; not to exceed 2 ml/kg/d.

22.6.1 ENERGY

In general, the energy requirement for a steady growth during total parenteral nutrition is 85 to 95 kcal/kg/d, because the energy loss related to absorption is bypassed and there is no energy loss through stooling. About half of the calories are provided from glucose, 30 to 40% from lipids, and the rest from amino acids. Nonprotein energy intake should be at least 60 to 70 kcal/kg/d.

22.6.2 GLUCOSE

The typical glucose concentration is 12.5 to 15%. Peripheral administration cannot be more than 12.5% solution, because of the risk of sclerosis from extravasation. If higher delivery is needed, a central line should be placed. This provides a glucose delivery of 6 to 8 mg/kg/min, which is usually sufficient to maintain normoglycemia. Extremely low-birthweight infants frequently show glucose intolerance in the first few days of life [56]. If glucose delivery is minimized by the lowest possible glucose concentration (4 to 5%), insulin may be helpful and appears to be safe in these infants [57].

22.6.3 PROTEIN

The initial goal immediately after birth, besides providing caloric intake to maintain basal metabolic processes, is to prevent nitrogen loss. Protein should be started early, preferably on the first day, to prevent negative nitrogen balance. Providing at least 1 g/kg/d of protein from day 1 can maintain protein balance without any adverse effects. Paisley et al. reported a group of infants who were started at 3 g/kg/d, finding it efficacious and safe. Protein can be increased in daily increments of 0.5 to 1.0 g/kg up to 3.5 mg/kg/d, or not more than 10 to 12% of total energy intake. Rising BUN may be a sign of intolerance, and the increase may need to be held until nitrogen clearance improves. Protein is provided as a mixture of crystalline amino acids. Cysteine, an essential amino acid for the neonate, is added to the commercial preparation later (40 mg/g/AA), because it is unstable in solution. Cysteine has been shown to enhance nitrogen balance [58].

22.6.4 LIPIDS

The currently used lipid preparations are derived from safflower oil or soybean oil. They are available in 10 and 20% concentrations. LBW neonates tolerate the 20% concentration better and show lower serum levels when given this preparation [59]. Lower serum levels may be explained by the lower phospholipid concentration in the 20% solution, because the phospholipid component competes for the lipoprotein lipase, therefore decreasing its clearance. Lipids are usually started at 0.5 to 1.0 g/kg/d and gradually increased to 3.5 to 4.0 g/kg/d or not more than 40% of total calories. To prevent essential fatty acid deficiency, the minimal intake should be 0.5 g/kg/d. In small infants, daily measurements are necessary during advancement to ensure proper lipid clearance, and the dose must be held or decreased if the triglyceride level is over 180 to 200 mg/dl. Intravenous lipids are better tolerated if infused over prolonged periods (at least 20 hours).

22.6.5 VITAMINS AND TRACE ELEMENTS

Vitamins and trace elements are added to the preparation from commercial formulas. See Table 22.6.

22.6.6 COMPLICATIONS

The complications of parenteral nutrition are related to the content of the solution (metabolic), associated with the route of delivery, or both. The most common metabolic complications are metabolic bone disease and liver dysfunction. Providing calcium intake that is comparable to intrauterine accretion rates is impossible through intravenous nutrition, because of precipitation at higher concentrations. Therefore, infants maintained on TPN for a prolonged time will develop metabolic bone disease to some extent. Currently, there are no good clinical markers of metabolic bone disease. Increasing alkaline phophatase levels, which signify extensive bone remodeling, are the best practical tools to monitor the evolving disease, because serum electrolyte levels are maintained at the expense of bone reabsorption. The most prevalent sign of liver dysfunction is cholestasis. Signs usually develop after a few weeks of parenteral nutrition. Elevated direct bilirubin is a late sign but probably the most cost-effective way to monitor periodically. The prognosis is good; the process is typically reversible once enteral feeding is started. Every effort should be made to advance these infants to at least some partial feeding. Periodic monitoring is needed to minimize and monitor complications while a patient is on parenteral nutrition (Table 22.7).

Catheter-related complications include tip misplacement, thrombosis, extravasation, and sepsis or bacteremia. These complications can be minimized by proper sterile technique, use of heparin to prevent clot formation in the lumen or hub, avoidance of multiple manipulation of the dressing, and breaking up the continuity of the line.

In infants maintained on parenteral nutrition, special attention should be paid to the possibility of metabolic acidosis, mainly because most of the salts are given in chloride form. Partial replacement of chloride with acetate can prevent this problem [60].

22.7 FEEDING THE PRETERM INFANT

Although the suck reflex may be observed in many premature infants, the coordination of sucking, swallowing, and breathing is not present until 32 to 34 weeks of postconceptional age [61]. Other factors affecting the feeding ability of the premature infant include delayed gastric emptying, low stomach volume, and weak esophageal sphincter, leading to an almost universal gastroesophageal reflux [62–64]. If the infant is unable to feed per os, an oro- or nasogastric tube is placed to initiate feedings. Gastric feeding can be continuous or bolus. Continuous feeding, although it is not physiologic, is more energy efficient and allows reaching higher volumes than bolus feedings [65,66]. A subgroup of infants cannot tolerate even continuous gastric feeding. For them, transpyloric feeding may be an option until gastric emptying improves. This should be a last resort only,

TABLE 22.7
Suggested Monitoring during Parenteral Nutrition

Component	Initial	Later
Weight	Daily	Daily
Length	Weekly	Weekly
Head circumference	Weekly	Weekly
Na, K, Cl, CO_2	Daily until stable	Weekly
Glucose	Daily	PRN
Triglycerides	With every lipid change	Weekly or biweekly
Ca, PO_4	Daily until stable	Weekly or biweekly
Alkaline phosphatase	Initial	Weekly or biweekly
Bilirubin	Initial	Weekly or biweekly
Mg	Initial	Weekly or biweekly
Ammonia	PRN	PRN
Gamma GT	Initial	Weekly or biweekly
ALT/AST	Initial	Weekly or biweekly
Complete blood count	Initial	Weekly or PRN

TABLE 22.8
Commonly Used Feeding Practices

Method	Advantages	Disadvantages
Nipple	Simple; physiologic; hormonal, digestive, and neurologic benefit	Consumes energy; possible aspiration; not feasible on CPAP or ventilator
Orogastric–nasogastric	Suck–swallow not required; can be used in intubated patients; decreased risk of aspiration; conserves energy	Inadvertent tracheal intubation; blocks nasal passage and increases airway resistance; vagal stimulation and gagging
Intermittent bolus	Mimics nipple feeding with possible enteric hormone benefits	Gastric residuals, reflux, abdominal distention
Constant infusion	Better tolerated by infants with delayed gastric emptying; possible larger milk intake	Not physiologic; loss of cyclic hormonal effect
Transpyloric	Fewer residuals and less reflux in infants with poor gastric emptying; possible larger milk intake	Multiple x-rays; catheter misplacement and complication; alters gut flora
Gastrostomy	Indicated for patients with severe neurologic damage	Morbidity/mortality with the procedure

Source: Adapted from Dweck HS, *Clin. Perinatol.*, 1975, 2:183-202.

because it does not seem to provide much advantage in weight gain or caloric intake but exposes the infant to a lot more radiation [67]. Table 22.8 shows characteristics of the commonly used feeding practices.

Because of the concern about vascular compromise with the use of intra-arterial catheters, such as umbilical arterial catheters, there appears to be a variation in feeding when these lines are in place. The potential of vascular compromise to the gut and subsequent risk of necrotizing entercolitis (NEC) have not been studied well in randomized, controlled trials. In a recent survey, Tiffany et al. found that most of the units they surveyed used some kind of enteral feeding with umbilical lines in place [68]. Although physicians were more liberal with feedings when only umbilical venous catheters (UVCs) were left in place, the majority were also using trophic feedings with umbilical arterial catheters (UACs) still present.

Studies published in the recent years show the benefit of providing minimal feeding for the preterm infant on parenteral nutrition to prevent atrophy of villi and to promote gut maturation [69,70]. The usual amount of feeding in these studies was ≤ 20 ml/kg/d. The studies demonstrated a shorter time to reach full volume of feeds, a decreased incidence of feeding intolerance without an increase in the incidence of NEC [71–73].

Berseth et al. compared minimal feeding (where feeding was held at 20 ml/kg/d) and advancing feeding over a 10-day period. They showed an increased risk of NEC in the group in which feedings were advanced [74].

Although we have more and more evidence to support early feeding, the controversy is not resolved. This is reflected in recent reviews in the Cochrane Database that concluded that there is still not enough clinical evidence to promote the universal use of early feeding in high-risk infants. [75,76]. Therefore, the most common approach is to hold feeding in high-risk infants for a few days, start slowly with low volumes, and advance slowly (≤ 20 ml/kg/d) [77]. These infants require a high index of suspicion to withhold feeding, but feedings can be restarted if symptoms subside.

Human milk, although is still not widely used for preterm infants, is superior to formula in several aspects. Preterm human milk has a higher content of nitrogen, sodium, vitamins, and lipids than mature milk. Also, human milk contains several important immunologic factors and has been shown to be protective against NEC. Table 22.5 shows a comparison of preterm and term human milk [78]. During the first few weeks, preterm human milk can provide enough nutrients to meet the requirements for LBW infants, but later, especially for babies with < 1800 g birth weight, supplementation may be required. Preterm human milk can be fortified by mixing 1:1 with a preterm formula or commercially available human-milk fortifiers. Commercial formulas designed for preterm infants provide more protein, fat, sodium, calcium, phosphorus, vitamins, and trace minerals than human milk [79]. These formulas come in preparations of 22 kcal/oz (for infants less than 2500 g) and 24 kcal/oz (for infants less than 1800 g).

Soy-based formulas are not recommended for preterm infants, because the phytic acid can bind calcium, lowering its absorption. Infants fed soy-based formula also showed less nitrogen retention, lower levels of serum albumin and total protein, and diminished weight gain [79].

22.8 FEEDING THE TERM INFANT

Term infants admitted to NICU are usually too unstable to be fed enterally or orally. The initial nutrition, therefore, must be intravenous. When the infant becomes more stable and the gut function is appropriate (good bowel sounds, no distention, regular stooling pattern), enteral feeding can be started, even when the infant is on the ventilator. If the infant's condition allows, feeding can be advanced faster than in preterm infants. Once feasible, oral feeding is started. Most term infants are able to nipple after a short intensive care course. A subgroup of infants who had more prolonged illness (such as CDH, post-ECMO) frequently shows suck–swallow dysfunction and gastroesophageal reflux. These infants stay on tube feeding for a longer time, which may prolong their length of stay [80].

The American Academy of Pediatrics strongly recommends the use of breast milk [81]. Every effort should be made to provide support for a mother to pump while her baby is critically ill and to allow her to visit and nurse whenever possible. If breast milk is not available, most NICUs use term, cow milk–based formulas. If one encounters malabsorption, as seen in short-gut syndrome, a more elemental formula can be used (e.g., Neocate).

22.9 SPECIAL CONSIDERATIONS

Glutamine has received some attention in the past few years. Although not considered an essential amino acid, it is the primary fuel for the enterocyte and is the most abundantly found amino acid in the body. Regular diet sufficient in protein provides enough glutamine, and supplementation is not needed. In conditions involving stress and catabolic processes or intestinal disease, glutamine has been shown to be "conditionally" essential [82]. Glutamine is not supplied during parenteral nutrition, so preterm infants maintained on prolonged TPN are high risk for gut atrophy and may benefit from glutamine supplementation. A randomized clinical trial in premature infants receiving parenteral nutrition is underway. Neu et al. conducted a randomized trial in 68 VLBW infants (< 1250 g), in which they used a formula supplemented with 0.3 g/kg/d of glutamine. Decreased hospital-acquired infections, improved tolerance to enteral feeds, and decreased hospital costs were found in the glutamine-supplemented group, without any safety concerns [83]. In a later study, Vaughn et al. found no difference in nosocomial sepsis using the same dose of supplementation [84]. Tubman and Thompson reviewed the current literature for the Cochrane Database and concluded that there is not enough evidence in the randomized trials so far to support universal supplementation for preterm infants [85]. Larger studies are needed before recommending routine use of glutamine in infants' diet.

Corticosteroids became widely used in 1990s to improve respiratory outcome in infants with severe respiratory failure. Later in that decade, reports appeared on follow-up studies showing abnormal neurodevelopment, especially in infants treated with early and prolonged corticosteroid regimens. Steroids also have a profound effect on many aspects of the metabolism. Administration of pharmacological doses promotes protein catabolism, with subsequent protein wasting, and induces lipid and glucose intolerance. These alterations can put an extra burden on the metabolic needs of the preterm infant and further compromise growth. The benefit of using steroids should be strongly weighed against the risks and complications, and their use should be restricted to very special circumstances, as recently suggested by an AAP policy statement [86].

22.10 POSTDISCHARGE FEEDING OF THE PREMATURE INFANT

The challenge of providing appropriate nutritional support for preterm infants continues beyond their hospital stay. Providing the currently recommended energy and protein intake might not be sufficient to replicate intrauterine growth rate.

Ehrenkranz et al. published data from a large cohort of preterm infants (birth weight 500 to 1500 g) regarding their postnatal growth [6]. These infants accrued a considerable amount of nutritional deficit during their first few weeks. They were frequently unstable initially; parenteral and enteral nutrition advanced slowly because of concerns about complications. Therefore, full nutrition support might not be reached before the second or even third week of life. Despite some catch-up growth in the second month of their hospitalization, most infants born between 24 and 29 weeks did not reach the median weight of the reference fetus of the same gestational age. This "extrauterine growth restriction" seems to continue into the second year of life. The incidence of failure to thrive in infants less than 1000 g in the Neonatal Research Cohort was more than 30% at 18 months corrected age [87].

Lucas et al. conducted a randomized, double-blind study of preterm infants fed fortified formula after discharge to see if postdischarge growth deficit can be improved with higher caloric intake in the first nine months post term [88]. Significant increases in linear growth and weight gain were observed in the infants who received the enriched diet. There was no increase in diet-related complications in the group with the modified formula.

Carver et al. compared 22 kcal/oz enriched formula diet with regular term formula, feeding up to 12 months of corrected age [89]. They found improved growth in the group fed nutrient-enriched formula, with the highest benefit for infants less than 1250 g birth weight.

Several studies have now been published demonstrating the benefit of long-chain polyunsaturated fatty acids in the posthospital discharge period. In a recent study, infants randomized to DHA (17 mg/100 kcal) and ARA (34 mg/100 kcal) demonstrated greater weight gain than unsupplemented infants from 6 to 18 months of age; these infants also had greater lengths at 79 and 92 weeks postmenstrual age [90]. Innis et al. demonstrated that preterm infants fed DHA (0.14%) and AA (0.27%) gained weight significantly faster than unsupplemented infants and had weight-to-length ratios similar to those of term breast-fed infants at 48 and 57 weeks postmenstrual age [42]. In addition, visual acuity and neurodevelopmental benefits have been demonstrated. Based on these data, it seems prudent to maintain low-birthweight formula-fed infants on enriched formulas up to 6 to 9 months of corrected age.

22.11 SUMMARY

For the term infant, the growth and biochemical responses of a healthy infant breast fed by a healthy mother remain the gold standard. Over the past few decades, continued improvement in formulas have been made with the addition of iron, alteration of whey-to-casein ratio and the fat blends, and addition of taurine, nucleotides, and, most recently, DHA and ARA. The American Academy of Pediatrics and the Canadian Pediatric Society strongly recommend that breast feeding be the preferred feeding for all infants. In the absence of human milk, currently available formulas are appropriate substitutes for feeding full-term infants during the first year of life. Although we strive to increase breastfeeding rates in the United States, we need to continue to improve available formulas to be as close to human milk as possible. For the preterm infant, a continuous strategy to nourish the infant from birth, through the hospitalization period, and beyond must be continually improved to enhance the growth and development of this increasing cohort of infants. We need to continue to advocate human-milk feedings, appropriately fortify them as needed, and continue to make improvements in the commercially available formulas. The current generation of premature infant formulas was designed for the "larger" preterm infant and may not be the ideal formulation for the very small premature infant.

The strategies in feeding term and preterm infants differ and must be individualized. Although reliance on evidence should guide us in nourishing these infants, feeding infants is also an art based on experience. Experience should then be molded by evidence to enhance our nutritional care of these fragile infants.

REFERENCES

1. American Academy of Pediatrics, Committee on Nutrition. Nutritional needs of low-birth-weight infants. *Pediatrics* 1985, 75: 976.
2. Ziegler EE, O'Donnell AM, Nelson SE, Fomon SJ. Body composition of the reference fetus. *Growth* 1976, 40: 239.
3. Babson SG, Benda GI. Growth graphs for the clinical assessment of infants of varying gestational ages. *J. Pediatr.* 1976, 89: 814.
4. Lubchenco L, Hansman C, Boyd E. Intrauterine growth in length and head circumference as estimated from live births at gestational ages from 26 to 42 weeks. *Pediatrics* 1966, 37: 403.
5. Alexander GR, Himes JH, Kaufman RB, Mor J, Kogan M. A United States national reference for fetal growth. *Obstet. Gynecol.* 1996, 87: 163–168.
6. Ehrenkranz RA, Younes N, Lemons JA. Longitudinal growth of hospitalized very low birth weight infants. *Pediatrics.* 1999, 104, 2 (Pt 1): 280–289.
7. American Academy of Pediatrics, Committee on Nutrition. Nutritional needs of the preterm infant, *Pediatric Nutrition Handbook*, 5th edition, 2003, 23–54.
8. Hay WW Jr. (ed.). *Nutritional Requirement of the Extremely Low-Birth-Weight Infant.* Mosby Year Book, St. Louis, MO, 1991.
9. Sauer PJJ, Dane HF, Visser HKA. Longitudinal studies on metabolic rate, heat loss, and energy cost of growth in low birth weight infants. *Pediatr. Res.* 1984, 18: 254.

10. Ziegler EE, Thureen PJ, Carlson SJ. Aggressive nutrition of the very low birth weight infant. *Clin. Perinatol.* 2002, 29: 225–244.

11. Tsang RC et al. (eds.) *Nutritional Needs of the Preterm Infant: Scientific Basis and Practical Guidelines.* Williams & Wilkins, Pawling, NY 1993.

12. Brunton JA, Saigal S, Atkinson SA. Nutrient intake similar to recommended values does not result in catch-up growth by 12 mo of age in very low birth weight infants (VLBW) with bronchopulmonary dysplasia (BPD). *Am. J. Clin. Nutr.* 1997, 66: 221 (abs. 102).

13. Butte NF, Garza C, Smith EO, Nichols BL. Human milk intake and growth in exclusively breast-fed infants. *J. Pediatr.* 1984, 104(2): 187–195.

14. Garza C, Butte NF. Energy intakes of human milk-fed infants during the first year. *J. Pediatr.* 1990, 117(2 Pt 2): S124–S131.

15. Lorenz JM, Kleinman LI, Ahmed G, Markarian K. Phases of fluid electrolyte homeostasis in the extremely low birth weight infant. *Pediatrics* 1995, 96: 484.

16. Schaffer SG, Meade V. Sodium balance and extracellular volume regulation in very low birth weight infants. *J. Pediatr.* 1989, 115: 285–290.

17. Hartnoll G, Betremieux P, Modi N. Randomized controlled trial of postnatal sodium supplementation on oxygen dependency and body weight in 25–30 week gestational age infants. *Arch. Dis. Child Fetal Neonatal Ed.* 2000, 82 :F19–F23.

18. Costarino AT, Gruskay JA, Corcoran L, et al. Sodium restriction versus daily maintenance replacement in very low birth weight premature neonates: a randomized, blind therapeutic trial. *J. Pediatr.* 1992, 120: 99–106.

19. Sulyok E, Kovacs L, Lichardus B, et al. Late hyponatremia in premature infants: role of aldosterone and arginine vasopressin. *J. Pediatr.* 1985, 106: 990–994.

20. Baumgart S, Costarino AT. Water and electrolyte metabolism of the micropremie. *Clin. Perinatol.* 2000, 27: 131–146.

21. Gruskay J, Costarino AT, Polin RA, et al. Non-oliguric hyperkalemia in the premature infant weighing less than 1000 grams. *J. Pediatr.* 1988, 113: 381–386.

22. Rutter N, Hull D. Water loss from the skin of term and preterm babies. *Arch. Dis. Child.* 1979, 54: 858–868.

23. Parish A, Bhatia J. Nutritional considerations in the intensive care unit: neonatal issues. In: *Nutritional Considerations in the Intensive Care Unit: Science, Rationale and Practice.* Shikora SA, Martindale RG, Schwaitzberg SD, eds. ASPEN, Kendall/Hunt, Dubuque, IA, 2002. 297–310.

24. MacLean WC Jr., Fink BB. Lactose malabsorption by premature infants: magnitude and clinical significance. *J. Pediatr.* 1980, 97(3): 383–388.

25. Mobassaleh M, Montgomery RK, Biller JA, Grand RJ. Development of carbohydrate absorption in the fetus and neonate. *Pediatrics.* 1985, 75(1 Pt 2): 160–166.

26. Kashyap S, Schulze KF, Forsyth M, Zucker C, Dell RB, Ramakrishnan R, Heird WC. Growth, nutrient retention, and metabolic response in low birth weight infants fed varying intakes of protein and energy. *J. Pediatr.* 1988, 113(4): 713–721.

27. Schulze KF, Stefanski M, Masterson J, Spinnazola R, Ramakrishnan R, Dell RB, Heird WC. Energy expenditure, energy balance, and composition of weight gain in low birth weight infants fed diets of different protein and energy content. *Pediatrics* 1987, 110(5): 753–759.

28. Bhatia J, Rassin DK, Cerreto MC, et al. Effect of protein/energy ratio on growth and behavior of premature infants: preliminary findings. *J. Pediatr.* 1991, 119: 103–110.

29. Zlotkin SH, Bryan MH, Anderson GH. Intravenous nitrogen and energy intakes required to duplicate *in utero* nitrogen accretion in prematurely born human infants. *J. Pediatr.* 1981, 99(1): 115–120.

30. Hoffman DR, Birch EE, Birch DG, Uauy R, Castaneda YS, Lapus MG, Wheaton DH. Impact of early dietary intake and blood lipid composition of long-chain polyunsaturated fatty acids on later visual development. *J. Pediatr. Gastroenterol. Nutr.* 2000, 31(5): 540–553.

31. Makrides M, Neumann MA, Jeffrey B, Lien EL, Gibson RA. A randomized trial of different ratios of linoleic to alpha-linolenic acid in the diet of term infants: effects on visual function and growth. *Am. J. Clin. Nutr.* 2000, 71(1): 120–129.

32. Carlson SE et al. Visual acuity and fatty acid status of term infants fed human milk and formulas with and without docosahexanoate and arachidonate from egg yolk lecithin. *Pediatr. Res.* 1996, 39: 882–888.

33. San Giovanni JP, Berkey CS, Dwyer JT, Colditz GA. Dietary essential fatty acids, long-chain poly-unsaturated fatty acids, and visual acuity in healthy fullterm infants: a systematic review. *Early Hum. Dev.* 2000, 57: 165–188.

34. Birch EE, Garfield S, Hoffman DR, Uauy R, Birch DG. A randomized controlled trial of early dietary supply of long-chain polyunsaturated fatty acids and mental development in term infants. *Dev. Med. Child Neurol.* 2000, 42(3): 174–181.

35. Agostini C, Trojan S, Bellu R, et al. Neurodevelopmental quotient of healthy term infants at 4 months and feeding practice: the role of long-chain polyunsaturated fatty acids. *Pediatr. Res.* 1995, 38: 262–266.

36. Wilatts P, Forsyth JS, DiMadugno MK, et al. Effect of long-chain polyunsaturated fatty acids in infant formulas on problem solving at 10 months of age. *Lancet* 1998, 352: 688–691.

37. Makrides M et al. Are long-chain polyunsaturated fatty acids essential nutrients in infancy? *Lancet* 1995, 345: 1463–1468.

38. Markides M et al. A critical appraisal of the dietary long-chain polyunsaturated fatty acids on neural indices of term infants: a randomized controlled trial. *Pediatrics* 2000, 105: 32–38.

39. Auestad N et al. Growth and development in term infants fed long-chain polyunsaturated fatty acids: a double-masked, randomized, parallel, prospective, multivariate study. *Pediatrics* 2001, 108: 372–381.

40. Lucas A et al. Efficacy and safety of long-chain polyunsaturated fatty acid supplementation of infant-formula milk: a randomized trial. *Lancet* 1999, 354: 1948–1954.

41. O'Connor DL, Hall R, Adamkin D, Auestad N, et al. Growth and development in preterm infants fed long-chain polyunsaturated fatty acids: a prospective, randomized controlled trial. *Pediatrics* 2001, 108(2): 359–371.

42. Innis SM, Adamkin DH, Hall RT, Kahlan SC, Lair C, Lim M, et al. Docosahexanoic acid and arachadonic acid enhance growth with no adverse effects in preterm infants fed formula. *J. Pediatr.* 2002, 140: 547–554.

43. Clandinin M, VanArde J, Antonson D, Lim M, Stevens D, Merkel K, Harris J, Hansen J. Formulas with docosahexanoic acid [DHA] and arachadonic acid [ARA] promote better growth and develop-mental scores in very-low-birth-weight infants [VLBW]. *Ped. Res.* 2002, 51(4): 1092.

44. Fewtrell MS, Morley R, Abbott RA, Singhal A, Isaacs EB, Stephenson T, MacFadyen U, Lucas A. Double-blind, randomized trial of long-chain polyunsaturated fatty acid supplementation in formula fed to preterm infants. *Pediatrics* 2002, 110(1 Pt 1): 73–82.

45. Simmer K. Longchain polyunsaturated fatty acid supplementation in preterm infants. *Cochrane Data-base Syst Rev.* 2000, 2: CD000375. Review.

46. Simmer K. Longchain polyunsaturated fatty acid supplementation in infants born at term. *Cochrane Database Syst Rev.* 2001, 4: CD000376. Review.

47. Koo WWK, Gupta JM, Nayanar VV, et al. Skeletal changes in preterm infants. *Arch. Dis. Child.* 1982, 57: 447–452.

48. American Academy of Pediatrics, Committee on Nutrition. Iron supplementation. *Pediatrics* 1976, 58: 765.

49. Rao R, Georgieff MK. Neonatal iron nutrition. *Semin. Neonatol.* 2001, 6(5): 425–435.

50. Carnielli VP, Da Riol R, Montini G. Iron supplementation enhances response to high doses of recombinant human erythropoietin in preterm infants. *Arch. Dis. Child. Fetal Neonatal Ed.* 1998, 79: F44–F48.

51. Ohls RK, Ehrenkrantz RA, Wright LL, Lemons JA, Korones SB, Stoll BJ, et al. Effects of early erythropoietin therapy on the transfusion requirements of preterm infants below 1250 grams birth-weight: a multi-center, randomized controlled trial. *Pediatrics* 2001, 108: 934–942.

52. Shenai JP, Chytil F, Stahlman. Vitamin A status of neonates with bronchopulmonary dysplasia. *Pediatr. Res.* 1985, 19: 185.

53. Oski FA, Barnes LA. Vitamin E deficiency: a previously unrecognized cause of hemolytic anemia in the premature. *J. Pediatr.* 1967, 70: 211.

54. Zlotkin SH. Assessment of trace element requirements [zinc] in newborns and young infants, including the infant born prematurely. In: *Trace Elements in Nutrition of Children II*. Chandra RK, ed. Raven Press, New York, 1991, 49–64.

55. Bhatia J, Bucher C, Bunyapen C. Feeding the preterm infant. In: *Handbook of Nutrition and Food*. Berdanier CD, ed. CRC Press, Boca Raton, FL, 2002, 203–218.

56. Lilien DP, Rosenfeld RL, Baccaro MM, et al. Hyperglycemia in stressed, small premature infants. *J. Pediatr.* 1979, 94: 454–459.

57. Collins JW Jr, Hoppe M, Browne K, et al. A controlled trial of insulin infusion and parenteral nutrition in extremely low birth weight infants with glucose intolerance. *J. Pediatr.* 1991, 118: 921–927.

58. Rivera A, Jr., Bell EF, Steginic LD, Ziegler EE. Effect of intravenous amino acids on protein metabolism of preterm infants during the first three days of life. *J. Pediatr.* 1989, 115: 465.

59. Haumont D, Deckelbaum RD, Richelle M, et al. Plasma lipid and plasma lipoprotein concentration in low birth weight infants given parenteral nutrition with 20% compared to 10% intralipid. *J. Pediatr.* 1989, 115: 787.

60. Sugiura S, Inagaki K, Noda Y, Nagai T, Nabeshima T. Acid load during total parenteral nutrition: comparison of hydrochloric acid and acetic acid on plasma acid–base balance. *Nutrition* 2000, 16(4): 260–263.

61. Broussard DL. Gastrointestinal motility in the neonate. *Clin. Perinatol.* 1995, 22: 37.

62. Ittman PI, Amarnath I, Berseth CL. Maturation of antroduodenal activity in preterm and term infants. *Dig. Dis. Sci.* 1992, 37: 14.

63. Siegel M, Lebenthal E, Krantz B. Effect of caloric density on gastric emptying in premature infants. *J. Pediatr.* 1984, 104: 118.

64. Cavell B. Gastric emptying in preterm infants. *Acta Paediatr. Scand.* 1979, 68: 725–730.

65. Grant J, Denne SC. Effect of intermittent versus continuous enteral feeding on energy expenditure in premature infants. *J. Pediatr.* 1991, 118: 928.

66. Robertson AF, Bhatia J. Feeding premature infants. *Clin. Pediatr.* 1993, 31: 36.

67. Laing IA, Lang MA, Callaghan O, et al. Nasogastric compared with nasoduodenal feeding in low birthweight infants. *Arch. Dis. Child.* 1986, 61: 138–141.

68. Tiffany KF, Burke, BL, Collins-Odoms C, Oelberg DG. Current practice regarding the enteral feeding of high-risk newborns with umbilical catheters *in situ. Pediatrics* 2003, 112: 20–23.

69. Berseth CL. Effect of early feeding on maturation of the preterm infant's small intestine. *J. Pediatr.* 1992, 120: 947–953.

70. Berseth CI, Nordyke C. Enteral nutrients promote postnatal maturation of intestinal motor activity in preterm infants. *Am. J. Phys.* 1993, 264: G1046–G1051.

71. Slagle TA, Gross SJ. Effect of early low-volume enteral substrate on subsequent feeding tolerance in very low birth weight Infants. *J. Pediatr.* 1988, 113: 526–531.

72. Troche B, Harvey-Wilkes K, Engle WD, Nielsen HC, Frantz ID 3rd, Mitchell ML, Hermos RJ. Early minimal feedings promote growth in critically ill premature infants. *Biol. Neonate* 1995, 67(3): 172–181.

73. Ostertag SG, LaGamma EF, Reisen CE, et al. Early enteral feeding does not affect the incidence of necrotizing enterocolitis. *Pediatrics* 1986, 77: 275–280.

74. Berseth CL, Bisquera JA, Paje VU. Prolonging small feeding volumes early in life decreases the incidence of necrotizing enterocolitis in very low birth weight infants. *Pediatrics* 2003, 111: 529–534.

75. Kennedy KA, Tyson JE, Chamnanvanikij S. Early versus delayed initiation of progressive enteral feedings for parenterally fed low birth weight or preterm infants. *Cochrane Database Syst. Rev.* 2000, 2: CD001970.

76. Tyson JE, Kennedy KA. Minimal enteral nutrition for promoting feeding tolerance and preventing morbidity in parenterally fed infants. *Cochrane Database Syst. Rev.* 2000, 2: CD000504.

77. La Gamma EF, Browne LE. Feeding practices for infants weighing less than 1500 gm at birth and the pathogenesis of necrotizing enterocolitis. *Clin. Perinat.* 1994, 21: 271–306.

78. Jensen RG (ed). *Handbook of Milk Composition.* Academic Press, San Diego, 1995.

79. Schanler RJ, Cheng SF. Infant formulas for enteral feeding. In: *Neonatal Nutrition and Metabolism.* Hay WW Jr. (ed). Mosby Year Book, St. Louis, 1991, 303.

80. Van Meurs KP, Robbins ST, Reed VL, Karr SS, Wagner AE, Glass P, Anderson KD, Short BL. Congenital diaphragmatic hernia: long-term outcome in neonates treated with extracorporeal membrane oxygenation. *J. Pediatr.* 1993, 122(6): 893–899.

81. American Academy of Pediatrics, Committee on Nutrition. Encouraging breast-feeding. *Pediatrics* 1980, 65: 657.

82. Lacey JM, Wilomre DW. Is glutamine a conditionally essential amino acid? *Nutr. Rev.* 1990, 48: 397–409.

83. Neu J, DeMarco, V, Weiss M. Glutamine supplementation in low-birth-weight infants: mechanism of action. *JPEN* 1999, 23: S49–S51.
84. Vaughn P, Thomas P, Clark R, Neu J. Enteral glutamine supplementation and morbidity in low birth weight infants. *J. Pediatr.* 2003, 142(6): 662–668.
85. Tubman TR, Thompson SW. Glutamine supplementation for prevention of morbidity in preterm infants. *Cochrane Database Syst. Rev.* 2001, 4: CD001457.
86. Friedman S, Shinnell ES. Prenatal and postnatal steroid therapy and child neurodevelopment. *Clin. Perinatol.* 2000, 31: 529–544.
87. Clark RH, Wagner CL, Merritt RJ, Bloom BT, Neu J, Young TE, Clark DA. Nutrition in the neonatal intensive care unit: how do we reduce the incidence of extrauterine growth restriction? *J. Perinatol.* 2003, 23(4): 337–344.
88. Lucas A, Bishop NJ, King FJ, et al. Randomized trial of nutrition for preterm infants after hospital discharge. *Arch. Dis. Child.* 1992, 67: 324–327.
89. Carver JD, Wu PY, Hall RT, Ziegler EE, et al. Growth of preterm infants fed nutrient-enriched or term formula after hospital discharge. *Pediatrics* 2001, 107(4): 683–689.
90. Clandinin M, Vanaerde J, Antonson P, et al. Formulas with docosahexanoic acid (DHA) and arachadonic acid (ARA) promote better growth and development score in very-low-birth-weight infants (VLBW). *Pediatr. Res.* 2002, 51: 187A–188A.

23 Pediatrics

Lori Kowalski and Anita Nucci
Children's Hospital of Pittsburgh

CONTENTS

23.1 INTRODUCTION

Provision of adequate nutritional support to infants and children in the intensive care unit (ICU) should initially focus on minimizing the effects of the acute phase of critical illness. It has been estimated that 15 to 20% of all pediatric patients admitted to the ICU have preexisting malnutrition.[1] Malnutrition is associated with the depletion of protein and fat stores, reduced immunocompetence, increased risk of infection, poor wound healing, and increased morbidity and mortality.[2] Protracted catabolic stress in children who have reduced body stores, higher baseline energy requirements, or malnutrition may have devastating effects. Secondary goals should include the provision of adequate protein to promote positive nitrogen balance and to preserve lean muscle tissue. Finally, nutritional support should be designed to promote anabolism and growth in the convalescent stage of critical illness. This is one of the key differences in the care of critically ill children and adults.

23.2 METABOLIC CONSEQUENCES OF CRITICAL ILLNESS

The hypermetabolic state that exists after acute illness or trauma has been well documented in adults. This metabolic state causes a rapid turnover of protein, fat, and carbohydrate, which makes substrate available for wound healing, tissue repair, and immune response. It is usually divided into phases: an "ebb" phase and a "flow" phase.

The *ebb phase*, for the first 24 to 48 hours, consists of hyperglycemia, hypovolemia, decreased temperature and insulin levels, with a rise in catecholamines, glucose, lactate, and free fatty acid secretion and production. The *flow* or *catabolic phase* usually begins after fluid and volume resuscitation is complete. Hypermetabolism, protein catabolism, negative nitrogen balance, and an active inflammatory process are the hallmarks of this phase (see Chapter 1). Skeletal muscle protein is broken down, and there is a loss of lean body mass, with nitrogen being wasted in the urine (in proportion to the severity of the injury or stress). This muscle breakdown is not decreased by the introduction of glucose. Branch-chain amino acids (leucine, isoleucine, and valine) from gluconeo-genesis are preferentially utilized as an energy source. This lean body mass loss may impact children more quickly than adults because of their initial lower body weight and surface area. Protein synthesis is reprioritized to produce acute-phase reactants (C-reactive protein [CRP], alpha-1-acid glycoprotein), which are necessary for immune response and wound healing rather than secretory proteins (albumin, prealbumin [PAB] and transferrin). The stress response causes an increase in the rate of gluconeogenesis, which is also not suppressed by exogenous glucose administration. The normal glucagon–insulin ratio is increased, and insulin resistance occurs. Ketone production and utilization, typical in starvation states, are decreased, and there is a greater clearance and utilization of free fatty acids, glycerol, and triglycerides. During this initial phase, water and sodium are retained because of increased levels of antidiuretic hormone, aldosterone, and renin. Increased requirements have also been shown for vitamin C, thiamin, zinc, copper, and pyridoxine. The level of the stress response is usually proportional to the magnitude, nature, and duration of the injury or illness. In adults, this process causes an increase in resting energy expenditure that is significantly greater than the normal resting nonstressed state.[3]

Children generally have higher baseline energy requirements than adults, with an inverse relation of higher energy needs at a decreased body weight and surface area. In healthy children, it has been shown that resting energy expenditure (REE) accounts for 65 to 70% of total energy expenditure. The other 30 to 35% of REE is the energy for physical activity and growth. In stressed children, during this acute phase of injury, meeting activity and growth requirements may not be essential. Children are frequently sedated or paralyzed in the intensive care unit, which causes a drastic reduction in their activity level. Insensible energy losses may also be reduced for children who are mechanically ventilated and have a decreased work of breathing. Warm, humidified air that is used in ventilators may decrease insensible losses by one-third.[4]

Until the precipitating factors of infection, fractures, or wounds are treated, the catabolic phase will continue. This may have a greater impact on children because of their limited lean muscle and tissue reserves. The catabolism of skeletal muscle for glucose production is good in the short term, but serious depletion of lean body mass and fat stores may occur when the course of critical illness is protracted. Children who become critically ill on top of a chronic disease state may be further at risk. Once the convalescent stage of illness is established, growth and activity energy requirements may become important. At this point, an appropriate mixed fuel system of nutritional support can result in anabolism and continued growth in children.

23.3 NUTRITIONAL ASSESSMENT

Appropriate nutritional assessment of infants, children, and adolescents is imperative and serves as the basis of a comprehensive nutritional care plan. Identifying the children who are potentially at risk for malnutrition, growth restriction, or other nutritional deficiencies is the primary goal of assessment. Components of pediatric nutritional assessment include:

- Medical history evaluation
- Laboratory assessment
- Growth pattern and development, as compared to children of the same age
- Medications, including drug–nutrient interactions
- Evaluation of the adequacy of the child's typical nutrient intake

This information is usually gathered in a critical care setting by baseline screening, collection, and interpretation of medical, physical, and nutritional data and followed by the initiation and monitoring of individualized nutritional therapy.

23.3.1 MEDICAL HISTORY

Many medical conditions common to pediatric patients, such as cystic fibrosis, pulmonary disease, congenital heart disease, and short bowel syndrome, among others, require specific nutritional intervention. Acute conditions, such as infection, fever, surgery, and respiratory distress, superimposed on these conditions can increase the risk of malnutrition.

23.3.2 LABORATORY ASSESSMENT

Laboratory parameters, such as prealbumin, albumin, and hemoglobin/hematocrit, may be helpful in pediatric nutritional assessment (see Chapter 5). In critically ill patients, visceral protein status is easily altered by hydration. Levels should be evaluated in the context of other parameters and may have more meaning when done serially. Iron-deficiency anemia and macrocytic anemia may be evaluated by measures of mean corpuscular volume, mean corpuscular hemoglobin, and mean corpuscular hemoglobin concentration. Requests for laboratory data in pediatric patients should be made with consideration for how often blood draws must be done, especially in infants.

23.3.3 GROWTH HISTORY

Anthropometric assessment is probably the most crucial factor in pediatric assessment. Body weight, recumbent length or height, and head circumference (from birth to 36 months) are the most important indices of growth. Weight, length or height, and head circumference are plotted on charts based on age and sex. The Centers for Disease Control and Prevention have recently revised these charts to provide a more up-to-date, ethnically diverse set of standards for comparison.[5] By plotting individual parameters over time, growth curves and velocity can be evaluated.

In general, weight is the most basic parameter for evaluation of nutritional status. Weight is affected more quickly than length or height when under- or overnutrition is present. Length or height may be delayed with persistent inadequate intake of protein or calories. Children are frequently admitted to an intensive care setting with "estimated" weights and no height or head circumference measurement. Parents or caregivers can be helpful with this information. Also, once the patient's clinical status is at least stabilized, measurements can be done at the bedside. Weight may continue to be a difficult measure to evaluate if hydration, fluid status, or edema persists.

23.3.4 MEDICATION HISTORY

Medications should be evaluated for their influence on energy requirements, gastrointestinal function, and nutrient intake. Medications often used in pediatric intensive settings include steroids, neuromuscular blocking agents, antiseizure medications, ionotropic agents, and immunosuppressants. Knowledge of an individual medication's effect on nutrient absorption and utilization is important to ensure adequate delivery of all nutrients to the child.

23.3.5 NUTRIENT INTAKE HISTORY

Finally, an adequate diet history is very important in both nutritional assessment and recommendations in the ICU setting. A typical pediatric ICU will include many children who were previously well-nourished, as well as patients on chronic enteral or parenteral nutrition. Speaking with parents or caregivers will help to set a baseline to support the nutritional therapy that is needed critically. Important points to consider include:

- Has the child been without food or fluid > 3 to 5 days?
- Does the child have food allergies or intolerances?
- Has the child been on home tube feedings or parenteral nutrition, and has this been adequately supporting him or her?
- Is the child on chronic tube feedings?
- Does the child receive adequate vitamin and mineral supplements?
- What is the status of the gastrointestinal tract?

23.4 NUTRITIONAL REQUIREMENTS

23.4.1 ENERGY REQUIREMENTS

The calculation or measurement of energy requirements for critically ill children is probably the most studied factor in pediatric critical care nutritional support. Children's energy requirements are variable and are dependent on age, clinical factors, and phase of illness,[3] including the resumed need for growth and physical activity later in the course of care. Careful appraisal of energy needs is required because of the risks of over- and underfeeding. Overfeeding has been linked to diet-induced thermogenesis and fatty deposition in the liver, as well as to increased carbon dioxide production, which may delay extubation from mechanical ventilation.[6] Conversely, underfeeding may lead to depletion of protein and fat reserves and, eventually, malnutrition. Depletion of skeletal muscle mass may also lead to respiratory compromise, with the loss of diaphragmatic and intercostal muscle mass.

Actual measured energy expenditure (MEE) has been shown to be less than previously assumed.[3] In children, mechanical ventilation decreases both heat loss and the work of breathing. These in turn decrease the energy expenditure for thermoregulation. Sedation has been shown to decrease muscle activity by 10 to 15%.[7] In addition, neuromuscular blockade decreased REE by 10% in a study of 20 children being mechanically ventilated.[8] There may also be a reduction in nonessential or facultative metabolism, which may reduce growth, neurotransmitter synthesis, and catecholamine secretion.[9,10]

Most sources agree that the best measurement of pediatric energy expenditure is indirect calorimetry using a portable metabolic cart.[3,11,12] Serial measurements are especially helpful as children move through the various stages of illness. Errors may be introduced with metabolic cart measurements in patients who experience large ventilatory air leaks or high rates of FIO2 and in small infants and other patients who cannot remain in a steady state during the measurement period. Despite the advantages and precision of indirect calorimetry, MEE in clinical practice is not common. Machines are expensive and require extensive validation. Accurate testing also requires a skilled technician or respiratory therapist to administer the test.

Many predictive equations have been developed to help identify energy expenditure when indirect calorimetry is not available (Table 23.1). These equations include a modified Harris–Benedict, Schofeld, recommended dietary allowances (RDA), WHO, Talbot, and basal metabolic rate

TABLE 23.1
Caloric Guidelines for Pediatric Critical Care

Age (Years)	Recommended Calorie Intake (kcal/kg)
0–1	90–100
1–3	75–90
4–7	70–80
7–10	55–70
11–15	45–55
> 15	35–45

(BMR) with added stress factors.[13–17] Many of these equations may overestimate calorie require-ments, especially in the critically ill. Briassoulis et al. found that in 77 measurements made in 37 children, 50 to 60% had MEE less than 90% of predicted values using the Schofeld equation and 20 to 25% had MEE greater than 110% of the equation.[3] White et al. have also developed an equation using age, weight, and body temperature that has a close correlation to measured values.[11]

Serial measurement of CRP has been suggested as a key to the end of the acute-phase response. PAB levels will decrease in the acute phase, and CRP will increase in a proportional manner to the severity of illness or injury.[18] CRP then will decrease and PAB will rise with an end of this response with adequate nutrition provision.

23.4.2 PROTEIN REQUIREMENTS

The provision of adequate protein to critically ill children may be the single most important nutritional intervention that is made in their care. Adequate levels of protein in nutritional support help to maximize protein synthesis, facilitate wound healing and the inflammatory response, and preserve skeletal muscle protein stores. When comparing the macronutrient metabolic reserves of children vs. adults in terms of percentage of body weight, most often carbohydrate and lipid reserves are similar. However, protein will be present in a far greater amount in adults. As stated previously, a child's limited skeletal muscle mass will provide enough precursors for gluconeogenesis in the short term but is then severely limited in protracted catabolic stress. Nitrogen balance will be negative in two to three days after trauma and will usually level off after the stress response ends. A lack of adequate protein has been associated with respiratory failure, muscle weakness, and sepsis.[19]

Protein requirements will vary with the age of the patient and can be as high as 2 to 2 ½ times the RDA in critical illness or trauma (Table 23.2). Protein retention is also enhanced by the provision of adequate energy. Assurance of adequate protein intake is difficult in children. Nitrogen balance studies are often hard to complete. Insensible losses of nitrogen from stool, skin, and wounds make balances hard to quantify. Protein losses can also be significant with chest tubes and other drains and fistulas that are common in pediatric critical care. It has also been suggested that hospitalized children under metabolic stress be given 1.5 g/kg/d of protein.[20] Acute-phase proteins, such as CRP, and secretory proteins, such as PAB, are commonly used to measure the adequacy of protein intake and energy intake when adequate nutrients are provided. PAB levels usually will increase and CRP levels will decrease as the initial stress of illness subsides and anabolism returns.

23.4.3 FLUID REQUIREMENTS

Fluid requirements for children are routinely estimated using a formula developed in 1957 (Table 23.3).[21] They vary with the age and the weight of the child. Fluid limitations commonly occur in pediatric patients with high intracranial pressure, renal failure, congenital heart disease,

TABLE 23.2
Protein Guidelines for Pediatric Critical Care

Age (Years)	Protein (g/kg)
0–1	2.0–3.5
1–6	2.0–2.5
> 6	1.5–2.0

Source: From Persinger, M., Pediatric nutrition support in critical care, in *Pediatric Manual of Clinical Dietetics*, Nevin-Folino, N.L., Ed., Pediatric Nutrition Practice Group of the American Dietetic Association, 2003, chap. 34. With permission.

TABLE 23.3
Fluid Guidelines for Pediatric Patients

Weight (kg)	Volume (ml/d)
0–10 kg	100 ml/kg
11– 20 kg	1000 ml + 50 ml/kg for each kg > 10 kg
> 20 kg	1500 ml + 20 ml/kg for each kg > 20 kg

and bronchopulmonary dysplasia.[22] Parenteral nutrition and intravenous solutions may need to be concentrated for patients who need to be fluid restricted to provide optimum calories. Enteral nutrition solutions can also be given at higher calorie concentrations if necessary. The osmolarity of these solutions should be monitored carefully to ensure adequate tolerance and to avoid the risk of dehydration. Fever may also increase fluid requirements, with extra losses from respiration and though the skin. It has been suggested that for each degree of temperature above 38°C, insensible water loss is increased by 5 ml/kg over 24 hours.[23]

23.4.4 MICRONUTRIENT REQUIREMENTS

Although absolute micronutrient requirements have not been established for critically ill children, nutritional recommendations should include an intake sufficient for growth. Because vitamins, minerals, and trace minerals are considered essential, it is important to provide at least the minimum estimated requirements to prevent both deficiency and toxicity. The risk of toxicity is probably greater for fat-soluble vitamins (vitamins A, D, E, and K), which have the potential for storage, and for the trace elements. Daily vitamin, mineral, and trace element guidelines for oral and parenteral nutrition have been outlined by the National Advisory Group on Standards and Practice Guidelines for Parenteral Nutrition and the Food and Nutrition Board (Table 23.4 through Table 23.6).[15,24,25] Changes in the supplementation of certain nutrients may be necessary for specific disease states. Copper and manganese should be monitored carefully in children with either cholestasis.[26] Providing half of the daily dose or every-other-day doses of these nutrients may help to avoid deficiency in some patients. Selenium, chromium, and molybdenum are excreted by the kidney and may need to be decreased in renal disease.[27] High ileostomy drainage or persistent diarrhea may indicate a need for extra zinc supplementation.[28]

TABLE 23.4
Daily Vitamin and Mineral Requirements in Children with Normal Organ Function

	Infants/Children		Adolescents	
	Parenteral Dose/day	Oral Dose/day	Parenteral Dose/day	Oral Dose/day
Vitamin				
A (retinol) μg	700	375–700	1000	800–1000
E mg	7	3–7	10	8–10
K μg	200	5–30	2–4 mg/week	45–65
D μg	10	5	5	5
C mg	80	30–45	100	50–60
Thiamin mg	1.2	0.2–0.9	3	0.9–1.3
Riboflavin mg	1.4	0.3–0.9	3.6	0.9–1.3
Pyridoxine mg	1	0.1–1	4	1–1.3
Niacin mg	17	2–12	40	12–16
Pantothenate mg	5	1.7–4	15	4–5
Biotin μg	20	5–20	60	20–25
Folate μg	140	65–300	400	300–400
B_{12}	1	0.4–1.8	5	1.8–2.4
Mineral				
Sodium (mEq)	2–6	5.2–21.7	60–150	21.7
Potassium (mEq)	2–3	12.8–51.3	70–180	51.3
Chloride (mEq)	2–5	5.1–21.2	60–150	21.2
Magnesium (mEq)	0.3–0.5	2.47–19.7	10–30	19.7–33.7
Calcium (mEq)	1–2.5	10.5–65	10–20	65
Phosphorous (mmol)	0.5–1	3.2–40	10–40	40

Sources: From Parenteral: National Advisory Group on Standards and Practice Guidelines for Parenteral Nutrition.[24] Oral: Food and Nutrition Board.[15,25]

TABLE 23.5
Daily Parenteral Trace Element Requirements for Children with Normal Organ Function

Trace Element	Neonates (kg/d)	<5 Years Old (kg/d)	≥5 Years to Adolescents
Zinc	300 μg	100 μg	2–5 mg/d
Copper	20 μg	20 μg	200–500 μg/d
Manganese	1 μg	2–10 μg	50–150 μg/d
Chromium	0.2 μg	0.14–0.2 μg	5–15 μg/d
Selenium	2–3 μg	2–3 μg (max 40 μg/d)	30–40 μg/d

23.5 NUTRITIONAL DELIVERY ROUTES

23.5.1 ENTERAL NUTRITION

Enteral feeding should always be considered initially in pediatric critical care patients.[28] Benefits to enteral feeding include maintenance of mucosal integrity, limitation of bacterial translocation,

TABLE 23.6
Daily Oral Trace Element Requirements for Children with Normal Organ Function

Trace Element	Neonates (kg/d)	≤5 Years Old (kg/d)	≥5 Years to Adolescents
Zinc (mg/d)	5	10	12–15
Copper (µg/d)	400–700	700–2000	1500–2500
Manganese (µg/d)	300–1000	1000–3000	2000–5000
Chromium (µg/d)	10–60	20–200	50–200
Molybdenum (µg/d)	15–40	25–150	75–250
Selenium (µg/d)	10–15	20–30	40–50

decreased septic morbidity, and a blunting of the metabolic response.[29] It has also been shown that enteral feeding can be achieved safely in children within 24 hours of admission, even with mechanical ventilation and neuromuscular blockade.[30]

Selecting an appropriate formula for children in intensive care requires knowledge of the underlying disease state, current medical condition, and the patient's absorptive capacity, fluid allowances, and nutritional requirements.[31] Formulas for children are divided into two categories (Table 23.7):

• Polymeric — Composed of intact nutrients
• Elemental — Composed of nutrients with lower molecular weights

Polymeric formulas may have other characteristics, such as being fiber enriched or lactose free. These formulas are usually easily tolerated by patients with a functional gastrointestinal tract or patients who are not sensitive or allergic to individual nutrients. Elemental formulas are composed of amino acids or short-chain peptides, alone or in combination; medium-chain and long-chain triglycerides to help avoid essential fatty acid deficiency; and glucose polymers as a carbohydrate source. They may be an appropriate choice for those patients who have not tolerated intact nutrient formulas, have severe food or protein allergies, or who have limited intestinal surface area for absorption because of malabsorptive conditions or short gut syndrome.

Infant formulas may also be used for enteral feeding in the critical care unit for infants younger than 12 months. They come in a variety of forms that include cow's milk–based, soy, elemental, and formulas specifically designed for prematurity and follow-up care (Table 23.8). For special circumstances, low-carbohydrate and metabolic formulas are also available. Currently, the large variety of disease-specific formulas that are available for adult patients are not available for pediatric patients. Standard dilution of infant formulas is usually 20 kcal/oz; however, they can be concentrated to 24 to 27 kcal/oz and then further concentrated with modular components in conditions that require fluid restriction. Careful monitoring for signs of dehydration is necessary with concentrated formulas (Table 23.9). Urine output, serum electrolytes, and weight changes should be watched.

Adult formulas may also be used in older children or adolescents when pediatric formula does not meet the patient's specific requirements. Care should be taken with adult formulas to ensure proper vitamin, mineral, and fluid provision to meet a child's requirements.

The use of nasojejunal (NJ) vs. nasogastric (NG) feedings has not been well studied in children. It is generally felt that feeding into the stomach is more physiological and allows for larger boluses or osmotic loads. Feedings can be given as a bolus or provided continuously via the gastric route. Nasogastric feedings are contraindicated with persistent emesis, delayed gastric emptying, neuromotor impairment, or severe gastroesophageal reflux. Nasojejunal feedings are often better tolerated when these conditions exist. Feeding into the small intestine must be done continuously because it has no reservoir capacity and is unable to push along a bolus of feeding. The small intestine is also more sensitive to concentration changes. Nasojejunal feeding tube placement is usually accomplished with fluoroscopy but has also been tried with other methods, such as prokinetic drugs. Nasojejunal feeding may also provide critical care patients with a better overall nutritional intake because of the frequent practice of holding of NG feeds for extubation attempts, tests, and procedures.

In cases in which nutritional goals cannot be met by enteral feedings within 72 hours, parenteral nutrition (PN) should be considered. Trophic enteral feeds should still be tried (< 20% of calorie goals) along with the PN to help maintain gut mucosal integrity.[32]

23.5.2 PARENTERAL NUTRITION

Parenteral nutritional support is used extensively in pediatric critical care when enteral nutrition cannot meet nutritional requirements, is contraindicated, or has failed. Indications include severe ischemic injuries, pancreatitis, severe pulmonary problems, necrotizing enterocolitis, and other types of surgery or trauma to the bowel.

Pediatric PN is usually designed as a nonstandard formula rather than the standardized formulas many hospitals have for their adult patients. Ranges of calories from specific nutrients for metabolic support have been suggested as 20% protein, 20 to 50% fat, and 20 to 60% carbohydrate.[33] Overall energy needs are provided at 10 to 15% below enteral needs based on the lack of digestive or absorptive losses.[34] The glucose infusion rate (GIR) helps to guide the initial percentage of dextrose ordered for a pediatric patient. The usual starting point is 5 to 6 mg/kg/min, with advancement over several days to 14 to 15 mg/kg/min as a maximum intake. Critically ill children may exhibit glucose intolerance at a level of hepatic glucose production, and they usually respond well to a decrease in GIR. Dextrose concentrations > 12.5% must be infused through a central vein. Peripheral infusion should be kept to < 900 mOsm/l to avoid sclerosing of the blood vessel. Ten to 12.5% dextrose peripheral solutions, which are usually well tolerated in younger children, should be used with caution in adolescent patients because of the risk of vein sclerosis.

Protein and lipid requirements are also increased in a stepwise manner, usually starting at 1.0 g/kg/d and advancing as high as 3.5 g/kg/d with protein and 3 to 4 g/kg/d with fat. It is recommended that nonprotein calorie-to-nitrogen ratios for general pediatric patients range from 150:1 to 250:1.[34] This may decrease to as low as 100:1 in critically ill patients, because of the need for greater amounts of protein.[33] The lower limit for lipid provision should be 0.5 g/kg/d to avoid essential fatty acid deficiency. Lipids are also occasionally limited to 1 g/kg/d in cases of poor pulmonary gas exchange, hyperbilirubinemia (> 10 mg/dl), sepsis, and thrombocytopenia.[35,36]

23.6 MONITORING NUTRITION SUPPORT

Regular monitoring of nutritional support is required to ensure an appropriate response to the prescribed enteral or parenteral nutrition program and for early detection of complications.

Monitoring of enteral nutritional support usually centers on gastrointestinal and metabolic complications. Vomiting, aspiration, and diarrhea may be signs of a hyperosmolar formula, a too rapid advancement of feedings, delayed gastric emptying, or, in the worst case, obstruction (see Chapter 19). Metabolic complications can include dehydration, overhydration, and electrolyte imbalances. Abdominal distention, high gastric residuals (except in jejunal feedings), and stool output should be monitored. Often, a decrease in rate or osmolarity of the formula for a short period of time will help overall formula tolerance. Feeding tubes may also be placed in the duodenum or transpylorically to help with formula tolerance. The same symptoms may also signify an intolerance to the nutrient composition of a formula. Adjustments in formula content for the presence of cow's milk protein, lactose medium-chain triglycerides or long-chain triglycerides, and fiber may need to be made to enhance the patient's tolerance.

TABLE 23.7
Pediatric Enteral Formulas

Product	g/100 ml			mg/100 ml					mOsm kg H_2O
	Cho	Pro	Fat	Na	K	Ca	PO_4	Fe	
Polymeric									
Compleat Pediatric (Novartis) (1.0 cal/ml) 4.4 g fiber/l	12.6 cst, veg, fruit	3.8 beef, ca	3.9 sf, s mct (20%)	68	152	100	100	1.3	380
Kindercal Oral (Mead Johnson) (1.0 cal/ml)	13.5 su, ma	3.0 m	4.4 cn, sf, mct, c	37	131	101	85	1.1	440 520 — choc
Kindercal Tube Feeding (Mead Johnson) (1.0 cal/ml)	13.5 ma, su	3.4 m	4.4 cn, sf, mct, c	37	131	101	85	1.1	345
Modulen IBD (Nestlé) (1.03 cal/ml)	10.8 cs, su	3.6 ca	4.6 m, mct, c, s	34	120	89	60	1.1	370
Nutren Junior (Nestlé) (1.0 cal/ml) w/fiber — 6 g/l	11 ma, su	3.0 m, w	5.0 s, mct, cn, s	46	132	100	80	1.4	350
Pediasure Oral (Ross) (1.0 cal/ml) w/fiber — 4.8 g/l	11 su, ma	3.0 ca, w	5.0 sa, s, mct	38	131	97	80	1.4	430 520 — choc 440 — fiber
Pediasure Enteral Formula (Ross) (1.0 cal/ml) w/fiber – 3.2 g/l	13.2 ma, su, d	3.0 m	4.0 sa, s, mct	38	131	97	80	1.4	335 345 — fiber
Resource Just For Kids (Novartis) (1.0 cal/ml) w/fiber – 6 g/l	11.0 cst, su	3.0 ca, w	5.0 sf, s, mct	59	114	114	80	1.4	390 440 — choc

Elemental

Elecare (Ross) (1.0 cal/ml)	10.7 cs	3.0 aa	4.8 sa, mct, s	45	150	108	81	1.8	551
Neocate 1+ (SHS) (1.0 cal/ml) Unflavored	14.6 cs	2.5 aa	3.5 co, cn, sa	20	93	62	62	0.8	610
Neocate Junior (SHS) (1.0 cal/ml) Unflavored	10.4 cs	3.0 aa	5.0 co, cn, sa	41	137	113	94	1.4	607
Pediatric E028 (SHS) (1.0 cal/ml)	14.6 ma, su	2.5 aa	3.5 co, cn, sa	20	93	62	62	0.8	820
Peptamen Junior (Nestlé) (1.0 cal/ml)	13.8 ma, cst	3.0 w	3.9 mct, s, cn, s	46	132	100	80	1.4	260
Pepdite One + (SHS) (1.0 cal/ml)	10.6 cs	3.1 pork, s	5.0 co, cn, sa	41	136	113	94	1.4	430
Vivonex Pediatric (Novartis) (0.8 cal/ml)	13.0 ma, ms	2.4 aa	2.4 mct, s	40	120	97	80	1.0	360

Note: aa: amino acids; c: corn; ca: caseinates; cn: canola; co: coconut; cs: corn syrup solids; cst: cornstarch; d: dextrose; m: milk; ma: maltodextrin; mct: mct oil; ms: modified cornstarch; s: soy; sa: safflower; sf: sunflower; su: sucrose; w: whey.

TABLE 23.8
Infant Enteral Formulas

Product	g/100 ml			mg/100 ml					mOsm kg H₂0
	Cho	Pro	Fat	Na	K	Ca	PO₄	Fe	
Prematurity									
Enfamil Premature 20* (Mead Johnson) (0.67 cal/ml)	7.4 cs, l	2.0 m, w	3.4 mct, s, sf, sa	39	66	110	56	1.2	240
Enfamil Premature 24* (Mead Johnson) (0.8 cal/ml)	8.8 cs, l	2.4 m, w	4.1 mct, s, sf, sa	46	78	132	66	1.4	300
Similac Special Care Advance 20* (Ross) (0.67 cal/ml)	7.1 cs, l	1.8 m, w	3.6 mct, s, co	29	82	121	67	1.2	235
Similac Special Care Advance 24* (Ross) (0.8 cal/ml)	8.5 cs, l	2.2 m, w	4.3 mct, s, co	34	103	144	80	1.4	280
Cow's Milk-Based									
Enfamil LIPIL (Mead Johnson) (0.67 cal/ml)	7.3 l	1.4 m, w	3.6 p, s, co, sf	18	72	52	36	1.2	300
Good Start Supreme (Nestlé) (0.67 cal/ml)	7.6 l, c, ma	1.5 w	3.5 p, s, co, sa	16	68	44	25	1.0	265
Similac Advance (Ross) (0.67 cal/ml)	7.2 l	1.4 m, w	3.6 sa, s, co	16	70	52	28	1.2	300
Soy									
Good Start Essentials Soy (Nestlé) (0.67 cal/ml)	7.4 c, ma, su	1.9 s	3.4 p, s, co, sa	24	78	70	42	1.2	200
Isomil Advance (Ross) (0.67 cal/ml)	6.9 cs, su	1.6 s	3.7 sa, s, co	29	72	70	50	1.2	200
Prosobee (Mead Johnson) (0.67 cal/ml)	7.1 cs	1.7 s	3.6 p, s, co, sf	24	80	70	56	1.2	200

Elemental

Product											
Alimentum Advance (Ross) (0.67 cal/ml)	6.8	su, t	1.8	ca, aa	3.7	sa, mct, s	30	79	70	50	1.2	370
Neocate (SHS) (0.67 cal/ml)	7.8	cs	2.5	aa	3.0	sa, co, s	25	104	83	62	1.2	353
Nutramigen LIPIL (Mead Johnson) (0.67 cal/ml)	6.9	cs, ms	1.9	ch, aa	3.6	p, s, co, sf	32	74	63	42	1.2	320
Pregestimil LIPIL (Mead Johnson) (0.67 cal/ml)	6.8	cs, d, ms	1.9	ch, aa	3.8	mct, s, c, sa	32	74	77	50	1.2	320

Follow-Up

Product											
Good Start 2 Essentials (Nestlé) (0.67 cal/ml) > 4 months of age	8.9	l, cs, c, ma	1.7	m	2.8	p, s, co, sa	26	91	81	54	1.3	326
Good Start 2 Essentials Soy (Nestlé) (0.67 cal/ml) > 4 months of age	8.0	c, ma, su	2.1	s	2.9	p, s, co, sa	25	79	90	60	1.2	200
Similac 2 Advance (Ross) (0.67 cal/ml) Toddlers	7.1	l	1.4	m, w	3.7	sa, s, co	16	70	79	43	1.2	300
Isomil 2 Advance (Ross) (0.67 cal/ml) Toddlers	6.9	cs, su	1.6	s	3.6	sa, co, s	30	72	90	60	1.2	200

Note: aa: amino acids; c: corn; ca: caseinates; ch: casein hydrolysate; cn: canola; co: coconut; cs: corn syrup solids; cst: cornstarch; d: dextrose; l: lactose; m: milk; ma: maltodextrin; mct: mct oil; ms: modified cornstarch; p: palm; s: soy; sa: safflower; sf: sunflower; su: sucrose; t: tapioca; w: whey.

* Also comes in low iron.

TABLE 23.9
Modular Additives

	kcal/g	g/Tbsp	Source	Comments
Carbohydrate				
Cornstarch	3.8	8	Corn	Slow release of carbohydrate
Fructose	4	12	Fructose	Monosaccharide
Polycose, liquid	2 kcal/ml	—	Glusose polymers	50 g Cho/100 ml
Polycose, powder	3.8	6	Glucose polymers	94 g Cho/100 g
Sucrose	4	12	Cane or beet sugar	Disaccharide
Protein				
Casec	3.8	4.4	Caseinate, soy lecithin	1 Tbsp = 4 g protein
ProMod	4.2	4.0	Whey protein, soy lecithin	1 Tbsp = 3 g protein
Fat				
MCT Oil	8.3	14	Coconut oil	Does not contain essential fatty acids
Corn Oil	8.3	14	Corn	
Microlipid	4.5 kcal/ml	—	Safflower oil, soy lecithin	50% fat emulsion, high in linoleic acid

Parenteral nutrition monitoring is usually done to detect metabolic complications. During the early phase of parenteral nutrition, while the patient is adjusting to the nutrient load, laboratory studies may be more frequent. In children, where a rapid or frequent withdrawal of a large volume of blood may be detrimental, studies may need to be done in increments over a period of a few days.

Laboratory monitoring should include baseline glucose levels; electrolytes and blood urea nitrogen; calcium, phosphorus, and magnesium; albumin, prealbumin of C-reactive protein; triglycerides; ALT (SGPT); and direct and indirect bilirubin. Glucose, electrolytes, and BUN should be checked daily to weekly to assess a need for changes in the PN solution. Dextrose levels of PN should be kept in a range to help prevent hyperglycemia. The glucose infusion rate (GIR) is often calculated for the dextrose in PN. In infants and children this rate should be < 14 to 15 mg/kg/min to help prevent overfeeding of carbohydrate and its symptoms: increased carbon dioxide production and hepatic steatosis.[37] The maximum GIR in adolescents may be closer to the normal rates listed for adults. The use of insulin to help manage hyperglycemia in children varies with the institution. However, when insulin is used it is rarely included in the PN solution because of widely varying dose response in children. It is usually given in a separate infusion and then increased or decreased in small increments as needed.

Hypertriglyceridemia is also a common side effect of PN in the critically ill child. Metabolic stress, organ dysfunction, and underlying malnutrition all can influence the ability to metabolize fat. Various recommendations are given in the literature for an acceptable upper limit, from as low as 150 to as high as 400 mg/dl.[38] If levels are high, it is generally recommended to discontinue lipids until serum levels normalize and then restart lipids at 0.5 g/kg/day to prevent essential fatty acid deficiency.

23.7 CONCLUSION

Critical illness in the pediatric population cascades into a sequence of metabolic changes that cause large turnovers of protein, fat, and carbohydrate in patients with very limited tissue reserves and high baseline requirements. Although very little data exist as to the proper amount of nutritional support for sick children, it is apparent that the careful administration of nutrients, particularly protein, can promote anabolism, wound healing, and growth. Patients should be monitored frequently to assess tolerance of nutritional support, especially in the critically ill patient, whose medical status may change rapidly. New studies on neural pathways and the effects of adequate analgesia on metabolic response, growth hormones, and inflammatory mediators such as cytokines may help in avoiding or tempering the response to injury in children.

23.8 CASE STUDY

M.A. is a 6-month-old female. Her medical history is significant for microvillus inclusion disease, PN-related cholestasis, hepatomegaly, and thrombocytopenia. MA has had problems with hypoglycemia. Microvillus inclusion disease is a progressive intestinal disease that is characterized by chronic, severe, watery diarrhea. It generally occurs in infants soon after birth. Signs and symptoms include dehydration, growth restriction, and developmental delay.

On physical examination, M.A. weighed 3.6 kg (< 3rd percentile weight for age), with a length of 53.5 cm (< 3rd percentile length for age). Weight to height measurement plotted at the 25th percentile. These measurements reveal M.A. to be severely growth restricted, with the weight age of a two-week-old and the height age of a one-month-old. Her nutritional history includes PN since birth. She also has been trialed with Pregestimil formula by mouth but has not been able to tolerate more than 15 ml four to five times per day (because of increased stool output). She averages nine stools (300 to 500 ml) per day. Laboratory assessment shows an elevated total bilirubin level of 17.1 mg/dl, an albumin level of 3.0 mg/dl, and an increased PT, PTT, and INR.

23.8.1 QUESTIONS

1. What are M.A.'s protein and calorie requirements?

   Calorie requirements for this patient would be estimated based on the RDAs for the patient's weight age because of her growth restriction. If the patient were receiving PN alone, the calories may be reduced by 10% because of the central infusion of nutrients. Protein intake would also be based on the RDAs for weight age. In a patient such as M.A. who already shows some signs of cholestasis (elevated bilirubin, milk jaundice), the protein may be limited in an effort to improve the liver function.

2. Given the condition of this patient, would you suggest any additions or deletions of vitamins, minerals, or electrolytes from the PN solution?

   With evidence of cholestasis, many centers are eliminating copper and manganese from the PN solution because they are excreted through the biliary system. This should be done cautiously and with occasional serum testing to avoid problems with copper deficiency in patients on chronic PN. Zinc may also be increased in this patient's PN in case of increased zinc loss with excessive stool output. The patient's elevation in PT and PTT may also point to a need for additional vitamin K, which can be given in the PN daily.

3. Should the PN be cycled in this patient?

   Cycling PN in patients with intestinal failure and PN-associated liver disease is a common practice. The theory is to provide a short, daily rest for the liver from the metabolism of parenteral nutrients. In this patient, her young age and history of hypoglycemia may make cycling difficult.

4. Should there be any changes made to the enteral formula the patient has been taking?

   The patient has a fairly high stool output with the small amount of Pregestimil formula she is taking. A change to an amino acid–based formula may help. Also, a fiber supplement such as Benefiber or pectin could be added to improve stool consistency and hopefully decrease stool output.

REFERENCES

1. Pollack, M.M., Wiley, J.S., and Holbrook, P.R., Early nutritional depletion in critically ill children, *Crit. Care Med.*, 9, 580, 1981.
2. Pollack, M.M., Ruttimann, U.E., and Wiley, J.S., Nutritional depletions in critically ill children: associations with physiologic instability and increased quantity of care, *J. Parenter. Enteral Nutr.*, 9, 309, 1985.
3. Briassoulis, G., Venkataraman, S., and Thompson, A.E., Energy expenditure in critically ill children, *Crit. Care Med.*, 28, 1166, 2000.
4. ASPEN Board of Directors and the Clinical Guidelines Task Force, Guidelines for the use of parenteral and enteral nutrition in adult and pediatric patients, *J. Parenter. Enteral Nutr.*, 26 (1 suppl.), 126SA, 2002.
5. Kuczmarski, R.J. et al., *CDC Growth Charts: United States. Advance Data from Vital Health Statistics, No. 314.* National Center for Health Statistics, Hyattsville, MD, 2000.
6. Chwals, W.J., Overfeeding the critically ill child: fact or fantasy?, *New Horiz.*, 2, 147, 1994.
7. Bishop, M.J., Hemodynamic and gas exchange effects of pancuronium bromide in sedated patients with respiratory failure, *Anesthesiology*, 60, 369, 1984.
8. Vernon, D.D. and Witte, M.K., Effect of neuromuscular blockade on oxygen consumption and energy expenditure in sedated, mechanically ventilated children, *Crit. Care Med.*, 28, 1569, 2000.
9. Fahey, J.T. and Lister, G., Response to low cardiac output: developmental differences in metabolism during oxygen deficit and recovery in lambs, *Pediatr. Res.*, 26, 180, 1989.
10. Lister, G., Metabolic response to hypoxia, *Crit. Care Med.*, 21, S340, 1992.
11. White, M.S., Shepard, J.A., and McEniery, J.A., Energy expenditure in 100 ventilated, critically ill children: improving the accuracy of predictive equations, *Crit. Care Med.*, 28, 2307, 2000.
12. Coss-Bu, J.A. et al., Resting energy expenditure in children in a pediatric intensive care unit: comparison of Harris–Benedict and Talbot predictions with indirect calorimetry values, *Am. J. Clin. Nutr.*, 67, 74, 1998.
13. Harris, J.A. and Benedict, F.G., *A Biometric Study of Basal Metabolism in Man*, Carnegie Institute, Washington, DC, 1919.
14. Schofield, W.N., Predicting basal metabolic rate: new standards and review of previous work, *Hum. Nutr. Clin. Nutr.*, 39 (suppl. 1), 5, 1985.
15. Food and Nutrition Board. National Academy of Sciences: National Research Council, *Recommended Dietary Allowances*, 10th ed., National Academy Press, Washington, DC, rev. 1989.
16. World Health Organization, *Energy and Protein Requirements: Report of a Joint FAO/WHO/UNU Expert Consultation, Technical Report Series 724*, World Health Organization, Geneva, 1972.
17. Talbot, F.B., Basal metabolism standards for children, *Am. J. Dis. Child.*, 55, 455, 1938.
18. Chawals, V.J. and Bistrian, B.R., Predicted energy expenditure in critically ill children: problems associated with increased variability (letter), *Crit. Care Med.*, 28, 2655, 2000.
19. Deitch, E., Ma, W.J., and Ma, L., Protein malnutrition predisposes to inflammatory-induced gut-origin septic states, *Ann. Surg.*, 211, 560, 1990.
20. Shew, S.B. and Jaksic, T., The metabolic needs of critically ill children and neonates, *Semin. Pediatr. Surg.*, 8, 131, 1999.
21. Holliday, M.A. and Segar, W.E., The maintenance need for water in parenteral fluid therapy, *Pediatrics*, 19, 823, 1957.
22. Henry, B.W., Pediatric parenteral nutrition support, in *Pediatric Manual of Clinical Dietetics*, Nevin-Folino, N.L., Ed., Pediatric Nutrition Practice Group of the American Dietetic Association, 2003, chap. 32.
23. Ellis, K.J., Shypailo, R.J., and Wong, W.W., Measurement of body water by multi-frequency bioelectrical impedance spectroscopy in a multiethnic pediatric population, *Am. J. Clin. Nutr.*, 70, 847, 1999.
24. National Advisory Group on Standards and Practice Guidelines for Parenteral Nutrition, Safe practices for parenteral feeding formulations, *J. Parenter. Enteral Nutr.*, 22, 49, 1998.
25. Food and Nutrition Board, *Dietary Reference Intake: Recommended Levels for Individual Intake*, Institute of Medicine, National Academy Press, Washington, DC, rev. 1998.
26. Fell, J.M.E. et al., Manganese toxicity in children receiving long-term parenteral nutrition, *Lancet*, 347, 1996.

27. Leung, F.Y., Trace elements in parenteral micronutrition, *Clin. Biochem.*, 28, 561, 1995.
28. DeLucas, C., et al., Transpyloric enteral nutrition reduces the complication rate and cost in the critically ill child, *J. Pediatr. Gastroenteral. Nutr.*, 30, 175, 2000.
29. Fuchs, G.J., Enteral support of the hospitalized child, in *Textbook of Pediatric Nutrition*, Suskind, R.M. and Lewinter-Suskind, L., Eds., Raven Press, New York, 239, 1993.
30. Chellis, M.J., et al., Early enteral feeding in the pediatric intensive care unit, *J. Parenter. Enteral. Nutr.*, 20, 71, 1996.
31. Klawitter, B.M., Pediatric enteral nutritional support, in *Pediatric Manual of Clinical Dietetics*, Nevin-Folino, N.L., Ed., Pediatric Nutrition Practice Group of the American Dietetic Association, 2003, chap. 31.
32. Meetze, W.H., et al., Gastrointestinal priming prior to full enteral nutrition in very low birth weight infants, *J. Pediatr. Gastroenterol. Nutr.*,15, 163, 1992.
33. Dimand, R.J., Parenteral nutrition in the critically ill infant and child, in *Pediatric Parenteral Nutrition*, Baker, R.D., Baker, S.S., and Davis, A., Eds., Chapman & Hall, New York, 1997, chap. 17.
34. Wesley, J.R. and Coran, A.G., Intravenous nutrition for the pediatric patient, *Semin. Pediatr. Surg.*, 1, 212, 1992.
35. Mitton, S.G., Amino acid and lipid in total parenteral nutrition for the newborn, *J. Pediatr. Gastroenterol. Nutr.*, 18, 25, 1993.
36. Friedman, S., et al., Rapid onset of essential fatty acid deficiency in the newborn, *Pediatrics*, 58, 640, 1976.
37. Cox, J.H. and Metbardis, I.M. Parenteral nutrition, in *Handbook of Pediatric Nutrition*, 2nd ed., Samour, P.Q., Hehn, K.K., and Lang, C.E., Eds., Aspen Publishers, Gaithersburg, MD, 1999, chap. 25.
38. Koretz, R.L., Lipman, T.O., and Klein, S., AGA technical review on parenteral nutrition, *Gastroenterology*, 4, 970, 2001.

24 Geriatrics

Alice E. Buchanan, Marie-Andrée Roy, and Gordon L. Jensen
Vanderbilt Center for Human Nutrition

CONTENTS

24.1 INTRODUCTION

It has been widely reported that the American population is getting older.[1] The proportion of older persons admitted to an intensive care unit (ICU) is estimated to be between 25 and 50% and is likely to grow as a result of the increasing age of the U.S. population.[2–4] Among hospitalized patients, the elderly constitute a majority of nutrition support users, and it is therefore essential to address their specific needs. However, there is a paucity of quality research concerning optimal nutrition support of critically ill older persons. Many of the current standards of care have been extrapolated from younger and middle-aged adults.

Unlike younger or middle-aged adults, the elderly are more likely to manifest chronic health conditions, such as diabetes, coronary heart disease (CHD), and cancer, prior to their admission to the ICU. In addition, older patients are at greater risk for presenting with nutritional deficiencies as a result of body composition, physiology, and lifestyle changes that occur with aging. Among many factors, social isolation, oral health problems, functional limitations, depression, and altered mental status can negatively impact the quantity and quality of dietary intakes. Polypharmacy may also exacerbate nutritional problems by interfering with nutrient intake or absorption.

Increasing age has been associated with a decline in muscle mass called sarcopenia.[5–7] This loss of muscle can adversely impact critical care outcomes secondary to decreased metabolic reserve for response to injury and inflammation. Older age is also associated with an increase in total body fat mass and deposition of intra-abdominal fat (visceral fat). Obesity is growing in prevalence among the U.S. older population. The NHANES 1999–2000 survey found that 38.1% of males and

42.5% of females between the ages of 60 and 69 were obese. The corresponding figures were 28.9% of males and 31.9% of females between the ages of 70 and 79 years. At 80 years or greater, the prevalence of obesity fell off precipitously.[8,9] Excess weight and obesity are associated with medical comorbidities such as hypertension, diabetes mellitus, dyslipidemia, and coronary artery disease in old age.[10]

Undernutrition syndromes, such as wasting, cachexia, failure to thrive, and protein energy undernutrition, are routinely observed among hospital older patients. The proportion of hospitalized older persons found to be undernourished may be over one-third or greater of all hospital admissions and may be even higher in a critical care setting.[11–13] Among these patients, undernutrition has been associated with an increased risk of adverse outcomes, such as poor wound healing, increased pressure ulcers, higher rate of infections, and longer length of hospital stay and recovery period.[14–17] Furthermore, nutritional status is likely to deteriorate as the catabolic response associated with critical illness takes place. It has been suggested that negative energy balance in critically ill patients puts these patients at particularly high risk for undernutrition.[18]

24.2 NUTRITION ASSESSMENT

It is important to undertake a comprehensive nutritional assessment of critically ill elderly patients to detect any suspected undernutrition syndrome or obesity. Based on this assessment, appropriate interventions and monitoring must be initiated to maintain optimal nutrition status throughout the hospital stay. Nutrition status at time of discharge is a strong predictor of early nonelective hospital readmission.[19,20]

24.2.1 ANTHROPOMETRIC MEASURES

Anthropometric measurements are fundamental components of nutrition assessment. They include weight history, weight, height, body mass index (BMI), skinfolds, and circumferences.

Although difficult to obtain from critically ill patients, weight history provides useful information regarding a patient's nutritional status. Caregivers, family members, and medical records can be helpful resources. Any weight loss of more than 5% of usual body weight in the last month or 10% in the past 6 months is prognostic of adverse clinical outcomes.[21,22] Weight should be closely monitored throughout the hospital stay, using bed scales for bed-bound patients if necessary. Note that fluid shifts and fluid retention can often mask lean body mass changes.

Height is useful for the calculation of anthropometric indices, such as BMI. For bed-bound patients, height can be estimated by doubling the arm span measurement (from the patient's sternal notch to the end of the longest finger) or by using knee height (measured with a caliper device) in the following formulas:[23]

Men:

$$\text{Stature (cm)} = [2.02 \times \text{knee height (cm)}] - (0.04 \times \text{age}) + 64.19$$

Women:

$$\text{Stature (cm)} = [1.83 \times \text{knee height (cm)}] - (0.24 \times \text{age}) + 84.88$$

In older persons, including the seriously ill elderly, BMI values under the 15th percentile (using cutoff points in the NHANES follow-up studies) have been associated with a higher risk of mortality.[24,25] According to the latest National Institute of Health (NIH) guidelines on body size, a BMI (defined as weight [kg]/height [m^2]) under 18.5 places the patient at high risk for being undernourished.[26]

Reduced skinfold thickness and midarm circumference have been associated with risk of adverse outcomes in hospitalized elderly patients.[14,16] Changes in body composition, skin elasticity, and muscle tone that occur with aging limit the reliability of these measurements, and only trained clinicians should consider their use. Monitoring changes over time, using each patient as his or her own control, is the optimal way of using these measurements. A detailed description of procedures for anthropometric measurements can be found in the NHANES III Anthropometric Procedures video.[27]

24.2.2 LABORATORY DATA

Laboratory data are generally evaluated as part of routine nutritional assessment. In the critically ill elderly, laboratories can be affected by many factors unrelated to nutrition and should be interpreted with caution. They should also be used in combination with clinical judgment and with other indicators of nutritional status.

Serum albumin levels are generally well preserved among healthy older persons. Hypoalbuminemia is particularly useful as an indicator of risk of adverse outcomes among hospitalized patients. It has been linked with an increased length of hospital stay, complications, readmissions, and mortality.[11,19,28] In the critical care setting, the prognostic value associated with hypoalbuminemia is related to cytokine-mediated response to injury, disease, and inflammatory conditions.[14,29–31] Serum albumin levels less than 35 g/l are often seen in the critically ill elderly and are associated with adverse outcomes.[29,32] Transthyretin (prealbumin) may be a better indicator of short-term visceral protein status than albumin but otherwise suffers many of the same limitations as an indicator of nutritional status.[14,33] Prealbumin is highly sensitive to changes in dietary intakes and disease activity. It would therefore be a better indicator for nutrient intake adequacy during the recovery phase of an acute illness.[14]

Hypocholesterolemia (< 160 mg/dl) is often observed among undernourished older persons presenting with serious underlying disease.[34,35] It is a nonspecific indicator of poor health status that has been associated with increased complications and mortality. In many clinical settings, such as in the ICU, low cholesterol levels are independent of dietary intakes and nutritional deprivation.[14,36] Most likely, they result from ongoing cytokine-mediated inflammatory response, particularly interleukin-6 (IL6).[37]

Undernutrition is also associated with a decline in many cell-mediated immune functions, including such indicators as total lymphocyte counts, helper/suppressor T-cell ratios, and skin test anergy. In the critically ill elderly, impaired immune response is, however, a nonspecific marker for undernutrition and is more likely to reflect a variety of other conditions, such as response to injury, underlying disease, and polypharmacy.[38–42]

24.2.3 NUTRITION SCREENING TOOLS

There are no established gold standard measures to assess nutritional status of older individuals. Over the past decade, researchers have attempted to develop multi-item nutrition risk–screening tools, particularly for application to geriatric populations.[43,44] However, for many of these tools, it is unknown whether they have appropriate specificity and sensitivity to identify undernourished persons correctly. This is particularly true in the critical care setting.[43,45] It also remains to be clarified whether people identified at high nutritional risk can be treated with interventions that result in more favorable outcomes.[45]

Table 24.1 summarizes nutrition screening tools and prediction equations that are commonly used in the hospital geriatric population.

TABLE 24.1
Nutrition Screening Tools

Tools	Purpose, Administration, and Description of Tool	Reference Measure and Validation Data

MNA-SF[a,70]	Assessment of nutritional status
	Trained clinician administered
	   Six items, including appetite, weight loss, mobility, psychological and neuropsychological status, dementia, BMI
		Standard MNA score[71]
		  Sensitivity: 97.9%
		  Specificity: 100%
		  PPV: 98.7%

MNA[b,72,73]	Assessment of nutritional status
	Trained clinician administered
	   18 items, including anthropometric and dietary assessment, weight loss, living environment, medication use, clinical global assessment, self-perception of health, and nutritional status
		Clinical status, dietary intakes, laboratory data[74–76]
		  Sensitivity: 96%
		  Specificity: 98%
		  Internal consistency ≥ 0.74
		  Intraclass correlation coefficient ≥ 0.89

NSI[c] — Level I Screen[77]	Assess for further evaluation and intervention Trained clinician administered 31 items, including measures of height and weight, weight change, dietary habits, functional status, and living environment	No data

NSI[c] — Level II Screen[77]	Collect diagnostic information for evaluation and intervention
	Trained clinician administered
	   46 items, including all items from level 1 plus additional biochemical and anthropometric measures, provision for more detailed evaluation of depression and mental status
		Hospital admissions[78]
		Eating problems and polypharmacy items
		  Sensitivity: 58%
		  Specificity: 56.3%
		  PPV: 17.9%
		Functional limitations[79]
		  Items found to be significant predictors of functional limitations: Age ≥ 75 y, use of ≥ 3 medications, albumin concentration < 35.0 g/l, poor appetite, eating problems, income < \$6000/y, eating alone, and depression

SGA[d,80]	Assess nutrition status
	Trained clinician administered
	   11 items, including weight loss, dietary intake, presence of gastrointestinal symptoms, functional capacity, physical assessment, subjective assessment of nutritional status
		Nutrition-related complications[81]
		  Sensitivity: 82%
		  Specificity: 72%

NRI[e,81]	Predict operative complications
	Predictive equation
	2 items:
	   [1.59 (albumin) + 0.417 (current or usual weight)] × 100
		Nutrition status using a combined index[82]
		  Sensitivity: 100%
		  Specificity: 46%
		  PPV: 87%

HPI[f,83]	Predict sepsis and mortality
	Predictive equation
	4 items:
	   0.91 (albumin) − 1.00 (delayed hypersensitivity) − 1.44 (presence or absence of sepsis) + 0.98 (presence or absence of cancer cachexia) − 1.09
		Sepsis and mortality[83]
		  Sensitivity: 74%
		  Specificity: 66%
		  PPV[g]: 72%

(continued)

TABLE 24.1 (CONTINUED)
Nutrition Screening Tools

Tools	Purpose, Administration, and Description of Tool	Reference Measure and Validation Data
PNI[h,84]	Predict operative complications Predictive equation 4 items: 158 – 16.6 (albumin in g/dl) – 0.78 (tricep skinfolds in mm) – 0.20 (transferring in mg/dl) – 5.8 (delayed hypersensitivity skin test)	Mortality[85] Sensitivity: 93% Specificity: 44%
PINI[i,86]	Predict mortality and risk of complication Predictive equation 4 items: (a1-acid glycoprotein) × (C-reactive protein)/(albumin) × (prealbumin)	Hospital mortality RR = 4.34 with PINI score ≥ 25 Chronic institutionalization RR = 2.04 with PINI score ≥ 25

[a] Mini nutritional assessment short form.
[b] Mini nutritional assessment.
[c] Nutrition screening initiative.
[d] Subjective global assessment.
[e] Nutrition risk index.
[f] Hospital prognostic index.
[g] Positive predictive value.
[h] Prognostic nutritional index.
[i] Prognostic inflammatory and nutritional index.

Source: Adapted from Reuben D.B., Greendale G.A., and Harrison G.G., *J. Amer. Ger. Soc.* 1995, 43: 415–425.

24.3 NUTRITIONAL REQUIREMENTS

24.3.1 ENERGY

With aging, there is a decrease in energy needs as a consequence of a decline in lean body mass and physical activity.[46] Energy requirements should be estimated to ensure adequate nutritional support and avoid complications associated with over- or underfeeding. Overfeeding has been linked with severe adverse events, such as difficulties in ventilator weaning, congestive heart failure, and refeeding syndrome.[47,48]

Several ways of estimating resting energy expenditure have been studied. Indirect calorimetry is considered the gold standard but is technically demanding and time consuming, and requires expensive equipment.[49,50] It is also not suitable for use with the high FIO_2 (> 60 mm Hg) requirements of many ventilated, critically ill patients.

The Harris–Benedict equation, which includes age as a variable in the estimation of energy requirements, is often used. Because this equation may underestimate energy needs of highly stressed persons, it should be adjusted to account for additional requirements imposed by critical illness. Using a correction factor between 1.00 and 1.55 is most likely to match true energy requirements of the critically ill elderly and avoid complications associated with overfeeding.[51] Another common approach is to estimate needs at 25 to 35 kcal/kg/d. An adjusted body weight must be used for obese individuals.

Harris–Benedict equation:[52]
In men:

$$BEE \text{ (kcal/d)} = 66.5 + (13.8 \times \text{weight [kg]}) + (5 \times \text{height [cm]}) - (6.8 \times \text{age [y]})$$

In women:

$$BEE \text{ (kcal/d)} = 655.1 + (9.6 \times \text{weight [kg]}) + (1.8 \times \text{height [cm]}) - (4.7 \times \text{age [y]})$$

24.3.2 PROTEIN

According to the latest Dietary Reference Intakes, protein requirements for the elderly would be 0.8 g/kg/d, which is the same as for middle-aged adults.[53] However, although these intakes would be sufficient to meet requirements of healthy elderly, they are likely to be insufficient for patients with acute illness or chronic disease. The hypercatabolic response to serious stress increases requirements to 1.5 g/kg/d among critically ill older persons.[54] Evaluation of muscle catabolism and adequacy of protein replacement can be monitored with urinary nitrogen excretion and determination of nitrogen balance. Note that certain conditions, such as renal or hepatic dysfunction, may require protein restriction.

Nitrogen balance calculation:

$$\text{Nitrogen balance (g/24 h)} = (\text{protein intake [g/24 h]}/6.25) - (\text{urine urea nitrogen [g/24 h]} + 4)$$

24.3.3 MICRONUTRIENT

The recommended dietary allowances (RDA) for micronutrients have been completely revised in the past few years.[53,55–57] The updated values now include life stages 51 to 70 years and 71 years and older and have been regrouped under the name of Dietary Reference Intakes (DRI), which includes 4 subdivisions:

- Recommended dietary allowance (RDA)
- Adequate intake (AI)
- Tolerable upper intake level (UL)
- Estimated average requirement (EAR)

Table 24.2 describes the DRI for older persons.

These reference values have been developed for healthy individuals, and they have yet to be specifically addressed in the critically ill population. Decreased food intakes that occur with aging can result in vulnerable nutritional status before hospitalization. Older persons are particularly at risk for developing nutrient deficiencies in calcium; vitamins D, B12, and B6; folate; and iron. Severe nutritional deficiencies may be even more likely to develop as a result of increased needs associated with critical illness and its treatment.[18] Note that recent trends favoring pharmacologic supplementation of vitamin A, vitamin C, vitamin E, and zinc, for patients with severe traumatic wounds or thermal injuries, should be approached with caution for older, critically ill patients.

24.3.4 FLUID

Dehydration is a common fluid and electrolyte disorder among elderly hospital patients. Aging has been associated with a decline in thirst drive, impaired response to fluid deprivation, and lower urine concentration after water deprivation.[58] Although there is no consensus on fluid requirements in the elderly, dehydration can be prevented with an intake of 30 ml/kg actual body weight/d or

TABLE 24.2
Dietary Reference Intakes (DRIs) for Micronutrients for Older Persons

Nutrient	Male 51–70 years	Male > 70 years	Female 51–70 years	Female > 70 years
Calcium (mg)	1200*	1200*	1200*	1200*
Phosphorus (mg)	700	700	700	700
Magnesium (mg)	420	420	320	320
Vitamin D (μg)	10*	15*	10*	15*
Fluoride (mg)	4*	4*	3*	3*
Thiamin (mg)	1.2	1.2	1.1	1.1
Riboflavin (mg)	1.3	1.3	1.1	1.1
Niacin (mg)	16	16	14	14
Vitamin B_6 (mg)	1.7	1.7	1.5	1.5
Folate (μg)	400	400	400	400
Vitamin B_{12} (μg)	2.4	2.4	2.4	2.4
Pantothenic acid (mg)	5*	5*	5*	5*
Biotin (μg)	30*	30*	30*	30*
Choline (mg)	550*	550*	425*	425*
Vitamin C (mg)	90	90	75	75
α-Tocopherol (mg)	15	15	15	15
Selenium (μg)	55	55	55	55

Note: Recommended dietary allowances (RDA) are presented in ordinary type, and adequate intakes (AI) are followed by an asterisk (*).

Sources: Adapted from *Dietary Reference Intakes for Calcium, Phosphorus, Magnesium, Vitamin D, and Fluoride*, National Academy Press, Washington, DC, 1997; *Dietary Reference Intakes for Thiamin, Riboflavin, Niacin, Vitamin B6, Folate, Vitamin B12, Pantothenic Acid, Biotin, and Choline*, National Academy Press, Washington, DC, 1998; and *Dietary Reference Intakes for Vitamin C, Vitamin E, Selenium, and Carotenoids*, National Academy Press, Washington, DC, 2000.

1 ml/kcal consumed.[59] Fluid needs may be higher when disease and infection are present or with the administration of medication such as diuretics and laxatives.

Fluid intakes should be closely monitored, and patients showing any sign of dehydration — such as rapid weight loss (greater than 3% of body weight), abnormal declines in orthostatic blood pressure, orthostatic pulse increases, decreased urine output, elevated body temperature, constipation, mucosal dryness, or mental confusion — should be treated promptly. The American Medical Association guidelines on the management of dehydration in older adults may be useful in this case.[59] Laboratory parameters (electrolytes, osmolality, creatinine, serum urea nitrogen [SUN], SUN–creatinine ratio, hematocrit, and hemoglobin) can also be used to determine hydration status, although these can be altered by other medical conditions in the elderly.[59] Alternatively, volume overload is common among critically ill older persons with conditions like cardiac, hepatic, or renal failure. In these states, fluid restriction may be indicated.

24.4 NUTRITIONAL INTERVENTION

24.4.1 INITIATING NUTRITIONAL SUPPORT

All elderly persons admitted to the intensive care unit should be considered at high risk for malnutrition, because many of these patients are malnourished upon admission.[60] Table 24.3 describes patients admitted to the ICU who would most likely benefit from early nutrition support.

TABLE 24.3
ICU Patient Who May Require Early Enteral Feeding

Respiratory failure requiring ventilatory support
Cerebrovascular accident, advanced dementia, head trauma
May have swallowing problems related to neurological injury, can be retrained to swallow, should be reevaluated often
Degenerative chronic diseases
Refusal or inability to sustain adequate intake of food
Acute hip fracture
Reduces rehabilitation time in undernourished patients hospitalized with acute hip fracture
Surgery, trauma, or acute disease states
Predicted intake to be inadequate for > 5 days

Sources: Adapted from Sullivan, D.H., Nelson, C.L., Bopp, M.M., Puskarich-May, C.L., and Walls, R.C., *Journal of the American College of Nutrition*, 17, 155, 1998; and Karkeck, J.M., *Nutrition in Clinical Practice*, 8, 211, 1993.

Elderly patients may deteriorate more rapidly due to decreased lean body mass and decreased nutritional reserves.[61] Nutrition support should be considered within two to three days of the onset of acute critical illness in elderly patients who are unable to eat adequately (less than 50% of their estimated needs) to avoid declines that contribute to increased morbidity, mortality, and prolonged hospital stays.[62] Nutritional support results in increased energy and nutrient intakes and may result in improvements in nutritional status and clinical and functional parameters in elderly patients.[63]

24.4.2 NUTRITION SUPPORT GUIDELINES

Total parenteral nutrition (TPN) should only be initiated if the patient's gastrointestinal tract is not functional or cannot be used for an extended period, greater than 7 to 10 days. In general, older patients without organ failure tolerate standard TPN formulations containing conventional amounts of macronutrients, electrolytes, and multivitamins with minerals. Adult-onset diabetes mellitus is common among older persons, so intensive insulin management and reduced dextrose loads should be considered among those with a history of diabetes or evident stress-related hyperglycemia.[64] Similarly, marked volume overload is common among critically ill older persons and should warrant consideration of concentrated TPN formulas.

Enteral nutrition is the preferred method of feeding for older critically ill persons and should be used whenever possible.[65,66] Standard enteral feeding formulations are generally well tolerated. Respiratory failure requiring ventilatory support is a common indication for enteral feeding in the intensive care setting. Patients with cerebrovascular accidents or with degenerative chronic diseases, such as Parkinson's disease or multiple sclerosis, will often require enteral nutritional support. Patients with surgery, trauma, or acute disease states that leave them with anticipated inadequate intakes for more than five days should be evaluated for enteral nutritional support.[32] Elderly patients hospitalized with acute hip fracture may benefit from early nutritional support. Enteral feeding may reduce rehabilitation time in undernourished patients hospitalized with acute hip fracture.[67]

Nasoenteric feeding tubes are undesirable for use longer than 4 to 6 weeks, which is a requirement characteristic of many older critically ill patients.[62] Patients with advanced dementia or otherwise altered mental status are not good candidates for nasoenteric tubes due to the risk of aspiration from self-extubation.[62] Restraints can be used to reduce the risk of self-extubation but are inappropriate for long-term use. Percutaneous endoscopic gastrostomy (PEG), percutaneous endoscopic jejunostomy (PEJ), or surgical gastrostomy or jejunostomy tubes may be the best option for many elderly patients. Patients receiving nutritional support through these types of tubes vs. nasoenteric tubes receive more of their prescribed feeds, suffer fewer treatment failures, and are often discharged earlier from the hospital.[68]

24.5 CONCLUSIONS

Unfortunately there has been only limited investigation of nutrition support for older critically ill persons. Many of the current standards of care have been extrapolated from younger and middle-aged adults. Changes in body composition, physiology, and lifestyle factors that occur with aging place many older persons at nutritional risk. An individualized approach to nutrition screening, assessment, and intervention is recommended. Nutrition support should be considered early in the critical care course, with the level of care guided by advanced directive.

24.6 CASE STUDY*

A 100-year-old woman residing in a nursing home presented with fever, abdominal pain, and vomiting. Her past medical history was remarkable for coronary heart disease with Class II angina pectoris, hypothyroidism, a paratracheal mass, organic brain syndrome, and fecal and urinary incontinence.

In the emergency department, she exhibited generalized marasmus. Her abdomen was distended. Laboratory results were within normal limits, except for an albumin level of 2.8 g/dl (normal range: 4 to 5) and a white blood cell count of $13.2 \times 100/mm^2$ (normal range: 4.5 to 11). Obstruction series radiographs showed dilated loops of small bowel with air–fluid levels consistent with small bowel obstruction.

The patient was deemed a high-risk surgical candidate; therefore, conservative treatment measures were selected. Unfortunately, her condition did not improve. Peripheral intravenous nutrition was initiated on the fifth hospital day. A frank discussion was held with family members regarding risks and benefits, and the patient was taken to the operating room on the ninth hospital day. Exploratory laparotomy revealed a high-grade small bowel obstruction caused by adhesive bands of fibrous tissue. Lysis of adhesions was performed, and no other abnormalities were identified. Peripheral parenteral nutrition was continued in anticipation of return of bowel function. By the fourth postoperative day, anasarca developed and bowel function had not resumed.

The nutrition support service was consulted for further nutritional assessment and intervention. The patient had taken nothing by mouth for about 2 weeks. Her albumin level had decreased to 1.8 g/dl. The anasarca was attributed to the extravasation of fluids into the extracellular compartments due to hypoalbuminemia. TPN was recommended in view of deteriorating nutritional status, volume constraints imposed by fluid overload, and exhaustion of peripheral venous access. Actual body weight was 59 kg and height was 155 cm (corresponding ideal body weight: 58 kg). Preoperative weight was unrecorded but was estimated to be 50 kg. Based on a protein intake of 1.5 g/kg/d and 25 to 30 kcal/kg/d, her nutritional needs were calculated at 87 g protein and 1500 kcal daily.

A central venous catheter was placed, and TPN was cautiously begun. Fluid intake and output, weight, and electrolyte levels were closely monitored. Her bowel function gradually returned to baseline. She remained on TPN for a total of 10 days and then resumed oral intake. Following the 24-day hospitalization, the patient returned to the nursing home in her usual state of health.[69]

REFERENCES

1. U.S. Census Bureau, Vol. 2003, United States Department of Commerce, 2000.
2. Fedullo, A.J. and Swinburne, A.J., *Critical Care Medicine*, 11, 155, 1983.
3. Chelluri, L., Grenvik, A., and Silverman, M., *Archives of Internal Medicine*, 155, 1013, 1995.
4. Dragsted, L. and Qvist, J., *International Journal of Technology Assessment in Health Care*, 8, 395, 1992.

---

* This case study is reproduced with the permission of Talabiska, D.G. and Jensen, G.L., *News Lines*, 4, 1, 1995.

5. Evans, W.J. and Campbell, W.W., *Journal of Nutrition*, 123 (Suppl 2), 465, 1993.
6. Visser, M., Kritchevsky, S.B., Goodpaster, B.H., Newman, A.B., Nevitt, M., Stamm, E., and Harris, T.B., *Journal of the American Geriatrics Society*, 50, 897, 2002.
7. Kamel, H.K., *Nutrition Reviews*, 61, 157, 2003.
8. National Center for Health Statistics, Vol. 2003, U.S. Department of Health and Human Services, Centers for Disease Control and Prevention, 1999.
9. Flegal, K.M., Carroll, M.D., Ogden, C.L., and Johnson, C.L., *Journal of the American Medical Association*, 288, 1723, 2002.
10. Stevens, J., Cai, J., Pamuk, E.R., Williamson, D.F., Thun, M.J., and Wood, J.L., *New England Journal of Medicine*, 338, 1, 1998.
11. Constans, T., Bacq, Y., Brechot, J.F., Guilmot, J.L., Choutet, P., and Lamisse, F., *Journal of the American Geriatrics Society*, 40, 263, 1992.
12. Mowe, M. and Bohmer, T., *Journal of the American Geriatrics Society*, 39, 1089, 1991.
13. Sullivan, D.H., Moriarty, M.S., Chernoff, R., and Lipschitz, D.A., *Journal of Parenteral and Enteral Nutrition*, 13, 249, 1989.
14. Sullivan, D.H., Bopp, M.M., and Robertson, P.K., *Journal of General Internal Medicine*, 17, 923, 2002.
15. Sullivan, D.H., Patch, G.A., Walls, R.C., and Lipschitz, D.A., *American Journal of Clinical Nutrition*, 51, 749, 1990.
16. Potter, J., Klipstein, K., Reilly, J.J., and Roberts, M., *Age and Ageing*, 24, 131, 1995.
17. Naber, T.J., Schermer, T., de Bree, A., Nusteling, K., Eggink, L., J.W., K., Bakkeren, J., van Heereveld, H., and Katan, M.B., *American Journal of Clinical Nutrition*, 66, 1063, 1997.
18. Klipstein-Grobusch, K., Reilly, J.J., Potter, J., Edwards, C.A., and Roberts, M.A., *British Journal of Nutrition*, 73, 323, 1995.
19. Friedmann, J.M., Jensen, G.L., Smiciklas-Wright, H., and McCamish, M.A., *American Journal of Clinical Nutrition*, 65, 1714, 1997.
20. Sullivan, D.H., *Journal of the American Geriatrics Society*, 40, 792, 1992.
21. Stanley, K.E., *Journal of the National Cancer Institute*, 65, 25, 1980.
22. Dewys, W.D., Begg, C., Lavin, P.T., Band, P.R., Bennett, J.M., Bertino, J.R., Cohen, M.H., Douglass, H.O., Jr., Engstrom, P.F., Ezdinli, E.Z., Horton, J., Johnson, G.J., Moertel, C.G., Oken, M.M., Perlia, C., Rosenbaum, C., Silverstein, M.N., Skeel, R.T., Sponzo, R.W., and Tormey, D.C., *American Journal of Medicine*, 69, 491, 1980.
23. Chumlea, W.C., Roche, A.F., and Steinbaugh, M.L., *Journal of the American Geriatrics Society*, 33, 116, 1985.
24. Cornoni-Huntley, J.C., Harris, T.B., Everett, D.F., Albanes, D., Micozzi, M.S., Miles, T.P., and Feldman, J.J., *Journal of Clinical Epidemiology*, 44, 743, 1991.
25. Galanos, A.N., Pieper, C.F., Kussin, P.S., Winchell, M.T., Fulkerson, W.J., Harrel, F.E., Teno, J.M., Layde, P., Connors, A.F., Phillips, R.S., and Wenger, N.S., *Critical Care Medicine*, 25, 1962, 1997.
26. National Institute of Health, Bethesda, MD, 1998.
27. U.S. Department of Health and Human Services, Government Printing Office, 1988.
28. D'Erasmo, E., Pisani, D., Ragno, A., Romagnoli, S., Spagna, G., and Acca, M., *American Journal of the Medical Sciences*, 314, 17, 1997.
29. Doweiko, J.P. and Nompleggi, D.J., *Journal of Parenteral and Enteral Nutrition*, 15, 476, 1991.
30. Rall, C., Roubenoff, R., and Harris, T., in *Nutritional Assessment of Elderly Populations: Measure and Function*, I.H. Rosenberg, Ed., Raven, New York, 1991.
31. Rothschild, M.A., Oratz, M., and Schreiber, S.S., *Hepatology*, 8, 385, 1988.
32. Karkeck, J.M., *Nutrition in Clinical Practice*, 8, 211, 1993.
33. Ingenbleek, Y. and Young, V., *Annual Review of Nutrition*, 14, 495, 1994.
34. Noel, M.A., Smith, T.K., and Ettinger, W.H., *Journal of the American Geriatrics Society*, 39, 455, 1991.
35. Rudman, D. and Feller, A.G., *Journal of the American Geriatrics Society*, 37, 173, 1989.
36. Goichot, B., Schlienger, J.L., Grunenberger, F., Pradignac, A., and Aby, M.A., *American Journal of Clinical Nutrition*, 62, 547, 1995.
37. Ettinger, W.H., Jr., Harris, T., Verdery, R.B., Tracy, R., and Kouba, E., *Journal of the American Geriatrics Society*, 43, 264, 1995.
38. Bistrian, B.R., Blackburn, G.L., Scrimshaw, N.S., and Flatt, J.P., *American Journal of Clinical Nutrition*, 28, 1148, 1975.

39. Law, D.K., Dudrick, S.J., and Abdou, N.I., *Annals of Internal Medicine*, 79, 545, 1973.
40. Seltzer, M.H., Fletcher, H.S., Slocum, B.A., and Engler, P.E., *Journal of Parenteral and Enteral Nutrition*, 5, 70, 1981.
41. Mitchell, C.O. and Lipschitz, D.A., *American Journal of Clinical Nutrition*, 36, 340, 1982.
42. Kaiser, F.E. and Morley, J.E., *Journal of the American Geriatrics Society*, 42, 1291, 1994.
43. Jones, J.M., *Journal of Human Nutrition and Dietetics*, 15, 59, 2002.
44. Reuben, D.B., Greendale, G.A., and Harrison, G.G., *Journal of the American Geriatrics Society*, 43, 415, 1995.
45. Rush, D., *Annual Review of Nutrition*, 17, 101, 1997.
46. Shock, N.W., *Normal Human Aging: The Baltimore Longitudinal Study of Aging*, NIH Publication, Washington, DC, 1994.
47. Weinsier, R.L. and Krumdiek, C.L., *American Journal of Clinical Nutrition*, 34, 393, 1981.
48. Solomon, S.M. and Kirby, D.F., *Journal of Parenteral and Enteral Nutrition*, 14, 90, 1990.
49. Weissman, C., Kemper, M., Askanazi, J., Hyman, A.I., and Kinney, J.M., *Anesthesiology*, 64, 673, 1986.
50. Makk, L.J., McClave, S.A., Creech, P.W., Johnson, D.R., Short, A.F., Whitlow, N.L., Priddy, F.S., Sexton, L.K., and Simpson, P., *Critical Care Medicine*, 18, 1320, 1990.
51. Mann, S., Westenskow, D.R., and Houtchens, B.A., *Critical Care Medicine*, 13, 173, 1985.
52. Harris, J.A. and Benedict, F.G., *A Biometric Study of Basal Metabolism in Man*, Carnegie Institution of Washington, Washington, DC, 1919.
53. Institute of Medicine, *Dietary Reference Intakes for Energy, Carbohydrate, Fiber, Fat, Fatty Acids, Cholesterol, Protein, and Amino Acids*, National Academy Press, Washington, DC, 2002.
54. McMahon, M.M. and Bistrian, B.R., *Disease-a-month*, 36, 373, 1990.
55. Institute of Medicine, *Dietary Reference Intakes for Calcium, Phosphorus, Magnesium, Vitamin D, and Fluoride*, National Academy Press, Washington, DC, 1997.
56. Institute of Medicine, *Dietary Reference Intakes for Thiamin, Riboflavin, Niacin, Vitamin B6, Folate, Vitamin B12, Pantothenic Acid, Biotin, and Choline*, National Academy Press, Washington, DC, 1998.
57. Institute of Medicine, *Dietary Reference Intakes for Vitamin C, Vitamin E, Selenium, and Carotenoids*, National Academy Press, Washington, DC, 2000.
58. Phillips, P.A., Rolls, B.J., Ledingham, J.G., Forsling, M.L., Morton, J.J., Crowe, M.J., and Wollner, L., *New England Journal of Medicine*, 311, 753, 1984.
59. Weinberg, A.D. and Minaker, K.L., *Journal of the American Medical Association*, 274, 1552, 1995.
60. Mowe, M., Bohmer, T., and Kindt, E., *American Journal of Clinical Nutrition*, 59, 317, 1994.
61. Gariballa, S.E., *The Journal of Nutrition, Health, and Aging*, 4, 25, 2000.
62. Lipschitz, D.A., in *Geriatric Medicine*, C.H. Cassel C.K., Larson E.B., Meier D.E., Resnick N.M., Rubenstein L.Z., and Sorenson L.B., Eds., Springer, New York, 801.
63. Volkert, D., Hubsch, S., Oster, P., and Schlierf, G., *Aging Clin Exp Res*, 8, 386, 1996.
64. van den Berghe, G., Wouters, P., Weekers, F., Verwaest, C., Bruyninckx, F., Schetz, M., Vlasselaers, D., Ferdinande, P., Lauwers, P., and Bouillon, R., *New England Journal of Medicine*, 345, 1359, 2001.
65. Anding, R., *Critical Care Nursing Quarterly*, 19, 13, 1996.
66. Opper, F.H. and Burakoff, R., *Critical Illness in the Elderly*, 10, 31, 1994.
67. Sullivan, D.H., Nelson, C.L., Bopp, M.M., Puskarich-May, C.L., and Walls, R.C., *Journal of the American College of Nutrition*, 17, 155, 1998.
68. Norton, B., Homer-Ward, M., Donnelly, M.T., Long, R.G., and Holmes, G.K.T., *BMJ*, 312, 13, 1996.
69. Talabiska, D.G. and Jensen, G.L., *News Lines*, 4, 1, 1995.
70. Rubenstein, L.Z., Harker, J.O., Salva, A., Guigoz, Y., and Vellas, B., *Journals of Gerontology Series A: Biological Sciences and Medical Sciences*, 56, M366, 2001.
71. Cohendy, R., Rubenstein, L.Z., and Eledjam, J.J., *Aging (Milano)*, 13, 293, 2001.
72. Guigoz, Y., Vellas, B., and Garry, P.J., *Nutrition Reviews*, 54 (1 Pt 2), S59, 1996.
73. Vellas, B., Guigoz, Y., Garry, P.J., Nourhashemi, F., Bennahum, D., Lauque, S., and Albarede, J.L., *Nutrition*, 15, 116, 1999.
74. Vellas, B., Lauque, S., Andrieu, S., Nourhashemi, F., Rolland, Y., Baumgartner, R., and Garry, P., *Current Opinion in Clinical Nutrition and Metabolic Care*, 4, 5, 2001.
75. Vellas, B., Guigoz, Y., Baumgartner, M., Garry, P.J., Lauque, S., and Albarede, J.L., *Journal of the American Geriatrics Society*, 48, 1300, 2000.

76. Bleda, M.J., Bolibar, I., Pares, R., and Salva, A., *Journal of Nutrition, Health and Aging*, 6, 134, 2002.

77. Nutrition Screening Initiative, *Nutrition Interventions Manual for Professionals Caring for Older Americans*, Washington, DC, 1992.

78. Jensen, G.L., Friedmann, J.M., Coleman, C.D., and Smiciklas-Wright, H., *American Journal of Clinical Nutrition*, 74, 201, 2001.

79. Jensen, G.L., Kita, K., Fish, J., Heydt, D., and Frey, C., *American Journal of Clinical Nutrition*, 66, 819, 1997.

80. Detsky, A.S., McLaughlin, J.R., Baker, J.P., Johnston, N., Whittaker, S., Mendelson, R.A., and Jeejeebhoy, K.N., *Journal of Parenteral and Enteral Nutrition*, 11, 8, 1987.

81. The Veterans Affairs Total Parenteral Nutrition Cooperative Study Group, *New England Journal of Medicine*, 325, 525, 1991.

82. Pablo, A.M., Izaga, M.A., and Alday, L.A., *European Journal of Clinical Nutrition*, 57, 824, 2003.

83. Harvey, K.B., Moldawer, L.L., Bistrian, B.R., and Blackburn, G.L., *American Journal of Clinical Nutrition*, 34, 2013, 1981.

84. Buzby, G.P., Mullen, J.L., Matthews, D.C., Hobbs, C.L., and Rosato, E.F., *American Journal of Surgery*, 139, 160, 1980.

85. Dempsey, D.T. and Mullen, J.L., *Journal of Parenteral and Enteral Nutrition*, 11 (Suppl 5), 109S, 1987.

86. Ingenbleek, Y. and Carpentier, Y.A., *International Journal for Vitamin and Nutrition Research*, 55, 91, 1985.

Section V

Physiology Stress

25 Trauma

Rosemary A. Kozar
University of Texas — Houston Medical School

Margaret M. McQuiggan
Memorial Hermann Hospital

Frederick A. Moore
University of Texas — Houston Medical School

CONTENTS

25.1 INTRODUCTION

The purpose of this chapter is to briefly review the following:

- Clinical trials supporting early enteral nutrition
- Trials supporting the use of immune-enhancing diets
- An evidence-based enteral nutrition protocol
- Complications and controversies relevant to ICU patients

25.2 ENTERAL ROUTE PREFERRED

Three prospective randomized controlled trials (PRCTs) and one meta-analysis published in the late 1980s and early 1990s had significant impact on clinical practice in trauma ICUs.[1-4] The first PRCT enrolled trauma patients who required an emergency laparatomy and had an abdominal trauma index (ATI > 15).[1] The study group (n = 31) received early (beginning 12 hours postoperatively) total enteral nutrition (TEN), and the control group (n = 32) received delayed total parenteral nutrition (TPN), starting on day 6 if oral intake was inadequate (30% received TPN). Those who received early TEN had better nitrogen balance, higher lymphocyte counts, and fewer major infections.

In a follow-up study, patients having an ATI of 15 to 40 were randomized to receive early TEN (n = 29) or early TPN (n = 30), formulated to be comparable to the enteral diet.[2] Despite a slight advantage in protein–caloric intake with TPN, there was no significant difference in nitrogen balance. In regard to clinical outcome, there was a significant decrease in the incidence of major infections (one [3%] patient in the TEN group vs. six [20%] in the TPN group).

The third study (done by different investigators) confirmed these observations. Patients with an ATI >15 were randomized to receive early TEN (< 24 hrs, n = 51) or early TPN (n = 45) with a comparably formulated TPN solution.[3] Again, it was observed that patients who received early TEN experienced significantly fewer major septic complications than those receiving TPN (TEN = 14% vs. TPN = 38%).

In the same year, a meta-analysis was published that combined data from eight PRCTs (six published, two not published) conducted to assess the nutritional equivalence of TEN compared to TPN in high-risk trauma and/or postoperative patients.[4] The same enteral formula was compared to similar TPN formulations, and septic complications were recorded prospectively by similar definitions. The eight studies' contributing data enrolled 230 patients; 118 were randomized to TEN and 112 to TPN. One or more infections developed in twice as many TPN as TEN patients (TPN = 35% vs. TEN = 16%). When patients with catheter-related sepsis were removed from the analysis, a significant difference in infections between groups remained (TEN = 16% vs. TPN = 35%).

Taken together, the preceding PRCTs provide convincing evidence that TEN is preferred to TPN in patients sustaining major torso trauma.

25.3 ROLE OF IMMUNE-ENHANCING DIETS

The previously described PRCTs documenting improved outcomes with enteral nutrition utilized elemental formulas, a standard of practice in that era. More recent trials suggest that additional benefits can be achieved by utilizing polymeric immune-enhancing diets (IEDs). IEDs include a variety of potential immune-enhancing agents (e.g., arginine, glutamine, fish oil, and nucleotides):

Arginine is a semiessential amino acid that is important for T cell function and wound healing. Endogenous production is insufficient during periods of metabolic stress, and exogenous supplementation is required for maximal function of the immune system. It also is a powerful secretagogue, increasing the production of growth hormone, prolactin, somatostatin, insulin, and glucagon. Additionally, arginine is the chief precursor of nitrous oxide and has been shown to increase protein synthesis and improve wound healing.[5]

Glutamine is acknowledged to be the preferred fuel of the enterocyte and stimulates lymphocyte and monocyte function. The demand for glutamine is increased during stressed states, and supplementation at pharmacologic doses may be required. It also promotes protein synthesis, is a precursor for nucleotides and glutathione, and is thought to play a role in maintaining gut integrity.[6]

Although traditional enteral products contain a high proportion of omega-6 polyunsaturated fatty acid (PUFA), diets with a low omega-6 PUFA and high omega-3 PUFA content more favorably alter the fatty acid composition of membrane phospholipids toward reduced inflammation.[7]

Finally, nucleotides (purines and pyrimidines) are needed for DNA and RNA synthesis and may be necessary in stressed states to maintain rapid cell proliferation and responsiveness.[8] In the setting of increased demand, most tissues can increase intracellular *de novo* synthesis of nucleotides. Lymphocytes, macrophages, and enterocytes, however, rely on increased salvage from the extracellular pool, which may be depleted during stress.

A number of commercially available formulas contain two or more of these agents. Two formulas, Immun-Aid and Impact, have been to shown in clinical studies to improve patient outcome (principally, reduced infections and improved wound healing). The others have not been adequately tested and are dissimilar enough from the tested formulas that no conclusions can be made about their use in trauma patients.

Numerous PRCTs have tested the efficacy and safety of IEDs in a variety of clinical settings, with the majority demonstrating improved patient outcome with the use of IEDs.[9] These data have also been analyzed by meta-analysis and, overall, demonstrate improved patient outcome.[10–12] Five of these studies have been performed specifically in trauma patients.[13–17] The first study, by Brown et al., documented that patients who received IEDs had fewer nosocomial infections (16% vs. 56%) than those randomized to standard enteral diets (SEDs).[13] This study, however, has several methodologic flaws, including:

- Nonspecific entry criteria
- TEN was started late (IED = 3.5 days and SED = 5.0 days)
- Patients who received the IED had more jejunostomy tubes and were fed earlier

The second study, a multicenter study by Moore et al., showed a reduction in intra-abdominal abscesses (IED = 0% vs. SED = 11%) and multiple organ failure (MOF) (IED = 0% vs. SED = 11%) in patients receiving the IED.[14] This study has been criticized because the control group received an elemental diet that had a lower nitrogen content than the IED. This concern was addressed in a follow-up by Kudsk et al., who used the same IED, but the control diet was isonitrogenous and polymeric.[15] The results showed a similar reduction in intra-abdominal abscess (IED = 6% vs. SED = 35%), as well as a decrease in days of therapeutic antibiotic usage and length of hospital stay. The fourth study, by Mendez et al., failed to demonstrate any outcome improvement and suggested that the IED may exacerbate organ failure.[16] This study had several methodologic flaws, including:

- TEN was started late
- There was a 25% dropout rate
- The IED and SED groups were not comparable

The IED patients were a decade younger (IED = 25 vs. SED = 35 years) and, prior to starting TEN, they had a higher incidence of ARDS (IED = 31% vs. SED = 14%). The last study, by

Weimann et al., demonstrated a decrease in the number of days of SIRS and a decrease in MOF.[17] Analysis of these individual studies provides convincing evidence that IEDs provide additional benefits, compared to SEDs, in patients sustaining major torso trauma.

25.4 COMPLICATIONS AND CONTROVERSIES RELEVANT TO ICU PATIENTS

25.4.1 ACUTE RENAL FAILURE

Approximately 1% of trauma patients will have underlying chronic renal insufficiency and, for a variety of reasons, trauma places patients at high risk for acute renal failure. Nutritional support of hypermetabolic trauma patients with renal failure is challenging. Increasingly, these patients are treated with continuous venous–venous hemodialysis (CVVHD). Intermittent hemodialysis is generally reserved for those whose hypermetabolism has resolved and in whom hemodynamic stability has been achieved. Although more labor intensive, CVVHD is better tolerated from a hemodynamic perspective and allows for greater volume, urea, and electrolyte clearance. As a result, standard enteral formulas with high protein loads and normal electrolytes are employed.

The usage of high-volume postfilter dextrose solutions delivers considerable dextrose calories (approaching 300 g daily) and should be considered as part of the total kilocalories.[18] Hyperglycemia often results, so using sterile water as the vehicle should be coordinated with the nephrologist.[19] Standard nutritional assessment parameters are of limited utility in acute renal failure. Measurements of urine urea nitrogen (UUN) become less reliable when creatinine clearance is below 50 ml/min, whereas prealbumin and transferrin can be misleading in the acute stages of renal failure. Additionally, renal failure has variable effects on energy expenditure. Indirect calorimetry, if feasible, is recommended. Kilocalorie level should match needs, and increasing kilocalorie loads are associated with a decreased protein catabolic rate.[20] An estimate of protein catabolic rate can be obtained during intermittent dialysis by urea kinetic modeling. Generally, 30 kcal/kg in normal weight and 25 kcal/kg adjusted weight in obesity and 1.6 to 1.8 g protein/kg in the patient with continuous dialysis are appropriate. Once the patient makes the transition to intermittent hemodialysis, a specialty renal enteral formula is employed, with the addition of a modular protein component.

25.4.2 COMORBID DISEASES

Comorbid conditions may be present in up to 20% of severely injured patients.[21,22] This will influence the patient's specific nutritional goal (Table 25.1). Obesity and morbid obesity are increasingly encountered in the trauma patient and may also increase risk for morbidity and mortality.[23] Trauma patients with a body mass index (BMI) > 31 were found to have an eightfold higher rate of mortality following blunt trauma, frequently due to pulmonary complications.[24] Although controversial, hypocaloric feeding in the obese patient has been suggested to lessen infectious complications secondary to hyperglycemia. Comparable nitrogen balance is achieved in this patient population when hypocaloric feeds are administered.[24] General recommendations are to provide a high-protein (2 g/kg IBW/d) but low-caloric (10 to 20 kcal/kg adjusted weight/d in morbid obesity; 20 to 25 kcal/kg adjusted weight in obesity) diet. Monitoring for clinical evidence of overfeeding (hypercapnea, hyperglycemia, insulin resistance, hypertriglyceridemia, diarrhea, and distention) is used to refine predictions.

25.4.3 REFEEDING SYNDROME

Refeeding syndrome can occur with rapid and excessive feeding of patients with severe malnutrition due to starvation, alcoholism, delayed support, anorexia nervosa, and insufficient intracellular ions.[25]

TABLE 25.1
Comorbid Conditions that Influence Nutritional Support

Comorbid Condition	Global Nutritional Assessment	Action
Elderly	Reduced muscle mass	Early nutrition intervention; weight bearing and resistance activity
	Decreased serum creatinine masks declining renal function	Measure creatinine clearance; reduced electrolyte formulas
	Decline in testosterone in aging males	Assess hormonal status; consider oxandrolone
Obesity	Increased risk of aspiration	Postpyloric feeding
	Increased insulin resistance	Hypocaloric feedings
		Indirect calorimetry
		Insulin protocol
	Increased infectious morbidity	Tight glucose control
	Decreased substrate mobilization in elderly obese	Ensure positive nitrogen balance when hypocaloric regimens are used
Diabetes mellitus type 2	Increased insulin resistance	Indirect calorimetry; insulin protocol
	Increased infectious morbidity	Tight glucose control
		Strict catheter site hygiene
	Gastroparesis	Postpyloric feeding; avoid high-fat intragastric feedings
Liver disease	Urine urea nitrogen, prealbumin, and transferrin are inaccurate indicators of nutritional status	Indirect calorimetry to assess nutritional status
	Chronic severe malnutrition	Anticipate refeeding syndrome
	Hepatic encephalopathy	Limit protein if needed to assess neurologic status or to aid in ventilator weaning

As a result of ion fluxes into the cell with refeeding, serum phosphate, magnesium, potassium, and calcium levels can drop precipitously. Due to blunted basal insulin secretion, severe hyperglycemia may arise. Symptoms include cardiac arrhythmias, confusion, respiratory failure, and even death. This can be prevented by initiating nutritional replacement, whether it is TPN or enteral feeds, at approximately two-thirds of the required goal. Caloric intake can then be gradually increased over the next five to seven days, while anticipating and correcting electrolyte abnormalities. Exogenous insulin may be required.

25.4.4 HYPERGLYCEMIA

Critical illness is accompanied by increased plasma counter regulatory hormone levels that have multiple effects on glucose homeostasis. The end result is hyperglycemia with resistance to insulin, a common entity in critically ill patients. Other factors that contribute to "stress diabetes" include obesity, systemic inflammatory response syndrome, advanced age, exogenous steroids or catecholamines, increased free fatty acids, and nutritional support (TPN > TEN). The resulting hyperglycemia can adversely affect outcome through several mechanisms, including glycosuria and inappropriate diuresis, increased risk of infection (by impairing neutrophil and immunoglobulin function), and exacerbation of cerebral edema. Van den Berghe et al. have recently demonstrated, in a prospective randomized fashion, a reduction in mortality in critically ill surgical patients from 8 to 4.6% when glucose levels were strictly controlled between 80 and 110 mg/dl vs. conventional therapy (120 to 180 mg/dl).[26] In a follow-up analysis, the same investigators demonstrated that the reduction in critical illness polyneuropathy, bacteremia, inflammation, and mortality was related to the lowering of blood glucose levels and not the amount of infused insulin *per se*.[27] These data support the maintenance of normoglycemia.

25.4.5 JEJUNOSTOMY-RELATED COMPLICATIONS

The largest study examining the safety of needle catheter jejunostomies (NCJs) in patients undergoing major elective and emergency abdominal operations documented an incidence of major complications of 1% and minor complications of 1.7%.[28] When feeding jejunostomy–related complications in trauma patients were reviewed by Holmes et al., the overall major complications rate was 4% (9/122).[29] However, the majority of complications (10%) occurred in patients with a standard, open jejunostomy (typically a 14 French catheter), with only a 2% rate with 5 to 7 French needle catheter jejunostomy. In fact, the only difference between patients with and without major complications was the type of feeding access. Major complications included small bowel perforation, volvuli with infarction, intraperitoneal leaks, and nonocclusive small bowel necrosis. The first three of these complications can be minimized by improved technique and the last minimized by more judicious feeding.

25.4.6 NONOCCLUSIVE BOWEL NECROSIS

Failure to recognize and appropriately manage intolerance can lead to a rare but frequently fatal condition known as nonocclusive bowel necrosis (NOBN). Though clinical reports are derived from retrospective case reports, the consistent association of NOBN with enteral nutrition implicates the inappropriate administration of nutrients into a dysfunctional gut. The incidence is less than 1%, with a mortality in excess of 50%.[30] No specific gastrointestinal symptoms associated with this entity were identified, though distention was common and occurred late in the course. Additional symptoms associated with NOBN are abdominal pain and tenderness, vomiting, and high nasogastric output — all frequently encountered indicators of intolerance. No accurate predictors of impending bowel necrosis have been identified.

The precise etiology of NOBN remains unclear. Though a number of hypotheses have been proposed to explain its development, all focus on the role of secondary gut mucosal hypoperfusion. Hypotheses have included an increase in the metabolic demand (imposed by the administration of nutrients to an already metabolically stressed gut) and abdominal distention (from either hyperosmolar formulas or bacterial overgrowth). Signs and symptoms can range from mild abdominal distention, vomiting, or diarrhea to full-thickness necrosis and death if not promptly recognized.

25.4.7 ANABOLIC COMPOUNDS

Trauma and immobilization are associated with a progressive loss of body cell mass that may become extraordinary in prolonged illness, despite aggressive nutrition care. Interest in anticatabolic strategies has included trials of anabolic compounds. The four major classes of anabolic compounds include:

- Recombinant human growth hormone (rhGH)
- Insulinlike growth factor (IGF-1)
- Anabolic steroids
- High-dose insulin

These drugs have been tested most extensively in burn patients. rhGH is the most tested compound and has powerful anabolic effects on most body cells, either directly or by stimulating IGF-1 secretion. Relatively small trials have demonstrated accelerated donor site healing, improved muscle protein synthesis, decreased length of hospital stay, and improved mortality in trauma patients.[31] A recent large, multicenter, European trial employing growth hormone early after cardiac or abdominal surgery, multiple trauma (8% of the subjects), or respiratory failure demonstrated significantly higher morbidity and mortality in the treated group.[32,33] Although there is no explanation for this increased mortality, enthusiasm for using rhGH has been tempered in nonburned ICU patients. In fact, current ASPEN practice guidelines recommend against the routine use of anabolic agents (growth hormone, oxandrolone) in burn patients.[34]

Oxandrolone (Oxandrin) is a synthetic testosterone analog with high anabolic and relatively low androgenic potential. It preserves body cell mass in burn patients, restores muscle mass in AIDS, and accelerates wound healing. Gervasio et al. administered 10 mg twice daily to trauma patients with injury severity scores ≥25, beginning within 5 days of admission and lasting up to 28 days.[35] There was no significant difference in length of hospital stay, ICU length of stay, frequency of pneumonia, sepsis, ARDS, or MOF. No studies are reported evaluating the use of Oxandrin in patients who are no longer in the acute-phase response but demonstrate failure to become anabolic.

25.5 ENTERAL NUTRITION PROTOCOL (DEVELOPED AND UTILIZED AT MEMORIAL HERMAN HOSPITAL TRAUMA ICU)

25.5.1 RATIONALE

Although trauma patients benefit from receiving early TEN, many clinicians lack specific training and experience in administering TEN. Current feeding protocols were empirically developed in centers to perform studies in specific subgroups of high-risk patients. When clinicians apply these protocols to broader groups of patients, not surprisingly, they are less successful. But more disturbingly, there are case reports of nonocclusive bowel necrosis that suggest that caution is warranted when administering early TEN to certain patients. The clinical presentation of this devastating complication is similar to neonatal necrotizing enterocolitis, and its pathogenesis is undoubtedly multifactorial. However, the consistent association with TEN indicates that the inappropriate administration of nutrients into a dysfunctional gut plays a pathogenic role. In order to provide a systematic, evidence-based approach to enteral nutrition and minimize complications, an enteral protocol was devised in 1997.[36] The protocol streamlines the decision-making process related to enteral feeding, accelerates initiation and advancement of feedings, and serves as a multidisciplinary learning tool. It has been successfully exported to other trauma ICUs.

25.5.2 PATIENT SELECTION

Identification of patients who are candidates for nutritional support is based on ASPEN guidelines.[37] Potential candidates are identified within the first day of ICU admission and early enteral nutrition begun in high-risk patients.

25.5.3 POSTPYLORIC FEEDING ACCESS

Clinical experience and experimental evidence demonstrate that gastric motility is attenuated in critically ill patients.[38–40] Studies specifically addressing the optimal site for enteral feedings are limited.[41–44] Based on a review of the literature and clinical experience, early TEN is best delivered into the proximal small intestine. Enteral feeding access should be obtained at the time of initial laparotomy, or subsequent laparotomy if damage control is initially performed. The NCJ is the preferred method of access, and a commercially available kit containing a silastic 7 French catheter is available. Critically injured patients who do not undergo immediate laparotomy should have a nasojejunal (NJ) tube placed, preferably in the first 24 hours after injury. This procedure is first attempted by the bedside nurse who makes one attempt to blindly place a "push" NJ tube (Corpak Medsystems, Wheeling IL). This is successful in approximately half of cases. The remaining patients receive an endoscopically placed NJ by the ICU procedure team in a 10-minute bedside procedure. The technique involves passage of a 8 French nasobiliary drainage catheter (Wilson, Winston-Salem, NC) through the biopsy channel of a flexible endoscope that has been advanced into the duodenum.[45] NJ feeding may be done indefinitely, but if the need for long-term access becomes apparent, the NJ tube can be converted into a jejunal extension tube through a percutaneous endoscopic gastrostomy (PEG-J).

25.5.4 GASTRIC FEEDING

Although we advocate post–ligament of Treitz feeding in high-risk patients, we acknowledge the logistic difficulties of obtaining this access. A gastric feeding protocol is currently being tested in patients in whom the risk of aspiration is low (Figure 25.1).[46] Our focus of clinical research is directed at better understanding and monitoring of gastric emptying, with the goal of safely extending the indications for gastric feeding in our shock trauma ICU. Nasogastric output should be < 500 ml/12 h at the initiation of feeds. Sepsis and hyperglycemia should be well controlled prior to starting gastric feeds, because these factors have been shown to decrease gastric emptying. Maintaining the head of the bed at least 30 degrees is essential for minimizing pulmonary aspiration of stomach contents. Feedings should be held 4 hours prior to undergoing an anesthetic for an operative procedure but may be restarted immediately postoperatively at the previous rate. Feedings are held 4 hours prior to endotracheal extubation. Historically, practices regarding checking gastric residual volumes (GRVs) and cessation of feeds have greatly varied.[47] Because salivary and gastric secretions proximal to the pylorus normally approach 200 cc/h, there is no need to respond to GRV less than 200 cc. Feedings should be discontinued for GRV > 500 cc and postpyloric feeding started.

25.5.5 FORMULA SELECTION

The selection criteria for enteral formulas are depicted in Table 25.2. We use IEDs in patients at high risk for infectious morbidity, but after 10 days switch to a cheaper polymeric high-protein formula. Elemental formulas are reserved for patients with pancreatitis or high risk for intolerance to enteral feeding.

25.5.6 ADMINISTRATION OF FEEDS

Once resuscitation is judged to be complete (generally 24 hours after admission) and enteral access has been obtained, feeding is initiated at 15 cc/h of full-strength formula and advanced by 15 cc/h every 12 hours if no moderate or severe symptoms of intolerance exist, to a set goal of 60cc/h. To assure tolerance, this rate is maintained for 24 hours and then advanced by 15cc/h every 12 hours to a patient-specific targeted goal determined by the ICU dietitian. A registered dietitian assesses the patient within 72 hours of admission. Physical assessment of the patient includes evaluation of body composition, edema, wound healing, nutrient composition of fluid losses through wounds or drains, indirect calorimetry, and review of the lab and medication profile. A height and preadmission weight are obtained, and information on chronic disease, medications, previous dietary restrictions, and drug and tobacco patterns is elicited. Patient-specific nutritional goals are initially based on body weight (see Table 25.3). Actual body weight is used when the patient is ≤120% of ideal body weight and an adjusted body weight for patients > 120%, employing the formula:

$$\text{Adjusted weight} = [(\text{actual weight} - \text{ideal weight}) \times 25\%] + \text{ideal body weight}$$

Initially, protein is provided at 1.5 to 1.75 g/kg actual or adjusted body weight.

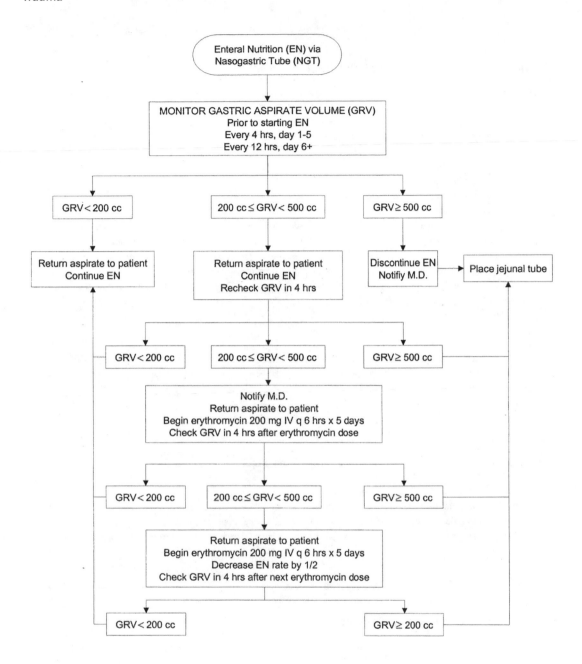

FIGURE 25.1 Gastric feeding protocol.

25.5.7 Monitoring Tolerance and Managing Intolerance

Tolerance parameters are assessed and documented on an enteral tolerance flow sheet by the bedside ICU nurse every 12 hours and are reviewed by the ICU team daily. The decision to advance feeding is based on objective data. Specific criteria to identify and manage intolerance (see Table 25.4) have also been developed and are managed per protocol. Current indicators of intolerance are vomiting, abdominal distention or cramping/tenderness, diarrhea, and high nasogastric tube output. Symptoms are graded as mild, moderate, or severe.

TABLE 25.2
Formula Selection in an Enteral Nutrition Protocol

A. Immune-enhancing diet: These formulas should be used in patients sustaining major torso trauma who are at known risk for major septic complications and MOF:
  1. Combined flail chest/pulmonary contusion anticipated to require prolonged mechanical ventilation
  2. Major abdominal trauma defined by an Abdominal Trauma Index >18
  3. Two or more of the following:
     a. > 6 unit transfusion requirement
     b. Major pelvic fracture
     c. Two or more long bone fractures
  4. Nontrauma patients at risk for major septic morbidity:
     a. Moderately malnourished patients (albumin < 3.5 g/dl) undergoing major elective procedures of the esophagus, stomach, pancreas (with or without duodenum), hepatobiliary tree or abdominal–perineal resection
     b. Severely malnourished patients (albumin < 2.8 g/dl) undergoing colonic or proximal rectal anastamosis
B. Polymeric high-protein formula: These formulas should be used in patients who do not meet the criteria for immune-enhancing diets but have normal digestive and absorptive capacity of the GI tract and are believed to have increased nitrogen requirements due to the presence of:
  1. Major torso trauma
  2. Major head injuries
  3. Major upper GI surgery
  4. Obese patients with moderate caloric but high protein needs
C. Elemental formulas: These should be used in patients who have:
  1. Proven intolerance to the first formula used
  2. Not been fed enterally starting hospital day #7
  3. Pancreatitis
  4. Short gut
  5. High output distal colonic or ileal fistula
  6. Persistent, severe diarrhea > 48 hours while on polymeric formula
  7. Moderate distention > 24 hours and/or girth increase > 2 inches
     Maintain elemental feeding minimum 72 hours
D. Renal failure formula: Renal failure requiring intermittent hemodialysis degree of injury may merit dilution of formula to Ω strength to reduce viscosity and the addition of Promod (protein powder) to meet protein needs

TABLE 25.3
Nutritional Goals in Trauma Patients

Admit Weight	Total kcal/kg	Indirect Calorimetry	Protein (g/kg)
Normal weight 80–120% IBW	30	REE × 1.0	1.75
Obesity > 120% IBW or BMI 30–40	20–25 adjusted weight	REE ×.85	1.75 adjusted weight
Morbid obesity > 200% IBW or BMI ≥ 40	10–20 adjusted weight	REE ×.75	1.75 adjusted weight
Underweight < 80% IBW	40	REE × 1.2	1.75

Note: IBW = ideal body weight; BMI = body mass index; REE = resting body weight.

TABLE 25.4
Grading and Management of Intolerance to Enteral Nutrition

Indicator	Severity	Definition	Treatment
Vomiting	Occurrence	> 1 time/12 h	Place NG suction catheter, check function
			Check existing NG function
			Decrease TF infusion rate by 50%
Abdominal distention,	Mild	Hx and/or PE	Maintain TF infusion rate
			Re-examine in 6 h
cramping or tenderness	Moderate	Hx and/or PE	Stop TF infusion
			Order abdominal x-ray to assess for small bowel obstruction
			Re-examine in 6 h; if moderate distension for > 24 h, switch to elemental formula for 72 h
	Severe	Hx and/or PE	Stop TF infusion
			Hydrate
			Consider CBC, lactate, ABG, Chem7, and CT scan abdomen
Diarrhea	Mild	1–2× per shift or 100–200 cc/12 h	Maintain or increase TF infusion rate per protocol
	Moderate	3–4× per shift or 200–300 cc/12 h	Maintain TF infusion rate
			Re-examine in 6 h
	Severe	> 4× per shift or >300 cc/12 h	Decrease TF infusion rate by 50%
			Give Diphenoxylate/Atropine (Lomotil) 10 cc q 6 h via feeding tube
			Review medications
			Send stool for fecal leukocytes and toxins; if persists >48 h, Δ to elemental feeding
High NG output (for jejunal feeds)	Measured		Verify postpyloric placement of tube
			Check NG aspirate for glucose
			If glucose present and feeding tube postpyloric, hold TF
			Retest NG aspirate for glucose 12 h
Medication contraindications	Inotropic agents		Discontinue feeds
	Paralytics		Discontinue feeds
	Vasopressor		Discontinue feeds

Note: NG = nasogastric; Hx = history; PE = physical exam; TF = tube feeds.

25.5.8 RESULTS OF PROTOCOL

The incidence of enteral tolerance while using the protocol was analyzed in a prospective multi-institutional study.[48] Early tolerance (during advancement of enteral feeds to a goal of 60 cc/h) was good in 84% (41/49) of patients and moderate in 16% (8/49). No patients experienced poor tolerance or complete intolerance. Late tolerance (after standard goal rate met) was good in 80% (39/49), moderate in 16% (8/49), and poor in 4% (2/49) of patients. The site of feeding (gastric vs. jejunal) was not dictated by the protocol. Moderate intolerance was primarily due to high gastric output in patients fed via the stomach. All patients were successfully maintained on early enteral nutrition using this standardized protocol.

25.5.9 MONITORING RESPONSE TO SUPPORT

A weekly 12-hour urine urea nitrogen (UUN) is obtained in all patients with creatinine clearance > 50 ml/min, without cirrhosis or acute spinal cord injury. A UUN is not obtained in patients with

TABLE 25.5
Serum Proteins that Aid in Nutritional Assessment

Protein	Synthetic Site	Clinical Significance	Half-Life	Limitations	Interpretation
Albumin (g/dl)	Liver	Relates to outcomes; relates to edema	20–21 d	Best-case scenario for hepatic production — 12–25gm/24 h; dilutional effects; long half-life; used alone, sensitivity poor	Normal: < 3.5 Mild depletion: 2.8–.5 Moderate: 2.2–2.8 Severe: < 2.2
Prealbumin (mg/dl)	Liver	Indicates nutritional deficits before albumin	2–4 d	Short half-life	Normal: > 18 Mild depletion: 10–18 Moderate: 5–10 Severe: < 5
Transferrin (mg/dl)	Liver	More sensitive than albumin; relatively useful in liver disease compared with albumin; can calculate from TIBC	8–10 d	Poor marker of early repletion; sensitive to changes in body iron	Normal: > 200 Mild depletion: 150–200 Moderate: 100–150 Severe: < 100
C-Reactive protein (mg/dl)	Liver	Increases abruptly after injury; early and reliable indicator of disease injury/severity	48–72 h		Baseline normal: < 3 Bacterial infection: 30–35 Viral infection: < 20 Posttrauma: 20–35

spinal cord injury and paralysis because obligatory losses are generally extraordinary regardless of the level of support and persist for up to seven weeks post injury.[49] One may estimate the protein needed to achieve optimal nitrogen dosage by:

$$[24 \text{ h UUN (g)} + 2 \text{ g N insensible losses} + 5] \times 6.25 = \text{amount of protein (g)}$$

The serum proteins that correlate with nutritional status can be assessed (see Table 25.5). We obtain a C-reactive protein obtained within 72 hours of admission and then weekly, along with serum prealbumin. C-reactive protein is a sensitive acute-phase reactant that increases from a normal level near zero up to 20 to 30 within 48 to 72 hours of injury. It can be used as an indicator of the severity of injury, inflammation, and sepsis. Only when this level begins to decline will the liver begin to synthesize constitutive proteins such as albumin, prealbumin, and transferrin. Once the level falls below 10 to 15 mg/dl, a prompt increase in prealbumin typically occurs. If not, the clinician should reevaluate the adequacy of the support regimen or investigate other factors that may thwart anabolism. Prealbumin is an accessible and inexpensive indicator of anabolic activity. A half-life of 2 to 4 days increases its utility in the critical care setting. Once the acute-phase response has subsided, increases in prealbumin are typically 0.5 to 1.0 mg/dl daily in the patient with adequate support.

Indirect calorimetry is obtained on an as-needed basis and may be performed on the mechanically ventilated patient with an $FiO_2 < 60\%$ and PEEP < 10. Studies are helpful when:

- Overfeeding would be undesirable (as in diabetes, obesity, or COPD)
- Underfeeding would be especially detrimental (renal failure, large wounds)
- Patients have physical or clinical factors that promote energy expenditure deviant from normal

- Drugs are used that may significantly alter energy expenditure (paralytic agents, beta-blockers, corticosteroids)
- Patients do not respond as expected to calculated regimens
- Body habitus makes energy expenditure predictions challenging (morbid obesity, quadriplegia)[49]

REFERENCES

1. Moore, E.E. and Jones, T.N. Benefits of immediate jejunal feeding after major abdominal trauma: a prospective randomized study. *J. Trauma*, 26, 874, 1986.
2. Moore, F.A., Moore, E.E., and Jones, T.N. TEN versus TPN following major abdominal trauma reduced septic morbidity. *J. Trauma*, 29, 916, 1989.
3. Kudsk, K.A., Croce, M.A., Fabian, T.C., et al. Enteral versus parenteral feeding: effects on septic morbidity following blunt and penetrating abdominal trauma. *Ann. Surg.*, 215, 503, 1992.
4. Moore, F.A., Feliciano, D.V., Andrassy, R.J., et al. Early enteral feeding, compared with parenteral, reduces postoperative septic complications: the results of a meta-analysis. *Ann. Surg.*, 216, 62, 1992.
5. Barbul, A., Lazarou, S.A., and Efron, D.T. Arginine enhances wound healing and lymphocyte immune responses in humans. *Surgery*, 108, 331, 1990.
6. Wilmore, D.W. and Shabert, J.K. Role of glutamine in immunologic responses. *Nutrition,* 14, 618, 1998.
7. Alexander, J.W., Saito, H., Ogle, C.K., et al. The importance of lipid type in the diet after burn injury. *Ann. Surg.*, 1986, 204, 1, 1986.
8. Van Buren, C.T., Kulkarni, A., Fanslow, W.C., et al. Dietary nucleotides, a requirement for helper/inducer T lymphocytes. *Transplantation*, 40, 694, 1985.
9. Moore, F.A. Effects of immune-enhancing diets on infectious morbidity and multiple organ failure. *J. Parenter. Enteral Nutr.*, 25, S36, 2001.
10. Heys, S.D., Walker, L.G., Smith, I., and Eremin, O. Enteral nutrition supplementation with key nutrients in patients with critical illness and cancer. *Ann. Surg.*, 229, 467, 1999.
11. Beale, R.J., Bryg, D.J., and Bihari, D.J. Immunonutrition in the critically ill: a systematic review of clinical outcome. *Crit. Care Med.*, 27, 2799, 1999.
12. Heyland, D.K., Novak, F., Drover, J.W., et al. Should immunonutrition become routine in the critically ill patient? *JAMA*, 286, 944, 2001.
13. Brown, R.O., Hunt, H., Mowatt-Larssen, C.A., et al. Comparison of specialized and standard enteral formulas in trauma patients. *Pharmacotherapy*, 14, 314, 1994.
14. Moore, F.A., Moore, E.E., Kudsk, K.A., et al. Clinical benefits of an immune-enhancing diet for early postinjury enteral feeding. *J. Trauma*, 37, 607, 1994.
15. Kudsk, K.A., Minard, G., Croce, M.A., et al. A randomized trial of isonitrogenous diets following severe trauma: an immune-enhancing diet reduces septic complications. *Ann. Surg.*, 1996; 224, 531, 1996.
16. Mendez, C., Jurkovich, G.J., et al. Effects of an immune-enhancing diet in critically injured patients. *J. Trauma*, 42, 933, 1997.
17. Weimann, A., Bastian, L., Bischoff, W.E., et al. Influence of arginine, omega-3 fatty acids and nucleotide-supplemented enteral support on systemic inflammatory response syndrome and multiple organ failure in patients after severe trauma. *Nutrition*, 14, 165, 1998.
18. Cacheco, R., Milham, F.H., and Wedel, S. Management of the trauma patients with preexisting renal disease. *Crit. Care Clin.*, 10, 523, 1994.
19. Frankenfield, D.C., Reynolds, H.N., and Badellino, M.M. Glucose dynamics during continuous hemo-diafiltration and total parenteral nutrition. *Intens. Care Med.*, 21, 1016, 1995.
20. Macias, W.L., Alaka, K.J., and Murphy, M.H. Impact of the nutritional regimen on protein catabolism and nitrogen balance in patients with acute renal failure. *J. Parenter. Enteral Nutr.*, 20, 56, 1996.
21. Sauaia, A., Moore, F.A., Moore, E.E., et al. Multiple organ failure can be predicted as early as 12 hours after injury. *J. Trauma*, 45, 291, 1998.
22. Baulanger, B.R., Milzman, D.P., Rodriguez, A., et al. Obesity. *Crit. Care Clin.*, 10, 613, 1994.
23. Smith-Choban, P., Weireter, L.J., and Maynes, C. Obesity and increased mortality in blunt trauma. *J. Trauma*, 31, 1253, 1991.

24. Smith-Choban, P., Burge, J.C., and Scales, D. Hypoenergetic nutrition support in hospitalized obese patients: a simplified method for clinical application. *Am. J. Clin. Nutr.,* 66, 546, 1997.
25. Crook, M.A., Hally, V., and Pantelli, J.V. The importance of the refeeding syndrome. *Nutrition,* 17 (7–8), 632, 2001.
26. Van den Berghe, G., Wouters, P., Weekers, F., et al. Intensive insulin therapy in critically ill patients. *N. Engl. J. Med.,* 345(19), 1359, 2001.
27. Van den Berghe, G., Wouters, P.J., Boullion, R., et al. Outcome benefit of intensive insulin therapy in the critically ill: insulin dose versus glycemic control. *Crit Care Med.,* 31, 359, 2003.
28. Myers, J.G., Page, C.P., Stewart, R.M., et al. Complications of needle catheter jejunostomy in 2,002 consecutive applications. *Am. J. Surg.,* 170, 551, 1995.
29. Holmes, J.H., Brundage, S.I., Hall, R.A., et al. Complications of surgical feeding jejunostomy in trauma patients. *J. Trauma,* 47, 1009, 1999.
30. Marvin, R.G., McKinley, B., McQuiggan, M., et al. Nonocclusive bowel necrosis occurring in critically ill trauma patients receiving enteral nutrition manifests unreliable signs for early detection. *Am. J. Surg.,* 179, 7, 2000.
31. Peterson, S.R., Holaday, N.J., Jeevanandam, M. Enhancement of protein synthesis efficiency in parenterally fed trauma victims by adjuvant recombinant human growth hormone. *J. Trauma,* 36, 726, 1994.
32. Takala, J., Ruokonen, E., Webster, N.R. Mortality associated with growth hormone treatment in critically ill adults. *N. Engl. J. Med.,* 341, 785, 1999.
33. ASPEN. Guidelines for the use of parenteral and enteral nutrition in adult and pediatric patients. *J. Parenter. Enteral Nutr.,* Supp 26 (1), 88SA, 2002.
34. Gervasio, J.M., Dickerson, R.N., Swearingen, J., et al. Oxandrolone in trauma patients. *Pharmacotherapy,* 20, 1328, 2000.
35. McQuiggan, M.M., Marvin, R.G., McKinley, B.A., et al. Enteral feeding following major torso trauma: from theory to practice. *New Horizons,* 7, 131, 1999.
36. Guidelines for the use of parenteral and enteral nutrition in adult and pediatric patients. *J. Parenter. Enteral Nutr.,* 17 (Suppl), 15A, 2002.
37. Ott, L., Young, B., Phillips, R., et al. Altered gastric emptying in the head-injured patient: relationship to feeding intolerance. *J. Neurosurg.,* 74, 738, 1991.
38. Ritz, M.A., Fraser, R., Edwards, N., et al. Delayed gastric tying in ventilated critically ill patients: measurement by 13C-octanoic acid breath test. *Crit. Care Med.,* 29, 1744, 2001.
39. Tournadre, J.-P., Barclay, M., Fraser, R., et al. Small intestinal motor patterns in critically ill patients after major abdominal surgery. *Am. J. Gastroenterol.,* 96, 2418, 2001.
40. Kortbeek, J.B., Haigh, P.I., and Doig, C. Duodenal versus gastric feeding in ventilated blunt trauma patients: a randomized controlled trial. *J. Trauma,* 37, 581, 1994.
41. Adams, G.F., Guest, D.P., Ciraulo, D.L., et al. Maximizing tolerance of enteral nutrition in severely injured trauma patients: a comparison of enteral feedings by means of percutaneous endoscopic gastrostomy versus percutaneous endoscopic gastrojejunostomy. *J. Trauma,* 48, 459, 2000.
42. Heyland, D.K., Drover, J.W., MacDonald, S., et al. Effect of postpyloric feeding on gastroesophageal regurgitation and pulmonary microaspiration: results of a randomized controlled trial. *Crit. Care Med.,* 29, 1495, 2001.
43. Dunham, C.M., Frankenfield, D., Belzberg, H., et al. Gut failure: predictor of or contributor to mortality in mechanically ventilated blunt trauma patients? *J. Trauma,* 37, 30, 1994.
44. Reed, R.L., Eachempati, S.R., Russell, M.K., et al. Endoscopic placement of jejunal feeding catheters in critically ill patients by a "push" technique. *J. Trauma,* 45, 388, 1998.
45. McClave, S.A., Sexton, L.K., Spain, D.A., et al. Enteral tube feeding in the intensive care unit: factors impeding adequate delivery. *Crit. Care Med.,* 27, 1252, 1999.
46. Mentec, H., Dupont, H., Bocchetti, M., et al. Upper digestive intolerance during enteral nutrition in critically ill patients: Frequency, risk factors, and complications. *Crit. Care Med.,* 19, 1955, 2001.
47. Kozar, R.A., McQuiggan, M.M., Moore, E.E., et al. Postinjury enteral tolerance is reliably achieved by a standardized protocol. *J. Surg. Res.,* 104, 70, 2002.
48. Rodriguez, D.J., Clevenger, F.W., Osler, T.M., et al. Obligatory negative nitrogen balance following spinal cord injury. *J. Parenter. Enteral Nutr.,* 15, 319, 1991.
49. McClave, S.A. and Snider, H.L. Understanding the metabolic response to critical illness: factors that cause patients to deviate from the expected pattern of hypermetabolism. *New Horizons,* 2, 139, 1994.

26 Burns and Wound Healing

Theresa Mayes and Michele M. Gottschlich
Shriners Hospital for Children

CONTENTS

26.1 BURNS AND WOUND HEALING

Wounds originate from a variety of sources. Burns, surgery, infectious disease, trauma, radiation therapy, decubiti, and diabetic or vascular ulcers are only a few of the many causes of tissue destruction. Normal progression of tissue repair requires conditions that maximize vascular sufficiency, aseptic state, immunity, and nutritional balance. This chapter focuses on the metabolic alterations produced by burns and wounds, the nutritional components of tissue repair, methods for assessment of nutritional adequacy, and therapeutic modalities that maximize anabolism and thus the promotion of healing, despite wound etiology.

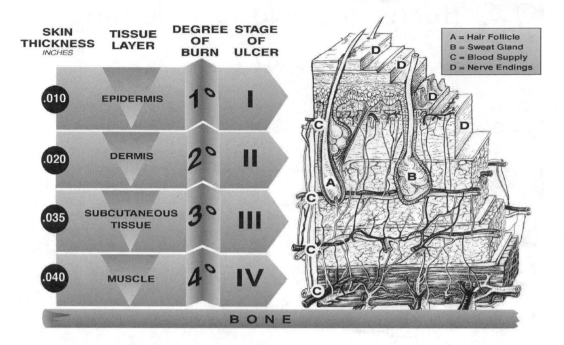

FIGURE 26.1 Interpretation of wound classification based on damage to the integument.

26.2 METABOLIC CONSEQUENCES

Wounds are classified according to size and depth of skin-layer injury (Figure 26.1). Alterations in metabolism positively correlate with the assessment of both of these parameters. Wound specification in this manner allows the clinician to determine the degree of heat, fluid, and nutrient losses, as well as the comorbid risk of infection and mortality.

The classic injury response, as described by Cutherbertson and Tilstone, is most obvious following a burn that covers a large surface area.[1] Table 26.1 describes the dominant factors of the ebb and flow phases and how these responses are characterized clinically. The ebb phase is typically present for 24 to 48 hours postburn but can last up to 5 days. The transition to the flow response is primarily driven by an increase in the catabolic hormones epinephrine and norepinephrine, their metabolites, glucocorticoids, and glucagon. The synergistic effects of these hormones accelerate proteolysis, gluconeogenesis, lipolytic activity, and, most profoundly, energy expenditure.[2] The effects of these hormones on metabolic rate and catabolism are present until the wound achieves closure and the patient enters the adaptive or convalescent state.

The etiology of hypermetabolism is driven not only by hormonal alterations but also by a number of additional contributing factors. Increased evaporative water and heat loss from the burn wound appear to increase the metabolic response.[3] In addition, significant sleep pattern disruption in burn patients has been reported, suggesting that lack of deep sleep in the acute postburn period may contribute to hypermetabolism.[4] Furthermore, early enteral feeding has also been proposed as a means to reduce the postinjury surge in metabolism.[5–7] Finally, cytokines appear to affect metabolic rate indirectly by stimulating the endocrine system to release increased concentrations of the catecholamines, cortisol, and glucagons.[8,9]

Gradual wound closure provides the greatest effect on decreasing metabolic rate. Reduction in wound size serves to decrease catabolic hormone production, enhance sleep, and diminish evaporative heat loss. Prevention of systemic infection and providing adequate pain and anxiety relief are also important factors in lessening the metabolic response.

TABLE 26.1
Metabolic Alterations Produced by Burns

		Flow Response	
	Ebb Response	Acute Phase	Adaptive Phase
Dominant factors	Loss of plasma volume	Increased total body blood flow	Stress hormone response
	Poor tissue perfusion	Elevated catecholamines	subsiding
	Shock	Elevated glucagon	Convalescence
	Low plasma insulin levels	Elevated glucocorticoids	
		Normal or elevated serum insulin	
		High glucagon–insulin ratio	
Metabolic	Decreased oxygen	Catabolism	Anabolism
and clinical	consumption	Hyperglycemia	Normoglycemia
characteristics	Depressed resting energy	Increased respiratory rate	Energy expenditure
	expenditure	Increased oxygen consumption and	diminished
	Decreased blood pressure	hypermetabolism	Bone demineralization
	Cardiac output below normal	Increased carbon dioxide production	Nutrient requirements
	Decreased body temperature	Increased body temperature	approaching preinjury
		Redistribution of polyvalent cations,	needs
		such as zinc and iron	
		Increased urinary excretion of	
		nitrogen, sulfur, magnesium,	
		calcium, phosphorus, potassium,	
		and creatinine	
		Accelerated gluconeogenesis	
		Fat mobilization	
		Increased use of amino acids as	
		oxidative fuels	

Source: Adapted from Gottschlich MM, Alexander JW, and Bower RH, in *Enteral and Tube Feeding*, vol. 1, WB Saunders, Philadelphia, 1990, 307.

26.3 MACRONUTRIENTS

26.3.1 PROTEIN

The role of protein in tissue repair is irrefutable. Adequate protein ensures cell multiplication and collagen and connective tissue formation. Intact protein, particularly of whey source, has been proved superior to free amino acids in maintaining body weight and nitrogen retention.[10–12]

Protein requirements positively correlate with the total body surface area (TBSA) affected and the depth of injury. Patients with burn injuries affecting greater than 25% TBSA benefit from approximately 23% of total calories as protein.[13] Given the hypermetabolic state of the burn patient, this may translate to 3 to 5 g/kg/d. Evidence-based guidelines are lacking for protein provision in patients with less than 25% open area. It is generally prudent, however, to begin protein replacement at slightly above the RDA, at 1.2 to 1.5 g/kg/d for the adult patient that presents with less than 10% TBSA wound (as with small burns, decubitus,[14] amputations, etc.) and upwards of 2 g/kg/d in patients whose wounds affect areas approaching the 20% TBSA marker (as with moderate burns). Increasing protein intake beyond 1.5 g/kg/d for smaller wounds may not increase protein synthesis, particularly in the elderly, and may predispose to dehydration.[15] Despite etiology, size, and depth of the wound, the amount of protein should be modified based on routine evaluation of parameters noted in Section 26.5.

26.3.1.1 Arginine

Arginine has a role in wound healing.[16–19] In addition to tissue repair, arginine augments the immune system through enhanced lymphocyte activity and stimulates the release of anabolic hormones such as insulin, growth hormone, and insulinlike growth factor-1. The recommended dose of arginine replacement is at 2% of overall calories in burns.[20] The application of arginine replacement in other wound types, trauma, and sepsis, is also gaining acceptance.

26.3.1.2 Glutamine

Glutamine enhances proliferation of fibroblasts and macrophages, both of which are integral components of the wound-healing process. Fibroblasts use glutamine as energy to produce collagen. Macrophages require glutamine for their role in growth factor production. Oral glutamine has been shown to improve healing of colonic anastomoses in rats.[21] In addition, Zhou and colleagues report attenuated intestinal permeability and decreased early rise in plasma endotoxin levels, leading to improved wound healing and reduced length of stay.[22]

Glutamine is also the major fuel source for immune cells and enterocytes, providing a protective effect on gut barrier function.[23–25] The optimal amount and form of glutamine required to achieve beneficial results is unknown. Recently Gottschlich and colleagues[24] performed a prospective, randomized, double-blind study examining the clinical effect of adding 14.3 g of glutamine per liter of tube feeding vs. control tube feeding lacking glutamine in pediatric patients with large burns. Four percent of patients in the control group experienced bowel necrosis, and an additional 4% required laparotomy, whereas no patient in the treated group experienced such morbid outcome. In addition, the treated group had significantly fewer positive blood cultures for Gram-negative bacteria. Trends toward reduced incidence of diarrhea, provision of exogenous albumin and insulin, and use of parenteral nutrition were associated with glutamine supplementation. The authors concluded that the decreased morbidity associated with glutamine enrichment may be the result of improved gut integrity, hemodynamic stability, or immune function. Glutamine supplementation is safe for patients (except those with hyperammonemia or hepatic or renal failure) and may be worth trialing as an adjunctive intervention, especially in patients with large, nonhealing wounds.

26.3.2 Carbohydrate and Fat

Energy demands also positively correlate with the size and depth of the wound. Energy in sufficient quantity to spare the increased protein requirement of wound healing is essential. The appropriate source of energy, either carbohydrate or fat, to be provided in the greatest quantity has been debated. Glucose is utilized efficiently as an energy source in tissue repair, and fat is a necessary component of cell membranes. A deficiency of essential fatty acids suppresses tissue repair. However, there is evidence that low-fat, high-carbohydrate provision enhances wound healing, suggesting that carbohydrate may be the preferred energy fuel.[26,27]

Lipid is an essential component of wound healing, because it comprises cell membranes and acts as a carrier of the fat-soluble vitamins. Delayed wound healing has been shown in fatty acid deficiency.[28] Although the clinician may be attracted to fat as a concentrated means of supplying calories to the hypermetabolic patient, large amounts of fat have proved detrimental in wound recovery. A number of studies correlate high fat intake with a poor immune response.[26,27,29] In addition, fat does not stimulate insulin production or assist with protein sparing. Mochizuki and colleagues recommend a diet containing 5 to 15% of nonprotein calories as fat in order to assist optimally in the recovery from burn injury.[27]

In addition to the amount of fat, the type of fat provided to support wound healing is an essential component of the nutrition care plan.[30] Arachidonic acid is formed from linoleic acid and further metabolizes to the 1 and 2 series of prostaglandins, thromboxane, prostacyclin, and leukotrienes. These metabolites are associated with immunosuppression, inflammation, and proteolysis, thus with impairment of the healing process. For these reasons, the diet of the patient with an open wound should be limited in linoleic acid, the precursor of arachidonic acid.

Eicosapentanoic acid, a derivative of alpha-linolenic acid, and docosahexanoic acid are precursors of the triene prostaglandins and series 5 leukotrienes. These metabolites are known to have anti-inflammatory, immune-enhancing properties and, furthermore, to prevent the linoleic to PGE1 and PGE2 cascade. The clinical contribution of Gottschlich and colleagues supports the laboratory work of Alexander and associates, deducing that an enteral diet that is low in fat and linoleic acid and supplemented with omega-3 fatty acids improves the immune response significantly, decreasing morbidity, wound infection, and length of stay.[26,30]

Choosing the appropriate enteral formula for the patient with large body surface area burns from the myriad products available on the market takes a bit of scrutiny. For practical purposes, the formula should provide 20 to 25% of calories as protein, be low in linoleic acid, contain omega-3 fatty acids, (if not marketed as such, evaluate the linolenic acid content), and have fairly low fat content (as low as 12 to 15% of calories, although most products are in the 20 to 30% range). Patients with wounds of any etiology covering less than 10% body surface area do not usually undergo a huge inflammatory response (unless other trauma is invoked, e.g., smoke inhalation, fracture, blunt trauma), thus the primary nutrition objective is provision of sufficient calories, protein, and micronutrients.

26.4 MICRONUTRIENTS

Most micronutrients function as coenzymes and cofactors that permit protein and calories to be utilized more efficiently. The role of various micronutrients in wound healing is outlined in Table 26.2. Inadequate intake, increased loss via wound exudate, malabsorption, and heightened metabolism affect micronutrient status postinjury. Experience suggests that, for some nutrients, intake beyond that found in a standard multivitamin–mineral provision is beneficial to wound healing. For this reason, vitamins A and C and zinc are most commonly supplemented in burns, according to the standards listed in Table 26.3.

Clinical reports of prolonged hypocalcemia, hypomagnesemia, and hypophosphatemia following burn injury are prevalent in the literature.[32–42] Recently, depressed vitamin D status has been confirmed in the postburn state as well.[43–46] Reduced stores of these nutrients may partially account for reports of decreased bone density, increased fracture risk, and pediatric growth delay in the burns.[44,47–53]

In other, less catabolic wound types, supplementation of micronutrients in patients without clinical symptoms of deficiency is contended. Supplementation of zinc, for example, should consider the interaction between zinc and copper.[54] Caution toward supplementation is prudent because data supports reduced copper status in patients receiving zinc for an extended period of time. Copper is also important for wound homeostasis; therefore, decisions to supplement should be made only after a thorough review of intake from all sources (oral, enteral, and parenteral), confounding medical condition (e.g., malabsorptive diseases, preexisting malnutrition, medications), nutrient–nutrient interaction, and clinical manifestations of deficiency have been assessed. Routine multivitamin–mineral supplementation is suggested for identified high-risk patients or patients with low serum nutrient value.[55] Patients receiving corticosteroids should be considered for vitamin A supplementation because evidence suggests a protective effect against the negative consequences of such medication on wound healing.[56,57]

26.5 NUTRITIONAL ASSESSMENT

The process of nutritional assessment should include physical assessment of the condition of the skin. Changes in skin condition of the at-risk, long-term care resident, surgical patient, and burn

TABLE 26.2
Micronutrient Summary Pertinent to Wound Healing

Micronutrient	Function in Wound Healing	Food Sources	Deficiency Symptoms	Test to Determine Deficiency State[31]
Vitamin A	Enhances tissue regeneration by aiding in glycoprotein synthesis; cofactor for collagen synthesis and crosslinkage	Liver, fish liver oils, enriched dairy products, egg yolk, carrots, sweet potato, squash, apricots, peaches, and dark green leafy vegetables	Xerophthalmia (night blindness, conjunctival xerosis, Bitot's spots), respiratory ailments (pneumonia, bronchopulmonary dysplasia), affects epithelial tissues of the gut	Serum vitamin A
Thiamin (B_1)	Cofactor in collagen crosslinking	Brewer's yeast, unrefined cereal grains, organ meats, pork, legumes, nuts, seeds	Beriberi, anorexia, fatigue, peripheral neuropathy, foot and wrist drop, cardiomegaly, hyperlactatemia	Serum or 24-hour urinary thiamin
Riboflavin (B_2)	Cofactor in collagen crosslinking	Broccoli, spinach, asparagus, turnip greens, meat, poultry, fish, yeast, egg whites, dairy products, milk, fortified grain products	Cheilosis, angular stomatitis, glossitis, scrotal dermatitis, cessation of growth, photophobia	Serum erythrocyte glutathione reductase
Pyridoxine (B_6)	Coenzyme that activates protein synthesis	Chicken, fish, kidney, liver, pork, bananas, eggs, soy beans, oats, whole wheat products, peanuts, walnuts	Irritability, depression, stomatitis, glossitis, cheilosis, seborrhea of the nasal labial folds, normochromic, microcytic or sideroblastic anemia	Serum erythrocytic glutamic–oxalo acetic transaminase (EGOT) and serum erythrocytic glutamic–pyruvic transaminase (EGPT)
Cobalamin (B_{12})	Coenzyme for protein and DNA synthesis	Meat and meat products, fish, shellfish, poultry, eggs	Megaloblastic anemia, loss of appetite, weight loss, fatigue, glossitis, leukopenia, thrombocytopenia, achlorhydria	Serum cobalamin
Vitamin C	Necessary for hydroxylation of lysine and proline in collagen formation as well as crosslinking; protects tissue from superoxide damage; enhances tissue regeneration	Citrus fruits, green vegetables, potatoes	Fatigue; anorexia; muscular pain; scurvy (characterized by anemia, hemorrhagic disorders, weakening of collagenous structures in bone cartilage, teeth, and connective tissue; degeneration of muscle; gingivitis; capillary weakness; and rheumatic leg pain)	Serum vitamin C

Nutrient	Function	Food Sources	Signs of Deficiency	Laboratory Assessment
Vitamin D	Regulates the synthesis of several structural proteins, including collagen type I	Fortified dairy products, eggs, butter, fortified margarine	Bone demineralization	Serum 25 (OH) vitamin D
Vitamin E	Antioxidant properties promote cell membrane integrity	Wheat germ, rice germ, vegetable oil, dark green leafy vegetables, nuts, legumes	Increased platelet aggregation, decreased red blood cell survival, hemolytic anemia, neurologic abnormalities, decreased serum creatinine levels, excessive creatinuria	Serum vitamin E
Vitamin K	Essential for coagulation, which is a prerequisite for wound healing	Green leafy vegetables, dairy products, meat, eggs, cereals, fruits	Hemorrhage	Plasma vitamin K, prothrombin time
Magnesium	Cofactor for enzymes involved in protein and collagen synthesis	Nuts, legumes, unmilled grains, green vegetables, bananas	Nausea, muscle weakness, irritability, mental derangement	Serum magnesium
Calcium	Both the remodeling process and the degradation of collagen are accomplished through the action of various collagenases, all of which require calcium	Dairy products, sardines, oysters, kale, greens, tofu	Osteoporosis	Serum calcium
Copper	Promotes the crosslinking reactions of collagen and elastin synthesis; scavenges free radicals	Whole grain breads and cereals, shellfish (especially oysters), organ meats, poultry, dried peas and beans, dark green leafy vegetables	Skeletal demineralization, impaired glucose tolerance, anemia, neutropenia, leukopenia, changes in hair and skin pigmentation	Serum copper or ceruloplasmin
Iron	Necessary for hydroxylation of lysine and proline in collagen synthesis, as well as transportation of oxygen to the wound bed	Egg yolk, red meats, dark green leafy vegetables, enriched breads and cereals, legumes, dried fruits	Anemia, cheilosis, glossitis, atrophy of the tongue, hair loss, brittle fingernails, koilonychia, pallor, tissue hypoxia, exertional dyspnea, heart enlargement	Serum ferritin, hemoglobin, hematocrit
Selenium	Reduces intracellular hydroperoxides, thereby protecting membrane lipids from oxidant damage	Seafood, kidney, liver, meats, grains	Growth retardation, muscle pain and weakness, myopathy, cardiomyopathy	Serum or plasma selenium
Zinc	A cofactor in over 100 different enzyme systems that promote protein synthesis, cellular replication, and collagen formation	Oysters, dark-meat turkey, liver, lima beans, pork	Hair loss, dermatitis, growth retardation, delayed sexual maturation, testicular atrophy, decreased appetite, depressed smell and taste acuity, depression, diarrhea, decreased dark adaptation	Serum or plasma zinc

Source: Adapted from Mayes T and Gottschlich MM, *American Society for Parenteral and Enteral Nutrition, The Science and Practice of Nutrition Support*, Kendall Hunt Publishing, Dubuque, IA, 2001, 391–392.

TABLE 26.3

Micronutrient Guidelines after Thermal Injury

Adults and Children	Children
≥ 3 years of age	< 3 years of age
> 40 lbs	≤ 40 lbs
≥ 20% burn	≥ 10% burn
1 multivitamin (qd)	1 children's multivitamin (qd)
500 mg ascorbic acid (bid)	250 mg ascorbic acid (bid)
10,000 IU vitamin A (qd)	5000 IU vitamin A (qd)
220 mg zinc sulfate (qd)[a]	110 mg zinc sulfate (qd)[a]

Note: qd: everyday; bid: twice a day.

[a] Recommended delivery in suspension for tube feeding, because orally administered zinc in large doses may precipitate nausea or vomiting.

Source: Adapted from Mayes T, Gottschlich M, Warden GD, *J. Burn Care Rehabil.* 18, 365–368, 1997.

victim provide essential information about the adequacy of nutrition support. A thorough evaluation of skin condition is an essential component of nutritional adequacy and therefore should be completed each week at a minimum.

26.5.1 ENERGY

The provision of sufficient calories for wound repair is a major component of healing. Multiple equations exist to assist the clinician in the assessment of energy requirements for the burn patient (Table 26.4).[58–76] For other types of wounds, the use of a basal estimate calculation like the Harris–Benedict[64] with added factors for activity, wound healing, and other variables is common practice. The reliability of equations is questioned, because confounding factors that influence metabolic rate are not wholly inherent in any calculation. For example, formulas cannot accurately predict energy needs if weight is skewed by edema, amputation, or wound dressing or if additional stress factors are present, such as fractures, smoke inhalation injury, head trauma, surgery, or infection.

For these reasons, indirect calorimetry remains the preferred method of determining energy needs for any stressed patient. Indirect calorimetry determines energy needs inherently, accounting for changes in weight and wound size, the presence or absence of infection or inhalation injury, and other extraneous variables. For the burn patient, a factor of 20 to 30% should be added to measured resting energy expenditure to account for increased demands from physical therapy, wound dressing changes, temperature spikes, anxiety, pain, and other conditions that serve to increase energy requirement but are not accounted for at the time of the resting measurement. For the mechanically ventilated, severely burned, or hospitalized patient presenting with open wound, indirect calorimetry is recommended 2 to 3 times per week. Spontaneously breathing patients with wounds who require enteral nutrition support should have indirect calorimetry repeated a minimum of once per week. The nutrition support regimen should be routinely adjusted in accordance with the metabolic cart measurement.

Respiratory quotient (RQ) is an assessment tool that accompanies standard indirect calorimetry measurements. RQ is helpful to the clinician as a means of determining overfeeding or underfeeding, both of which have deleterious stresses on the patient. Table 26.5 provides an interpretive tool to assist in the clinical application of RQ.

TABLE 26.4
Formulas for Calculating Energy Requirements of Burn Patients

Reference	Age	% BSAB	Calories/Day
Curreri[58–60]	0–1 yr	< 50	Basal + (15 × % BSAB)
	1–3 yr	< 50	Basal + (25 × % BSAB)
	4–15 yr	< 50	Basal + (40 × % BSAB)
	16–59 yr	Any	25W + (40 × % BSAB)
	> 60 yr	Any	Basal + (65 × % BSAB)
Davies and Liljedahl[61]	Adult	Any	20W + (70 × % BSAB)
	Child	Any	60W + (35 × % BSAB)
Long modification[62,63] of the Harris–Benedict[64] equation	Adult Male	Any	$(66.47 + 13.7W + 50H - 6.76A) \times$ (activity factor) × (injury factor)
	Adult Female	Any	$(655.1 + 9.56W + 1.85H - 6.68A) \times$ (activity factor) × (injury factor)
Hildreth[65–67]	< 15 yr	> 30	$(1800/m^2 \text{ BSA}) + (2200/m^2 \text{ burn})$
Hildreth[68]	< 12 yr		$(1800/m^2 \text{ BSA}) + 1300/m^2 \text{ burn}$
Mayes[69]	0–3 yr	10–50	108 + 68W + (3.9 × % BSAB)
	5–10 yr		818 + 37.4W + (9.3 × % BSAB)
Parks[70]	Adult	Any	$(1800/m^2 \text{ BSA}) + (2200 \text{ kcal}/m^2 \text{ BSAB})$
Molnar[71]	Adult	Any	2 × BMR
Pruitt[72]	Adult	Any	$2000–2200/m^2 \text{ BSA}$
Soroff[73]	Adult	Any	$3500/m^2 \text{ BSA}$
Sutherland[74]	Adult	Any	20W + (70 × % BSAB)
Troell and Wretlind[75]	Adult	Any	40–60W
Wilmore[76]	Adult	Any	$2000/m^2 \text{ BSA}$

Note: BSAB: body surface area burned; BSA: body surface area; W: weight in kg; A: age in years; H: height in cm.

Source: Adapted from Kagan RJ, Gottschlich MM, Jenkins ME, in *Problems in General Surgery*, vol. 8, JB Lippincott, Philadelphia, 1991, 65.

In addition, the practicality of using commercially available handheld devices that estimate energy needs should be considered. This technology is relatively inexpensive in comparison to the larger indirect calorimetry machines. The handheld devices are limited to use in spontaneously breathing patients and do not indicate RQ, but, for the convalescing burn patient, postoperative surgical patient, or the noncombative long-term care resident with decubitus ulcer, the technology can assist in accurate energy assessment.

Acute and chronic wounds require nutrition support that is tailored to meet the individual requirement of the patient. Indirect calorimetry provides the optimal means of individualizing the nutrition care plan; however, it is recognized that not all institutions are privy to this technology. For this reason, estimates from equations are a practical alternative for projecting calorie needs. In either method of energy assessment, the nutrition support regimen should be reevaluated regularly and alterations made concomitant with other assessment parameters.

26.5.2 ANTHROPOMETRICS

Accurate height and weight assessment is important. These two variables are crucial in the initial assessment of calorie and protein requirement of any patient. Trends in weight are especially important because they provide insight into the adequacy of calorie provision. For this reason, weekly weights are recommended for any burn patient or long-term care resident with greater than second-stage pressure ulcer. As in any patient, caution is presumed in the assessment of weight

TABLE 26.5

Braden Scale for Predicting Pressure Sore Risk

Client's Name _____ Evaluator's Name _____ Date of Assessment _____

	1	2	3	4				
Sensory perception Ability to respond meaningfully to pressure-related discomfort	1. Completely limited: Unresponsive (does not moan, flinch, or grasp) to painful stimuli, due to diminished level of consciousness or sedation. OR Limited ability to feel pain over most of body surface.	2. Very limited: Responds to only painful stimuli. Cannot communicate discomfort except by moaning or restlessness. OR Has a sensory impairment that limits the ability to feel pain or discomfort over half of body.	3. Slightly limited: Responds to verbal commands but cannot always communicate discomfort or need to be turned. OR Has some sensory impairment that limits ability to feel pain or discomfort in 1 or 2 extremities.	4. No impairment: Responds to verbal commands. Has no sensory deficit which would limit ability to feel or voice pain or discomfort.				
Moisture Degree to which skin is exposed to moisture	1. Constantly moist: Skin is kept moist almost constantly by perspiration, urine, etc. Dampness is detected every time patient is moved or turned.	2. Moist: Skin is often but not always moist. Linen must be changed at least once a shift.	3. Occasionally moist: Skin is occasionally moist, requiring an extra linen change approximately once a day.	4. Rarely moist: Skin is usually dry; linen requires changing only at routine intervals.				
Activity Degree of physical activity	1. Bedfast: Confined to bed.	2. Chairfast: Ability to walk severely limited or nonexistent. Cannot bear down weight and/or must be assisted into chair or wheelchair.	3. Walks occasionally: Walks occasionally during day but for very short distances, with or without assistance. Spends majority of each shift in bed or chair.	4. Walks frequently: Walks outside the room at least twice a day and inside room at least once every 2 hours during waking hours.				
Mobility Ability to change and control body position	1. Completely immobile: Does not make even slight changes in body or extremity position without assistance.	2. Very limited: Makes occasional slight changes in body or extremity position but unable to make frequent or significant changes independently.	3. Slightly limited: Makes frequent though slight changes in body or extremity position independently.	4. No limitations: Makes major and frequent changes in position without assistance.				

	1. Very poor:	2. Probably inadequate:	3. Adequate:	4. Excellent:
Nutrition Usual food intake pattern	Never eats a complete meal. Rarely eats more than one-third of any food offered. Eats two servings or less of protein (meat or dairy products) per day. Takes fluids poorly. Does not take a liquid dietary supplement. OR Is NPO[a] and/or maintained on clear liquids or IV[b] for more than 5 days.	Rarely eats a complete meal and generally eats only half of any food offered. Protein intake includes only three servings of meat or dairy products per day. Occasionally will take a dietary supplement. OR Receives less than optimum amount of liquid diet or tube feeding.	Eats over half of most meals. Eats a total of four servings of protein (meat or dairy products) each day. Occasionally refuses a meal, but will usually take a supplement if offered. OR Is on a tube feeding or TPN[c] regimen, which probably meets most of nutritional needs.	Eats most of every meal. Never refuses a meal. Usually eats a total of four or more servings of meat and dairy products. Occasionally eats between meals. Does not require supplementation.
Friction and shear	1. Problem: Requires moderate to maximum assistance in moving. Complete lifting without sliding against sheets is impossible. Frequently slides down in bed or chair, requiring frequent repositioning with maximum assistance. Spasticity, contractures, or agitation leads to almost constant friction.	2. Potential problem: Moves feebly or requires minimal assistance. During a move, skin probably slides to some extent against sheets, chair, restraints, or other devices. Maintains relatively good position in chair or bed most of the time but occasionally slides down.	3. No apparent problem: Moves in bed and in chair independently and has sufficient muscle strength to lift up completely during move. Maintains good position in bed or chair ant all times.	

Total Score

Note: The maximum possible score is 23. A lower score reflects higher risk for pressure ulceration. The cutoff score to denote risk for pressure ulceration is ≤16.

[a] NPO = Nothing by mouth.
[b] IV = Intravenously.
[c] TPN: Total parenteral nutrition.

Source: Reprinted from Braden B and Bergstrom N, *Res. Nurs. Health,* 1994, 17, 459–470. With permission.

fluctuation, due to the impact of edema. Burn patients exhibit fluid retention well into their acute course, at times lasting for 4 to 6 weeks (or longer). Varying medical conditions inherently cause chronic edema as well. The effects of such must be considered in the weight assessment.

Guidelines for initiating intervention based on weight fluctuation have been established in the long-term care setting (Table 26.6). In addition, maintenance of 90 to 110% of preburn weight is recommended for the burn patient. Furthermore, burned children have been reported to exhibit long-term growth delays — up to two years post burn.[53] This knowledge should be factored into the assessment of the pediatric burn patient in the outpatient setting.

TABLE 26.6
Formulas for Calculating Energy Requirements of Burn Patients

Reference	Age	% BSAB	Calories/Day
Curreri[58–60]	0–1 yr	<50	Basal + (15 × % BSAB)
	1–3 yr	<50	Basal + (25 × % BSAB)
	4–15 yr	<50	Basal + (40 × % BSAB)
	16–59 yr	Any	25W + (40 × % BSAB)
	>60 yr	Any	Basal + (65 × % BSAB)
Davies and Liljedahl[61]	Adult	Any	20W + (70 × % BSAB)
	Child	Any	60W + (35 × % BSAB)
Long modification[62,63] of the Harris-Benedict[64] equation	Adult Male	Any	$(66.47 + 13.7W + 50H - 6.76A) \times$ (activity factor) × (injury factor)
	Adult Female	Any	$(655.1 + 9.56W + 1.85H - 6.68A) \times$ (activity factor) × (injury factor)
Hildreth[65–67]	<15 yr	>30	$(1800/m^2\ BSA) + (2200/m^2\ burn$
Hildreth[68]	<12 yr		$(1800/m^2\ BSA) + 1300/m^2\ burn$
Mayes[69]	0–3 yr	10–50	108 + 68W + (3.9 × % BSAB)
	5–10 yr		818 + 37.4W + (9.3 × % BSAB)
Parks[70]	Adult	Any	$(1800/m^2\ BSA) + (2200\ kcal/m^2$ BSAB)
Molnar[71]	Adult	Any	2 × BMR
Pruitt[72]	Adult	Any	$2000–2200/m^2\ BSA$
Soroff[73]	Adult	Any	$3500/m^2\ BSA$
Sutherland[74]	Adult	Any	20W + (70 × % BSAB)
Troell and Wretlind[75]	Adult	Any	40–60W
Wilmore[76]	Adult	Any	$2000/m^2\ BSA$

Note: BSAB = body surface area burned; BSA = body surface area; W = weight in kg; A = age in years; H = height in cm.

Source: Adapted with permission from Kagan RJ, Gottschlich MM, Jenkins ME, Nutritional support in the burn patient. IN: Robin AP (ed), *Problems in General Surgery*, vol. 8, Philadelphia; JB Lippincott, 1991:65.

26.5.3 LABORATORY INDICES

Different labs are important in the nutritional assessment of patients with wounds, depending on severity and etiology. Patients with large burn wounds exhibit extremely low levels of albumin due to plasma leaks across the microvasculature. Exogenous albumin supplementation is routine in large burns, although guidelines have been established that have lowered the albumin threshold, thus decreasing the supplement requirement.[77]

Due to the marked, immediate impact of the burn injury itself and other burn-mediated factors, such as edema, surgery, excessive hydration, and blood loss, on serum albumin and because the plummet is related to injury conditions — not the adequacy of nutrition support — albumin is not routinely used in the nutritional assessment of the acutely burned individual. Due to its long half-life (essentially three weeks) and insensitivity to acute changes in nutrition status, albumin is a more effective indicator of nutrition status during the rehabilitation phase of burn or in the long-term care resident. Albumin serves the clinician in monitoring long-term trends in nutrition status or in determining the impact of initiating or withdrawing nutrition intervention over time.

Prealbumin is an additional indicator of visceral protein synthesis. The half-life of prealbumin is two days, making it a more sensitive indicator of nutrition status than albumin. Prealbumin is also an acute-phase reactant, so levels react to the stresses of acute burn injury and have negligible nutrition relevance. Surgery, wound exudate, fluid shifts, blood transfusions, and infection all negatively impact prealbumin level. Inclusion of prealbumin in the nutrition assessment is better suited for the convalescent stage of burn recovery or to monitor acute changes in the intake, weight, or skin condition of the long-term care resident.

Nitrogen balance is most often used in the acute setting following surgical stress or burn injury. Twenty-four-hour nitrogen intake and urinary nitrogen losses must be calculated precisely to determine balance and thus the degree of anabolism or catabolism. The standard equation used to estimate nitrogen balance (24 h nitrogen intake [g] – 24 h urinary urea nitrogen [g] + factor for insensible losses) is modified to account for nitrogen losses in wound exudate following a burn injury.[78] As an option, completing nitrogen balance studies in patients with burns in excess of 25% TBSA using the preceding equation and targeting a goal (unadjusted for wound size) at +5 to +10 clinically supports wound healing (the larger the percent burn, the higher the nitrogen balance goal in the noted range).

26.5.4 SPECIAL CONDITIONS

The presence of diabetes is the most common condition that attenuates wound healing. Factors including wound hypoxia from poor circulation and increased infection risk are recognized in the diabetic patient. An elevated serum glucose is indicative of failure of glucose to enter the cells. This interferes with aerobic and anaerobic metabolism. Insulin deficiency suppresses collagen deposition in wounds. Recently, the work of Van den Berghe et al. has indicated that tighter glucose control via increase insulin provision reduces infectious episodes and mortality.[79]

Pressure ulcers are a common wound-care issue in the immobilized elderly. Inadequate energy, protein, and fluid intake; significant weight loss; and urinary and fecal incontinence contribute to development. The Braden scale is typically employed in the long-term care setting by the interdisciplinary team to predict a resident's risk of pressure ulcer development (Table 26.7).[80] This assessment tool includes a nutrition component that identifies residents requiring nutrition intervention. It is recommended that the interdisciplinary assessment of ulcer risk be completed monthly for long-term care residents, so that timely interventions to prevent ulcer development or minimize size and depth can be initiated.

TABLE 26.7
Potential Factors Affecting Metabolic Rate in Patients with Burns

Activity
Age
Anxiety
Application and removal of allograft
Body composition
Body temperature
Catecholamine production
Circadian rhythm
Dry heat loss (ambient temperature)
Energy cost of protein synthesis
Energy cost of respiratory stress
Extent of injury
Evaporative heat loss (wound coverage)
Gender
Graft loss
Immediate vs. delayed feeding
Infection
Medications
Pain
Sedation
Sleep vs. wakefulness
Specific dynamic action of food
Surgery
Wound healing

Source: Adapted from Gottschlich et al, *J Am Diet Assoc* 97:132, 1997.

26.6   ANABOLIC AGENTS

Pharmacologic agents, such as anabolic steroids, recombinant growth hormone, and growth factors, reportedly have positive effects on wound healing. Oxandrolone, a testosterone analog, when combined with a high protein diet, enhances weight gain and closure of previously nonhealing wounds.[81–83] Also, a positive relationship has been established between recombinant human growth hormone provision and earlier donor site healing in patients with large burns that required multiple donor site reharvests.[84,85] Shortened donor site reharvest time translates to reduced length of stay and thus decreased cost. Furthermore, evidence supports reduced muscle catabolism and preserved bone density with long-term growth hormone therapy.[86] The success of growth hormone has been overshadowed by evidence of increased infectious morbidity and mortality in critically ill and burn patients treated with growth hormone.[87] Nevertheless, growth hormone supplementation, particularly in young children with severe burns, remains a suitable adjunct option for improved healing time. Finally, growth factors are a subgroup of cytokines that distinctively proliferate cells. Altered growth factor production has also been associated with poor wound healing. Numerous studies have demonstrated the ability of these cytokines to assist in tissue repair.[88–92] The effect of growth factors on healing remains controversial: clinical trials in the burn population have not produced consistent evidence to support application of such to routine care.[93,94] Risks to growth factor use include the possibility for increased scarring from enhanced granulation tissue accumulation and potentially malignant transformation. Growth factors have the potential for making significant enhancements to clinical care, although application guidelines must be refined.

26.7 NUTRITION SUPPORT GUIDELINES

Oral nutrition can usually be enhanced to increase calories and protein to a level that supports healing in previously well-nourished individuals who have acute wounds involving less than 20% open area. Combining provision of food preferences, supplementing with high-calorie, high-protein commercial products, and concealing protein and carbohydrate modules in foods and beverages are useful in increasing calorie and protein intake.

26.7.1 ENTERAL

Enteral nutrition is the preferred route of nutrient administration and is indicated in patients or residents exhibiting characteristics listed in Table 26.8, assuming that ethical issues related to sustaining quality of life have been addressed (Chapter 39). Increased intestinal blood flow, preserved gastrointestinal function, decreased mucosal atrophy, and reduced bacterial translocation are associated with feeding the gut.[95,96]

Acute wounds, such as burns, may be associated with gastric ileus, and the tendency may be to withhold enteral support or initiate parenteral nutrition in response. Although the stomach may be affected by posttraumatic ileus, the small intestine maintains its functional and absorptive capabilities and therefore remains a viable alternative postburn. Gastric feedings are not supported in the patient with large burns, because ileus often prevents the initial advancement and optimal delivery of enteral feedings. In addition, heightened aspiration risk is recognized in the burn patient, due to multiple position changes during daily dressing changes, physical therapy sessions, and various postoperative position needs (e.g., prone, neck hyperextension, etc.). Furthermore, small bowel feedings permit minimal interruption of the nutrition regimen, thereby limiting chronic nutrient deficiencies, and preclude the need to withhold enteral feedings for respiratory treatments, intravenous line changes, or surgery, thus maximizing nutrient intake. Gastric feedings also interrupt the normal hunger response and therefore affect the oral intake of foodstuff. For the long-term care resident or stable surgical patient who is not subject to the multiple aspiration risks of a burn patient, routine gastric feedings via gastrostomy tube or nasogastric tube, respectively, are acceptable.

TABLE 26.8
Implications of Respiratory Quotient (RQ)

RQ	Significance
<0.70	Oxidation of alcohol
	Oxidation of ketones
	Carbohydrate synthesis
	Measurement problem
0.70–0.75	Mostly lipid oxidation
	Possible starvation
0.85–0.95	Mixed substrate oxidation
	Calories adequate
>1.00	Lipogenesis
	Primarily carbohydrate oxidation
	Hyperventilation
	Measurement problem

Source: Reprinted with permission, Mayes T, Gottschlich M, Burns and wound healing. In: *Contemporary Nutrition Support Practice.*

Regardless of placement, alterations in the nutrition support regimen should occur (i.e., withhold feeds at meals or nocturnal feeds only) to maximize the oral intake of oriented individuals.

26.7.1.1 Feeding during Resuscitation

Feeding tube placement in the third segment of the duodenum to just beyond the ligament of Treitz is recommended for the burn patient. Continuous drip feedings are initiated within hours of admission. The initial hourly infusion should begin at one-half the goal and advance by 5 to 20 ml/h, dependent on age. Advancement of the feeding rate in this manner applies to admission, the postoperative period, and other irregular procedures that necessitate lengthy interruption of the enteral schedule.

There is no need to withhold feeds during the resuscitation period of the burn patient.[97] The tube feeding rate is simply run above total hourly fluid requirements until the shock phase has ended, typically by 48 hours postinjury. At this time, the tube feeding rate is incorporated into the hourly total fluid goal. As a precautionary means of preserving gastrointestinal integrity, if a patient arrives at the burn unit and is clearly underresuscitated (as evidenced by poor urine output or poor edemetous response) or if a patient is placed on inotropic agents during resuscitation or throughout the acute course, enteral feeds should be provided at trophic rate (10 to 20 ml/h) sufficient to stimulate the gut but providing minimal nutrition support.[98]

26.7.1.2 Perioperative

Multiple studies support the role of nutrition and wound healing in the postoperative period.[99–105] However, it is common practice to allow patients nothing by mouth, with enteral feedings withheld, preceding and following surgical procedures. As a result, negligible nutrient intake is realized at a time when the body is most stressed, catabolic, and in need of nutrients that appropriately support healing.

Several authors have successfully accomplished continuous enteral feedings during operative procedures.[99,100,106] A significant reduction in caloric deficit, accompanied by less need for exogenous albumin to maintain serum levels and decreased wound infection, was noted in burn patients fed continuously through surgery. Strict guidelines must be in place to ensure diligent monitoring of feeding tube position and gastric reflux throughout the operative procedure.

26.7.2 PARENTERAL

Instituting parenteral nutrition as standard in patients with a functional gastrointestinal tract is unwarranted and not without complication. Parenteral nutrition is associated with a host of negative implications, including increased prevalence of blood-borne pathogens and suppressed immunity.[107,108] As a result, parenteral feeds are reserved for patients whose intestines are non- or low-functioning. Examples of such conditions include, but are not limited to, the following:

- Persistent intestinal ileus
- Abdominal trauma
- Intractable diarrhea
- Stress ulceration of the stomach or duodenum
- Pseudo-obstruction of the colon
- Superior mesenteric artery syndrome

Parenteral nutrition should be viewed as a backup means of nutrition support, with enteral nutrition always given primary consideration. When intravenous nutrition is necessitated, promotion of the following is recommended:

- Gut stimulation via trophic feeds
- Conservative fat provision, due to its hyperlipidemic and immunosuppressive effects
- Routine attempts to progress enteral feeds, thereby limiting intravenous support

26.8 SUMMARY

Wound healing is a multifactorial, complex process aided by appropriate nutrition support and the application of assessment methods that ensure that wound healing progression is maximized. Studies undoubtedly support the role of high-protein, high-calorie intake in wound healing. Burn wounds require further diet alteration, with research suggesting a regimen consisting not only of increased calories and protein but high-carbohydrate, low-fat, and omega-3 fatty acid supplementation. Micronutrient provision is to be carefully considered. Supplementation of vitamins A and C and zinc is fairly standard in large burns; however, it is beneficial to be prudent with supplementation of such in patients with other wound types. Given the positive effects on immunity, enteral feeding remains the preferred method of nutrient delivery in wound management. The role of nutrition support in wound healing has progressed significantly in the past 20 years. Appropriate nutrient provision is recognized as an intricate component to wound repair and, as such, should remain an irrefutable priority in the multidisciplinary plan of care.

26.9 CASE STUDY

26.9.1 HISTORY AND PHYSICAL

T.K. is a 30-year-old male admitted to the burn unit 4 hours postburn from a trailer fire. He was intubated at the scene and is reliant on mechanical ventilation. Upon exam, the patient appears neurologically intact and has suffered 60% TBSA burns to face and upper and lower extremities, with 45% full thickness. Adequate urine output is established, using the Parkland formula.[109] The patient is hemodynamically stable, weighs 86 kg and is 185 cm tall. Past medical history is unremarkable. A nasogastric tube is connected to low wall suction.

26.9.2 NUTRITION SUPPORT INITIATION

By postburn hour 6, the wounds have been cleansed and dressed and fluoroscopy is used to place the feeding tube just beyond the ligament of Treitz. Once tube placement is confirmed, a 1 cal/ml high–intact protein, moderately low-fat, linolenic acid– and arginine-enriched enteral formula is initiated. The initial goal rate is established using the recommended dietary allowance[110] for energy for a normal, healthy adult because the patient will remain in the ebb response until approximately 48 hours postburn. T.K.'s RDA is established at 3200 calories per day. It is estimated that dextrose in the maintenance fluid used following resuscitation will provide an additional 500 calories per day. As a result, the energy necessary from tube feeding is estimated at 2700 calories per day. The tube feeding rate will begin at one half of this goal, or 65 ml/h, and advance by 20 ml/h to a goal rate of 135 ml/h. Indirect calorimetry is performed approximately 30 hours postburn, and resting energy expenditure with a 30% activity/stress factor confirms the current goal of 3200 calories/d. The protein goal is established at 184 g/d (23% of total calories or 2 g/kg/d). Modular whey protein is added to the enteral formula to ensure protein provision at this level. A multivitamin–mineral supplement, vitamin C, and zinc are provided, according to guidelines listed in Table 26.3. Baseline transferrin and prealbumin labs are obtained. Twenty-four-hour urinary urea nitrogen lab tests are initiated the following morning and will continue daily until the urinary catheter is discontinued.

26.9.3 SURGERY

T.K. is taken to the operating room postburn day 3 for excision of all clearly demarcated full thickness areas. The following day, approximately 20% of the wounds are autografted and 25% of the wounds are covered in allograft. The allograft will remain on the wound until the donor site can be reharvested in approximately 10 to 14 days. T.K. requires two additional excision and grafting procedures before his wounds are covered by autograft. The enteral feeding regimen is not interrupted for any surgery and remains at goal rate postoperatively each time.

26.9.4 SEPSIS

Approximately 5 days postop, T.K. presents with a septic episode, for which a ten-day course of antibiotics is initiated. Indirect calorimetry is routinely completed two times per week. The latest test indicates energy needs have soared to 4500 calories per day; RQ is low at 0.80, and the tube feeding rate is adjusted upward. Mean nitrogen balance over the past week has been steady around +3. The tube feeding rate increase provides additional protein at approximately 3 g/kg/d; therefore, nitrogen balance into postburn week 2 has improved appropriately to +7. As expected, transferrin and prealbumin decline during this septic period, due to hepatic reprioritization to synthesizing inflammatory markers rather than visceral proteins.

26.9.5 DIARRHEA

Noninfectious, sepsis/antibiotic-induced diarrhea develops on postantibiotic day 4. Once the patient stool is confirmed to be *Clostridium difficile*–negative, scheduled antidiarrheal medications are administered every 4 to 6 hours. Loose stools are controlled by postantibiotic day 6, with no adjustment to the enteral regimen.

26.9.6 PROGRESSION TOWARD DISCHARGE

Over the next 7 weeks, T.K. progresses well, and his wounds are now > 95% healed. His tolerance of the enteral regimen (rate determined by biweekly indirect calorimetry) is good. T.K. is now free of edema, and his weight status is good at 95% of preburn weight. A gradual improvement in weekly transferrin and prealbumin levels is noted. T.K. is removed from the ventilator postburn week 5, and an oral diet is initiated two days later. As T.K.'s oral intake has improved, tube feeding is tapered accordingly: held 2 hours at meals when oral intake averages 25% of goal; held 7 A.M. to 7 P.M. when oral intake averages 50% of goal; and eventually discontinued postburn week 7, when oral intake consistently meets 75% of goal with the aid of a supplement. Indirect calorimetry was discontinued when the feeding tube was discontinued. T.K. is discharged postburn day 62 (1.03 days per percent burn) on a regular diet without need for further protein or micronutrient enhancement as all wounds are covered. The standard length of stay per percent burn is generally accepted at 1.0. He is now 93% of preburn weight. He will be monitored in the Outpatient Department for the next month for weight fluctuations and on an as-needed basis thereafter.

REFERENCES

1. Cuthbertson, D. and Tilstone, W.J., Metabolism during the post injury period, *Adv. Clin. Chem.*, 121, 1969.
2. Clowes, G.H.A., Metabolic responses to injury. Part 1: the production of energy, *J. Trauma*, 3, 149, 1963.
3. Harrison, H.N. et al., The relationship between energy metabolism and water loss from vaporization in severely burned patients, *Surgery*, 56, 203, 1964.

4. Gottschlich, M.M. et al., A prospective clinical study of the polysomno-graphic stages of sleep following burn injury, *J. Burn Care Rehabil.*, 15, 486, 1994.

5. Mochizuki, H. et al., Mechanisms of prevention of postburn hypermetabolism and catabolism by early enteral feeding, *Ann. Surg.*, 200, 297, 1984.

6. Dominioni, L. et al., Prevention of severe postburn hypermetabolism and catabolism by immediate intragastric feeding, *J. Burn Care Rehabil.*, 5, 106, 1984.

7. Jenkins, M. et al., An evaluation of the effect of immediate enteral feeding on the hypermetabolic response following severe burn injury, *J. Burn Care Rehabil.*, 15, 199, 1994.

8. Cerami, A., Inflammatory cytokines, *Clin. Immunopathol.*, 62, S3, 1992.

9. Tredgett, E.E. et al., Role of interleukin-1 and tumor necrosis factor on energy metabolism in rabbits, *Am. J. Physiol.*, 255, E760, 1988.

10. Prokop-Oliet, M. et al., Whey protein supplementation of complete tube feeding in the nutritional support of thermally injured patients, *Proc. Am. Burn Assoc.*, 15, 45, 1983.

11. Trocki, O. et al., Intact protein versus free amino acids in the nutritional support of thermally injured animals, *J. Parenter. Enteral Nutr.*, 10, 139, 1986.

12. Newport, M.M. and Henschel, M.M., Evaluation of the neonatal pig as a model for infant nutrition: effects of different proportion of casein and whey protein in milk on nitrogen metabolism and composition of digesta in the stomach, *Pediatr. Res.*, 18, 658, 1984.

13. Alexander, J.W. et al., Beneficial effects of aggressive protein feeding in severely burned children, *Ann. Surg.*, 192, 505, 1980.

14. Bergstrom, N. et al., Treatment of pressure ulcers (Clinical Practice Guide, No. 15), *AHCPR*, Publication No. 95-0652, U.S. Department of Health and Human Services Public Health Service, Agency of Health Care Policy and Research, Rockville, MD, 1994.

15. Long, C.L. et al., A physiological basis for the provision of fuel mixtures in normal and stressed patients, *J. Trauma*, 30, 1077, 1990.

16. Kirk, S.J. et al., Arginine stimulates wound healing and immune function in elderly human beings, *Surgery*, 114, 155, 1993.

17. Barbul, A. et al., Arginine enhances wound healing and lymphocyte immune responses in humans, *Surgery*, 108, 331, 1990.

18. Kirk, S.J. and Barbul, A., Role of arginine in trauma, sepsis, immunity, *J. Parenter. Enteral Nutr.*, 14(5), 226S–229S, 226S, 1990.

19. Cui X et al., Effects of dietary arginine supplementation on protein turnover and tissue protein synthesis in scald-burn rats, *Nutrition*, 15(7/8), 563, 1999.

20. Saito, H. et al., Metabolic and immune effects of dietary arginine supplementation after burn, *Arch. Surg.*, 122, 784, 1987.

21. Raeder da Costa, M.A. et al., Oral glutamine and the healing of the colonic anastomoses in rats, *J. Parenter. Enteral Nutr.*, 27, 186, 2003.

22. Zhou, Y. et al., The effect of supplemental enteral glutamine on plasma levels, gut function and outcome in severe burns: a randomized, double-blind, controlled clinical trial, *J. Parenter. Enteral Nutr.*, 27, 241, 2003.

23. O'Dwyer, S.T. et al., Maintenance of small bowel mucosa with glutamine-enriched parenteral nutrition, *J. Parenter. Enteral Nutr.*, 13, 579, 1989.

24. Gottschlich, M.M. et al., Effect of enteral glutamine supplementation on selected outcome variables in burned children, *Proc. Am. Burn Assoc.*, 25, 572, 2004.

25. Tazuke, Y. et al., Alanyl-glutamine supplemented parenteral nutrition prevents intestinal ischemia-reperfusion in rats, *J. Parenter. Enteral Nutr.*, 27, 110, 2003.

26. Gottschlich, M.M. et al., Differential effects of three enteral dietary regimens on selected outcome variables in burn patients, *J. Parenter. Enteral Nutr.*, 14, 225, 1990.

27. Mochizuki, H. et al., Optimal lipid content for enteral diets following thermal injury, *J. Parenter. Enteral Nutr.*, 8, 638, 1984.

28. Garrell, D.R. et al., Improved clinical status and length of care with low-fat nutrition support in burn patients, *J. Parenter. Enteral Nutr.*, 19, 482, 1995.

29. Hulsey, T.K. et al., Experimental wound healing in essential fatty acid deficiency, *J. Pediatr. Surg.*, 15, 505, 1980.

30. Alexander, J.W. et al., The importance of lipid type in the diet after burn injury, *Ann. Surg.*, 204, 1, 1986.

31. Sauberlich, H.E., *Laboratory Tests for the Assessment of Nutritional Status*, 2nd ed., CRC Press, Boca Raton, FL, 1, 486, 1999.

32. Klein, G.L. et al., Dysregulation of calcium homeostasis after severe burn injury in children: possible role of magnesium depletion, *J. Pediatr.*, 131, 246, 1997.

33. Murphey, E.D. et al., Up-regulation of the parathyroid calcium-sensing receptor after burn injury in sheep: a potential contributory factor to postburn hypocalcemia, *Crit. Care Med.*, 28, 3885, 2000.

34. Loven, L., Nordstrom, H., and Lennquist, S., Changes in calcium and phosphate and their regulating hormones in patients with severe burn injuries, *Scand. J. Plast. Reconstr. Surg.*, 18, 49, 1984.

35. Szytelbein, S.K., Drop, L.J., and Martyn, J.A., Persistent ionized hypocalcemia in patients during resuscitation and recovery phases of body burns, *Crit. Care Med.*, 9, 454, 1981.

36. Klein, G.L. and Herndon, D.H., Magnesium deficit in major burns: role in hypoparathyroidism and end-organ parathyroid hormone resistance, *Magnesium Res.*, 11, 103, 1998.

37. Klein, C.L., Langman, C.B., and Herndon, D.N., Persistent hypoparathyrodism following magnesium repletion in burn-injured children, *Pediatr. Nephrol.*, 14, 301, 2000.

38. Turinsky, J., Gonnerman, W.A., and Loose, L.D., Impaired mineral metabolism in postburn muscle, *J. Trauma*, 21, 417, 1981.

39. Broughton, A., Anderson, L.R.M., and Bowden, C.H., Magnesium deficiency syndrome in burns, *Lancet*, 1, 1156, 1968.

40. Lennquist, S. et al., Hypophosphatemia in severe burns, *Acta Chir. Scand.*, 145, 1, 1979.

41. Loven, L. et al., Serum phosphate and 2,3-diphosphoglycerate in severely burned patients after phosphate supplementation, *J. Trauma*, 26, 348, 1986.

42. Dickerson, R.N., et al., A comparison of renal phosphorus regulation in thermally injured and multiple trauma patients receiving specialized nutrition support, *J. Parenter. Enteral Nutr.*, 2225, 152, 2001.

43. Gottschlich, M.M. et al., Hypovitaminosis D in acutely injured pediatric burn patients, *J. Am. Dietet. Assoc.*, 104, 931, 2004.

44. Klein, G.L., Langman, C.B., and Herndon, D.N., Vitamin D depletion following burns in children: a possible factor in post-burn osteopenia, *J. Trauma*, 52, 346, 2002.

45. Wray, C.J. et al., Metabolic effects of vitamin D on serum calcium, magnesium and phosphorus in pediatric burn patients, *J. Burn Care Rehab.*, 23, 416, 2002.

46. Gottschlich, M.M. et al., Hypovitaminosis D in pediatric burn patients, *J. Burn Care Rehabil.*, 22, S60, 2001.

47. Klein, G.L. et al., Long-term reduction in bone mass after severe burn injury in children, *J. Pediatr.*, 126, 252, 1995.

48. Klein, G.L. et al., Histomorphometric and biochemical characterization of bone following acute severe burns in children, *Bone*, 17, 455, 1995.

49. Klein, G.L. et al., Burn-associated bone disease in sheep: roles of immobilization and endogenous corticosteroids, *J. Burn Care Rehabil.*, 17, 518, 1996.

50. Edelman, L.S. et al., Bone mineral density changes following burn injury, *J. Burn Care Rehabil.*, 23, S84, 2002.

51. Edelman, L.S. et al., Sustained bone mineral changes following burn injury, *J. Surg. Res.*, 114, 172, 2003.

52. Mayes, T. et al., A four-year review of burns as an etiologic factor in the development of long bone fractures in pediatrics, *J. Burn Care Rehabil.*, 24, 279, 2003.

53. Rutan, R.L. and Herndon, D.N., Growth delay in postburn pediatric patients, *Arch. Surg.*, 125, 392, 1990.

54. Brewer, G.J., Interactions of zinc and molybdenum with copper in therapy of Wilson's disease, *Nutrition*, 11, 114, 1995.

55. Ross, V., Micronutrient recommendations for wound healing, *Support Line*, 24, 3, 2002.

56. Wicke, C. et al., Effects of steroids and retinoids on wound healing, *Arch. Surg.*, 1355, 1265, 2000.

57. Anstead, G.M., Steroids, retinoids and wound healing, *Adv. Wound Care*, 6, 277, 1998.

58. Curreri, P.W. et al., Dietary requirements of patients with major burns, *J. Am. Diet. Assoc.*, 65(4), 415, 1974.

59. Day, T. et al., Nutritional requirements of the burned child: the Curreri junior formula, *Proc. Am. Burn Assoc.*, (abstract) 18, 86, 1986.

60. Adams, M.R. et al., Nutritional requirements of the burned senior citizen: the Curreri senior formula, *Proc. Am. Burn Assoc.*, (abstract) 19, 83, 1987.

61. Davies, J.W.L. and Liljedahl, S.L., Metabolic consequences of an extensive burn, in *Contemporary Burn Management*, Polk, H.C. and Stone, H.H. (eds.), Little, Brown, Boston, 1511, 1971.

62. Long, C.L., Energy expenditure of major burns, *J. Trauma*, 19(11 suppl), 904, 1979.

63. Long,C.L. et al., Metabolic response to injury and illness: estimation of energy and protein needs from indirect calorimetry and nitrogen balance, *J. Parenter. Enteral Nutr.*, 3(6), 452, 1979.

64. Harris, J.A. and Benedict, F.S., *Biometric Studies of Basal Metabolism in Man*, Pub. No. 279, Carnegie Institute of Washington, Washington, DC, 1919.

65. Hildreth, M. and Carvajal, H.F., Caloric requirements in burned children: a simple formula to estimate daily caloric requirements, *J. Burn Care Rehabil.*, 3, 78, 1982.

66. Hildreth, M.A. et al., Calorie needs of adolescent patients with burns, *J. Burn Care Rehabil.*, 10(6), 523, 1989.

67. Hildreth, M.A. et al., Evaluation of a caloric requirement formula in burned children treated with early excision, *J. Trauma*, 27(2), 188, 1987.

68. Hildreth, M.A. et al., Current treatment reduces calories required to maintain weight in pediatric patients with burns, *J. Burn Care Rehabil.*, 11(5), 405, 1990.

69. Mayes, T.M. et al., An evaluation of predicted and measured energy requirements in burned children, *J. Am. Diet. Assoc.*, 96(1), 24, 1996.

70. Parks, D.H., Carvajal, H.F., and Larson, D.L., Management of burns, *Surg. Clin. North Am.*, 57, 875, 1977.

71. Molnar, J.A. et al., Enteral nutrition in patients with burns or trauma, in *Enteral and Tube Feeding*, vol. 1, Rombeau, J.L. and Caldwell, F.T. (eds.), W.B. Saunders, Philadelphia, 307, 1990.

72. Pruitt, B.A., Metabolic changes and nutrition in burn patients, *Am. Chir. Plast.*, 24(1), 21, 1979.

73. Soroff, H.S., Pearson, E., and Artz, C.P., An estimation of nitrogen requirements for equilibrium in burned patients, *Surg. Gynecol. Obstet.*, 112, 159, 1961.

74. Sutherland, A.B., Nitrogen balance and nutritional requirements in the burn patients: a reappraisal, *Burns*, 2, 238, 1979.

75. Troell, L. and Wretlind, A., Protein and caloric requirements in burns, *Acta Chir. Scand.*, 122, 15, 1961.

76. Wilmore, D.W., Nutrition and metabolism following thermal injury, *Clin. Plast. Surg.*, 1(4), 603, 1974.

77. Greenhalgh, D.G. et al., Maintenance of serum albumin levels in pediatric burn patients: a prospective, randomized trial, *J. Trauma*, 39, 67, 1995.

78. Kien, C.L. et al., Increased rates of whole body protein synthesis and breakdown in children recovering from burns, *Ann. Surg.*, 187, 383, 1978.

79. Van den Berghe, G. et al., Intensive insulin therapy in critically ill patients, *N. Engl. J. Med.*, 345, 1359, 2001.

80. Braden, B. and Bergstrom, N., Predictive validity of the Braden Scale for pressure sore risk in a nursing home population, *Res. Nurs. Health*, 17, 459, 1994.

81. Demling, R.H. and Desanti, L., Oxandrolone, an anabolic steroid, significantly increases the rate of weight gain in the recovery phase after major burns, *J. Trauma*, 43, 47, 1997.

82. Demling, R.H. and Desanti, L., Involuntary weight loss and the nonhealing wound: the role of anabolic agents, *Adv. Wound Care*, 12(Suppl 1), 1, 1999.

83. Demling, D.H., Comparison of the anabolic effects and complications of human growth hormone and the testosterone analog, oxandrolone, after severe burn injury, *Burns*, 25, 215, 1999.

84. Herndon, D.N. et al., Effects of human growth hormone on donor site healing in severely burned children, *Ann. Surg.*, 212, 424, 1990.

85. Gilpin, D.A. et al., Recombinant human growth hormone accelerates wound healing in children with large cutaneous burns, *Ann. Surg.*, 220, 19, 1994.

86. Hart, D.W. et al., Attenuation of posttraumatic muscle catabolism and osteopenia by long-term growth hormone therapy, *Ann. Surg.*, 233, 827, 2001.

87. Takala, J. et al., Increased mortality associated with growth hormone treatment in critically ill adults, *N. Engl. J. Med.*, 341, 785, 1999.

88. Robson, M.C. et al., Platelet-derived growth factor BB for the treatment of chronic pressure ulcers, *Lancet*, 339, 23, 1992.

89. Mustoe, T.A. et al., A phase II study to evaluate recombinant platelet-derived growth factor-BB in the treatment of stage 3 and 4 pressure ulcers, *Arch. Surg.*, 129, 213, 1994.

90. Robson, M.C. et al., Safety and effect of transforming growth factor-beta$_2$ for treatment of venous stasis ulcers, *Wound Repair and Regeneration*, 3, 157, 1995.

91. Steed, D.L., The Diabetic Ulcer Group: clinical evaluation of recombinant human platelet-derived growth factor for the treatment of lower extremity diabetic ulcers, *J. Vasc. Surg.*, 21, 71, 1995.

92. Robson, M.C. et al., Safety and effect of topical recombinant human interleukin-1 in the management of pressure sores, *Wound Repair and Regeneration*, 2, 177, 1994.

93. Greenhalgh, D.G. and Rieman, M., Effects of basic fibroblast growth factor on the healing of partial-thickness donor sites: a prospective, randomized double-blinded trial, *Wound Repair and Regeneration*, 2, 113, 1994.

94. Barbul, A., The effects of interleukin-1 on the healing of split thickness donor sites, Reported at the 47th Annual Sessions of the Forum on Fundamental Surgical Problems at the Clinical Congress of the American College of Surgeons, Chicago, Oct. 20–25, 1991.

95. Saito, H., Trocki, O., and Alexander, J.W., Comparison of immediate postburn enteral vs parenteral nutrition, *J. Parenter. Enteral Nutr.*, 9, 115, 1985.

96. Saito, H., Trocki, O., and Alexander, J.W., The effect of route of nutrient administration on the nutritional state, catabolic hormone secretion, and gut mucosal integrity after burn injury, *J. Parenter. Enteral Nutr.*, 11, 1, 1987.

97. Gottschlich, M.M. et al., An evaluation of the safety of early vs delayed enteral support and effects on clinical, nutritional, and endocrine outcomes after severe burns, *J. Burn Care Rehabil.*, 23, 401, 2002.

98. Riegel, T. et al., Fluid resuscitation, inotropic agents and early feeding: is there a relation to bowel necrosis? *Proc. Am. Burn Assoc.*, 24, S61, 2003.

99. Jenkins, M.E., Gottschlich, M.M., and Warden, G.D., Enteral feeding during operative procedures in thermal injuries, *J. Burn Care Rehabil.*, 15(2), 199, 1994.

100. Buescher, T.M. et al., Perioperative enteral feedings, *Proc. Am. Burn Assoc.*, 22, 162, 1990.

101. Haydock, D.A. and Hill, G.L., Impaired wound healing in surgical patients with varying degrees of malnutrition, *J. Parenter. Enteral Nutr.*, 10(6), 550, 1986.

102. Kay, S.P., Moreland, J.R., Schmitter, E., Nutritional status and wound healing in lower extremity amputations, *Clin. Orthop.*, 217 (Apr), 253, 1987.

103. Casey, J. et al., Correlation of immune and nutritional status with wound complications in patients undergoing vascular operations, *Surgery*, 93(6), 822, 1983.

104. Haydock, D.A. and Hill, G.L., Improved wound healing response in surgical patients receiving intravenous nutrition, *Br. J. Surg.*, 74(4), 320, 1987.

105. Schroeder, D. et al., Effects of immediate postoperative enteral nutrition on body composition, muscle function, and wound healing, *J. Parenter. Enteral Nutr.*, 15(4), 376, 1991.

106. Pearson, K.S. et al., Continuous enteral feeding and short fasting periods enhances perioperative nutrition in patients with burns, *J. Burn Care Rehabil.*, 13(4), 477, 1992.

107. Herndon, D.N. et al., Failure of TPN supplementation to improve liver function, immunity and mortality in thermally injured patients, *J. Trauma*, 27(2), 195, 1987.

108. Lennard, E.S. et al., Association in burn patients of improved antibacterial defense with nutritional supplementation by the oral route, *Burns*, 1, 98, 1974.

109. Warden, G.D., Fluid resuscitation and early management, in *Total Burn Care*, Herndon, D.N. (ed.), W.B. Saunders, Philadelphia, 53, 1996.

110. Food and Nutrition Board and National Research Conference, *Recommended Dietary Allowances*, 10th ed., National Academy of Sciences, Washington, DC, 1989.

27 Solid Organ Transplantation

Jeanette Hasse and Srinath Chinnakotla
Baylor Institute of Transplantation Sciences

CONTENTS

27.1 TRANSPLANTATION BACKGROUND

The first successful kidney transplant was performed in 1954 by Dr. Joseph Murray in Boston. Since then, the field of organ transplantation has advanced rapidly. In 2002, more than 23,000 individuals received an organ transplant.[1] Almost 125,000 patients have undergone successful kidney transplantation in the United States alone; the worldwide experience exceeds a quarter of million kidney transplants.[2] The long-term survival after kidney transplantation is impressive: almost 70% of kidney transplant patients are alive 10 years after transplantation, and more that 50% of their primary grafts are still functioning.[3] The first isolated pancreas transplant was performed by Dr. Lillihei in 1966 at the University of Minnesota. In 2003, 406 adults received a pancreas transplant. The 1-year patient survival among recipients of a pancreas (without kidney) is 99%; 1-year graft survival is 81%.[1] In patients who are undergoing simultaneous pancreas and kidney (SPK) transplants, 1-year patient survival is 92%; 1-year pancreas survival is 84%.[1] Since the first liver transplant was performed by Dr. Starzl in 1963,[4] liver transplantation has achieved incredible success, with over 3600 liver transplants being performed annually in United States with a 1-year patient survival of 80%.[1] Heart transplants are now actively performed in more than 170 centers in United States, with a 1-year survival of more than 80% in lead centers.[2] Lung transplants are increasingly being performed with 1-year survival rates of 70%.[1] Advances in surgical techniques have broadened the indications for transplantation such that more patients have benefited. Combined advances in critical care immunosuppression are responsible for the vast improvements in allograft outcomes and, more importantly, prolonged patient survival.

27.1.1 IMPORTANCE OF NUTRITION IN CRITICALLY ILL TRANSPLANT PATIENTS

Nutrition support is an integral part of the management of critically ill transplant patients. Candidates with end-stage organ disease awaiting transplantation are often malnourished, and the operative stress of the transplant further decreases their metabolic stores.[5] The efficacy of nutrition support after transplantation in the ICU is well illustrated by three prospective, randomized clinical studies performed in liver transplant patients that are discussed later in this chapter.[6–8]

27.2 ROUTINE MEDICAL CARE OF UNCOMPLICATED TRANSPLANT PATIENTS

27.2.1 KIDNEY AND PANCREAS TRANSPLANTATION

The common indications for kidney transplantation are end-stage renal disease due to diabetes mellitus (DM), hypertension, and glomerulonephritis.[1] The primary indication for a pancreas transplant is DM. If individuals with type 1 DM also have associated end-stage renal disease, an SPK transplant may be performed.

In 60 to 70% of renal transplant recipients with grafts from deceased donors and virtually 100% of renal transplant recipients with grafts from living donors, the transplanted kidney will function immediately. In recipients of a living donor kidney, as much as 6 to 10 l of urine output can be produced in the first 24 hours post transplant. In this situation, accurate fluid balance and supplementation of potassium and other electrolytes is necessary. About 30 to 40% of patients with cadaveric donor transplants and a few patients with living donor transplants may develop delayed graft dysfunction due to acute tubular necrosis as a result of preservation injury. These patients will have oliguria or anuria and will require hemodialysis until the graft function improves.

All kidney transplant grafts are placed in an extraperitoneal location so bowel function returns upon recovery from anesthesia. Therefore, oral diet is initiated as early as the first day post transplant. The SPK transplant operation is significantly larger in scope than the kidney transplant. It is usually performed in an intraperitoneal fashion. There is more dissection and bowel manipulation during the operation. The return of bowel function often is delayed for several days. Also, many of these patients may have associated diabetic gastroparesis and a prolonged ileus. If the exocrine secretions of the pancreas graft are drained via the bladder, the transplant recipients also may lose a significant amount of fluids, due to loss of exocrine secretions rich in bicarbonate. Uncomplicated SPK patients typically do not require nutrition support; however, if they have a prolonged ileus, nutrition support may be indicated.

27.2.2 LIVER TRANSPLANTATION

The common indications for liver transplantation in the U.S. are cirrhosis of the liver due to hepatitis C and Laennec's (alcoholic) cirrhosis, as well as cholestatic diseases such as primary biliary cirrhosis and primary sclerosing cholangitis.[1] After a successful liver transplant, liver function usually steadily improves, and most patients achieve "good" liver function quickly. Once the new liver graft's physiologic makeup is sufficiently intact to handle basic synthesis and clearance of metabolic wastes, the intensive care unit (ICU) management mainly consists of replacing ongoing fluid losses and avoiding injury to the graft liver during the period of recovery. Advances in liver transplant surgical techniques have resulted in shortened ICU stay (median ICU stay for a liver transplant recipient at our center is one day) with early resumption of oral diet.[9] The liver transplant operation usually does not involve a bowel anastamosis, except in patients with primary sclerosing cholangitis who undergo a Roux-en-Y bile duct anastamosis. Thus, the return of bowel function occurs with in one or two days. Based on a global assessment of patient nutritional status, the majority of liver transplant recipients demonstrate moderate to severe malnutrition.[10] A practice in some transplant programs is to place a nasojejunal feeding tube at the time of the liver transplant operation so that enteral feeding can be initiated within 12 hours after transplantation. Oral diet is initiated after return of bowel function. Once a patient has adequate oral calorie intake, the feeding tube is removed.

27.2.3 SMALL BOWEL TRANSPLANTATION

The common indications for small bowel transplantation are short gut syndrome and congenital atresias.[11] In all small bowel transplant recipients, the distal transplant bowel is always brought out as an ostomy. After the operation, the small bowel starts functioning within the first few postoperative days. Ostomy losses of up to 100 ml/kg are acceptable and can be compensated for with supplemental intravenous fluids. Enteral nutrition is provided as soon as there is a return of intestinal function. In the absence of other clinical complications, enteral feedings are started on the third to fifth postoperative day.

27.2.4 HEART TRANSPLANTATION

The *sine qua non* consideration for heart transplantation is refractory congestive heart failure and severe functional limitation despite maximal medical therapy. Ischemic heart disease has become the number-one indication after idiopathic cardiomyopathy. Most patients require inotropic support for the first 12 to 24 hours after heart transplantation. Oral diets may begin as early as one to two days postoperatively.[12]

27.2.5 LUNG TRANSPLANTATION

Common indications for lung transplantation include cystic fibrosis, chronic obstructive pulmonary disease, bronchiectasis, and pulmonary hypertension.[12] A single- or double-lung transplant may be done. Patients with cystic fibrosis and broncheictasis are at high risk of malnutrition due to increased calorie needs from increased work of breathing and malabsorption.[12] An oral diet is usually initiated following extubation. Prolonged ventilation necessitates the initiation of tube feedings.

27.3 NUTRITION THERAPY

27.3.1 MALNUTRITION

Malnutrition is a risk factor for surgery and transplantation.[13,14] It is known to prolong posttransplantation ventilatory support and increase posttransplant hospital length of stay, infection rates, and mortality before and after transplantation.[14–19]

27.3.2 NUTRITION SUPPORT INDICATIONS

Although nutrition support is not necessary for transplant recipients who recover from surgery quickly and begin eating, it is almost always necessary for the critically ill, ICU-bound transplant patient. Transplant recipients who require ICU care are likely to be suffering from organ (possibly multiorgan) failure, sepsis, neurologic compromise, or all of these. A few of these patients may be allowed to eat or drink if they are not intubated, but even in this situation, oral intake usually is not adequate.

If a patient is well nourished and is expected to eat in less than three days, it is probably acceptable to wait to start nutrition support. However, many transplant recipients are malnourished, and nutrition support should not be delayed in those patients. Figure 27.1 outlines a decision tree to determine the need for nutrition support in critically ill transplant recipients.

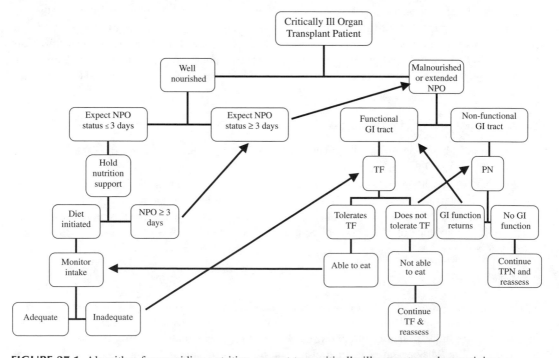

FIGURE 27.1 Algorithm for providing nutrition support to a critically ill organ transplant recipient.

The mode of nutrition support depends on gastrointestinal (GI) function. Parenteral nutrition is reserved for patients without GI function (e.g., ileus, high-output fistula, GI bleeding). Small bowel transplant recipients require PN until the transplanted graft recovers.[20–22] Although the goal is to establish enteral and oral nutrition in small bowel transplant recipients, PN may need to be reinstituted for severe intestinal graft rejection, major lymphatic leak, cytomegalovirus (CMV) enteritis, and graft dysmotility.[21,22] Increased stomal output and severe diarrhea may improve with administration of antidiarrheal agents, such as kaolin–pectin, loperamide, and opiates.[22] In fact, 50 to 75% of small bowel transplant recipients will require one of these drugs.[21] At the other end of the spectrum, prokinetics may help gastroparesis when it occurs.[22] D-xylose absorption and fecal excretion are used by some to monitor allograft function.[11]

Tube feeding (TF) is indicated for early postoperative feedings or supplementation when oral intake is not adequate (Figure 27.1). For small bowel transplant patients, TF can be initiated and PN tapered as TF and oral diet advance. The ideal TF formula for small bowel transplant recipients is yet to be determined. Some suggest using a semielemental formula; others use isotonic, intact-protein formulas with or without fiber. Glutamine may help promote epithelial and villous regeneration of a transplanted bowel.[23] It has been suggested to add 30 g glutamine/d (10 g powder mixed in water three times daily) to small bowel transplant recipients.[23] Some transplant centers also support the idea of giving insoluble fiber to small bowel transplant recipients (to help reduce bacterial translocation) as well as soluble fiber (to promote the restoration of villous functional capacity).[23]

Other types of transplant recipients tolerate a standard isotonic formula well. A high-nitrogen formula may be needed to meet protein needs, a concentrated formula may be helpful if a patient is hyponatremic or needs fluid restriction, and a fiber-containing formula may be helpful if a patient has constipation or diarrhea.[24]

Short-term TF access for critically ill transplant recipients is usually achieved with a nasoenteral tube. Feedings can be administered into the stomach if there is adequate gastric function. However, a majority of transplant patients may require a feeding tube placed into the small intestine because of reduced gastric emptying. A main cause of end-stage renal disease (ESRD) leading to kidney transplantation is DM. Because gastroparesis is common in these patients, postpyloric placement of an enteral feeding tube may be necessary. Likewise, patients undergoing pancreas transplantation usually have type 1 DM and often have gastroparesis. In one report of ten patients who underwent heart and lung transplantation, there also was an 83% incidence of symptomatic gastroparesis.[25] Postpyloric tubes are also preferred in immediate postoperative liver and small bowel transplant recipients. In small bowel transplant recipients, the nasointestinal route may be used, whereas other centers will surgically place a feeding jejunostomy or gastrostomy.[23]

Case reports illustrate the use of posttransplant tube feeding.[26,27] Lee et al. described the use of endoscopically placed nasogastrojejunal (NGJ) tubes for gastric decompression and jejunal feeding.[28] In 12 patients in the report who had undergone liver transplantation, no aspiration occurred and complications were self-removal, tube clogging, and migration of tube. Several randomized trials show that TF is tolerated in liver transplant recipients.[6–8,29] Wicks et al. randomized 24 patients to receive either PN or TF within 18 to 24 postoperative hours; PN and TF were tolerated well.[6] The number of days until diet initiation was not different between the PN and TF groups. Hasse et al. randomized 50 patients to receive either intravenous fluid (IVF) or postoperative TF.[7] There was a significant reduction in viral infections and a clinically relevant reduction in bacterial infections in the tube-fed group vs. the control group. More recently, a transplant group evaluated the effect of probiotics and TF in liver transplant recipients.[8] Thirty-two patients (group 1) were enterally fed with a 1.0 kcal/ml formula along with small bowel decontamination. Thirty-one patients (group 2) received a fiber-containing formula and *Lactobacillus plantarum* 299. Thirty-two patients (group 3) received the same fiber-containing formula with a placebo probiotic.[8] Infection rates were 48% in group 1, 34% in group 3, and 13% in group 2.

Providing enteral nutrition and probiotics to organ donors has also been proposed.[30] Five small bowel donors received a tube feeding formula containing arginine, glutamine, and n-3 fatty acids, along with *Lactobacillus plantarum* 299. Tube feeding continued after transplantation. The idea behind this protocol is to reduce infection by building a biologic shield from pathogenic organisms.[30]

Parenteral nutrition is used less frequently than enteral nutrition in transplant recipients. Indications for PN include ileus, high-output fistula, GI bleeding, and small bowel transplant failure. Only two studies in the literature evaluated PN in transplant recipients.[6,31] The study by Wicks et al. was discussed earlier. In the investigation by Reilly et al., 28 liver transplant patients were divided into three groups:[31]

- One group received no specific nutrition therapy
- The second received standard PN with 35 kcal/kg/d
- The third received PN with a branched chain–enriched amino acid solution

At the end of seven days, the PN groups had superior nitrogen balance, required a shorter period of posttransplant mechanical ventilation, and had shorter ICU stays. Also, the total hospital charges were the greatest in the group that received no nutrition support. It is unfortunate that this well designed study did not include a treatment arm that used TF, which could be delivered at a fraction of the cost of PN. Nevertheless, this study demonstrated the benefits of nutrition support in the ICU.

27.3.3 NUTRIENT NEEDS

Nutrient needs of transplant recipients have been outlined for the immediate posttransplant phase. However, nutrient requirements have not been delineated in transplant patients who develop medical or surgical complications and require ICU care. One could conjecture that the nutrient needs in a transplant patient during critical illness would mimic those of other types of patients with a critical illness (Table 27.1).[32–35]

TABLE 27.1
Nutrient Considerations in the Critically Ill Organ Transplant Recipient

Nutrition Recommendation	Comments
1.5 to 2.0 g protein/kg/d	Protein is needed for postoperative recovery and wound healing.
	Surgical stress and corticosteroids increase protein catabolic rate.
	Consider protein losses from surgical drains, fistulas, wounds, and dialysis.
	Glutamine may be helpful for small bowel transplant recipients. However, there is no research evaluating supplementation of arginine or glutamine in critically ill transplant patients.
130 to 150% of calculated basal energy expenditure (BEE)	If estimating calories, provide the upper limit of calories for underweight patients; provide the lower limit for overweight patients.
	Measure energy needs by indirect calorimetry in critically ill patients.

(continued)

TABLE 27.1 (CONTINUED)
Nutrient Considerations in the Critically Ill Organ Transplant Recipient

Nutrition Recommendation	Comments
50 to 70% of nonprotein calories as carbohydrate	Metabolic stress, infection, and medications (e.g., corticosteroids, cyclosporine, tacrolimus) can elevate serum glucose levels.
	Attain glucose control with insulin if needed; consider insulin drip for blood glucose levels consistently >150 mg/dl.
	Long-term, a combination of long- and short-acting insulin may be required for glucose control.
	Oral hypoglycemic agents can be considered if the patient can absorb, metabolize, and excrete the drug.
	Control glucose levels before advancing nutrition support.
30 to 50% of nonprotein calories as lipid	Increased lipid concentrations may be helpful temporarily when hyperglycemia is severe and not yet under control with insulin.
	Patients with cystic fibrosis and patients immediate post–small bowel transplant may malabsorb fat.
	There is no research on supplementation of fish oil (ω-3 fatty acids) in critically ill transplant patients.
1 ml fluid per calorie; adjust based on output	Monitor losses from urine, drains, wounds, diarrhea, nasogastric tube suction, fistulas, para- or thoracentesis.
	Exocrine secretions from a pancreas drained via the bladder can be as high as 2 to 3 l/d.
	Ostomy output from a small bowel transplant can be as high as 4 l/d.
	Restrict fluid if hyponatremia or excess water exists.
2 to 4 g sodium per day	Restrict if ascites or edema is severe.
	Correct hyponatremia slowly with fluid restriction and/or hypertonic sodium solution. There is a strong association with rapid resolution of hyponatremia and central pontine myelinolysis.
Individualize potassium prescription	Serum levels may increase with administration of tacrolimus, cyclosporine, or potassium-sparing diuretics; renal insufficiency; or metabolic acidosis. Infusion of red blood cells and fresh frozen plasma can contribute to hyperkalemia, as can hemolysis.
	Metabolic acidosis may also contribute to hyperkalemia.
	Serum levels may decrease with administration of potassium-wasting diuretics or amphotericin, refeeding syndrome, diarrhea, or fistulas.
	University of Wisconsin (UW) solution is an organ-preservation solution high in potassium. The solution is usually washed out of the liver before reperfusion but can still contribute to hyperkalemia.
1000 to 1500 mg calcium per day	Renal and hepatic disease lead to abnormal pretransplant calcium metabolism. If large amounts of citrated blood products are given to patients, there may be a low serum ionized calcium level.
Individualize phosphorus prescription	Serum levels may increase with renal insufficiency.
	Serum levels may decrease with refeeding syndrome or administration of corticosteroids.
Individualize magnesium prescription	Hypomagnesemia can occur due to:
	Increased GI losses from diarrhea, NG suction, fistula
	Increased urinary losses during diuretic phase of ATN and from calcineurin inhibitors
	Refeeding syndrome
	Losses from continuous renal replacement therapy
	Redistribution as in sepsis, massive blood transfusions
	Hypermagesemia occurs less often and is usually iatrogenic (e.g., administration of magnesium-containing antacids or renal insufficiency)
Evaluate acid–base status	Serum levels of bicarbonate often decrease due to exocrine losses of transplanted pancreas (bladder drainage) or losses from transplanted small intestine.

27.3.3.1 Calories

Measuring caloric needs via indirect calorimetry is preferred over estimating caloric needs. Underfeeding can lead to weight loss, muscle wasting (including respiratory muscles), and reduced immune defense. Overfeeding may lead to hyperglycemia and potentiate increased infection rates in an immunosuppressed host. Providing excess energy may also cause steatosis or difficulty in weaning from the ventilator.

27.3.3.2 Protein

Critically ill transplant patients have heightened protein requirements (up to 1.5 to 2.0 g/kg). Protein catabolic rate increases with surgical stress and administration of corticosteroids. Protein needs are also increased owing to losses from open wounds, surgical drains or chest tubes, dialysis, ostomy output, and para- or thoracentesis. Nitrogen balance studies may be helpful if renal function is adequate and it is possible to collect all losses.

27.3.3.3 Carbohydrate

Patients undergoing transplantation may have preexisting DM. As discussed earlier, DM is the primary indication for pancreas transplantation and is one of the leading causes of renal failure resulting in transplantation. In addition, patients with cystic fibrosis awaiting lung transplantation may have DM. DM is considered a comorbid condition that may complicate transplantation, but by itself is not a contraindication for transplantation.

Even in patients without previous DM history, posttransplant hyperglycemia frequently occurs, in part due to a metabolic stress response. However, immunosuppressive medications also cause hyperglycemia. Calcineurin inhibitors (tacrolimus and cyclosporine) decrease insulin secretion, increase insulin resistance, and exert a direct toxic effect on the beta cell.[36] Corticosteroids precipitate hyperglycemia by causing insulin resistance and perhaps through decreasing insulin receptor affinity, impairing peripheral glucose uptake in muscle, or activating glucose and free fatty acids.[36]

Tight glucose control has been shown to reduce mortality in critically ill patients.[37] One could theorize that tight glucose control would be important in transplant recipients who are prone to hyperglycemia and are at increased risk of infection (and increased mortality from infection) because of their immunosuppressed status. However, when the Van den Berghe paper is studied carefully, tight glucose control vs. standard glucose control did not reduce mortality in transplant recipients.[37]

27.3.3.4 Lipid

No studies in critically ill transplant patients have evaluated effects of different levels or types of enterally or parenterally administered fats. One potential benefit of an increased-fat diet would be better glucose control (due to the lower carbohydrate content). A theoretical downside would be further immune impairment and inflammatory state caused by n-6 fatty acids. A few studies evaluated n-3 fatty acids in stable transplant recipients.[38–42]

Supplementation of fish oil vs. corn oil for two months improved renal hemodynamics in liver transplant recipients maintained on a cyclosporine regimen.[43] In kidney transplant recipients, fish oil supplementation has been shown to improve renal transplant graft function and reduce adverse nephrotoxic effects of cyclosporine.[38–40] In addition, serum triglyceride concentrations, platelet aggregation, and blood pressure were reduced.[38–40]

Alexander et al. evaluated the effect of the combination of canola oil and arginine on kidney transplant function in 95 stable kidney transplant recipients.[42] Half of the study group ingested an arginine supplement (2% of energy) and canola oil (15% of energy of an 1800-calorie diet). All patients received cyclosporine-based immunosuppression. Of the patients who received kidneys

TABLE 27.2
Vitamin and Mineral Considerations for Critically Ill Transplant Recipients

Nutrient	Considerations
Fat-soluble vitamins	Possible deficiency due to fat malabsorption and bile diversion
	Vitamin A necessary for wound healing
	Active form of vitamin D may be deficient with prior liver or renal failure
	Vitamin K is necessary for normal blood clotting; short-term supplementation (e.g., 3 days) may be necessary after liver transplantation
B vitamins and folate	Hyperhomocysteinemia in kidney transplant recipients is correlated with renal function and folate, vitamin B_6, and vitamin B_{12} status
	Alcoholism can cause deficiency of B vitamins
Vitamin C	Necessary for wound healing

from deceased donors, 37% of the control group experienced rejection, compared with 7% of the supplemented group. This study evaluated only kidney transplant recipients taking cyclosporine (vs. another type of transplant immunosuppression regimen), and these patients were not critically ill. However, this research suggests that immunomodulation via nutrients can affect transplant outcomes. In addition, although these studies show some promise in stable patients, expecting similar results in critically ill patients with varying types of organ transplants would be pure conjecture.

Another consideration of lipids relates to fat absorption. In the initial stages after small bowel transplantation, fat malabsorption will occur, due to disruption of the lymphatic system. Regeneration of the lymphatic vessels occurs over time, but a low-fat diet is recommended for the first 4 to 6 weeks after intestinal transplantation.[20] If a liver transplant patient's bile is being diverted away from the intestine (such as via an external biliary drain), fat absorption may be impaired. Lung transplant recipients with cystic fibrosis may have malabsorption of long-chain fatty acids. In all of these instances, providing some fat as medium-chain triglycerides (MCTs) may improve caloric absorption.

27.3.3.5 Fluid

General fluid needs are approximately 30 ml/kg, but determination of fluid rates must be individualized. Fluid restriction is indicated for cases of volume overload, reduced urine output, and hyponatremia. Fluid resuscitation is necessary if a patient has increased losses (from ostomy, drains, chest tubes, high urine output, gastric tube output, emesis, diarrhea) or hypernatremia.

27.3.3.6 Vitamins and Minerals

There are no studies delineating vitamin requirements for stable transplant recipients, let alone critically ill patients. Nutrient levels are affected by original diagnosis, prehospitalization condition, medication therapy, and comorbid conditions. General considerations are outlined in Table 27.2.

27.3.4 DRUG–NUTRIENT CONSIDERATIONS

One cannot discuss nutrition therapy for transplant recipients without reviewing the nutritional implications of immunosuppressive drugs. Although immunosuppressive drugs are mandatory, the type and combination of drugs are individualized according to transplant type, patient characteristics, and transplant center protocols. Table 27.3 outlines the major immunosuppressive drugs and their nutritional ramifications.

TABLE 27.3
Major Side Effects of Commonly Used Immunosuppressive Medications

	Antilymphocyte serum	Azathioprine	Basiliximab	Daclizumab	Corticosteroids	Cyclosporine	Muromonab-CD3	Mycophenolate mofetil	Sirolimus	Tacrolimus
Anorexia							✔			
Bone marrow suppression		✔						✔	✔	
Diarrhea	✔	✔					✔	✔		
Dysgeusia		✔								
Fever and chills	✔						✔			
Gastrointestinal distress								✔	✔	✔
Hyperglycemia					✔	✔				✔
Hyperkalemia						✔				✔
Hyperlipidemia					✔	✔			✔	
Hyperphagia					✔					
Hypertension					✔	✔				✔
Hypomagnesemia						✔				✔
Impaired wound healing					✔				✔	
Macrocytic anemia		✔								
Nausea and vomiting	✔	✔					✔			✔
Neurotoxicity						✔				✔
Osteoporosis					✔					
Pancreatitis		✔			✔					
Sodium retention					✔					
Sore throat/mucositis		✔								
Ulcers					✔					
No known nutrition side effect			✔	✔						

Source: Adapted from Hasse J. and Robien K. Nutrition support guidelines for therapeutically immunosuppressed patients. In: Pichard C. and Kudsk K.A., Eds. *Update in Intensive Care and Emergency Medicine: From Nutrition Support to Pharmacologic Nutrition in the ICU.* Springer-Verlag, Heidelberg, 2000, 361–383.

27.4 COMPLICATIONS AND NUTRITION CONSIDERATIONS IN CRITICALLY ILL TRANSPLANT RECIPIENTS

Although the medical course of each transplant patient cannot be fully predicted, several potential complications can occur. Transplant patients are at risk for graft dysfunction and rejection, infection, renal failure, respiratory failure, GI complications, hyperglycemia, and other complications.

27.4.1 GRAFT DYSFUNCTION

27.4.1.1 Medical Considerations

The causes of graft dysfunction can be classified into early and late causes. The common early causes include:

- Primary nonfunction
- Preservation injury
- Vascular thrombosis
- Acute rejection

The late causes include:

- Chronic rejection
- Recurrence of primary disease
- Posttransplant lymphoproliferative disorder

Primary nonfunction is defined as a transplant that has not functioned. These patients will have severe organ failure. For example, a patient with primary nonfuction after liver transplantation will manifest failure to regain consciousness and sustained elevation in transaminases (increasing coagulopathy, acidosis, and poor bile production). Primary nonfunction is rarely seen since improved organ preservation solutions, such as the University of Wisconsin (UW) solution, have been introduced. The treatment of primary nonfunction is retransplantation with a new organ.

Preservation injury is associated with preservation of an organ to transport it from donor to recipient. After procurement from a deceased donor, the organs are transported in cold UW solution. The time from the organ procurement to the implantation into a recipient is called the *cold ischemia time*. The optimal cold ischemia time for a kidney or pancreas is < 24 h, < 12 h for liver, < 4 h for heart, < 6 h for lungs, and < 12 h for small intestine. Longer cold ischemia times can result in organ dysfunction, due to preservation injury.

Vascular thrombosis often presents acutely, and immediate surgical operative intervention is required. Acute rejections are common in all organs. The first line of treatment for acute rejection often is the administration of high-dose corticosteroids (e.g., 1 g of methylprednisolone for 3 d). If this fails, antibody preparations, such as muromonab CD3 or antithymocyte globulin, may be used.

Chronic rejection is less common but is difficult to treat; retransplantation is the solution in most patients. Recurrent disease can be addressed with standard medical therapy but may require retransplantation. Due to the prolonged immunosuppression, transplant patients are prone to lymphomas. The B cell lymphomas are driven by the Epstein–Barr virus. The treatment of posttransplant lymphomas can be successfully treated with reduction or withdrawal of immunosuppression and specific chemotherapy.[44]

There are several immunosuppressive drug protocols in use in solid organ transplantation. They usually are developed by an individual center, taking into account local experience and preferences. Most protocols will include a calcineurin inhibitor (tacrolimus or cylcosporine) and steroids. Mycophenolate mofetil (MMF) and sirolimus are increasingly being used as third agents. The side effects of the various drugs are listed in Table 27.3.

MMF causes significant GI side effects, such as diarrhea and nausea. The GI side effects are dose dependent (as established in the renal transplantation trials). When these side effects are significant and other etiology is ruled out, the first step would be to adjust the drug dose by giving the same daily dose by dividing it into three or four doses per day. This step alone frequently reduces the GI side effects. If the change in dosing frequency does not result in improvement of side effects, reducing the dosage by 50% is advised. Most patients tolerate a dose reduction; discontinuation of the drug is rarely necessitated for control of side effects.

27.4.1.2 Nutritional Considerations

If a patient experiences primary nonfunction or complete graft failure, end-stage organ failure is present and nutrition therapy guidelines should correspond to those for the specific organ dysfunction. For example, if a kidney transplant graft fails, dialysis will be required and potassium and phosphorus restriction may be needed. If a small bowel transplant fails, PN needs to be resumed. If pancreas transplantation fails, then insulin therapy must be resumed.

Preservation injury may cause delayed graft function. For example, if urine output is low following renal transplantation due to delayed graft function, intake may need to be limited as well. Because preservation injury will resolve given enough time, there is no permanent nutrition therapy adjustment needed in these instances.

As mentioned earlier, when a transplant graft rejects, the traditional rejection therapy is to heighten corticosteroid doses over a few days, starting with a high dose and tapering down to a maintenance dose. As mentioned earlier, this results in protein catabolism and increased protein needs. Adding or changing immunosuppressive drugs may create GI symptoms or cause other drug or nutrient interactions (see Table 27.3).

If chronic rejection ensues, the patient may exhibit symptoms of organ dysfunction. If organ dysfunction is great enough, nutrition therapy may need to be adjusted. For example, chronic rejection of a kidney will lead to dialysis and nutrition therapy adjustments for hyperkalemia, hyperphosphatemia, and reduced urine output.

27.4.2 INFECTION/SEPSIS

27.4.2.1 Medical Considerations

Infections continue to be the leading cause of mortality in solid organ transplantation. Immunosuppression is the main risk factor. A well defined temporal sequence of infections is present in the posttransplant period.[45] The typical time table is divided into three parts: first month, 1 to 6 months, and the late period. In the first month after transplant, the major infectious complications include postsurgical bacterial and *Candida* wound infections, postoperative pneumonia, and central line infections. These infectious complications are later followed by others, unique to the transplant patients, which include viral infections, mainly cytomegalovirus (CMV), Epstein–Barr virus, herpes simplex virus, *Pneumocystis carinii*, and *Cryptococcus neoformans*. Cytomegalovirus infection usually presents with fever, malaise, leukopenia, and pneumonitis.[46] Invasive CMV of the gastrointestinal tract may present with diarrhea. Confirmation is obtained by doing a blood PCR and for invasive gastrointestinal disease; a biopsy of the stomach or colon will reveal diagnostic CMV inclusion bodies.

A very aggressive approach is used for treatment of infections in transplant recipients. Intravenous antibiotics, with a broad spectrum covering both Gram-positive and -negative bacterial organisms, are initiated immediately; upon receipt of culture reports and sensitivities, specific antibiotics are used. Fungal prophylaxis is also used in high-risk patients. Cytomegalovirus infections are treated with intravenous ganciclovir for 2 to 4 weeks. Drugs such as sulfamethoxazole/trimethoprim are commonly used for prophylaxis of *Pneumocystis carinii*. Fluconazole, caspofungin, and amphotericin B are the commonly used antifungal agents.

27.4.2.2 Nutritional Considerations

Malnourished patients have an increased risk of developing infection. In addition, many antimicrobial agents cause GI symptoms, including diarrhea, nausea, and vomiting. Antidiarrheal agents, fiber, or pectin-containing substances (such as banana flakes) may help minimize diarrhea and potential skin breakdown.

27.4.3 ACUTE RENAL FAILURE

27.4.3.1 Medical Considerations

Acute renal failure is usually defined as an abrupt decrease in glomerular filtration rate caused by intrinsic renal disease or alteration in intrarenal hemodynamics, resulting in the accumulation of waste products (urea, creatinine, and potassium) in the blood. Renal failure complicates the medical management of the transplant patient, leading to increased morbidity and mortality.[47] The causes of renal failure may be prerenal (dehydration, fluid losses, or surgical hemorrhage), renal (drug toxicity from immunosuppression with tacrolimus or cylcosporine or acute tubular necrosis), or, usually, a combination of both.

Infection may also indirectly contribute to renal failure. The treatment will depend on the etiology — fluid resuscitation and correction of hypovolemia in dehydration and, in case of drug toxicity, stopping the offending drug. Temporary dialysis is often necessary, especially when hypervolemia, hyperkalemia, metabolic acidosis, or uremic symptoms occur.

27.4.3.2 Nutritional Considerations

When a critically ill transplant recipient develops renal insufficiency, adjustments in nutrition therapy may be required. Acid–base and electrolyte requirements may be altered. If hemodialysis is employed, restrictions of fluid, potassium, and phosphorus may be needed. If continuous renal replacement therapy (RRT) is used, patients may actually need additional potassium, magnesium, or phosphorus. Fluid restriction may not be necessary if the renal replacement therapy can remove adequate fluid amounts. Occasionally, renal failure may not require RRT, but potassium, phosphorus, magnesium, or fluid restrictions may be necessary. Generally, transplant patients who develop acute renal failure are catabolic and protein is not restricted.

27.4.4 RESPIRATORY FAILURE

27.4.4.1 Medical Considerations

Patients after liver, small bowel, pancreas, heart, and lung transplantation are usually received from the operating room to the ICU intubated. Often, after an uncomplicated posttransplant recovery, patients are extubated within 24 to 48 hours. However, if patients develop graft dysfunction or sepsis and hemodynamic instability, they may require prolonged respiratory support. The other indications for respiratory support include primary lung infections, like severe bacterial pneumonia, CMV pneumonia, and acute respiratory distress syndrome as part of sepsis. It is important to note that prolonged use of propofol for sedation in a patient who is being ventilated can cause severe hyperlipidemia.

27.4.4.2 Nutritional Considerations

When patients require mechanical ventilation, TF will be required. If mechanical ventilation is prolonged, it may be prudent to have a swallow evaluation prior to allowing a patient to eat. If aspiration occurs, pneumonia will develop and further compromise the patient's respiratory status.

27.4.5 GASTROINTESTINAL COMPLICATIONS

If an ileus develops in a critically ill patient who requires nutrition support, PN should be initiated. An active GI bleed, high-output fistula, or nonfunctioning transplanted intestinal graft would also warrant PN. Diarrhea can occur as a result of MMF, antibiotics, or other drugs. Diarrhea is common following small bowel transplantation, due to rapid transit from loss of the ileocecal valve or extrinsic neuronal control, as well as malabsorption and bacterial overgrowth.[21] Treatment of diarrhea in a transplant patient may include changing medications; adding antidiarrheal medications, fiber, or pectin; and replacing fluid and electrolyte losses.

27.4.6 ACID–BASE BALANCE DISORDERS

Acid–base disorders are caused by clinical circumstances that lead to biochemical dysfunction and accumulation of acid or loss of base. The most common acid–base balance disorder in transplant patients is metabolic acidemia of septic shock, where there is failure to supply tissue with sufficient blood flow and oxygen to meet the mitochondrial aerobic metabolism.[48] The treatment is to correct the etiology of septic shock and, if the pH is less than 7.2, give a slow intravenous infusion of bicarbonate. Acidosis can also occur from loss of sodium salt in a fluid with high bicarbonate, such as with the loss of exocrine secretions in pancreas transplant or with severe diarrhea or losses from ostomy in a small bowel transplant. The treatment is replacement of bicarbonate.[48] Metabolic alkalosis can occur in patients with prolonged vomiting or nasogastric drainage. When gastric juices rich in hydrochloric acid are lost and extracellular water and sodium become depleted, hormonal responses increase aldosterone. With more of the mineralcorticoid influence, more bicarbonate is transported to the already alkalemic plasma. This alkalosis problem is easily corrected by infusion of saline solution to restore intravascular volume and the administration of supplemental potassium chloride if potassium levels are low.[48]

27.4.7 HYPERGLYCEMIA

27.4.7.1 Medical Considerations

As mentioned several times, immunosuppressed patients are at increased risk for infection. When infection occurs, it is a serious complication. Poorly controlled glucose levels are a risk factor for infection.

Causes of hyperglycemia include drugs (discussed earlier) and metabolic distress. Type 2 DM is common in transplant patients, especially in renal transplant patients who may have required a kidney transplant for end-stage renal disease due to diabetic nephropathy.

27.4.7.2 Nutritional Considerations

Adequate glucose control is imperative. If a patient has a persistently high glucose level, an insulin drip may be necessary. Otherwise, a combination of long-acting insulin and short-acting insulin should be used to treat hyperglycemia. Oral agents can be considered if patients have the ability to absorb, metabolize, and excrete them normally.

27.5 CASE STUDY

27.5.1 HISTORY AND BACKGROUND

The case study patient is a 52-year-old male with Laennec's cirrhosis who presented for liver transplant evaluation. He was diagnosed with hepatopulmonary syndrome (HPS) and had been receiving a continuous intravenous infusion of epoprosterol (Flolan; Glaxo SmithKline, Research Park Triangle, NC) for 6 months. He had been abstinent from alcohol for 1 1/2 years and had been actively attending Alcoholics Anonymous meetings three times per week.

At his initial evaluation, the patient weighed 241 pounds (height, 69 inches). His usual weight was 282 pounds, but the patient had been intentionally losing weight for approximately two years. He reported that his appetite had decreased since the epoprosterol was initiated. He also complained of frequent nausea, early satiety, and diarrhea. These symptoms were consistent with side effects of epoprosterol and end-stage liver failure. The patient and his wife were counseled on a 2 g sodium diet. Because the patient was consuming < 1000 calories per day (based on a dietary recall), emphasis was placed on improving the patient's calorie and protein intake.

The patient was assigned a MELD score of 29 (Model for End-stage Liver Disease to determine waiting list priority, based on a scale of 6 to 40), based on the exception criteria for HPS. He returned home and was under the care of his primary-care physician. He presented two months later to the transplant center, when a suitable donor liver was available, to undergo liver transplantation. During the two months prior to transplantation, he lost an additional 40 pounds unintentionally due to anorexia, dysgeusia, early satiety, nausea, and diarrhea.

In order to qualify for transplantation, the patient's mean pulmonary pressure had to remain < 30 to 35 mm Hg. Prognosis is poor for patients undergoing transplantation whose mean pressures exceed this range.[49] The patient was admitted to the ICU in order to check pulmonary pressures prior to being prepared for surgery. A Swan–Ganz catheter was placed; mean pulmonary pressures were between 28 and 30 mm Hg. These readings were acceptable, so the patient was sent to the operating room to undergo liver transplantation with a liver from a deceased donor.

27.5.2 POSTOPERATIVE DAYS 1 TO 3 — IMMEDIATE POSTSURGICAL PERIOD

The patient tolerated the 3 1/2-hour operation well and was transported to the ICU in a stable but critical condition. To prevent rejection, the immunosuppressive drugs tacrolimus and prednisolone were initiated. To prevent infection, antimicrobial agents including ganciclovir, imipenem/cilastin, and fluconazole were added to the patient's medication regimen. Epoprosterol infusion continued.

Nutrient needs were calculated to be 2400 calories (130% basal energy expenditure calculated by Harris–Benedict equation) and 135 g pro/day (1.5 g pro/kg). On postoperative day 1, tube feedings were initiated via a nasoduodenal tube that was placed during surgery (Table 27.4). An elevation in liver function tests (LFTs) reflected mild preservation injury from the organ preservation solution (see Table 27.5 for laboratory values). The patient was hypotensive, and phenylephrine hydrochloride (neosynephrine) infusion was required. One day later, the patient was extubated and alert. The patient required no pressors. A transfer from the ICU to the nursing ward was planned; however, the patient developed a fever (102.5°F) and his urine output dropped dramatically. Therefore, transfer was halted. It was originally felt that the patient was volume contracted from overdiuresis. A 500 ml bolus of normal saline was given intravenously. He was awake and was requiring 4 l oxygen via a face mask. His oxygen saturation was 90 to 95%. Later in the day, the patient's oxygen saturation dropped; ultimately, he required reintubation. Propofol and doxacurium infusions were begun to sedate the patient. A Swan–Ganz catheter was inserted, and the mean pulmonary pressure was 42 mm Hg. A continuous infusion of bumetanide was begun to help diurese the patient, who was now felt to be volume overloaded.

27.5.3 POSTOPERATIVE DAYS 4 TO 14 — SEPSIS AND MULTIORGAN DYSFUNCTION

By postoperative day 4, the patient spiked a temperature of 101.5°F and had nonoliguric acute renal failure and a sudden onset of hypotension. Phenylephrine hydrochloride infusion was restarted. Because sepsis was suspected, blood and urine cultures were drawn, a bronchoscopy was performed to look for a source of infection, and the patient returned to the operating room for exploratory laparotomy and wash out. The patient received gentamicin and piperacillin/tazobactam empirically. Prior to the return to the operating room, the patient was receiving a 1.2 cal/ml, high-nitrogen formula at 60 ml/h via his feeding tube (providing 1728 calories, 80 g protein).

TABLE 27.4

Nutrition Support Regimen in a Critically Ill Transplant Case Study Patient

Post-Transplant Day	Tube Feeding Formula and Rate	Tube Feeding Intake (Calories/g protein)	Oral Intake (Calories/g protein)	Comments
1	1.2 cal/ml high-nitrogen formula @ 20 ml/h	576/27		Immediate postoperative tube feeding protocol
2	1.2 cal/ml high-nitrogen formula @ 40 ml/h	1152/54		Advancement per protocol
3	1.2 cal/ml high-nitrogen formula @ 60 ml/h	1728/80		Advancement per protocol
4	1 cal/ml high-nitrogen formula @ 10 ml/h	240/15		Patient returned to surgery; propofol providing 588 calories
7	1 cal/ml high-nitrogen formula @ 90 ml/h	2160/136		Increased stooling; probiotic added; propofol discontinued
13	1.2 cal/ml high-nitrogen formula @ 100 ml/h	2880/134		Measured resting energy expenditure: 2914 calories
15	1.2 cal/ml high-nitrogen formula @ 60 ml/h × 24 h; then to 90 ml/h	1728/80		Tube feeding infused via nasojejunal tube; formula coming out nasogastric tube; rate reduced and x-ray ordered to check placement of tubes
19	1.2 cal/ml high-nitrogen formula at 75 ml/h	2160/101		Measured resting energy expenditure = 2200 calories
23	1.2 cal/ml, high-nitrogen, fiber-containing formula @ 85 ml/h	2448/114		Fiber added to add bulk to stools
28	1.2 cal/ml, high-nitrogen, fiber-containing formula @ 75 ml/h	2160/101	325/6	Full liquid diet with honey-thick liquids initiated
29	Feeding tube displaced; patient refuses replacement		385/20	Diet advanced to mechanical soft diet with honey-thick liquids; oxandrolone prescribed
30			1020/40	
31			900/35	
32			860/64	Diet changed to regular with thin liquids; high-calorie shakes added
33			1200/39	
34			1315/37	Fiber, banana flakes, multivitamin, and vitamin C added
35			1800/87	
37			2400/128	
38			2135/90	
39			3155/116	Patient discharged the next day

TABLE 27.5
Serum Laboratory Values in a Critically Ill Liver Transplant Case Study Patient

Post-operative Day	Total Bilirubin (0.2–1.3 mg/dl)	Alkaline Phosphatase (40–129 U/l)	Aspartate Amino-transferase (10–50 U/l)	Alanine Amino-transferase (10–50 U/l)	γ-Glutamyl Transpep-tidase (8–61 U/l)	Sodium (136–145 mEq/l)	Potassium (3.6–5.0 mEq/l)	Blood Urea Nitrogen (9–20 mg/dl)	Creatinine (0.7–1.2 mg/dl)	Glucose (75–110 mg/dl)
0	5.4	73	871	423	36	140	4.8	37	1.2	170
4	9.6	98	53	195	213	147	5.1	148	2.9	183
8	8.3	175	54	47	262	135	3.9	71	2.0	130
12	4.3	260	197	175	273	133	4.2	89	1.2	101
16	1.8	381	22	31	189	146	4.9	91	0.8	129
20	2.6	486	32	49	300	143	3.6	74	0.7	134
24	1.8	312	24	30	123	152	5.0	98	1.8	116
32	1.5	154	23	24	79	136	2.8	24	0.6	78
40	1.4	81	19	36	49	138	4.8	30	0.9	85

Following reoperation, the patient was sedated with propofol (providing 588 cal/d). His serum glucose levels were elevated, requiring about 15 units of regular insulin via a sliding scale per day. NPH insulin was initiated — 14 units in the morning and 10 units at night. He required intermediate-acting insulin for only 3 days; glucose was controlled thereafter with subcutaneous regular insulin injections based on a sliding scale. The tube feeding was changed to a 1 cal/ml, high-nitrogen formula to meet estimated needs more closely while receiving propofol.

On postoperative day 5, the patient was in septic shock. He had respiratory failure, requiring mechanical ventilation (FiO_2 of 90%), and renal failure, requiring the initiation of continuous veno–venous hemodiafiltration (CVVHDF). The patient was sedated and unresponsive; pulmonary infiltrates suggesting pneumonia or acute respiratory distress syndrome (ARDS) were identified on postoperative day 6. The patient appeared to have septic inflammatory response syndrome (SIRS) with preservation injury of the liver. The FiO_2 on the ventilator was reduced to 70%, suggesting some improvement in the pulmonary process; unfortunately, the FiO_2 level still exceeded the upper limit of acceptable values to be able to perform indirect calorimetry. The propofol was discontinued, and an ativan infusion was initiated for sedation. The tube feeding formula was infusing at 90 ml/h, providing 2160 calories and 136 g protein.

The next day, the FiO_2 was increased to 90%, a temperature of 101.3°F was measured, and hypotension required the patient to receive two pressors. Serum levels of bilirubin and γ-glutamyl transpeptidase increased (Table 27.5). Although it was felt that the elevation in LFTs was due to sepsis, a liver biopsy was performed to rule out rejection. The biopsy did not show any signs of rejection, just signs of nonspecific portal infiltrates. The patient continued to have respiratory failure, requiring mechanical ventilation, and renal failure, requiring CVVHDF. The patient began to have diarrhea; stool cultures were sent for analysis. Medications that could have been responsible for the onset of diarrhea included antibiotics and MMF. A probiotic product was added to the patient's regimen to combat the negative effects of antibiotics on the gut flora. The patient continued to have fevers and be hypotensive; a third pressor was added on postoperative day 10. *E. coli* and *Hemophilus influenzae* were cultured from the sputum. Treatment included imepenem, vancomycin, and gentamicin. By this time (postoperative days 11 and 12), the ventilator settings were reduced and the patient required only one pressor. Then, the patient had an upper GI bleed with "coffee grounds" being suctioned out of the nasogastric tube. This resolved in 24 hours. LFTs were elevated again, suggesting either rejection or shock liver. The *Clostridia difficile* culture from 4 days earlier was negative, and the patient was having soft stools.

27.5.4 POSTOPERATIVE DAYS 15 TO 23 — RECOVERY

Finally, by POD 15, the patient was more arousable. He developed high-output acute tubular necrosis (ATN), and CVVHDF was discontinued. Pressors and sedating agents were also discontinued. A metabolic cart study was performed (FiO_2 of 30%). The measured resting energy expenditure was 2914 calories (32 cal/kg). The tube feeding formula was changed to a 1.2 cal/ml, high-nitrogen formula at 100 ml/h (2880 calories, 134 g protein). Although the patient appeared to awake, he was not alert. A CT scan of his head on postoperative day 18 revealed no abnormalities. A CT of the abdomen and pelvis on the same day showed no abscess, but a chest CT revealed pulmonary infiltrates. The patient began to wake up and was following commands but was yet too obtunded to extubate. Pressors and epoprosterol were discontinued on day 19. A metabolic cart study was repeated. The REE had decreased to 2200 calories, suggesting a lowered metabolic rate with improvement in the patient's condition. The tube feeding rate was reduced to provide 2160 calories and 100 g protein. Free water was added as water flushes via the feeding tube, and IV dextrose solution to treat hypernatremia (serum sodium level — 150 mg/dl). The tip of the dialysis catheter was cultured and found to be positive for staphalococcus, and the tip of the Swan–Ganz catheter grew Gram-positive coccobacilli. Epoprosterol was restarted on postoperative day 20. The patient was awake and afebrile and had a stable blood pressure and good urine output. His sepsis, respiratory failure, and acute renal failure were resolving, and he was extubated the next day.

27.5.5 POSTOPERATIVE DAYS 23 TO 41 — REHABILITATION

On postoperative day 23, the patient was transferred out of the ICU to the transplant ward. The patient required 2 to 3 l oxygen via nasal cannula and remained on epoprosterol. He had a stage 4 sacral decubiti. Enterostomal therapy specialists were managing care of the wound. The tube feeding formula was changed to a high-fiber formula to add bulk to the stools. The patient's mental status improved, and a bedside swallow evaluation was performed by a speech therapist on postoperative day 26. The patient had a delayed swallow and showed inconsistent signs and symptoms of aspiration. A dysphagiagram was performed the next day; it revealed that the patient silently aspirated thin and nectar-thickened liquids. He was not able to clear penetrated material with a cough. The speech therapist recommended the patient begin to eat a mechanical soft diet and honey-thickened liquids using swallowing precautions (sit at a 90-degree angle, eat small bites, and take medications in applesauce). The patient began to eat a honey-thick-consistency liquid diet. He did not like the thickened liquid and was eating < 350 calories per day. His feeding tube was displaced; the patient was scheduled to have the feeding tube replaced. However, the patient asked for a "second chance" to see if he could eat adequately. High-calorie, high-protein shakes were provided. A consult was placed for a physical medicine physician to review the patient's case and determine his qualification for transfer to a rehabilitation hospital. On day 29, the physical medicine physician did not feel that the patient had adequate strength to participate in the rigorous physical therapy provided at the rehabilitation hospital. Oxandrolone (an anabolic steroid) was administered to help the patient regain lean body mass.

A neurology consult was ordered on postoperative day 30 because the patient was experiencing some right arm paresis. The neurologist felt that the patient had myopathy, likely due to cortico-steroids and deconditioning. The patient's history of alcohol abuse may have contributed to this neuropathy. The recommendation was made to continue with physical medicine and rehabilitation. The patient participated in physical therapy and was making progress with his strengthening. On postoperative day 33, his dysphagiagram was repeated. Aspiration occurred only if the patient took large sips of thin liquids with a straw. The patient was allowed to eat a regular diet and any liquid consistency, provided he took small sips. His oral intake improved steadily (see Table 27.5). The physical medicine physician reevaluated the patient; the patient was able to tolerate longer periods of physical therapy and qualified to transfer to the rehabilitation hospital. He was placed on a waiting list for a bed at the rehabilitation hospital. His LFTs and renal function were adequate. His stage 4 decubitis caused pain but was healing and granulating.

Over the next several days, the patient continued to work with physical therapy. By postoperative day 42, the patient's physical status had improved sufficiently to allow him to discharge to the transplant outpatient housing and receive outpatient physical therapy without need to transfer to the rehabilitation hospital. He was eating 2100 to 3100 calories and 90 to 130 g protein daily. The patient continued to be seen by a physician in the liver transplant clinic 1 to 2 times weekly. His appetite remained adequate. He and his wife attended a series of required outpatient transplant nutrition classes.

Three months after his transplant, he was discharged home to be under the medical care of his primary-care physician. The epoprosterol infusion continued until 5 months after the liver transplant. He remains in excellent health, with good liver allograft function 7 months after transplantation.

27.6 SUMMARY

Providing nutrition care to transplant recipients is challenging. When a transplant patient becomes critically ill, the challenges heighten. Not only does the transplant team need to consider the nutritional status and nutrient needs of the critically ill transplant patient, they must also consider all of the alterations in nutrient metabolism, requirements, and delivery that are affected by graft function, immunosuppressive drugs, infection, and other organ failures.

REFERENCES

1. United Network for Organ Sharing web site. Available at http://www.unos.org. Accessed January 8, 2004.
2. URREA, UNOS. *2002 Annual Report of the U.S. Organ Procurement and Transplantation Network and the Scientific Registry of Transplant Recipients: Transplant Data 1992–2001* [Internet]. HHS/HRSA/OSP/DOT, Rockville, MD, 2003 [modified 2003 Feb 18; cited 2003 Nov 4]. Available from http://www.optn.org/data/annualReport.asp.
3. Held, P. et al., The impact of HLA mismatches on the survival of the first cadaveric kidney transplant, *N. Engl. J. Med.,* 331, 765, 1994.
4. Starzl, T.E. et al., Orthotopic homotransplantations of the human liver, *Ann. Surg.,* 168, 392, 1968.
5. Lochs, H. and Plauth, M., Liver cirrhosis: rationale and modalities for nutritional support — the European Society of Parenteral and Enteral Nutrition consensus and beyond, *Curr. Opin. Clin. Nutr. Metab. Care,* 2, 345, 1999.
6. Wicks, C. et al., Comparison of enteral feeding and TPN after liver transplantation, *Lancet,* 344, 837, 1994.
7. Hasse, J.M. et al., Early enteral nutrition support in patients undergoing liver transplantation, *J. Parenter. Enteral Nutr.,* 19, 437, 1995.
8. Rayes, N. et al., Early enteral supply of lactobacillus and fiber versus selective bowel decontamination: a controlled trial in liver transplant recipients, *Transplantation,* 74, 123, 2002.
9. Levy, M.F. et al., Readmisson to the intensive care unit after liver transplantation. *Crit. Care Med.,* 29, 18, 2001.
10. Hasse, J.M., Nutritional implications of liver transplantation, *Henry Ford Hosp. Med. J.,* 14, 386, 1990.
11. Gilroy, R. and Sudan, D., Liver and small bowel transplantation: therapeutic alternatives for the treatment of liver disease and intestinal failure, *Semin. Liver Dis.,* 20, 437, 2000.
12. Pahwa, N. and Hedberg, A.-M., Adult heart and lung transplantation, in *Comprehensive Guide to Transplant Nutrition,* Hasse, J.M. and Blue, L.S., Eds., American Dietetic Association, Chicago, 2002, 31.
13. Merli, M. et al., Malnutrition is a risk factor for cirrhotic patients undergoing surgery, *Nutrition,* 18, 978, 2002.
14. Schwebel, C. et al., Prevalence and consequences of nutritional depletion in lung transplant candidates, *Eur. Respir. J.,* 16, 1050, 2000.
15. Hade, A.M. et al., Both under-nutrition and obesity increase morbidity following liver transplantation, *Ir. Med. J.,* 96, 140, 2003.
16. Pikul, J. et al., Degree of preoperative malnutrition is predictive of postoperative morbidity and mortality in liver transplant recipients, *Transplantation,* 57, 469, 1994.
17. Snell, G. et al., BMI as a predictor of survival in adults with cystic fibrosis referred for a lung transplant, *J. Heart Lung Transplant.,* 17, 1097, 1998.
18. Madill, J. et al., Nutritional assessment of the lung transplant patient: body mass index as a predictor of 90-day mortality following transplantation, *J. Heart Lung Transplant.,* 20, 288, 2001.
19. Plochl, W. et al., Nutritional status, ICU duration, and ICU mortality in lung transplant recipients, *Intens. Care Med.,* 22, 1179, 1996.
20. Weseman, R.A., Adult small bowel transplantation, in *Comprehensive Guide to Transplant Nutrition,* Hasse, J.M. and Blue, L.S., Eds., American Dietetic Association, Chicago, 2002, 106.
21. Dionigi, P., Alessiani, M., and Ferrazi, A., Irreversible intestinal failure, nutrition support, and small bowel transplantation, *Nutrition,* 17, 747, 2001.
22. Rovera, G.M. et al., Intestinal and multivisceral transplantation: dynamics of nutritional management and functional anatomy, *J. Parenter. Enteral Nutr.,* 27, 252, 2003.
23. Silver, H.J. and Castellanos, V.H., Nutritional complications and management of intestinal transplant, *J. Am. Diet. Assoc.,* 100, 680, 2000.

24. Hasse, J.M., Adult liver transplantation, in *Comprehensive Guide to Transplant Nutrition,* Hasse, J.M. and Blue, L.S., Eds., American Dietetic Association, Chicago, 2002, 58.

25. Sodhi, S.S. et al., Gastroparesis after combined heart and lung transplantation, *J. Clin. Gastroenterol.,* 34, 34, 2002.

26. Anbar, R. et al., The role of nutritional support in transplant recipients: two case reports, *Transplant. Proceedings,* 35, 614, 2003.

27. Sekido, H. et al., Impact of early enteral nutrition after liver transplantation for acute hepatic failure: report of four cases, *Transplant. Proceedings,* 35, 369, 2003.

28. Lee, S.S. et al., Endoscopically placed nasogastrojejunal feeding tubes: a safe route for enteral nutrition in patients with hepatic encephalopathy, *Am. Surg.,* 68, 196, 2002.

29. Mehta, P.L. et al., Nutrition support following liver transplantation: a comparison of jejunal versus parenteral routes, *Clin. Transplant.,* 344, 837, 1995.

30. Schultz, R.-J. et al., New dietary concepts in small bowel transplantation, *Transplant. Proceedings,* 34, 893, 2002.

31. Reilly, J. et al., Nutritional support after liver transplantation: a randomized prospective study, *J. Parenter. Enteral Nutr.,* 14, 386, 1990.

32. Hasse, J. and Robien, K., Nutrition support guidelines for therapeutically immunosuppressed patients, in *Update in Intensive Care and Emergency Medicine: From Nutrition Support to Pharmacologic Nutrition in the ICU,* Pichard, C. and Kudsk, K., Eds., Springer-Verlag, Heidelberg, 2000, 361.

33. Merritt, W.T., Metabolism and liver transplantation: review of perioperative issues, *Liver Transplant.,* 6, S76, 2000.

34. DeWolf, A.M., Intraoperative concerns when a liver recipient is critically ill, *Liver Transplant.,* 6, S10, 2000.

35. Whitmire, S.J., Fluid, electrolytes, and acid–base balance, in *Contemporary Nutrition Support Practice: A Clinical Guide,* 2nd ed., Matarese, L.E. and Gottschlich, M.M., Eds., Saunders, Philadelphia, 2003, 122.

36. Jindal, R.M., Posttransplant diabetes mellitus: a review, *Transplantation,* 58, 1289, 1994.

37. Van den Berge, G. et al., Intensive insulin therapy in critically ill patients, *N. Engl. J. Med.,* 345, 1359, 2001.

38. Homan van der Heide, J.J. et al., Dietary supplementation with fish oil modifies renal reserve filtration capacity in postoperative, cyclosporin A-treated renal transplant recipients, *Transplant. Int.,* 3, 171, 1990.

39. Homan van der Heide, J.J. et al., The effects of dietary supplementation with fish oil on renal function and the course of early postoperative rejection episodes in cyclosporine-treated renal transplant recipients, *Transplantation,* 54, 257, 1992.

40. Homan van der Heide, J.J. et al., Effect of dietary fish oil on renal function and rejection in cyclosporine-treated recipients of renal transplants, *N. Engl. J. Med.,* 329, 769, 1993.

41. Sweny, P. et al., Dietary fish oil supplements preserve renal function in renal transplant recipients with chronic vascular rejection, *Nephrol. Dial. Transplant.,* 4, 1070, 1989.

42. Alexander J.W., Role of immunonutrition in reducing complications following organ transplantation, *Transplant Proc.,* 32, 574, 2000.

43. Badalamenti, S. et al., Renal effects of dietary supplementation with fish oil in cyclosporine-treated liver transplant recipients, *Hepatol.,* 22, 1695, 1995.

44. Loren, A.W., et al., Post transplant lymphoproliferative disorder: a review, *Bone Marrow Transplant.,* 31, 145, 2003.

45. Rao, V.K., Post transplant medical complications, *Surg. Clin. N. Am.,* 78, 113, 1998.

46. Singh, N. et al., Infections with cytomegalovirus and other herpes viruses in 121 liver transplant recipients: transmission by donated organ and the effect of OKT3 antibodies, *J. Infect. Dis.,* 158, 124, 1988.

47. Lima, E.Q. et al., Risk factors for development of acute renal failure after liver transplantation, *Ren. Fail.,* 25, 553, 2003.

48. Adrogué, H.J. and Madias, N.E., Management of life threatening acid base disorders, *N. Engl. J. Med.,* 338, 26, 107, 1998.

49. Ramsey, M.A. et al., Severe pulmonary hypertension in liver transplant candidates, *L. Transpl. Surg.,* 3, 494, 1997.

Section VI

Specific Organ System Failure

28 Pulmonary Failure

Mary S. McCarthy
Madigan Army Medical Center

CONTENTS

28.1 INTRODUCTION

Nutritional support is an important adjunct to the care of the critically ill pulmonary patient in the intensive care unit (ICU). Although we have limited data to support disease-specific nutrition for the patient in pulmonary failure, we do know that there is a strong association between nutrition and lung function. It has been demonstrated that patients with protein-calorie malnutrition have an increased incidence of pneumonia, respiratory failure, and acute respiratory distress syndrome (ARDS).[1] In addition, malnutrition adversely affects lung function by diminishing respiratory muscle strength, altering ventilatory capacity, and impairing immune function.[2] Repletion of altered nutritional status and prevention of further malnutrition during critical illness results in improvement of altered function and may be important in improving outcome.

The critically ill patient with respiratory failure is especially vulnerable to complications of underfeeding or overfeeding. It is not uncommon for these patients to require intubation and mechanical ventilation, which may restrict nutrients by mouth for five days or longer. This interval is considered the maximum appropriate interval for lack of nutritional support, according to the guidelines published by the American Society for Parenteral and Enteral Nutrition (ASPEN).[3] The guidelines state that it is reasonable to recommend that some form of nutrition support be initiated after 5 to 10 days of fasting in patients who are likely to remain unable to eat for an unspecified period of time.[3] Whether the respiratory failure is acute or chronic, inadequate nutrition leads to further immunocompromise, respiratory muscle wasting, and ventilatory dysfunction, which may result in prolonged ventilator dependence or death.[1] Excessive nutrition may also be deleterious to the patient with respiratory failure as a result of increased carbon dioxide (CO_2) production and subsequent high ventilatory demands on a pulmonary organ system that is already compromised.

It is imperative that clinicians use available tools and resources to conduct a comprehensive nutritional assessment and recommend a safe, effective regimen of nutrition support for the critically ill pulmonary failure patient. Nutrition support for this high-risk population requires thorough knowledge of the underlying disease process and consideration of the potential benefits and risks of nutrition intervention. This chapter provides recommendations for nutrition support in critically ill patients with COPD, acute lung injury, acute respiratory distress syndrome, and lung transplantation, based on the most current literature available.

In today's healthcare environment, where quality is measured by outcomes, the goal of nutritional support for the critically ill pulmonary failure patient should be to provide sufficient energy to meet metabolic and protein requirements while limiting wasting of respiratory muscles, in order to restore health and baseline pulmonary function.

28.2 EFFECTS OF MALNUTRITION ON THE PULMONARY SYSTEM

Malnutrition is common in patients with lung disease. Impaired nutritional status can adversely affect pulmonary function in spontaneously breathing or mechanically ventilated patients with pulmonary disease by impairment of respiratory muscle function, ventilatory drive, response to hypoxia, and pulmonary defense mechanisms.[4]

In critical illness, protein catabolism occurs to provide energy. With inadequate caloric intake in critically ill patients, energy sources are derived from protein breakdown and glyconeogenesis. The muscle protein pool is susceptible to catabolism to provide fuel; both the diaphragm and the intercostal muscles are skeletal muscles at risk for catabolism. Malnutrition reduces diaphragmatic muscle mass in health and disease.[5]

When malnourished patients without lung disease were studied, respiratory muscle strength was reduced by 37%, maximum voluntary ventilation by 41%, and vital capacity was most affected, with a 63% reduction.[6] At autopsy, diaphragmatic muscle mass was reduced to 60% of normal in underweight patients who died of a variety of diseases.[5]

The chronic pulmonary disease patient is apt to develop malnutrition as an adaptive mechanism to decrease oxygen consumption and lower the work of breathing.[7] The interaction of nutrition and ventilatory drive appears to be a direct function of the effect of nutrition on metabolic rate. A parallel fall in metabolic rate and hypoxic ventilatory response has been documented in humans.[8] Consequences of decreased respiratory strength and decreased ventilatory drive could include decreased cough and an inability to mobilize secretions, leading to atelectasis and subsequent pneumonia in spontaneously breathing patients with any type of respiratory disease. The decrease in respiratory muscle strength and drive may prolong mechanical ventilation in patients who may otherwise be candidates for weaning. Extended mechanical ventilation and ICU stay may place the patient at risk for adverse outcomes, higher costs for hospitalization, and lengthy rehabilitation.

Sustained malnutrition alters host immune response and may contribute to chronic or repeated pulmonary infections. Along with diminished cell-mediated immunity is an alteration in immunoglobulin turnover, decreased surfactant production, and decreased ability for repair following lung injury.[9]

28.3 CAUSES OF PULMONARY FAILURE AND CONSIDERATIONS
FOR NUTRITIONAL INTERVENTION

The majority of patients who are critically ill with pulmonary failure are over 60 years of age and have underlying lung disease. Advanced age alone is associated with an increased risk of undernutrition and malnutrition and increased morbidity and mortality.[10] Although the prevalence of protein-calorie undernutrition among independent living elderly is 1 to 15%, it is 25 to 85% in institutionalized patients, and 35 to 65% in hospitalized older patients.[11–13] Undernutrition is associated with an increased risk of cardiac and respiratory problems, infections, deep-vein thrombosis and pressure ulcers, perioperative mortality, and multiorgan failure. Immune deficiency is caused by undernutrition, including a decrease in CD4 T-lymphocytes.[11,14]

The clinical and research data demonstrating a high incidence of malnutrition in lung disease are based on patients with chronic obstructive pulmonary disease (COPD), cystic fibrosis, idiopathic pulmonary fibrosis, or primary pulmonary hypertension — all of which can lead to eventual lung transplantation. Research over the last decade focusing on acute respiratory failure, acute lung injury, and ARDS has left us with some general guidelines for specialized nutritional support in critically ill patients experiencing these conditions. The next section will focus on the pathophysiology, nutritional assessment, and nutrition support recommendations for the subgroup of conditions mentioned previously.

28.3.1 Chronic Obstructive Pulmonary Disease (COPD)

28.3.1.1 Pathophysiology

COPD* is a generic term that includes emphysema, bronchitis, and chronic asthma. It is caused by an airflow obstruction during expiration secondary to airway smooth muscle contraction, bronchial inflammation and edema, loss of elastic recoil, or collapse of the airways and changes in lung volume. Precipitating factors include smoking, air pollution, occupational exposure, repeated respiratory infections, heredity, aging, and allergies.[10] Both ventilatory drive and the response to hypoxia are decreased in malnourished COPD patients. Hypercapnia is found in the majority of COPD patients when inspiratory pressures are approximately less than half of normal; it may be seen sooner when other mechanical abnormalities are present that increase the work of breathing.[1] Studies have shown that these abnormalities of respiratory muscle function and endurance may explain the tendency for respiratory failure in malnourished patients with COPD.

Malnutrition has long been established as a complication of COPD.[15] The incidence of altered nutrition status ranges from 19 to 74%, with a greater incidence in hospitalized COPD patients with acute respiratory failure.[2] A decrease in active cell mass estimated from bioelectrical impedance analysis has been reported to be associated with a high ICU mortality rate in patients with COPD with acute respiratory failure.[16] Several studies have shown that a low body weight, expressed as body mass index (BMI) or percentage of ideal body weight (IBW), is associated with an increased overall mortality, independently of degree of airway obstruction.[17–20]

A large study using the national database in France of COPD patients receiving long-term oxygen therapy found the highest survival and lowest hospitalization rates were observed in obese patients.[15] This trend was found in several other European studies that examined predictors of mortality, controlling for age, gender, use of home oxygen, and pulmonary parameters of FEV1 and vital capacity.[17–20] Although there is no clear reason why obesity should improve survival, it has been hypothesized that obese patients with COPD may be better protected from a decrease in body cell mass during periods of acute illness because of higher energy reserves.[18] One other hypothesis is that obesity contributes to low FEV_1, so that obese patients with COPD classified as having severe COPD may in fact have less severe airflow obstruction and therefore a better survival.[19]

Malnutrition has also been shown to be related to morbidity in acutely ill patients with COPD, resulting in an increased need for mechanical ventilation, increased risk for nonelective readmission in patients previously admitted for an exacerbation, and increased duration of ventilatory support

---

* The main goal in treating patients with COPD who suffer from hypoxemia, hypercapnia, and malnutrition is to correct the malnutrition without increasing the respiratory quotient and to minimize the production of carbon dioxide.

following lung transplantation or lung volume reduction surgery.[21–23] Perhaps of greater importance to the patient with COPD is the increase in severity of dyspnea, decreased exercise capacity, and greater impairment in health-related quality of life.[24–26]

Nutritional depletion secondary to the work of breathing has long been suspected as the primary cause of weight loss, but it is now known that weight-losing COPD patients are hypermetabolic. This demonstrates a poor adaptive response to weight loss. Most patients with other disease states will demonstrate a decrease in resting energy expenditure after weight loss.[1] Inadequate protein and calorie intake may further contribute to primary lung parenchymal disease, immunocompromise, and respiratory muscle dysfunction that result in the need for intubation and mechanical ventilation. Malnutrition, together with a loss of lean body mass, has been identified as a prognostic variable for greater morbidity and mortality in the patient with COPD, especially those with emphysema.[2] The effects of critical illness and malnutrition can be easily seen with failure to wean from mechanical ventilation.[9] Without adequate nutrient fuel, the inflammatory response of critical illness results in marked protein catabolism, which can lead to respiratory muscle impairment and decreased visceral proteins — these may be obstacles to successful weaning from ventilatory support.[3]

28.3.1.2   Nutrition Assessment

Comprehensive nutritional assessment using multiple parameters has been shown to be useful in identifying underlying malnutrition in the COPD patient with acute respiratory failure. If available, indirect calorimetry is recommended. Because of the physiologic derangements in oxygen consumption and CO_2 production in COPD, predictive equations may be inaccurate. For example, during critical illness, specifically with respiratory dysfunction, lung O_2 consumption may increase from 3 up to 31% of total body consumption.[27] Using equations with an assumed VO_2 could lead to under- or overfeeding. Assessment should include a thorough nutrition history, including evaluation of weight pattern, nutrient intake, and medication usage to help develop individualized nutritional goals. Albumin, transferrin, and prealbumin concentrations are typically decreased in COPD patients in pulmonary failure.

Malnourished, spontaneously breathing COPD patients have increased resting energy requirements, approximately 15% above values predicted by Harris–Benedict equations.[10] The relative hypermetabolism associated with COPD is explained by the increased energy needs of the ventilatory muscles. The energy cost of respiratory muscles can be estimated from the severity of lung hyperinflation. These factors will depend on whether the patient is breathing spontaneously or being mechanically ventilated. Nutritional support for the COPD patient who is spontaneously breathing should take into account the frequent reports of early satiety, anorexia, bloating, and fatigue. Thomas points out that the presence of cytokine-induced inflammatory markers in COPD patients suggests that interventions aimed at controlling cytokine production may be required to reverse the cachexia syndrome and improve functional status in older patients.[28]

28.3.1.3   Nutrition Support Recommendations

Studies conducted over the last decade have provided little evidence to suggest that special enteral or parenteral formulations are necessary for the critically ill COPD patient with pulmonary failure. As with all critically ill patients, complete nutritional support should be provided as early as feasible using the enteral route. Decreased CO_2 production and a lower RQ have been demonstrated when patients have 50% of nonprotein calories provided as lipid, compared with 100% glucose, in an overfed state.[2] Yet, when total calories are provided in moderate amounts, manipulation of the macronutrients to limit effects on pulmonary function is unnecessary.[28] Prevention of nutritionally related hypercapnia is the overall goal; if there are signs of worsening respiratory failure or difficulty weaning from the ventilator, a modification in the nutritional formulation, using fewer carbohydrate calories and more lipid calories, may be necessary. Formulas that have been marketed for the pulmonary failure patient include Pulmocare, Isosource, Novasource Pulmonary, Respalor, and Nutrivent. Protein requirements in the critically ill COPD patient are not significantly different from those in other patients. Optimal support would establish neutral or positive nitrogen balance, depending on the need for repletion. In the critically ill patient, this can be achieved with 1.0 to 2.0 g/kg/d of protein. This amounts to approximately 20% of total calories being administered as protein, carbohydrate providing 50% and lipid providing 30% of required calories.[1]

28.3.2 Acute Lung Injury (ALI) and ARDS

28.3.2.1 Pathophysiology

Acute lung injury results in an acute change in the gas exchange function of the lung. Injury to the alveolocapillary membrane inevitably disrupts the endothelial barrier, leading to the development of noncardiogenic pulmonary edema through increased vascular permeability. As the air spaces fill with fluid, the gas exchange and mechanical properties of the lung deteriorate. ARDS is the most severe form of acute lung injury, characterized by increasing pulmonary capillary permeability, pulmonary edema, increased pulmonary vascular resistance, and progressive hypoxemia. These abnormalities have been linked to the excessive release of arachidonic acid–derived inflammatory mediators and toxic oxygen radicals from activated macrophages and neutrophils. The amount of extravascular water in the lungs of ARDS patients is about three times the upper limit of normal, which is 500 ml.[11] Direct causes of both ALI and ARDS include aspiration of gastric contents, inhalation of toxic substances, high inspired oxygen, drugs, pneumonitis, pulmonary contusion, and radiation. Indirect causes include sepsis syndrome, multisystem trauma, shock, pancreatitis, pulmonary embolism, disseminated intravascular clotting, fat embolism, and bypass surgery.[11] Although the etiology of ARDS is multifactorial, sepsis is believed to be the predominant underlying cause. Inflammatory mediators, such as prostaglandins and leukotrienes derived from arachidonic acid metabolism, are implicated in ALI and ARDS.[2]

Therapeutic goals for both ALI and ARDS include the following:

- Improve oxygen delivery and provide hemodynamic support
- Reduce oxygen consumption
- Optimize gas exchange
- Individualize nutrition support

Positive pressure ventilation is used to reverse and prevent atelectasis and decrease the work of breathing. Improvements in pulmonary gas exchange and relief from excessive respiratory work provide an opportunity for the lungs and airways to heal.[12] All efforts must be directed at discontinuing ventilatory support as soon as possible, because complications are generally related to duration of support.

28.3.2.2 Nutrition Assessment

Nutritional assessment is the same as for any critically ill patient. As evident from the etiology of ALI and ARDS, patients may be young or old and may or may not have underlying lung disease. The severe metabolic and physiologic derangements associated with ALI and ARDS warrant indirect calorimetry if available. In general, the mean duration of mechanical ventilation in patients with ARDS is 10 to 14 days, whereas 10 to 20% remain ventilator-dependent for more than three weeks.[29] The hypermetabolism of this illness has many contributing factors, including fever, pain, anxiety, restlessness, work of breathing, and infection.

28.3.2.3 Nutrition Support Recommendations

Immune-enhancing diets (IEDs) have been available for over 10 years. Although varying results have been reported following prospective randomized clinical trials using IEDs, most researchers agree that they have a role in down-regulating the inflammatory response using n-3 polyunsaturated fatty acids (PUFAs). Omega-3 (n-3) PUFAs aid the immune system by competing with arachidonic acid for cyclooxygenase metabolism at the cell membrane. Although a ratio of n-3 to n-6 fatty acids is crucial to prevent adverse effects, the exact ratio of n-3 to n-6 fatty acids that best modulates lipid mediator production in critical illness remains to be determined. Morlion et al. observed that a ratio of 1:2 appears to modulate lipid mediator synthesis in the most beneficial manner.[30] The study most frequently cited for examining the effects of modified fat formulas on patients with ARDS was performed by Gadek et al.[31] The authors found beneficial effects of the experimental solution, when compared with the control solution, at 4 and 7 days after achieving target infusion rate regarding neutrophil recruitment, gas exchange, requirement for mechanical ventilation, length of ICU stay, and reduction in new organ failures.[31]

Metnitz and associates observed that the antioxidant status of patients with ARDS is severely depressed.[32] They hypothesized that the various antioxidants found in conventional enteral and parenteral nutrient solutions may be ineffective in restoring the antioxidant potential. Although further study is needed to define better the optimal supplementation of nutritive antioxidants, we do know that supplementation with vitamins A, C, and E has been beneficial.[31]

Fluid accumulation and pulmonary edema are common in patients with ARDS and have been associated with poor clinical outcome.[2] For this reason, it has been suggested that a fluid-restricted nutrient formula (e.g., 2 kcal/cc) be used for patients whose condition necessitates a volume restriction.

The electrolyte of greatest concern to the patient in pulmonary failure is phosphate. Phosphate is essential for the synthesis of ATP and 2,3 DPG, both of which are critical for normal diaphragmatic contractility and optimal pulmonary function. Length of hospital stay and duration of mechanical ventilation is increased in critically ill patients who become hypophosphatemic, when compared with those patients who do not have this electrolyte imbalance.[2]

In conclusion, patients with, or at risk for, ALI/ARDS are clearly candidates for an n-3 fatty acid–supplemented formula. The modified enteral formula should be instituted at the earliest manifestations of pulmonary dysfunction or systemic inflammation and continued throughout the period of ALI/ARDS, generally not longer than 2 to 3 weeks.[29] A number of enteral formulas are available that contain a modified n-3–n-6 fatty acid content: Crucial (Nestlé), Immun-Aid (McGaw), Isosource VHN and Novasource Pulmonary (Novartis), Respalor (Mead Johnson) and Oxepa (Ross). The one formula that has been extensively tested in the ALI/ARDS population is Oxepa (Ross). In patients with ALI/ARDS who need total parenteral nutrition (TPN) where intravenous n-3 fatty acid emulsions are not available, an alternate approach would be to limit intake of n-6 fatty acids to 2 or 3% of energy intake of fat, with the majority of calories provided as dextrose. When carbohydrate calories meet resting energy expenditure, the percentage of exogenously supplied lipids that are oxidized is believed to be relatively small, based on the theory that carbohydrates are the preferred substrate during critical illness.[31]

28.3.3 Lung Transplant

28.3.3.1 Pathophysiology

Lung transplantation has emerged as an established and accepted therapy for patients with end-stage pulmonary disease. Candidates for lung transplantation frequently have a diagnosis of cystic fibrosis, COPD, idiopathic pulmonary fibrosis, or primary pulmonary hypertension. Typically, patients awaiting lung transplant have severe airway obstruction with chronic hypercapnic respiratory failure. Many patients will die awaiting transplant, due to the limited number of organs available and the severity of their disease.[33] Lean body mass depletion has been identified as a risk factor for higher mortality while awaiting and following lung transplant; cystic fibrosis patients are affected most frequently.[34]

28.3.3.2 Nutritional Assessment

Very little information is available in the literature regarding specific nutritional needs of this population. However, the majority of candidates are malnourished when presenting for surgery. In one study of 78 lung transplant candidates, there was a high prevalence of nutritional depletion, with 54% of the candidates having an ideal body weight (IBW) < 90% and 49% having a body mass index (BMI) < 20 kg/m². Using the two criteria of body weight < 90% and creatinine–height index (CHI) < 60% predicted that 72% of the lung transplant candidates were severely depleted.[4] Studies conducted with patients having cystic fibrosis have found improved pulmonary function in conjunction with significant weight gain using long-term nocturnal enteral feedings.

Nutrition assessment in transplant patients is dependent on a carefully performed history and physical assessment. Objective measures such as body weight, anthropometric measures, and visceral protein levels may be less sensitive in detecting the degree of malnutrition as a result of fluid accumulation, organ dysfunction, and surgical stress. Immediately following transplantation, the goal of nutrition support is to promote wound healing, support the body's ability to fight infection, and allow for rehabilitation. Perioperative energy requirements are similar to those required to support similar uncomplicated surgical procedures. Most patients can be successfully fed with enteral nutrition. Parenteral nutrition should be reserved for severe complications, such as cytomegalovirus, esophagitis, and gastroenteritis; small bowel obstruction; fistula formation chylous ascites; gastrointestinal bleeding; and in the immediate postoperative period of small bowel transplantations.[2] Metabolic and nutritional complications post transplant may be related to underlying conditions, including obesity, hypertension, diabetes mellitus, and hyperlipidemia and should be treated with appropriate dietary and pharmacologic interventions.[2] It is critically important to avoid hyperglycemia postoperatively because elevated blood sugars can impair wound healing and increase the risk of infection. Hyperglycemia may occur following transplant due to insulin resistance associated with surgical stress, infection, and immune-modulating medications.

28.3.3.3 Nutrition Support Recommendations

Protein and energy requirements are affected by the stress of surgery, the use of immune-modulating medications, postoperative complications, and episodes of acute rejection. Protein requirements are elevated due to losses associated with surgical wounds, drains, fistulae, and the catabolism associated with steroid use. It has been suggested that 1.5 to 2.0 g/kg/d of protein be provided immediately following transplant, with a decrease to 1 g/kg/d as the dose of steroids is reduced to maintenance levels. Conservative carbohydrate administration is recommended to avoid contributing to metabolic complications. Supplemental arginine and n-3 PUFAs, alone and in combination, have been shown to improve survival in animal models. As with ARDS patients, the use of n-3 PUFAs can modulate the postsurgical inflammatory response with elaboration of less potent inflammatory cytokines, leukotrienes, and prostaglandins (see Chapter 4 and Chapter 11). Nucleotide-free diets have also been shown to enhance immunity and improve graft and recipient survival.[35]

28.4 CASE STUDY

Following presentation to the Emergency Department for shortness of breath, a 61-year-old obese female (D.S.) was admitted to the ICU service and intubated for impending respiratory failure secondary to suspected community-acquired multilobar pneumonia. Her O₂ saturation on admission was 83% on room air. Her chest radiograph showed almost "complete collapse of the right lung and decreased volume in the left lung with probable bilateral infiltrates" (medical record). She was

TABLE 28.1
Ventilator Settings Patient D.S.

Parameter	FiO$_2$	Vt	V$_E$	PEEP	PS	RR
Value	.35	370 ml	5 l/min	5 cm H$_2$O	20 cm H$_2$O	16 bpm

TABLE 28.2
Metabolic Cart Results Patient D.S. (Initial Study)

Parameter	FiO$_2$	VO$_2$	VCO$_2$	RQ	V$_E$	V$_T$	REE Predicted	REE Measured	Standard Deviation
Value	0.38	246 ml/min	174 ml/min	0.71	5.7 L/min	370 ml	1526 kcal	1708 kcal	±175 kcal

unresponsive due to severe hypercarbia and marked respiratory acidosis. Initial chemistries revealed hypokalemia, hypochloremia, hypomagnesemia, and mild hyperglycemia. Her course was complicated by hypotension requiring pressor agents, a urinary tract infection, and an inability to wean from mechanical ventilation. On day 15, a tracheostomy was performed. She received nutritional support via Dobhoff feeding tube, beginning 48 hours after admission.

D.S. had been in her previous state of generally good health until she experienced shortness of breath three days prior to admission. Her past medical history was significant for polio as a child, resulting in a nonambulatory status for the past five years. She was able to perform activities of daily living using a wheelchair and provided child care for her grandchildren. The polio resulted in altered thoracic anatomy and compromised lung volumes and ventilatory function with a baseline CO$_2$ of 50 to 60 mmHg. Past surgical history included multiple surgeries on her back, legs, and abdomen for polio, partial colectomy with ileostomy in 1975 for colon cancer, and partial thyroidectomy in 1990.

D.S. was 63 inches tall and weighed 199 pounds, with a body mass index of 35.2 (severe obesity). Prior to initiating full enteral feedings, a metabolic cart study was ordered. Mechanical ventilation settings at the time of the study are listed in Table 28.1.

The metabolic study was performed using a MedGraphics CCM mobile cart and Breeze® nutrition software (Medical Graphics Corp, St. Paul, MN). The patient had been receiving trophic enteral feedings using Jevity at 35 cc/h via Dobhoff tube for < 24 h. Results of the first study are listed in Table 28.2.

Results revealed that D.S. was hypermetabolic, with energy needs 110 to 120% above predicted needs. Her minute ventilation and tidal volumes were low, which is congruent with her pulmonary compromise from both the polio disease and her current multilobar pneumonia. Based on study results, the patient was ordered to have Jevity feedings infuse at 70 cc/h continuously, which provided approximately 1780 kcal and 72 g of protein per day. This feeding regimen was well tolerated for 3 weeks.

D.S. experienced much difficulty weaning from the ventilator. Her clinical condition was improved, yet she remained on the ventilator with CPAP support 3 weeks after admission. She remained confined to bed and expressed anxiety over the possibility of long-term ventilatory support. A second metabolic cart study was ordered to investigate whether the patient was being overfed or had an increased amount of deadspace ventilation. The second study results are listed in Table 28.3.

The deadspace estimation (V$_D$/V$_T$) was 0.30 to 0.40, which is within normal limits. The patient was clearly being overfed at this time. Her carbon dioxide production exceeded her oxygen consumption, resulting in an RQ > 1.0, which typically indicates overfeeding of carbohydrate

TABLE 28.3
Metabolic Cart Results Patient D.S. (Follow-up Study)

Parameter	FiO$_2$	VO$_2$	VCO$_2$	RQ	V$_E$	V$_T$	REE Predicted	REE Measured	Standard Deviation
Value	0.30	175 ml/min	185 ml/min	1.06	5.8 l/min	540 ml	1526 kcal	1309 kcal	±158 kcal

calories or total calories. The patient was quite sedentary and remained ventilated, so there was no expected increase in energy expenditure from her initial reading. But energy expenditure was actually lower than expected. Following this finding, the patient's tube feedings were decreased to 60 cc/h and she began to transition to some pureed foods while her tracheostomy remained in place. She was discharged to a long-term care facility 31 days after admission in good spirits.

REFERENCES

1. Pingleton, S.K., Enteral nutrition in patients with respiratory disease, *Eur. Respir. J.* 9, 364–370, 1996.
2. ASPEN, Board of Directors, Guidelines for the use of parenteral and enteral nutrition in adult and pediatric patients, *J. Parenter. Enteral Nutr.* 26, 1 (Suppl.), 90SA–92SA, 2002.
3. Radrizzani, D. and Iapichino, G., Nutrition and lung function in the critically ill patient, *Clin. Nutr.* 17, 7–10, 1998.
4. Braun, N., Arora, N., and Rochester, D., Respiratory muscle and pulmonary function in proximal myopathies, *Thorax* 38, 616–623, 1983.
5. Arora, N. and Rochester, D., Effect of body weight and muscularity on human diaphragm muscle mass, thickness and area, *J. Appl. Physiol.: Respirat. Environ. Exercise Physiol.* 52, 64–70, 1982.
6. Arora, N. and Rochester, D., Respiratory muscle strength and maximal voluntary ventilation in undernourished patients, *Am. Rev. Respir. Dis.* 126, 5–8, 1982.
7. Henessy, K.A. and Orr, M.E., Nutrition support nursing core curriculum, in *Respiratory Failure*, 3rd ed., Kovacevich, D. and Dechert, R., ASPEN, Silver Spring, MD, 1996, 14.
8. Askanazi, J., Rosenbaum, S.H., Hyman, A.I., et al., Effects of parenteral nutrition on ventilatory drive, *Anesthesiol.* 53 (Suppl. 1), 185, 1980.
9. Murphy, L.M. and Conforti, C.G., Nutritional support of the cardiopulmonary patient, *Crit. Care Clin. N. Am.* 5, 57–64, 1993.
10. Wilson, D.O., Rogers, R.M., and Pennock, B., Metabolic rate and weight loss in obstructive lung disease, *J. Parenter. Enteral Nutr.* 14, 7–11, 1990.
11. American Thoracic Society, Round table conference: acute lung injury, *Am. J. Respir. Crit. Care Med.* 158, 675–679, 1998.
12. Donohoe, M. and Rogers, R., Nutritional assessment and support in COPD, *Clin. Chest Med.* 11, 487–504, 1990.
13. Gadek, J., DeMichele, S., Karlstad, M., et al., Specialized enteral nutrition improves clinical outcomes in patients with or at risk for acute respiratory distress syndrome: a prospective, blinded, randomized, controlled multicenter trial, *Crit. Care Med.* 27, 1409–1420, 1999.
14. Omran, M. and Morley, J., Assessment of protein energy malnutrition in older persons. Part I: history, examination, body composition, and screening tools, *Nutrition* 16, 50–63, 2000.
15. Studley, H., Percentage of weight loss: a basic indicator of surgical risk in patients with chronic peptic ulcer, *Nutr. Hosp.* 16 (4), 141–143, 2001.
16. Lennard-Jones, J., *A Positive Approach to Nutrition and Treatment,* King's Fund, London, 1992.
17. Kaiser, F. and Morley, J., Idiopathic CD4+ T lymphopenia in older persons, *J. Am. Geriatr. Soc.* 42, 1291–1294, 1994.
18. Chailleux, E., Laaban, J., and Veale, D., Prognostic value of nutritional depletion in patients with COPD treated by long-term oxygen therapy, *Chest* 123, 1460–1466, 2003.

19. Wilson, D., Rogers, R., Wright, E., et al., Body weight in chronic obstructive pulmonary disease: The National Institutes of Health intermittent positive-pressure breathing trial, *Am. Rev. Respir. Dis.* 139, 1435–1438, 1989.

20. Gray-Donald, K., Gibbons, L., Shapiro, S., et al., Nutritional status and mortality in chronic obstructive pulmonary disease, *Am. J. Respir. Crit. Care Med.* 153, 961–966, 1996.

21. Shols, A., Slangen, J., Volovics, L., et al., Weight loss is a reversible factor in the prognosis of chronic obstructive pulmonary disease, *Am. J. Respir. Crit. Care Med.* 157, 1791–1797, 1998.

22. Landbo, C., Prescott, E., Lange, P., et al., Prognostic value of nutritional status in chronic obstructive pulmonary disease, *Am. J. Respir. Crit. Care Med.* 160, 1856–1861, 1999.

23. Faisy, C., Rabbat, A., Kouchakji, B., et al., Bioelectrical impedance analysis in estimating nutritional status and outcome of patients with chronic obstructive pulmonary disease and acute respiratory failure, *Intens. Care Med.* 26, 518–525, 2000.

24. Vitacca, M., Clini, E., Porta, R., et al., Acute exacerbations in patients with COPD: predictors of need for mechanical ventilation, *Eur. Respir. J.* 9, 1487–1493, 1996.

25. Pouw, E., Velde, G.T., Croonen, B., et al., Early nonelective readmission for chronic obstructive pulmonary disease is associated with weight loss, *Clin. Nutr.* 19, 95–99, 2000.

26. Sahebjami, H. and Sathianpitayakul, E., Influence of body weight on the severity of dyspnea on chronic obstructive pulmonary disease, *Am. J. Respir. Crit. Care Med.* 161, 886–890, 2000.

27. Shols, A., Mostert, R., Soeters, P., et al., Body composition and exercise performance in patients with chronic obstructive pulmonary disease, *Thorax* 46, 695–699, 1991.

28. Shoup, R., Dalsky, G., Warner, S., et al., Body composition and health-related quality of life in patients with obstructive airways disease, *Eur. Respir. J.* 10, 1576–1580, 1997.

29. Thomas, D., Dietary prescription for chronic obstructive pulmonary disease, *Clin. Geriatr. Med.* 18 (4), 835–839, 2002.

30. Headley, J., Indirect calorimetry, *AACN Clin. Iss.* 14 (2), 155–167, 2003.

31. Talpers, S., Romberger, D., Bunce, S., et al., Nutritionally associated increased carbon dioxide production: excess total calories vs. high proportion of carbohydrate calories, *Chest* 102, 551–555, 1992.

32. Morlion, B., Torwesten, E., Lessire, H., et al., The effect of parenteral fish oil on leukocyte membrane fatty acid composition and leukotriene-synthesizing capacity in patients with postoperative trauma, *Metabolism* 45, 1208–1213, 1996.

33. Gadek, J., DeMichele, S., Karlstad, M., et al., Effect of enteral feeding with eicospentaenoic acid, gamma-linolenic acid, and antioxidants in patients with acute respiratory distress syndrome, *Crit. Care Med.* 27, 1409–1420, 1999.

34. Mizock, B., Nutritional support in acute lung injury and acute respiratory distress syndrome, *NCP* 16, 319–328, 2001.

35. Schwebel, C., Pin, I., Barnoud, D., et al., Prevalence and consequences of nutritional depletion in lung transplant candidates, *Eur. Respir. J.* 16, 1050–1055, 2000.

36. Snell, G., Bennetts, K., Bartolo, J., et al., Body mass index as a predictor of survival in adults with cystic fibrosis referred for lung transplantation, *J. Heart Lung Transplant.* 17, 1097–1103, 1998.

37. Buren, C.V., Kulkami, A., Schandle, V., et al., The influence of dietary nucleotides on cell-mediated immunity, *Transplant* 36, 350–352, 1983.

29 Renal Failure

Tom Stone McNees
Clarian Nutrition Support/Methodist Hospital

CONTENTS

29.1 INTRODUCTION

The kidney regulates fluid, electrolyte, acid–base, and metabolite balance, and disorders of renal function will usually declare themselves with disruptions in homeostasis of these systems. Renal failure is often accompanied by hypoalbuminemia, which has been linked to malnutrition and, more recently, to inflammatory processes. In the critical care setting, as many as one in three admissions will develop some form of acute renal failure (ARF). Those cases severe enough to require renal replacement therapy (RRT) suffer high mortality, a condition which has persisted despite advances in medical technology and treatments. This discussion of renal failure will address ARF in particular, with consideration given to maintenance dialysis patients seen in critical care.

29.2 ACUTE RENAL FAILURE

Acute renal failure may be better understood as a syndrome rather than a disease in itself, which often becomes evident with uremia, electrolyte abnormalities, acid–base disturbances, or fluid overload.[1] Few patients may be admitted to the ICU solely on the basis of renal failure, yet sources estimate from 3 to 30% of these admissions will develop acute renal failure.[2] In Hoste et al., 16.2% of 185 septic patients developed ARF and 70% of these required renal replacement therapy (RRT).[3] This is concerning for high morbidity and mortality in this group. Researchers report 60 to 70% mortality in critically ill patients developing ARF severe enough to require RRT.[4–6]

There is also good news in these data, however. In a very large, multicenter study, Metnitz et al. showed by multivariate analysis that most interventions (including mechanical ventilation, vasoactive medications, cardiopulmonary resuscitation, treatment for complicated metabolic alkalosis or acidosis, and parenteral nutrition) were independently predictive of increased mortality.[5] In contrast, however, one of the interventions studied — enteral nutrition support — was associated with improved survival. The possibility that this could be due to a lower severity of illness in patients receiving enteral nutrition was ruled out by statistical analysis. In the authors' words, "Instead, our results demonstrate an additional effect of enteral nutrition on survival."[5]

29.2.1 CATEGORIES AND ETIOLOGY OF ACUTE RENAL FAILURE

Acute renal failure may be described as one of the following:[7]

- Prerenal — From causes related to hypovolemia or hypotension that lead to decreased renal perfusion
- Postrenal — Resulting from urinary obstruction
- Intrinsic — Due to disorders of renal physiology

Of all causes for ARF, three predominate, and all three are associated with acute tubular necrosis (ATN). Accounting for 65% of acute renal failure, in decreasing order of frequency, these three are:[4]

- Intraoperative ischemia or hypotension
- Nephrotoxin exposure
- Sepsis

29.2.2 DECREASED RENAL PERFUSION

Loss of blood or other intravascular fluid losses, including volume lost to extravascular space due to hypoproteinemia and low oncotic pressure, lead to decreased arterial blood volume and pressure. Hypotension associated with sepsis, cardiac failure, or other causes impairs delivery of blood and oxygen to the body's organs, including the kidneys. Regardless of cause, the effect is the same: decreased perfusion of the kidney and reduced glomerular filtration rate (GFR), with resulting impairment of renal function.[8]

29.2.3 NEPHROTOXIC MEDICATION

Toxic causes of acute renal failure have increased, but prognosis for survival in these cases is good — by one review, near 80%.[1] According to their mechanism of action, different drugs may impair renal function in different ways. It is possible for a medication to defeat intrinsic homeostatic mechanisms. With mild hypovolemia or hypotension, compensatory mechanisms may defend GFR,

TABLE 29.1
Medications that May Alter Glomerular Hemodynamics

Agent	Action	Predisposing Factors
NSAIDs	Inhibit prostaglandin-mediated renal vasodialation	CHF, cirrhosis, ASVD, CRF, hypovolemia
ACE inhibitors	Inhibit renal vasoconstriction	As with NSAIDs
Calcineurin inhibitors (tacrolimus, cyclosporine)	May induce preglomerular vasoconstriction	Hypovolemia, possible interaction with anti-hypertensives/anti-infectives
Amphotericin B	Disrupts tubular function, limiting urine concentration	Some diuretics, ↓ GFR
Radiographic contrast	Induces acute vasoconstriction	GFR < 35 ml/min, severe heart failure, diabetic nephropathy, large amounts of contrast
Cocaine	Induces vasoconstriction; rhabdomyolysis, acid–base, or electrolyte imbalance	Cocaine use

Note: NSAID: nonsteroidal anti-inflammatory drugs; CHF: congestive heart failure; ASVD: atherosclerotic vascular disease; CRF: chronic renal failure; GFR: glomerular filtration rate.

Source: Information from Albright, R.C., *Mayo Clin. Proc.*, 76, 67, 2001.[7]

but medications, including nonsteroidal anti-inflammatory drugs (NSAID), acetylcholine esterase (ACE) inhibitors, and angiotensin receptor blockers (ARB), may limit the ability to restore hemodynamics.[8]

Some drugs may impair intrarenal circulation and GFR by vasoconstriction in the kidney without affecting overall hemodynamics; these include the immunosuppressives tacrolimus and cyclosporine. (Sepsis and hypercalcemia, though not drugs, may reduce GFR and lead to ARF in the same manner.)[8]

Acyclovir nephrotoxicity was once relatively common but has become less so since high-dose bolus administration of the drug has been replaced by continuous infusions.[8] The nephrotoxic effects of cisplatin, amphotericin, and aminoglycoside antibiotics are related to cumulative dose history; the same is true for radiocontrast agents.[8] See Table 29.1 for a presentation of potentially nephrotoxic medications.

29.2.4 SEPSIS AND ARF

Hoste et al. studied the incidence of ARF in septic patients to identify characteristics of those patients who would later develop renal failure.[3] Patients who did develop ARF tended to have lower mean arterial blood pressure, despite normal or higher central venous pressure or pulmonary artery occlusion ("wedge") pressure. These patients were more likely to have received aggressive fluid loading and more likely to have received vasoactive medications.[3]

Looking at the patients who would go on to develop ARF, on the first day of sepsis they were six times more likely to have pH less than 7.35, and 7.5 times more likely to have serum creatinine greater than 1.0 mg/dl.[3]

29.2.5 NUTRITIONAL EFFECTS OF ACUTE RENAL FAILURE

From a nutrition standpoint, consider that some treatments a patient may receive in the early stages of renal insufficiency can lead to difficulty in subsequent ARF. Fluids and vasoactive medications intended to be therapeutic in early stages of renal insufficiency could become problematic. Fluid given with hope of increasing GFR and urine output may later be in excess.[2] Diuretics given to remove fluid can fail if the fluid has already escaped to the extravascular or "third space," due to decreased oncotic pressure from hypoalbuminemia. This may leave the patient intravascularly "dry" yet still fluid overloaded.

Hyponatremia is often seen with acute renal failure.[2] This may be dilutional, relating to fluid overload, but in cases of excessive fluid loss due to "third spacing" or gastrointestinal losses, a patient may exhibit hypovolemic hyponatremia.[2] Hyperkalemia is frequently present in ARF.[2] Accumulation of potassium may be due to impaired renal excretion secondary to nephrotoxic drugs or tissue damage or release of potassium from cells lost to catabolism or lysis, or it may simply result from excessive exogenous potassium delivery.[2] ARF interferes with homeostasis of phosphorous, calcium, and magnesium.[9] Phosphorous and magnesium can accumulate to high levels, which may be managed by limiting exogenous sources.[9]

Hypocalcemia is typical with ARF, and in many cases this will be mild to moderate.[10] Calcium supplementation will be indicated if hypocalcemia is severe, as may be the case with rhabdomyolysis or pancreatitis, or after the patient has received large amounts of bicarbonate.[9]

Impaired carbohydrate metabolism is characteristic of acute renal failure.[11,12] Hyperglycemia in ARF is often associated with insulin resistance and hyperinsulinemia;[2,11] insulin-mediated glucose uptake into skeletal muscle can be decreased by as much as 50%.[11] High serum glucose is exacerbated by accelerated gluconeogenesis, which is supported by catabolism and, unfortunately, cannot be suppressed by provision of exogenous glucose.[2,11,12]

Disturbances in lipid metabolism may lead to hypertriglyceridemia with ARF, due in large part to impaired lipolysis.[12] Serum levels of low and very low density lipoproteins are increased and high density lipoproteins commonly decreased.[11] Limits on lipid clearance have been shown to affect both long- and medium-chain triglycerides given as parenteral emulsions.[11,12]

Of all the nutrition-related factors associated with acute renal failure, a dominant feature is increased protein catabolism: "In ARF, hepatic gluconeogenesis is stimulated and increased skeletal muscle catabolism provides the amino acid substrates."[13] At the same time, protein synthesis is impaired, and amino acid transport into skeletal muscle is also inhibited.[13] An important catabolic stimulus in ARF is metabolic acidosis, and correction of acidosis is likely to improve protein and amino acid metabolism present in ARF.[13] Other causes also stimulate protein breakdown in acute renal failure. Catabolic hormones including catecholamines, glucagon, and glucocorticoids are released, as are inflammatory mediators such as tumor necrosis factor and interleukins, with hypercatabolic effect.[13]

The catabolic insult from ARF is exacerbated with renal replacement therapy. Not only are nutritional substrates (serum proteins, amino acids) lost to dialysis, but production of inflammatory mediators in response to bioincompatibility with dialyzer membranes can stimulate further breakdown of somatic proteins.[13]

Unfortunately, limits to catabolism that defend lean mass in fasting healthy individuals do not protect those with critical illness, trauma, or sepsis whose loss of serum, somatic, and visceral proteins may be very great.[14] If it is understood that net protein loss is obligatory and irreversible by administration of exogenous substrate proteins, then a primary goal of nutrition therapy should be to provide optimal support so that losses may be minimized.[13]

29.3 RENAL REPLACEMENT THERAPY

Renal replacement therapy may be indicated in acute renal failure with severe uremia, electrolyte imbalances, fluid overload, or metabolic acidosis.[8] RRT will not shorten the duration of renal failure; rather, it is utilized to ease metabolic consequences until renal recovery can take place.[8,9] Recovery will usually begin from 7 to 21 days following renal injury, but it may take as long as 6 months.[8]

Different modes of RRT have been developed to accomplish the same goals in significantly different ways.

29.3.1 MODES OF RRT

Intermittent hemodialysis (IHD) was the first mechanical form of RRT developed as an alternative to peritoneal dialysis (see following description) and a cornerstone of treatment in ARF for over 30 years.[9] IHD is usually applied 3 to 4 hours daily or on alternate days, depending on the needs of the patient.[8,9] The need to remove water and solutes in a relatively short time requires removal and processing of large volumes of blood, which can result in interdialytic hypotension.[8,9] This may be especially problematic in critically ill patients with concurrent hypoalbuminemia, intra-vascular fluid loss, and septic vasodilatation, leading to hypotension even without RRT. In these cases, a continuous treatment modality may be employed.

A number of continuous renal replacement therapies (CRRT) have been developed that vary in specific technical details of operation but share common features.[8] By removing and treating blood slowly over an extended period of time, these processes control uremia and fluid, electrolyte, and acid–base imbalances with minimal disruption of hemodynamic stability or plasma osmolality.[8]

Peritoneal dialysis (PD) is accomplished by infusion of fluid into the peritoneum that is relatively isotonic but contains a lower concentration of electrolytes that are to be removed so that uremic wastes and high-concentration electrolytes will diffuse across the peritoneal membrane, into the dialysate which is then drained to remove.[15] Like continuous RRT, PD takes place slowly and therefore is unlikely to cause hypotension.[8,15] Although use of PD has declined in contemporary acute care settings, it can be accomplished with the use of simpler technologies, which makes it practicable in remote or disadvantaged areas where IHD or CRRT may be less available.[8,9]

29.3.2 NUTRITIONAL EFFECTS OF RRT

Hemodialysis and hemofiltration remove amino acids at rates from 3 to 5 g/h,[16] and these losses have been considered in published nutrient recommendations for patients receiving RRT.[2,11,17,18] Bellomo reports that there is little information available regarding nutrient losses in critically ill patients receiving intermittent hemodialysis but has found support for recommendations in patients treated by continuous renal replacement therapies, or CRRT.[17] There is no significant loss of serum lipids in CRRT or in other forms of extracorporeal RRT.[12,17] If the replacement fluid used in RRT is rich in glucose (significantly higher in glucose concentration than blood levels), then the patient may be expected to gain approximately 500 kcal per day from glucose absorption at a dialysate flow rate of 1 l/h and proportionately more with higher flow rates or dialysate concentration.[17] Dialysate containing very low levels of glucose with patients receiving parenteral dextrose has resulted in a mean loss of infused glucose from the patient to the replacement fluid of 4%.[18] The use of lactate as a buffer in CRRT replacement fluid can contribute to caloric gain by the patient, estimated to be from 300 to 400 additional kcal/d, with this variable influenced not only by the rate of dialysate flow but also by the site of administration.[17]

29.4 NUTRITION MANAGEMENT IN ACUTE RENAL FAILURE

Dr. Wilfred Druml has written, "[T]here can be no doubt that nutritional therapy presents a cornerstone in the treatment of patients with ARF. Preexisting and/or hospital-acquired malnutrition have been identified as important factors contributing to the persisting high mortality in acutely ill patients with ARF."[11] Guidelines for nutrition management traditionally applied in cases of chronic renal failure have been replaced by an approach that is intended to address more specifically the needs of the patient with ARF.[11] Recommendations for nutrition support with patients in acute renal failure generally parallel those for other critically ill patients without ARF.[12] Table 29.2 compares

TABLE 29.2
Digest of Recommendations for Nutrition Support in Acute Renal Failure with RRT

Author	Publication Date	Protein/AA (g/kg)	Energy (kcal/kg)	Micronutrient Supplement	Notes
Druml[11]	2001	1.0–1.5	25–35	Water-soluble vitamins	Ascorbate < 200 mg
Bellomo[12]	2002	1.5–2.0	30–35	Ascorbate, B6, folate, Zn, Se	IED "yes"; early feeding "yes"; renal-specific formulas "no"
Scheinkestel[13]	2003	2.5	100% as measured or predicted		
Kapadia[2]	2003	1.5	35 (NPC)	Water-soluble vitamins	NPC: 60% CHO, 40% lipid IED "yes," as early as feasible

Note: RRT: renal replacement therapy.; IED: immune-enhancing diet; NPC: nonprotein calories.

several guidelines for nutrition support in ARF published since 2000 and reflects a significant departure from the traditional norm.

29.4.1 ENERGY

Recommendations for energy intake for patients with ARF published by Druml are among the most conservative.[11] The author points out that hypermetabolic conditions rarely exceed 130% of "calculated basic energy expenditure," and any complications there may be from slightly underfeeding would be less significant than those resulting from overfeeding. For this reason, it is advised that patients with ARF should receive 25 to 30 kcal per kilogram of body weight per day.[11] Kapadia et al. conclude that higher energy intakes are required in severe ARF than in isolated or uncomplicated disease and recommend 35 kcal/kg in addition to whatever energy may be contributed by protein.[2] Bellomo recommends early (and enteral) administration of 30 to 35 kcal/kg and does not specifically exclude the contribution of protein from calculations of energy provided.[17] Scheinkestel and colleagues determined energy requirements of acute renal failure patients in their study by direct measurement with a metabolic cart whenever possible, which they were able to do in 68% of subjects.[18] In the remaining 32%, energy needs were calculated by use of predictive equation. The group attempted to provide each patient with 100% of measured or calculated energy needs as early in their treatment as they could. They highlight the relationship between energy and nitrogen intakes and the likelihood that energy insufficiency will make achievement of positive or even neutral nitrogen balance very difficult. In the authors' words, "The difference between a surplus and a deficit in supplied energy may be critical in achieving a positive nitrogen balance."[18]

29.4.2 AMINO ACIDS AND PROTEIN

Given the hypercatabolic nature of severe ARF and the risk presented by loss of muscle and solid organ mass, protein requirements for these patients receive a great deal of attention. In 1998, Druml reviewed the literature of the time and found no support for delivery of protein in excess of 1.3 to 1.5 g/kg, except in cases of continuous hemofiltration or peritoneal dialysis, where an additional 0.2 g/kg were allowed, or up to a total of 1.7 g/kg.[13] He emphasizes that protein in excess of these recommendations would only increase uremia and need for dialysis, a position which is reinforced in a 2001 publication by the same author.[11] Nevertheless, study results show that protein losses in severe acute renal failure can exceed 150 g/d and increasing protein delivery from less than 1 to as much as 2.5 g/kg improves nitrogen balance in a nearly linear manner.[17] Macias et al. found that positive nitrogen balance could be achieved in patients with ARF receiving CRRT, but this requires protein delivery of 1.5 to 1.8 g/kg/d.[19] Kierdorf reports similar findings in groups receiving 1.5 and 1.74 grams of amino acids per kg per day and azotemia in these patients was well controlled by CRRT.[12] (Kierdorf's subjects in all groups received 30 nonprotein kcal/kg/d.)

In their study reported in 2003, Scheinkestel et al. tested nutrition support providing 1.5, 2.0, and 2.5 g of protein or amino acids per kilogram.[18] Recall that these subjects, as described earlier, were provided energy as close as possible to their measured or calculated needs. Nitrogen balance was assessed as protein delivery was increased for each experimental subject. Investigators found that nitrogen balance was very significantly more likely to be achieved when protein intake was greater than 2 g/kg/d. Nitrogen balance in these subjects was not just a technical success but associated directly with positive hospital and ICU outcomes. In fact, statistical analysis in this study revealed that for every gram increase in daily nitrogen balance, the probability of patient survival increased by 21%.

29.4.3 MICRONUTRIENT SUPPLEMENTATION

Reports as late as 2002 find no controlled trials to provide firm support for micronutrient supplementation in ARF.[12,17,20] Given such lack of evidence, it may seem reasonable to provide at least the recommended dietary allowance (RDA) for vitamins and minerals.[17,20] Water-soluble vitamins are lost with RRT, and some sources recommend additional supplements.[2,11,12,17] Ascorbic acid, however, is a precursor of oxalic acid, and excessive vitamin C may lead to oxalosis, aggravating ARF.[11,12] Supplemental vitamin C doses should be limited; in general, recommendations are similar, but specifics for ascorbate in ARF range from "at least 100 mg"[17] to "less than 200 mg"[11] to not more than 250 mg.[12] Significant losses of folic acid and vitamin B6 have been documented with CRRT, and additional supplementation of these nutrients has been recommended.[17]

Levels of fat-soluble vitamins A, D, and E are found to be decreased in acute renal failure (for A and E this is unlike chronic renal failure, where levels tend to accumulate), whereas vitamin K may be normal or even higher.[11]

29.4.4 ENTERAL NUTRITION IN ARF

In a study of critically ill patients with ARF, enteral feeding has been singled out as the one factor independent of any other intervention that was clearly associated with improved outcomes.[18] Benefits of enteral feeding in the critically ill are well recognized and include preservation of intestinal barrier function and gut-mediated immunity;[16] risk for infectious complications is lower in patients who are enterally fed.[16] (For a more comprehensive treatment of this subject, see Chapter 12.) Enteral tube feeding has been shown to improve renal function when ARF is induced in experimental animals and is generally accepted as the preferred modality for nutrition support in critically ill patients with ARF.[21,22]

Commercially available enteral feeding formulas designed for renal failure patients on dialysis are included in Table 29.3, which provides a view of selected formula products. (See Chapter 16 for a more complete description of these and other enteral formulas.) In view of the preceding discussion regarding optimal protein and energy dosing for patients with ARF, review of the nutrient composition of available renal formulas presents a clinical challenge. The renal-specific formulas are similar in that they provide 2 kcal/ml and from 70 to 75 g of protein per liter. Feeding one of these formulas at a rate sufficient to provide 30 kcal/kg will deliver approximately 1.0 to 1.1 g of protein per kilogram. Increasing the feeding rate to provide 35 kcal/kg will yield only 1.2 to 1.3 g

TABLE 29.3
Selected Characteristics of Renal-Specific Enteral Formulas, a Standard Calorically Dense Formula, and an "Immune-Enhancing" Formula that Could Be Used for a Patient with ARF

Product	kcal/ml	Protein (per liter)	Potassium (per liter)	Phosphorous (per liter)	Water (per liter)	n-6:n-3 lipids
Nepro®a	2.0	70 g	27.1 mEq	695 mg	699 g	5.5:1
Novasource™ Renalb	2.0	74 g	21 mEq	650 mg	709 g	N/A
Nutri-Renal™c	2.0	70 g	32.2 mEq	700 mg	700 g	4.74:1
Magnacal® Renald	2.0	75 g	32.6 mEq	800 mg	710 g	4.8:1
TwoCal®HNa	2.0	83.5 g	63 mEq	1055 mg	701 g	9.1:1
Crucial® c*	1.5	125 g*	63.8 mEq*	1330 mg*	1025 g*	1.7:1

* The caloric density of Crucial is 1.5 kcal/ml. To allow isocaloric comparison with 2 kcal/ml products, nutrient values for Crucial are per 1.33 l.

Sources: From manufacturers' published data. aRoss Products Division, Columbus, OH. bNovartis Nutrition Corp., Minneapolis, MN. cNestlé Clinical Nutrition, Deerfield, IL. dMead Johnson & Co., Evansville, IN.

of protein per kilogram, still substantially less than one might prefer based on recommendations ranging from 1.5 to 2.5 g of protein per kilogram.

To increase protein delivery, the clinician may add supplemental protein as a modular additive to the formula. Alternatively, protein may be mixed with water and delivered as a scheduled feeding tube flush, thereby maintaining the integrity of closed-system formula packaging. Five grams protein in 50 ml water given four times daily adds 0.3 g of protein per kilogram for the 70 kg patient; with a "renal" formula at 35 kcal/kg, the approximate combined yield is 1.5 to 1.6 g of protein per kilogram, within the range of contemporary guidelines (see Table 29.4).

Another option for enteral support is use of an immune-enhancing diet (IED) formula with 80 to 90 or more grams of protein per liter and 1.3 to 1.5 kcal energy per milliliter (see Chapter 11 and Chapter 16.) With an IED delivering 30 to 35 kcal/kg, the patient may approach or exceed a goal of 2 g of protein per kilogram. Supplemental arginine, which these products may contain, is a metabolic precursor to nitric oxide, which has been associated with increased renal perfusion and oxygenation.[23,24] The emerging view of ARF as an immune or toxic state rather than a hemodynamic one suggests other benefits may be derived from the antioxidant and immune-modulating properties of the IED.[25] Several contemporary authors have advocated use of IEDs in ARF.[2,17]

In some cases, a standard high-protein, isotonic, or calorically dense formula may provide effective metabolic support for the patient with ARF. Successful use of a standard formula will depend on patients' ability to tolerate the higher electrolyte concentrations found in these products. This will be a factor with the use of IED in renal failure as well; both immune-modulating and standard formulas provide sodium, potassium, magnesium, and phosphorous in amounts 50 to 100% greater than are found in renal-specific products. Because electrolyte intolerance is characteristic of renal failure, effective RRT should be available before use of standard or immune-modulating enteral formulas can be considered.

29.4.5 PARENTERAL NUTRITION IN ARF

In the event that metabolic needs cannot be met with enteral feeding, parenteral nutrition (PN) support may be indicated. In the previously discussed study reported by Scheinkestel et al., 54% of study patients with ARF were supported enterally, 30% with a combination of EN and PN, and in 16% of their subjects the authors conclude: "...the enteral route failed completely."[18] In a survey of Canadian ICU practices, 12% of patients on nutrition support received parenteral only.[26] Some patients inevitably will exhibit a degree of intolerance to enteral feeding, and for them it will be necessary to provide at least part of their metabolic needs by parenteral means.

Parenteral nutrition has the advantage of being readily adjustable to meet specific macro- or micronutrient needs of an individual patient and can be formulated to provide the balance of metabolic requirements when only very small volumes of enteral support are tolerated.

Preparation of a PN formula for the patient with ARF should take into account the volume status of the patient. If necessary, nutrients may be delivered in minimal volume or in a maximally concentrated form. Recall that patients with ARF typically exhibit some degree of carbohydrate intolerance.[11,12] To decrease the rate of parenteral dextrose infusion, a greater part of the nonprotein energy in the formula may be provided by lipid emulsion; however, exogenous insulin may still be necessary to control hyperglycemia.

Automatic compounding simplifies PN ordering, because specifications may be easily accommodated, but it is not available in every hospital. A model for renal PN has been suggested that is simply ordered: 500 ml each of glucose, lipids, and amino acids, concentration of each determined by patient requirements and capabilities of the compounding pharmacy.[11] Water- and fat-soluble vitamins are recommended daily, limiting total ascorbate to 200 mg or less.[11] Trace minerals twice weekly are recommended, and electrolytes and insulin should be added as needed.[11]

29.4.6 GLUTAMINE AND ARGININE IN ARF

The possibility that supplemental arginine or enteral formulas containing added arginine may be beneficial in various disease states has been the subject of study and debate for several years. Arginine and nitric oxide (NO), for which arginine serves as substrate, have been shown to improve renal function when impairment is related to vasoconstriction and reduced perfusion, and to reduce the nephrotoxic effects of cyclosporine.[24] On the other hand, inflammatory conditions may result in production of large amounts of NO sufficient to cause tissue damage. This is a key feature of the host response to infection but has raised questions about the appropriateness of arginine supplementation in ARF associated with inflammation, as in glomerulonephritis.[24,27] Schramm et al. found the pathological actions of NO were not related to supplemental arginine administration.[28]

With regard to glutamine, Druml reports that a *post hoc* analysis of data from a study in critically ill patients suggested that patients with ARF showed benefit most often.[11,29] Of the survivors in this study, patients with ARF were significantly more likely to show improvement leading to survival than were non-ARF patients when supplemental glutamine was administered.[11] Although these data are suggestive of benefit, firm recommendations await the publishing of conclusive clinical trials.[17]

Based on studies of antioxidant and glutamine use with critically ill patients and arginine with ARF, previously cited recommendations for use of immune-enhancing enteral formulas in critical care patients with renal failure are upheld.[2,17,24,30]

TABLE 29.4
Use of Modular Supplement to Increase Protein in Renal-Specific Formula, 70-kg Patient

Feeding Component	kcal/kg	Protein	Total Yield (Formula + Protein)
Renal-specific formula, 1 l	28	1.0 g/kg	
Modular protein, 5 g in 50 ml H₂O, qid (+20 g)	1.1	0.3 g/kg	29.1 kcal, 1.3 g protein per kilogram
Modular protein, 10 g in 100 ml H₂O, tid (+30 g)	1.7	0.4 g/kg	29.7 kcal, 1.4 g protein per kilogram

29.5 THE CHRONIC AND END-STAGE RENAL FAILURE PATIENT IN THE ICU

"The presence of renal disease in a critically ill patient should never lead to restrictions in nutritional support."[17] Recommendations from a 2002 report to the 6th International Conference on CRRT specify that full nutrition support should be provided to all patients with renal failure, including acute, chronic, and end-stage renal failure, who are critically ill.[17] Provision of recommended nutrients, especially protein, for these patients requires availability of appropriate dialysis therapy.

29.5.1 MAINTENANCE DIALYSIS AND ALBUMIN

The patient with severe chronic renal failure (CRF) or end-stage renal disease (ESRD), typically receiving maintenance dialysis treatments on a routine schedule prior to admission to the ICU, commonly exhibits both protein-energy malnutrition and multiple micronutrient deficiencies.[31,32] This state of being has been attributed to poor dietary intake, loss of substrate to RRT, hypermetabolism, and inflammatory response; it is also marked by hypoalbuminemia.[31] Albumin depletion in maintenance dialysis patients has been related less to protein intake or protein catabolic rate (PCR) than to inflammation as marked by C-reactive protein (CRP).[31] In Pifer et al., decreased serum albumin was independently associated with mortality, but protein intake or PCR was not.[33] This may support the use of serum albumin as a prognostic indicator in renal failure patients but not as a marker of nutrition status or adequacy of nutrition support.

29.5.2 NUTRIENT DEFICIENCIES AND RECOMMENDATIONS

Low serum albumin may indeed reflect decreased nutrient intake and reduced albumin synthesis, however.[34] The National Cooperative Dialysis Study reveals average protein and energy intake of dialysis patients is far less than recommended to maintain nitrogen and energy balance.[31,35]

Maintenance dialysis patients commonly suffer micronutrient deficiencies as well.[32] Most prominent among vitamin deficiencies are ascorbate, folate, B6, and calcitriol; trace element deficiencies of iron, zinc, and possibly selenium are noted in this population, and toxicity from aluminum and copper is seen.[32] If studies with dialysis patients suggest inadequate intake or if greater needs are frequently seen in this population, then this should be taken into account when the maintenance dialysis patient is seen in critical care. See Table 29.5 for micronutrient recommendations for the maintenance dialysis patient.

The provision of full nutrition support to chronic and end-stage renal failure patients in critical care, as recommended, requires prioritizing each patient's concurrent medical problems and designing the optimal nutrition care plan accordingly.[17] Traditionally, the necessity of severely limited fluid intake to prevent overload and protein restriction, hoped to reduce accumulation of nitrogenous wastes, created significant restraints on nutrition support. Contemporary renal replacement therapies enable control of fluid balance and azotemia so that metabolic needs of virtually all critically ill patients with renal failure can be more fully met.

29.6 MONITORING NUTRITION INTERVENTION IN ARF

If it is given that the exact cause of hypercatabolism in ARF cannot be clearly stated and that net nitrogen loss is unavoidable, then achieving the goal of minimizing protein loss requires some practicable method of measuring protein status in order to optimize nutrition support.[10,13] In some cases, it may be possible to monitor and track blood urea nitrogen levels as they respond to changes in protein intake and removal by RRT. A number of factors confound interpretation of serum protein levels in ARF. Fluid gains reduce measured serum levels and fluid losses increase them; in both cases, these changes are unrelated to protein nutriture and nitrogen balance. Suppression of albumin

TABLE 29.5
Micronutrient Daily Recommendations for Maintenance Dialysis (MD) Patients

Micronutrient	Daily Recommendation	Note
Vitamin B1	1.1–1.2 mg	Same as for non-MD patients
Vitamin B2	1.1–1.3 mg	Same as for non-MD patients
Pantothenic acid	5 mg	Same as for non-MD patients
Biotin	30 mg	Same as for non-MD patients
Niacin	14–16 mg	Same as for non-MD patients
Vitamin B6	10 mg	Removed by hemodialysis
Vitamin B12	2.4 mg	Same as for non-MD patients
Ascorbate	75–90 mg	Risk for oxalosis with excessive intake
Folic acid	1 mg	Removed by hemodialysis
Vitamin A	800–1,000 mg	Vulnerable to toxicity, do not exceed RDA
Vitamin D	0.25–1.0 mg	MD patients often deficient unless supplemented
Vitamin E	400–800 IU (optional)	Effectiveness uncertain, apparently safe
Vitamin K	Not specified	Supplement *if* not eating *and* receiving antibiotic therapy
Iron	Not specified	Deficiency common in MD patients, parenteral supplementation preferred
Zinc	RDA (15 mg enteral)	More definitive studies needed
Selenium	Not specified	Low serum levels typical in MD patients
Copper	Not specified	Essential, but excess can cause hemolytic anemia

Source: Information from Kalantar-Zadeh, K. and Kopple, J.D., *Adv. Ren. Replac. Ther.*, 10, 170, 2003.[32]

or prealbumin synthesis due to inflammation may occur despite provision of adequate protein, yet decreased renal clearance of proteins may lead to exaggerated serum levels and a false confidence with inadequate support.

With regard to nitrogen balance, it should be noted that nitrogen balance studies are limited in ARF due to loss of urinary nitrogen excretion.[15] Nevertheless, nitrogen balance is calculated and may provide a useful guide to therapy if results are interpreted with careful awareness of potentially confounding factors.

29.6.1 CALCULATION OF NITROGEN BALANCE

A method for assessing nitrogen balance is suggested in Suleiman and Zaloga, where nitrogen output is estimated from urea nitrogen appearance.[36]

To calculate urea nitrogen appearance, or UNA, sum:

- Urinary urea nitrogen (g/d) +
- Dialysate urea nitrogen (g/d) +
- Change in body urea nitrogen (CBUN), where CBUN (g/d) = SUN2 (g/l) − SUN1 (g/l) × BW2 × (0.6 l/kg) + (BW2 − BW1) × SUN2 × (1.0 l/kg)

In this equation, 1 (as in SUN1, BUN1) identifies the initial value for the study period and 2 is the final value. SUN, or serum urea nitrogen, is functionally equivalent to BUN, or blood urea nitrogen, and BW is weight in kilograms.

Once UNA has been calculated in this manner, then *total nitrogen output* is estimated to be the sum of UNA + 2.[36] The patient's net *nitrogen balance* = total nitrogen output − total nitrogen intake (where nitrogen intake is calculated from protein intake in grams by multiplying by 0.16).

29.7 CASE STUDY

The best measure of a patient's response to care is his or her outcome. In the following example, polycystic disease was later found to be underlying the patient's acute renal failure and affected the progress of her illness.

29.7.1 ASSESSMENT

Mrs. G. was 56 years of age, admitted from a smaller outlying hospital with hypotension and abdominal abscess that had progressed to extensive necrotizing fasciitis and sepsis. The nutrition support service found the patient on mechanical ventilation per endotracheal tube with Gram-positive cocci in the abdominal wound and the blood. Assessment revealed height 172 cm and weight 115 kg, from which an IBW of 64 kg and AdjBW of 77 kg were calculated.

PN was infusing, maximally concentrated in 2.4 l volume, delivering 3600 total kcal and 150 g amino acids (AA), or 46 kcal and 1.9 g AA per kilogram AdjBW per day. Regular insulin was infusing separately at a rate of 10 units per hour.

Laboratory values included albumin 1.4, sodium 145, potassium 3.8, chloride 107, CO_2 21, BUN 113, creatinine 3.9, glucose 355, ionized calcium 0.99, phosphorous 4.0, and triglycerides 457. The patient was nonoliguric with urine output greater than 50 ml/ h.

29.7.2 INTERVENTION

Macronutrient delivery was clearly exceeding the patient's ability to tolerate it, so the PN was adjusted to provide 25 kcal and 1.5 g AA per kilogram AdjBW. Because it would be 12 hours before a new PN formula was delivered, infusion rate of the existing PN was decreased to 55 ml/h, and a maintenance IV of 0.45% saline was initiated to maintain intravascular volume. The patient's nurse was advised to anticipate lower insulin needs, which would be evident at hourly blood sugar checks. It was documented that if triglyceride levels did not decrease as a result of these changes, all lipids would be removed from the PN until dyslipidemia resolved.

29.7.3 RESPONSE

By the next day, serum glucose was normal at 106 with an insulin infusion rate of 4 units per hour. Enteral nutrition was initiated by nasogastric tube at 5 ml/h. The day after that (intervention day 3), with the maintenance fluids at 125 ml/h and urine output from 70 to 125 ml/h, uremia had increased with BUN 120 and creatinine 4.5. Nephrology was consulted and intermittent hemodialysis was ordered. Triglycerides were acceptable at 275, and, with PN continuing, EN was increased to 10 ml/h.

The patient was weaned from mechanical ventilation the day after that, and on intervention day 5, sips of liquid PO were allowed. Enteral nutrition was increased to 15 ml/h, for combined support of 30 kcal and 1.7 g protein/AA per kilogram. On intervention day 6, the patient transferred to a progressive care unit, PN was discontinued, and EN was increased to provide 30 kcal and 1.5 g protein per kilogram. Serum triglycerides were acceptable at 186.

By the eighth day of nutrition support intervention, Mrs. G. was much more alert, still with only clear liquids by mouth but increasing intake tentatively while EN continued to meet metabolic needs. Uremia had improved but not resolved completely, with BUN 66 and creatinine 3.5. A new diagnosis of polycystic kidney disease was noted. The patient was still requiring IHD, but fasciitis and septic hypotension had resolved. The patient was in good spirits, visiting with family and anticipating transfer to long-term acute care for continuing treatment.

29.8 SUMMARY

In recent years, recommendations for the nutritional care of patients with ARF in intensive care have clarified the need for an approach that is not based on our experience with chronic renal failure. The need for protein and fluid restriction in ARF has been substantially reduced by effective renal replacement, allowing the patient a greater chance to escape the ravages of catabolic disease. The emerging appreciation of inflammatory processes related to renal failure leads to a new view of the interrelationships among biochemical markers, as well as to novel therapeutic approaches. The beneficial role of enteral nutrition is reemphasized in view of the special needs of the patient with acute renal failure. As awareness increases among clinicians, improvements in the standard of care may contribute to easing the historically high mortality among this patient population.

REFERENCES

1. Chew, S.L. et al., Outcome in acute renal failure, *Nephrol. Dial. Transplant*, 8, 101, 1993.
2. Kapadia, F.N., Bhojani, K., and Shah, B., Special issues in the patient with renal failure, *Crit. Care Clin.*, 19, 233, 2003.
3. Hoste, A.J. et al., Acute renal failure in patients with sepsis in a surgical ICU: predictive factors, incidence, comorbidity, and outcome, *J. Am. Soc. Nephrol.*, 14, 1022, 2003.
4. Chertow, G.M. et al., Prognostic stratification in critically ill patients with acute renal failure requiring dialysis, *Arch. Inern. Med.,* 155, 1505, 1995.
5. Metnitz, G.H. et al., Effect of acute renal failure requiring renal replacement therapy on outcome in critically ill patients, *Crit. Care Med.*, 30, 2051, 2002.
6. Clermont G. et al., Renal failure in the ICU: comparison of the impact of acute renal failure and end-stage renal disease on ICU outcomes, *Kidney Int.,* 62, 986, 2002.
7. Albright, R.C., Acute renal failure: a practical update, *Mayo Clin. Proc.*, 76, 67, 2001.
8. Lennon, A.-M., Coleman, P.L., and Brady, H.R., Management and outcome of acute renal failure, in *Comprehensive Clinical Nephrology*, Johnson, R.J. and Feehally, J., Eds., Harcourt Publishers, Edinburgh, 2000, chap. 19.
9. Brady, H.R. et al., Acute renal failure, in *Brenner and Rector's the Kidney*, Brenner, B.M., Ed., W.B. Saunders, Philadelphia, 2000, 1241.
10. Anderson, R.J and Schrier, R.W., Acute renal failure, in *Diseases of the Kidney and Urinary Tract*, 7th ed., Schrier, R.W., Ed., Lippincott, Williams & Wilkins, Philadelphia, 2001, 1119.
11. Druml, W., Nutritional management of acute renal failure, *Am. J. Kidney Dis.*, 37, S89, 2001.
12. Kierdorf, H.P., The nutritional management of acute renal failure in the intensive care unit, *New Horizons*, 3, 699, 1995.
13. Druml, W., Protein metabolism in acute renal failure, *Mineral and Electrolyte Metab.*, 24, 47, 1998.
14. Hoogerwerf, M., Nutritional aspects of acute renal failure, *EDTNA/ERCA J.*, Suppl. 2, 54, 2002.
15. Gennari, F.J. and Rimmer, J.M., The dialysis patient, in *Massry and Glassock's Textbook of Nephrology*, 4th ed., Massry, S.G. and Glassock, R.J., Eds., Lippincott, Williams & Wilkins, Philadelphia, 2001, 1387.
16. Cerra, F.B. et al., Applied nutrition in ICU patients: a consensus statement of the American College of Chest Physicians, *CHEST*, 111, 769, 1997.
17. Bellomo, R., How to feed patients with renal dysfunction, *Blood Purif.*, 20, 296, 2002.
18. Scheinkestel, C.D. et al., Prospective randomized trial to assess caloric and protein needs of critically ill, anuric, ventilated patients requiring continuous renal replacement therapy, *Nutrition*, 19, 909, 2003.
19. Macias, W.L. et al., Impact of the nutritional regimen on protein catabolism and nitrogen balance in patients with acute renal failure, *JPEN*, 20, 56, 1996.
20. Wolk, R., Nutrition in renal failure, in *The Science and Practice of Nutrition Support: A Case-Based Core Curriculum*, ASPEN, Silver Spring, MD, 2001, chap. 28.
21. Roberts, P.R., Black, K.W., and Zaloga, G.P., Enteral feeding improves outcomes and protects against glycerol-induced acute renal failure in the rat, *Am. J. Respir. Crit. Care Med.*, 156, 1265, 1997.

22. Druml, W. and Mitch, W.E., Enteral nutrition in renal disease, in *Enteral and Tube Feeding*, Rombeau, J.L. and Rolandelli, R.H., Eds., W.B. Saunders, Philadelphia, 1997, chap. 26.
23. Herselman, M., Protein and energy requirements in patients with acute renal failure on continuous renal replacement therapy, *Nutrition*, 19, 813, 2003.
24. Efron, D.T. and Barbul, A., Arginine and nutrition in renal disease, *J. Ren. Nutr.*, 9, 142, 1999.
25. Wan, L. et al., The pathogenesis of septic acute renal failure, *Curr. Opin. Crit. Care*, 9, 496, 2003.
26. Heyland, D.K. et al., Nutrition support in the critical care setting: current practice in Canadian ICUs—opportunities for improvement? *JPEN*, 27, 74, 2003.
27. Marletta, M.A. and Spierling, M.M., Trace elements and nitric oxide function, *J. Nutr.*, 133, 1431S, 2003.
28. Schramm, L. et al., L-arginine deficiency and supplementation in experimental acute renal failure and in human kidney transplantation, *Kidney Int.*, 61, 1423, 2002.
29. Griffiths, R.D., Outcome of critically ill patients after supplementation with glutamine, *Nutrition*, 13, 752, 1997.
30. Lovat, R. and Preiser, J.C., Antioxidant therapy in intensive care, *Curr. Opin. Crit. Care.*, 9, 266, 2003.
31. Burl, R.D., and Kaysen, G.A., Assessment of inflammation and nutrition in patients with end-stage renal disease, *J. Nephrol.*, 13, 249, 2000.
32. Kalantar-Zadeh, K. and Kopple, J.D., Trace elements and vitamins in maintenance dialysis patients, *Adv. Ren. Replac. Ther.*, 10, 170, 2003.
33. Pifer, T.B. et al., Mortality risk in hemodialysis and changes in nutritional indicators: DOPPS, *Kidney Intl.*, 62, 2238, 2002.
34. Kaysen, G.A. et al., Relationships among inflammation nutrition and physiologic mechanisms establishing albumin levels in hemodialysis patients, *Kidney Int.*, 61, 2240, 2002.
35. Schoenfeld, P.Y. et al., Assessment of nutritional status of the National Cooperative Dialysis Study population, *Kidney Intl. Suppl.*, Apr., 13, 1983.
36. Suleiman, M.Y. and Zaloga, G.P., Renal failure, in *Nutrition in Critical Care*, Zaloga, G.P., Ed., Mosby Year Book, St. Louis, 1994, chap. 36.

30 Nutrition for the Critically Ill Patient with Hepatic Failure

Adam D. Waller and Ayaz J. Chaudhary
Medical College of Georgia

CONTENTS

30.1 INTRODUCTION

The liver is responsible for providing the appropriate amount of substrate needed for the adequate function of other organ systems. To this end, the liver plays a major role in carbohydrate, protein, and fat metabolism; storage of nutrients; and regulation of substrate availability, as described in Table 30.1. Hepatic failure, which can be divided into two categories — acute, or fulminant, and chronic liver failure — can adversely affect any of these activities. In addition, the liver of patients with hepatic failure is often challenged by undernourishment due to the prevalence of malnutrition. Therefore, the provision of nutritional support to patients with hepatic failure can be a life-saving treatment modality. An important aspect of critically ill patients with hepatic failure, whether acute or chronic, is hepatic encephalopathy, primarily because of its relative protein intolerance.

30.2 ACUTE LIVER FAILURE

Acute liver failure (ALF) is an uncommon clinical syndrome characterized by severe impairment of liver function that results in jaundice, followed by hepatic encephalopathy within 8 weeks after the onset of disease.[1] This occurs in the absence of previous liver disease and often involves massive hepatocellular necrosis. The leading causes of ALF in the United States are acetaminophen toxicity, acute viral hepatitis, and idiosyncratic drug reactions.[2] Complications involving almost every organ system can occur, including cerebral edema, renal failure, respiratory failure, and cardiovascular collapse, with mortality ranging from 40 to 95%.[3] Higher mortality is associated with a longer interval between the onset of jaundice and the development of encephalopathy. To better predict prognosis, O'Grady et al. proposed categorizing ALF into:[4]

- Hyperacute liver failure — Jaundice-to-encephalopathy interval of less than 7 days
- Acute liver failure — Interval of 8 to 28 days
- Subacute liver failure — Interval greater than 28 days

30.2.1 CLINICAL PRESENTATION

The clinical presentation of ALF is characterized by an acute onset of severe hepatic dysfunction in a patient with no stigmata of chronic liver disease. Patients can present with nonspecific findings of fever, abdominal pain, fatigue, nausea, dark urine, and jaundice and, later, with hepatic encephalopathy, coagulopathy, and other clinical features found in Table 30.2. The mortality rate in ALF is high and is typically caused by infection, cerebral edema, bleeding, hypoglycemia, or multiple organ failure, which complicates massive liver injury.[5]

TABLE 30.1
Nutrition-Related Liver Functions

Galactose and fructose converted into glucose and stored as glycogen
Glycogenolysis when blood glucose levels become low
Synthesis of the vital plasma proteins
Fatty acids and adipose tissue converted to Acetyl-CoA by beta oxidation to produce energy
Synthesis of triglycerides, phospholipids, cholesterol, and bile salts
Storage, activation, and transport of fat-soluble vitamins, zinc, iron, copper, magnesium, vitamin B_{12}

TABLE 30.2
Clinical Features of Acute Liver Failure

Hepatic Encephalopathy
Cerebral edema

Hepatocellular Dysfunction
Coagulopathy
Hypoglycemia
Metabolic acidosis

Cardiovascular Abnormalities
Hypoxia
Hypotension

Renal Dysfunction
Acute tubular necrosis
Hepatorenal syndrome

Multiple Organ Dysfunction Syndrome

TABLE 30.3
Staging of Encephalopathy

Stage	Clinical Manifestations
0	No change in consciousness, no degree of encephalopathy present
1	Impaired attention, mild confusion, insomnia/sleep disturbance, agitation, euphoria or depression
2	Lethargy, disorientation, bizarre behavior, anxiety, slurred speech, personality change
3	Marked confusion, somnolence but arousable, asterixis
4	Stupor and coma, no response to painful stimuli

30.2.1.1 Hepatic Encephalopathy and Cerebral Edema

With progression of encephalopathy, increasing degrees of neurologic dysfunction are commonly graded on a numeric scale, as described in Table 30.3.[6] If the encephalopathy only progresses to stage 2, prognosis for recovery is excellent, whereas those patients who reach stage 3 or stage 4 tend to do worse because of the development of cerebral edema and raised intracranial pressure.[1] The pathogenesis of the cerebral edema appears to result from neurotoxins, not cleared by the injured liver, that alter cerebral blood flow and increase permeability of the blood–brain barrier.[7] Other theories to explain the development of encephalopathy are discussed later.

30.2.1.2 Hepatocelluar Dysfunction

Other clinical features of ALF may result from the loss of important hepatocellular functions. Coagulopathy can result from decreased synthesis of coagulation factors, as well as the consumption of clotting factors and platelets caused by disseminated intravascular coagulation (DIC).[8] This increases the patient's risk for gastrointestinal hemorrhage. Hypoglycemia results from diminished glucose synthesis and, eventually, depletion of glycogen stores in the liver. Metabolic acidosis can occur as a result of reduced clearance of lactic acid.

30.2.1.3 Sepsis

Approximately 80% of patients with ALF are at increased risk of infection with bacterial pathogens because of damage to hepatic macrophages (Kupffer cells), impaired polymorphonuclear leukocyte function, and low levels of circulating complement.[9] The environment of an intensive care setting also increases the patient's exposure to pathogens with the possible requirement of invasive procedures. Fungal infections, predominantly *Candida albicans*, are also seen and develop in up to one-third of patients with ALF.[10]

30.2.1.4 Cardiovascular Abnormalities

Cardiovascular changes seen in ALF are characterized by a decreased systemic vascular resistance and, despite a compensatory rise in cardiac output, tissue hypoxia and lactic acidosis develop.[11] This is often a prelude to the development of multiorgan failure. In addition, hypotension is a common finding in patients with advanced coma.

30.2.1.5 Renal Failure

Renal dysfunction is a common complication of ALF and is associated with a poor outcome.[12] It is often related to hepatorenal syndrome or acute tubular necrosis. In addition, acetaminophen toxicity can cause direct nephrotoxicity.

30.2.1.6 Multiple Organ Dysfunction Syndrome

The inflammatory response to massive liver injury can lead to widespread and progressive inflammatory injury. Frequently, sepsis contributes to this insult, with endotoxinemia leading to circulatory collapse, tissue hypoxia, and increased bacterial translocation across leaky intestinal mucosa.[5] Multiple organ failure can develop, which manifests as hypotension, pulmonary edema, renal failure, and DIC.

30.2.2 Medical Management of Acute Liver Failure

Medical care should be provided in an intensive care unit for all patients with ALF, with placement of venous and arterial lines, nasogastric tube to prevent aspiration, Foley catheter to monitor urinary output, and intracranial pressure monitors to guide cerebral edema therapy. It is generally recommended to start an intravenous H_2 receptor antagonist[13] with a broad-spectrum antibiotic to reduce the risk of gastrointestinal bleeding and prevent translocation of enteric organisms. If the patient is in stage 3 or 4 coma, endotracheal intubation and mechanical ventilation should be considered for airway protection. If the cause of the ALF can be identified, it should be treated specifically, such as acetaminophen toxicity treated with N-acetylcysteine. Blood glucose levels should be monitored frequently, because hypoglycemia commonly occurs. Cerebral edema can be treated with intravenous mannitol, which has been shown to reduce the elevated intracranial pressure and improve survival.[14] Because rapid clinical deterioration is common in patients with ALF, the patient's candidacy for liver transplantation should be decided early, with urgent transfer to a liver transplantation center if deemed a candidate. Orthotopic liver transplantation can be a life-saving remedy for patients who are not recovering from ALF. It has been clearly shown to improve both short-term and long-term survival in patients with grade 3 or grade 4 coma.

30.3 CHRONIC LIVER FAILURE

The liver is the only vital organ that has the capacity to significantly regenerate after it has been injured. This can be seen in patients who recover from acute liver failure; however, chronic liver

---

TABLE 30.4
Causes of Cirrhosis

Alcoholic liver disease
Chronic hepatitis C
Primary biliary cirrhosis
Primary sclerosing cholangitis
Autoimmune hepatitis
Chronic hepatitis B
Hereditary hemochromatosis
Wilson's disease
Alpha-1-antitrypsin deficiency
Budd–Chiari syndrome
Cryptogenic cirrhosis

---

injury seems to disrupt the mechanism of regeneration, as is seen in alcoholic liver disease, and results in the gradual development of fibrosis and cirrhosis.[15] Cirrhosis is the final stage of liver disease, with a variety of causes, as listed in Table 30.4. This degree of liver failure essentially becomes nonreversible and, similar to acute liver failure, has consequences that affect multiple organ systems. The major complications of cirrhosis include the development of portal hypertension, which can result in portal systemic shunting and esophageal and gastric varices that can rupture and bleed; ascites, which can be further complicated by spontaneous bacterial peritonitis; and hepatic encephalopathy. Other complications include thrombocytopenia, hepatorenal syndrome, hepatopulmonary syndrome, and hepatocellular carcinoma. Hepatic encephalopathy, a complication seen in both acute and chronic liver failure, deserves special recognition because of its unique nutritional considerations.

30.4 HEPATIC ENCEPHALOPATHY

Hepatic encephalopathy (HE), or portosystemic encephalopathy (PSE), reflects a spectrum of neuropsychiatric abnormalities seen in patients with liver dysfunction after exclusion of other known brain disease.[6] It is a reversible metabolic encephalopathy that occurs as a consequence of liver failure and resolves with improvement in liver function. HE is characterized by sleepiness, impaired mental function, and distinct motor abnormalities (asterixis) in its early stages, followed by confusion, lethargy, and, ultimately, unresponsiveness (Table 30.3). It is usually seen in patients with chronic liver disease, although it can occur in previously healthy patients presenting with acute liver failure. Classification of HE is based on the underlying liver disease and the duration and characteristics of the neurologic manifestations.

30.4.1 Pathogenesis

The exact pathogenesis of HE remains unclear. Several theories have been proposed to explain the syndrome and its clinical manifestations. The three most relevant theories involve ammonia metabolism, activation of inhibitory neurotransmitters, and the development of "false neurotransmitters." It appears that these theories are not mutually exclusive.[16]

The most likely theory designates ammonia as a cerebral toxin. Ammonia is the byproduct of nitrogen metabolism, which originates from several sources in the body. A significant portion of the ammonia is derived from bacterial degradation of intestinal protein. The ammonia is transported through the portal vein to the liver, where it undergoes conversion to urea and glutamine. Approximately 75% of the urea is then excreted by the kidneys, thus completing the process of ammonia disposal. In hepatic failure, the liver develops impaired ammonia metabolism, resulting in ammonia accumulation in the blood. In addition, a portal–systemic shunt, often seen in chronic liver disease, shunts blood flow away from the liver and further impairs hepatic clearance of ammonia. The circulating ammonia enters the brain and is thought to precipitate HE. This theory is supported by the fact that treatments that lower the serum ammonia level result in improvement of the HE.[17]

Several neurotransmitter systems have been implicated in the pathogenesis of HE.[18] Gamma-aminobutyric acid (GABA) is an inhibitory neurotransmitter with receptors throughout the central nervous system. Activated GABA-ergic tone is associated with neuronal depression and HE.[19] In addition, the GABA receptor complex involves a linked benzodiazepine receptor. An increase in benzodiazepine receptor ligands is found in states of HE,[20] and improvement in mental status after the administration of a benzodiazepine receptor antagonist has been observed.[21]

An altered amino acid profile theory has also been implicated in the pathogenesis of HE. Astrocytes within the brain detoxify ammonia by converting it to glutamine, which accumulates intracellularly and contributes to development of brain edema. The glutamine is later exchanged for an aromatic amino acid, which is influxed into the brain.[22] The exchange is facilitated by the fact that patients with liver failure have an increase in aromatic amino acids and a decrease in branched-chain amino acids (BCAA).[23] The excess of aromatic amino acids is thought to be responsible for the synthesis of "false neurotransmitters," resulting in ineffective neurotransmission and the induction of HE.

30.4.2 PRECIPITATING EVENTS

Any chronic liver failure patient with new-onset or worsening HE should be evaluated carefully for a precipitating event (Table 30.5). These clinical events precipitate HE either by raising blood ammonia levels (via an increase in nitrogenous substances) or by further impairing liver function, which may result in enhanced portosystemic shunting. In addition, drugs, toxins, and medications can directly suppress the central nervous system and its neurotransmitters. In an analysis of 100 patients with HE, azotemia, sedative use, and gastrointestinal (GI) bleeding accounted for nearly 75% of all admissions.[24] Effective therapy is based on recognition and treatment of these reversible causes of HE.

30.4.3 DIAGNOSIS

The diagnosis of HE is based primarily on recognition of the pattern of clinical neuropsychiatric changes in patients with chronic liver disease. Any change in mental status in a patient with cirrhosis should raise suspicion of the possibility of HE. With progression of encephalopathy, increasing degrees of neurologic dysfunction are commonly graded on a numeric scale, as described in Table 30.3.[6]

TABLE 30.5
Precipitating Events for Hepatic Encephalopathy

Clinical Event	Management
Azotemia	Prevent intravascular volume depletion, reduce diuretics, avoid nephrotoxic antibiotics and IV contrast
Sedatives	Avoid analgesics and sedatives, including antihistamines
GI hemorrhage	Control GI bleeding, purge blood from GI tract
Hypokalemic alkalosis	Correct acidosis, alkalosis, hypoxia, or electrolyte abnormalities
Dietary indiscretion	Avoid excessive protein intake
Infection	Screen for and pursue aggressive therapy of any infection
Constipation	Keep stools soft, prevent constipation

Liver injury tests will generally show changes consistent with the etiology of the liver disease but are not identifiers of HE. Some of the more common physical findings seen in cirrhosis include palmar erythema, spider angiomas, gynecomastia, ascites, and splenomegaly. Asterixis, or flapping tremor, is a nonspecific clinical sign that is generally present in the early stages of HE. Infrequently, additional tests may be necessary to confirm the diagnosis of HE.

30.4.3.1 Serum Ammonia

Blood ammonia levels are often very elevated in critically ill patients with HE,[25] but this elevation does not occur in all patients and, therefore, may not correlate with the severity of illness. Normal values do not exclude the diagnosis of HE.

30.4.3.2 Cerebrospinal Fluid Glutamine

Glutamine can be found in the cerebrospinal fluid and is considered a more specific marker of encephalopathy. It may be useful in cases in which the diagnosis of HE is uncertain; however, it is almost never used clinically because it requires lumbar puncture.

30.4.3.3 Neuropsychological and Neurophysiologic Tests

Assessment of abnormal cognition can be helpful in patients with subclinical HE, and several batteries of tests have been developed for this purpose (number-connection, line-drawing, serial dotting, and digital symbol tests).[26] Abnormal electroencephalographic readings are characteristic of HE. Patients generally show high-voltage and slow wave forms.[27]

30.4.3.4 Neuroimaging

Computed tomography (CT) is often indicated in encephalopathic patients to evaluate for organic brain disease or to document cerebral edema. However, CT does not depict specific abnormalities in HE. Magnetic resonance imaging (MRI) can reveal pallidal hyperintensity on T1-weighted images, possibly from manganese deposition, which is seen most frequently in cirrhotics with severe liver failure. Currently, CT and MRI are used to exclude structural causes of altered mental status, such as intracerebral bleeding. Proton magnetic resonance spectroscopy has been shown to be helpful in evaluating various metabolites, such as glutamine and myo-inositol, which are thought to be involved in the pathogenesis of HE.[28]

30.4.4 MEDICAL THERAPY OF HEPATIC ENCEPHALOPATHY

The development of HE is a complication of severe hepatic failure. Most episodes of HE occur in cirrhotics and have specific precipitating factors or events. Prevention or treatment of these precipitants is the important initial therapy. Other effective treatment involves ammonia-lowering therapy and providing adequate nutritional support (Table 30.6).

30.4.4.1 Lactulose

Lactulose is considered the mainstay of therapy for HE. This synthetic disaccharide is not absorbed in the upper gastrointestinal tract and passes unchanged into the cecum, where it is metabolized to acetic and lactic acids by the enteric bacteria.[29] The acidification within the lumen of the colon leads to the conversion of ammonia to ammonium ion and, ultimately, to an increase in fecal nitrogen excretion. This is reflected in a decrease in plasma levels of ammonia.[30]

Effective therapy with lactulose involves taking enough of the syrup to produce two to four bowel movements per day. The dose should be titrated to achieve this goal, because not all patients respond the same. In the critically ill patient, oral intake may not be possible, and the lactulose

TABLE 30.6
Treatment of Hepatic Encephalopathy

Treatment	Dose
Lactulose	Acute: 45 ml each hour until bowel movement
	Chronic: 15–45 ml bid or tid
Neomycin	Acute: PO: 3.6 g/d
	Chronic: PO: 1–2 g/d
Metronidazole	PO: 0.5 to 1.5 g/d
Flumazenil	IV: 1 mg

can be given rectally or by nasogastric tube (NGT), although there is an increased risk of aspiration with the obtunded patient. Excessive lactulose can cause severe diarrhea, with marked volume loss and electrolyte abnormalities, and thereby exacerbate the encephalopathy.

30.4.4.2 Neomycin

Neomycin has been used with some success in treating HE. However, no controlled studies have found it to be effective compared with standard treatment alone. Controlled trials comparing oral neomycin with oral lactulose have shown similar efficacies of the two drugs,[31–33] although one study, which compared neomycin to placebo, reported no difference in outcomes.[34] Neomycin does not cause diarrhea and may be used in patients who cannot tolerate lactulose, or it can be given as a supplement with lactulose. Unfortunately, it is highly nephrotoxic, and long-term use of this drug is not recommended.

30.4.4.3 Metronidazole

Metronidazole is an alternative to lactulose and neomycin. Although strong evidence of effectiveness in lowering serum ammonia is lacking, one controlled trial showed similar efficacies between metronidazole and neomycin.[35] Its usefulness in HE is further based on its tolerability and safety, because this antibiotic does not cause diarrhea and is not nephrotoxic. If the HE is poorly responsive to regular lactulose, metronidazole can also be added to the current use of lactulose. Of note, metronidazole has been associated with peripheral neuropathy when used as maintenance treatment for longer than two weeks.

30.4.4.4 Flumazenil

The hypothesis of enhanced GABA-ergic tone in HE led to the study of benzodiazepine antagonists. Flumazenil has shown a positive effect on HE in several randomized, controlled trials;[21,36–38] however, this was demonstrated as only transient improvement in mental state and no differences were seen 24 hours after the start of therapy.[36] Two meta-analyses found that treatment with flumazenil was associated with improvement in HE compared with placebo, but that benefit was short term and no improvement of recovery or survival was demonstrated.[39,40]

30.4.4.5 Other Treatments

Several drugs with possible beneficial effects for hepatic encephalopathy include vancomycin, rifaximin, ornithine–aspartate, zinc (a cofactor of urea cycle enzymes), benzoate, and bromocriptine. These have all shown variable responses but are not routinely used in the treatment of HE.

30.4.5 PORTOSYSTEMIC SHUNTS

Patients who have received a surgical portocaval shunt, such as a transjugular intrahepatic porto-systemic shunt (TIPS), are at increased risk of developing HE.[41] Most episodes of encephalopathy occur during the first two to three months after shunt placement and usually respond to treatment with lactulose. A small number of cases are refractory and may be considered for reduction in the diameter of the stent or stent occlusion.

30.4.6 LIVER TRANSPLANTATION

The development of HE in a patient with chronic liver disease indicates severe hepatic dysfunction and carries prognostic implications.[42] In addition, there is extensive impact on the quality of life in these patients.[43] Alternative therapy for HE includes a liver support device, such as the molecular absorbents reticulating system (MARS), which has been used with some success, or orthotopic liver transplantation. Improvement in HE manifestations after transplant has been reported.[44] Patients should be considered for liver transplantation with the development of recurrent or difficult-to-treat HE.

30.5 NUTRITION THERAPY IN HEPATIC FAILURE

Providing appropriate nutritional support for the critically ill patient with hepatic failure can be challenging. Most patients with liver failure have significant protein energy malnutrition and may present with muscle wasting, decreased fat stores, and overt cachexia.[45] Several factors contribute to the malnutrition in patients with liver failure. Patients with ascites have a decreased appetite as a result of early satiety, although they may present with substantial weight gain because of increasing ascites. Alcoholics routinely have inadequate protein intake as the percentage of total calories from ethanol increases. They are particularly at risk for thiamine, magnesium, and folate deficiency. Deficiency of the fat-soluble vitamins (A, D, E, and K) can be seen as a result of maldigestion and malabsorption, particularly in cholestatic liver disease and in cases of bacterial overgrowth. Needs for replacement of thiamine and other suspected vitamin deficiencies should be identified before feeding begins.

30.5.1 NUTRITION ASSESSMENT

Most of the traditional markers of nutritional status can be notably affected. Indicators of protein status, such as albumin, transferrin, prealbumin, and retinal binding protein, are often depressed due to impaired protein production. Further, the assessment of nutritional status may be imprecise because of possible concurrent ascites, edema, or renal insufficiency.[46]

30.5.2 NUTRITION REQUIREMENTS

30.5.2.1 Calories

Aggressive nutritional support in malnourished liver failure patients can lead to complications and has not been shown to reduce mortality.[47] These patients, particularly with alcoholism, are at risk for the refeeding syndrome, which is characterized by hypophosphatemia and hypomagnesemia.[48] Reduced calorie levels should be initiated slowly, and serum concentrations of electrolytes should be closely monitored.[49] Provision of calories significantly above energy expenditure will result in hyperglycemia, increase septic complications, and nullify any benefit of feeding.[50] Generally, it is recommended to provide calories of 15 to 20 kcal/kg/d for patients at refeeding risk, and 25 to 30 kcal/kg/d for maintenance caloric support. Patients with acute liver failure need 35 to 50 kcal/kg/d

TABLE 30.7
Nutrition Therapy in Hepatic Failure

Calories	
Refeeding risk	15–20 kcal/kg
Maintenance	25–30 kcal/kg
Catabolic (ALF)	35–50 kcal/kg

Protein	
Minimum intake	1.2 g/kg
Critically ill	1.5 g/kg
Vegetable protein	> 70% replacement
Branched-chain amino acids (consider for patients intolerant of standard protein intake)	

to meet resting metabolic demand. Nutrition therapy for hepatic failure and encephalopathy are summarized in Table 30.7.

30.5.2.2 Protein Requirements

Historically, the general recommendation for patients with HE has been to restrict protein intake to avoid any further ammonia production. However, severe restriction of protein can worsen nutritional deficits and liver function. Trials have demonstrated that patients with hepatic failure can tolerate normal or increased protein intake of up to 70 g/d without exacerbating encephalopathy.[51] It is important to provide adequate energy and protein to support liver function and to prevent any further breakdown of muscle mass.[50] A positive nitrogen balance can promote hepatic regeneration, and a minimum protein intake of 1.2 g/kg/d has been recommended to maintain this balance in cirrhotic patients.[52] Critically ill patients with major acute stress, such as those with gastrointestinal bleeding or infection, will have higher protein requirements and may require 1.5 g/kg/d, along with adequate lactulose therapy.[53]

30.5.2.2.1 Branched-Chain Amino Acids

BCAAs have been considered the alternative for protein intolerance in HE. They were initially administered to correct the abnormal amino acid profile and to prevent the formation of "false neurotransmitters." However, several randomized, controlled trials of BCAAs have not shown major beneficial effects. Many of the early studies compared parenteral BCAAs to lactulose or neomycin, and some found beneficial effect on encephalopathy with BCAAs.[54,55] Another trial, by Wahren et al., noted that parenteral BCAAs corrected the abnormal amino acid profile but did not show a beneficial effect on encephalopathy, with no decrease in mortality.[56] In a meta-analysis by Naylor et al., parenteral BCAAs did show reduction of the incidence of encephalopathy but did not show any survival benefit.[57] Overall, based on conflicting results and questionable benefit, recommendations have been made by the nutrition societies that both enteral and parenteral BCAAs be used only in those few patients with liver disease who are catabolic and intolerant of standard protein intake. However, more recently, Marchesini et al. reported a trial of 174 patients comparing outcomes after one year of dietary supplements of BCAAs vs. either lactoalbumin or maltodextrin, showing significantly lower mortality, decreased hospital admission, and shorter hospital stay in the BCAA arm of the study.[58] This study has been criticized,[59] but the results indicate the need for further investigation of BCAAs.

30.5.2.2.2 Vegetable Protein

Another option to provide nutrition support to refractory catabolic patients is the use of vegetable protein diets. The concept that vegetable protein causes less encephalopathy than animal protein has not been clearly proved. The data of multiple trials remain inconclusive; however, one study did show improvement in mental status with 70 to 90% replacement of vegetable protein.[60]

30.5.2.3 Fat Requirements

Cirrhosis is marked by impaired fat metabolism. Long-chain triglycerides, or dietary fat, are incompletely metabolized in liver failure. Therefore, overfeeding, regardless of the energy source, should be avoided, because excess calories can contribute to fat synthesis and accumulation in the liver. A range of 10 to 15% of calories as fat is generally recommended. If significant steatorrhea is present, replacement of some of the dietary fat with medium-chain triglycerides may be useful.

30.5.3 NUTRIENT DELIVERY METHODS

During the early period of acute encephalopathy with coma, the oral route of nutrition is usually avoided and glucose parenteral solutions are administered.[17] In most cases, the patient recovers in a few days, and the oral diet can be reinstituted. At this time, a moderate dose of protein (40 to 60 g/d) is given, and this is gradually increased until the maximum tolerance (usually 70 to 80 g/d) is reached. When the oral diet is reinstituted, effort should be made to optimize oral intake by avoiding long periods of nothing by mouth (NPO) and providing small meals and snacks during the day, which helps to reduce muscle breakdown during periods of fasting. If there is no improvement in mental status and coma is prolonged, it is critical to maintain a positive nitrogen balance through the use of enteral nitrogen supplements of amino acids.[61]

30.5.3.1 Enteral Nutrition

Enteral nutrition may be used to supplement oral feeding or to replace it entirely in patients who are unable to meet nutrient needs orally. It is safer and cheaper than parenteral nutrition and is the preferred route when the integrity of the GI tract is preserved. In acutely ill patients, early nutritional regimens using small bowel feedings may accelerate improvement and should be attempted whenever possible;[53] however, nutrient delivery by the enteral route may not initially fulfill needs, and the concomitant administration of parenteral nutrition may be needed.

Several enteral formulas appropriate for liver disease are available. When fluid restriction is indicated, formulas with higher energy content may be used. Most patients tolerate the protein in standard tube-feeding formulas without precipitation of HE;[53] therefore, specialized BCAA formulas should be reserved for patients intolerant of standard protein intake. Unfortunately, some patients may have diarrhea, electrolyte abnormalities, and volume overload from high osmotic loads, so daily monitoring of water balance, electrolytes, osmolality, and blood urea is recommended. In addition, enteral feeding tubes may cause variceal bleeding from erosion into esophageal varices.[53]

30.5.3.2 Parenteral Nutrition

Parenteral nutrition is generally reserved for patients who cannot receive enteral nutrition, as in cases of active gastrointestinal hemorrhage or small bowel obstruction. The parenteral route can be associated with serious complications related to mechanical aspects of line insertion, infections, and metabolic abnormalities from inappropriate nutrient formulations.

The use of central parenteral nutrition is preferred over peripheral because less fluid volume is required to provide calories and protein. It appears that parenteral protein is less likely to precipitate encephalopathy;[41] however, the vast majority of patients will tolerate standard tube-feeding formulas.

As with enteral feeding, parenteral BCAA solutions should be reserved for patients who have refractory HE.

REFERENCES

1. Trey, C. and Davidson, C., The management of fulminant hepatic failure, *Prog. Liver Dis.*, 3, 292, 1970.
2. Schiadt, F.V. et al., Etiology and prognosis for 295 patients with acute liver failure in the United States, *Gastroenterology*, 122, A1376, 1997.
3. Lee, W.M. et al., Acute liver failure, *N. Engl. J. Med.*, 329, 1862, 1993.
4. O'Grady, J.G. and Williams, R., Classification of acute liver failure, *Lancet*, 342, 743, 1993.
5. Riordan, S.M. and Williams, R., Fulminant hepatic failure, *Clin. Liver Dis.*, 4, 25, 2000.
6. Ferenci, P. et al., Hepatic encephalopathy: definition, nomenclature, diagnosis, and quantification: final report of the working party at the 11th World Congresses of Gastroenterology, Vienna, 1998, *Hepatology*, 35, 716, 2002.
7. Blei, A.T. and Larsen, F.S., Pathophysiology of cerebral edema in fulminant hepatic failure, *J. Hepatol.*, 31, 771, 1999.
8. Krasko, A., Deshpande, K., and Bonvino, S., Liver failure, transplantation, and critical care, *Crit. Care Clinics*, 19, 32, 2003.
9. Rolando, N. et al., Prospective study of bacterial infection in acute liver failure: an analysis of fifty patients, *Hepatology*, 11, 49, 1990.
10. Rolando, N. et al., Fungal infection: a common unrecognized complication of acute liver failure, *J. Hepatol.*, 12, 1, 1991.
11. Bihari, D. et al., Tissue hypoxia during fulminant hepatic failure, *Crit. Care Med.*, 13, 1034, 1985.
12. Ring-Larsen, H. and Palazzo, U., Renal failure in fulminant hepatic failure and terminal cirrhosis: a comparison between incidence, types, and prognosis, *Gut*, 22, 565, 1981.
13. Martin, L.F. et al., Continuous intravenous cimetidine decreases stress-related upper gastrointestinal hemorrhage without promoting pneumonia, *Crit. Care Med.*, 21, 19, 1993.
14. Canalese, J. et al., Controlled trial of dexamethasone and mannitol for the cerebral edema of fulminant hepatic failure, *Gut*, 23, 625, 1982.
15. Tsukamoto, H., Gaal, K., and French, S.W., Insights into the pathogenesis of alcoholic liver necrosis and fibrosis: status report, *Hepatology*, 12, 599, 1990.
16. Butterworth, R.F., The neurobiology of hepatic encephalopathy, *Semin. Liver Dis.*, 16, 235, 1996.
17. Cordoba, J. and Blei, A.T., Treatment of hepatic encephalopathy, *Am. J. Gastroenterol.*, 92, 1429, 1997.
18. Butterworth, R.F., Hepatic encephalopathy: a neuropsychiatric disorder involving multiple neurotransmitter systems, *Curr. Opin. Neurol.*, 13, 721, 2000.
19. Basile, A.S. and Jones, E.A., Ammonia and GABA-ergic neurotransmission: interrelated factors in the pathogenesis of hepatic encephalopathy, *Hepatology*, 25, 1303, 1997.
20. Basile, A.S. et al., Relationship between plasma benzodiazepine receptor ligand concentrations and severity of hepatic encephalopathy, *Hepatology*, 19, 112, 1994.
21. Barbaro, G. et al., Flumazenil for hepatic encephalopathy grade 3 and 4a in patients with cirrhosis: an Italian multicenter double-blind, placebo-controlled, cross-over study, *Hepatology*, 28, 374, 1998.
22. James, J.H. et al., Hyperammonemia, plasma amino acid imbalance, and blood-brain amino acid transport: a unified theory of portal-systemic encephalopathy, *Lancet*, 772, 1979.
23. Morgan, M.Y., Milson, J.P., and Sherlock, S., Plasma ratio of valine, leucine and isoleucine to phenylalanine and tyrosine in liver disease, *Gut*, 19, 1068, 1978.
24. Fessel, J.M. and Conn, H.O., An analysis of the causes and prevention of hepatic coma, *Gastroenterology*, 62, 191, 1972.
25. Vogels, B.A. et al., The effects of ammonia and portal-systemic shunting on brain metabolism, neurotransmission and intracranial hypertension in hyperammonaemia-induced encephalopathy, *J. Hepatol.*, 26, 387, 1997.
26. Weissenborn, K. et al., Neuropsychological characterization of hepatic encephalopathy, *J. Hepatol.*, 34, 768, 2001.
27. Quero, J.C. et al., The diagnosis of subclinical hepatic encephalopathy in patients with cirrhosis using neuropsychological tests and automated electroencephalogram analysis, *Hepatology*, 24, 556, 1996.

28. Laudenberger, J. et al., Proton magnetic resonance spectroscopy of the brain in symptomatic and asymptomatic patients with liver cirrhosis, *Gastroenterology*, 112, 1610, 1997.
29. Florent, C. et al., Influence of chronic lactulose ingestion on the colonic metabolism of lactulose in man (an *in vivo* study), *J. Clin. Invest.*, 75, 608, 1985.
30. Mortensen, P.B., The effect of oral-administered lactulose on colonic nitrogen metabolism and excretion, *Hepatology*, 16, 1350, 1992.
31. Atterbury, C.E., Maddrey, W.C., and Conn, H.O., Neomycin-sorbitol and lactulose in the treatment of acute portal-systemic encephalopathy: a controlled, double-blind clinical trial, *Am. J. Dig. Dis.*, 23, 398, 1978.
32. Conn. H.O. et al., Comparison of lactulose and neomycin in the treatment of chronic portal-systemic encephalopathy: a double blind controlled trial, *Gastroenterology*, 72, 573, 1977.
33. Orlandi, F. et al., Comparison between neomycin and lactulose in 173 patients with hepatic encephalopathy: a randomized clinical study, *Dig. Dis. Sci.*, 26, 498, 1981.
34. Strauss, E. et al., Double-blind randomized clinical trial comparing neomycin and placebo in the treatment of exogenous hepatic encephalopathy, *Hepatogastroenterology*, 39, 542, 1992.
35. Morgan, M.H., Read, A.E., and Speller, D.C., Treatment of hepatic encephalopathy with metronidazole, *Gut*, 23, 1, 1982.
36. Pomier-Layrargues, G. et al., Flumazenil in cirrhotic patients in hepatic coma: a randomized double-blind placebo-controlled crossover trial, *Hepatology*, 19, 32, 1994.
37. Gyr, K. et al., Evaluation of the efficacy and safety of flumazenil in the treatment of portal systemic encephalopathy: a double blind, randomized, placebo controlled multicenter study, *Gut*, 39, 319, 1996.
38. Cadranel, J.F. et al., Flumazenil therapy for hepatic encephalopathy in cirrhotic patients: a double-blind pragmatic randomized, placebo study, *Eur. J. Gastroenterol. Hepatol.*, 7, 325, 1995.
39. Als-Nielsen, B., Kjaergard, L.L., and Gluud, C., Benzodiazepine receptor antagonists for acute and chronic hepatic encephalopathy (Cochrane Review), *Cochrane Database Syst. Rev.*, 4, CD002798, 2001.
40. Goulenok, C. et al., Flumazenil vs. placebo in hepatic encephalopathy in patients with cirrhosis: a meta-analysis, *Aliment. Pharmacol. Ther.*, 16, 361, 2002.
41. Plauth, M. et al., Post-feeding hyperammonemia in patients with transjugular intrahepatic portosystemic shunt and liver cirrhosis: role of small intestinal ammonia release and route of nutrient administration, *Gut*, 46, 849, 2000.
42. Bustamante, J. et al., Prognostic significance of hepatic encephalopathy in patients with cirrhosis, *J. Hepatol.*, 30, 890, 1999.
43. Lockwood, A.H., Hepatic encephalopathy, *Neurologic Clinics*, 20, 1, 2002.
44. Powell, E.E. et al., Improvement in chronic hepatocerebral degeneration following liver transplantation, *Gastroenterology*, 98, 1079, 1990.
45. Nompleggi, D.J. and Bonkovsky, H.L., Nutritional supplementation in chronic liver disease: an analytical review, *Hepatology*, 19, 519, 1994.
46. DiCecco, S.R. et al., Assessment of nutritional status of patients with end-stage liver disease undergoing liver transplantation, *Mayo Clinic Proc.*, 64, 95, 1989.
47. Hirsch, S. et al., Controlled trial on nutrition supplementation in outpatients with symptomatic alcoholic cirrhosis, *J. Parenter. Enter. Nutr.*, 17, 119, 1993.
48. Solomon, S.M. and Kirby, D.F., The refeeding syndrome: a review, *JPEN*, 14, 90, 1990.
49. Havala, T. and Shronts, E., Managing the complications associated with refeeding, *Nutr. Clin. Pract.*, 5, 23, 1990.
50. Pomposelli, J.J. and Burns, D.L., Nutrition support in the patient with hepatic failure, in Shikora, S.A., Martindale, R.G., and Schwaitzberg, S.D., eds., *Nutritional Considerations in the Intensive Care Unit*, 199, Kenall/Hunt Publishing Company, Dubuque, IA, 2002.
51. Cabre, E. et al., Effect of total enteral nutrition on the short-term outcome of severely malnourished cirrhotics, *Gastroenterology*, 98, 715, 1990.
52. Kondrup, J. and Mueller, M.J., Energy and protein requirements of patients with chronic liver disease, *J. Hepatol.*, 27, 239, 1997.
53. Kearns, P.J. et al., Accelerated improvement of alcoholic liver disease with enteral nutrition, *Gastroenterology*, 102, 200, 1992.

54. Cerra, F.B. et al., Disease-specific amino acid infusion (F080) in hepatic encephalopathy: a prospective, randomized, double-blind, controlled trial, *J. Parenter. Enter. Nutr.*, 9, 288, 1985.

55. Rossi-Fanelli, F. et al., Effect of glucose and/or branched chain amino acid imbalance in chronic liver failure, *J. Parenter. Enter. Nutr.*, 5, 414, 1981.

56. Wahren, J. et al., Is intravenous administration of branched chain amino acids effective in the treatment of hepatic encephalopathy? A multicenter study, *Hepatology*, 3, 475, 1983.

57. Naylor, C.D., O'Rourke, K., and Baker, J.P., Parenteral nutrition with branched-chain amino acids in hepatic encephalopathy: a meta-analysis, *Gastroenterology*, 97, 1033, 1989.

58. Marchesini, G. et al., Italian BCAA Study Group. Nutritional supplementation with branched-chain amino acids in advanced cirrhosis: a double-blind, randomized trial, *Gastroenterology*, 127, 1792, 2003.

59. Charlton, M., Branched-chain amino acid-enriched supplements as therapy for liver disease: Rasputin lives, *Gastroenterology*, 124, 2003.

60. Bianchi, G.P. et al., Vegetable protein diet and hepatic encephalopathy, *J. Intern. Med.*, 233, 385, 1993.

61. Cabre, E. and Gasull, M.A., Nutritional support in liver disease, *Eur. J. Gastroenterol. Hepatol.*, 7, 528, 1995.

31 Nutrition for the Critically Ill Cardiac and Thoracic Patient

A. Christine Hummell
The Cleveland Clinic Foundation

CONTENTS

The purposes of nutrition therapy for critically ill, cardiac and thoracic patients are to provide adequate and appropriate nutrition to maintain lean body mass and visceral protein stores, to replenish nutrient losses, to promote wound healing, and to regain strength for participation in rehabilitation. In providing medical nutrition therapy to this critically ill patient population at risk for multisystem organ failure, the therapy must do no harm.

31.1 CARDIAC PATIENTS

There are numerous reasons for admission to a coronary intensive care unit (ICU): life-threatening arrhythmias, unstable angina, acute myocardial infarction, endocarditis, congestive heart failure, and cardiogenic shock. At their endpoints, these disorders result in heart failure.

Heart failure is the inability of the heart to work as a pump.[1] One or both sides of the heart can become impaired, and the location of the impairment can determine nutrition care. When the left ventricle becomes dysfunctional, blood backs up into the pulmonary circulation, causing pulmonary edema and possibly respiratory failure.[1] During right-sided failure, blood pools in the venous system, thus resulting in edema in the lower extremities, hepatomegaly, congested bowel, and distended jugular veins.[1] Consequently, the critically ill cardiac patient is at risk for developing multiple organ system failure.

31.1.1 NUTRITIONAL STATUS

The nutritional status of cardiac patients ranges from overnutrition to malnutrition upon admission to the ICU. Having a patient with morbid obesity or cardiac cachexia is not unusual in the coronary ICU. Patients with acute disorders, such as acute myocardial infarction, are more likely to be in good nutritional status than the person with chronic disease. Persons with endocarditis frequently have significant weight loss due to impaired oral intake and the adverse effects of antibiotics.

Nutritional assessment in the coronary ICU can be difficult, due to edema, the use of resuscitating fluids, and the inflammatory nature of myocardial infarctions and cardiogenic shock. An admitting weight should be obtained and then compared to subsequent weights while fluid intakes and outputs are monitored. Diuresis is frequently one goal of treatment in the coronary ICU. Patients who do not have congestive heart failure may know their usual weights. However, due to frequent fluid imbalances, the person with congestive heart failure most likely will not know his or her usual weight. Fluid overload and the stress of myocardial infarctions and cardiogenic shock will render serum albumin and other visceral proteins useless as nutritional parameters.

If possible, a brief diet history should be obtained from the patient or the family members. Usually, the person with an acute cardiac event was eating well prior to admission, whereas the person with chronic disease may have impaired oral intake due to illness and adverse effects of some cardiac medications.

A physical assessment can be performed, but edema and critical care medicine limit its value. Edema masks the loss of muscle mass and fat stores; temporal muscle wasting, if present, will be visible. Due to poor blood circulation in persons with chronic cardiac disease, persons who have been bedfast are at high risk for developing decubiti.

31.1.2 NUTRITION THERAPY FOR CRITICALLY ILL CARDIAC PATIENTS

Many patients are able to eat. The diet will frequently be a heart-healthy diet that is restricted in cholesterol, saturated fats, and total fat. A sodium restriction will be prescribed, ranging from 2 g for those with congestive heart failure to 4 g of sodium for those without significant edema. Other therapeutic diets may be necessary, such as a consistent carbohydrate diet for those with diabetes. Because heart failure can cause multiple organ failure, short-term modifications may be needed, such as restrictions during acute renal failure. Fluid restrictions are often prescribed in varying amounts, depending on the severity of fluid retention and the response to diuretics.

Adequacy of oral intake can vary. Some persons will eat well, whereas other patients will have nearly no appetite. Nausea, vomiting, diarrhea, anorexia, ascites, and early satiety can occur due to poor blood perfusion to the gastrointestinal tract during heart failure. Adjusting the cardiac medications may help improve gastrointestinal function. Cardiac medications may alter taste. For those who are not eating well, providing only the diet restrictions needed to promote recovery may assist in enhancing food palatability, increasing provision of nutrients and promoting patient satisfaction. For example, if the patient is eating very little food, there is no need for diet restrictions until oral intake significantly improves. Patients with poor appetites may benefit from liquid oral supplements and frequent, small meals. Lastly, critically ill cardiac patients may complain about the food, partly because of its blandness without salt and fat, but also due to their frustration and anger about being in the ICU.

Patients who are on mechanical ventilation will need alternate routes of nutrition. If the gastrointestinal tract is functioning, enteral nutrition should be initiated early during the ICU admission. Parenteral nutrition is utilized only if the gastrointestinal tract is dysfunctional. The concentration of the enteral formula and parenteral solutions is dependent on cardiac function. Those patients with congestive heart failure, pulmonary edema, New York Heart Association classification of III or IV, or ejection fraction of less than 25% will probably need 2 cal/ml tube-feeding products and concentrated TPN solutions.[2] Other cardiac patients may not need concentrated products, so standard 1 cal/ml tube feedings should be well tolerated. Patients with cardiac cachexia are particularly at risk for developing refeeding syndrome, so electrolytes and fluid status will require close monitoring. Because critically ill cardiac patients are at risk for multiple organ system failure, the nutrition support must take into account other organ dysfunction and its treatment, such as acute renal failure treated with dialysis.

TABLE 31.1
Caloric and Protein Requirements for Cardiac and Thoracic Patients

Disorder	Calories	Protein (g/kg Weight)
Congestive heart failure[4]	20–30% above BEE[a]	1.2–1.5
Cardiac surgery[11,12]	BEE[a] × 1.2–1.5	1.2–1.5
	BEE[a] × 1.2–1.6[b]	
Heart transplant[13,16,17]	130–150% of BEE[a]	1.0–1.5
	30–35 calories/kg weight	2.0[c]
Lung transplant[23]	BEE[a] × 1.3 - 1.5	1.2–2.0
	30–35 calories/kg weight	
	BEE[a] × 1.75[b]	

[a] BEE: basal energy expenditure.
[b] Infected patient.
[c] Preoperative malnutrition.

Congestive heart failure is an inflammatory, hypermetabolic state in which levels of tumor necrosis factor and proinflammatory cytokines are elevated.[3] Consequently, patients will have high caloric and protein requirements;[4] see Table 31.1 for nutritional requirements. Due to losses and possibly poor oral intake, a multivitamin supplement is recommended. Patients receiving thiazide diuretics may need potassium and magnesium supplementation.[5]

31.2 CARDIAC SURGERY PATIENTS

Most patients undergoing cardiac surgery will need cardiopulmonary bypass (CPB). CPB produces a systemic inflammatory response that harms most organs.[6] Most patients do well after cardiac surgery, but for the few who have difficulties and stay in the ICU, this is due to preoperative problems, the operation, and CPB.[6] Postoperative cardiac problems range from arrhythmias to poor cardiac output and hypotension.[6] Fluid accumulates during the surgery, promoting pulmonary edema.[6] Excessive bleeding, neurological disturbances, and gastrointestinal issues are more common after open heart surgery than any other major surgery.[6] Acute renal failure is common, and it is associated with a high mortality rate because these patients are at risk for infection.[6] CPB causes fluid and electrolyte shifts, resulting in water and sodium retention and excretion of potassium.[7] Lastly, CPB impacts glucose metabolism, because elevated levels of epinephrine promote insulin resistance and hyperglycemia.[7] Consequently, the person undergoing cardiac surgery is at risk for developing multiple organ system failure. See Table 31.2 for postoperative complications with nutritional implications.

31.2.1 NUTRITIONAL STATUS

Nutritional status of cardiac surgical patients at the time of surgery is identical to that of cardiac patients. Incidentally, some patients may have poor oral intake preoperatively due to anxiety about the upcoming surgery. Very elderly cachetic patients have an increased mortality rate.[8]

31.2.2 NUTRITION THERAPY FOR CARDIAC SURGERY PATIENTS

Most cardiac surgical patients are extubated within 24 to 48 hours of surgery. Small amounts of clear liquids are initiated, and then diet is usually advanced to a heart-healthy, 3 to 4 g sodium diet with a mild fluid restriction within 24 h of extubation. Other restrictions, depending on comorbidities,

TABLE 31.2
Complications of Cardiac Surgery[6] with Nutritional Implications

Complication	Nutritional Implications
Infection	Elevated nutritional requirements
Respiratory failure	If intubated, use enteral nutrition
Acute respiratory distress syndrome	If pulmonary edema is present, use concentrated products
Paralytic diaphragm	
Acute renal failure	Diet prescription/enteral or parenteral nutrition appropriate for acute renal failure
Perforated gastrointestinal ulcer	Use parenteral nutrition until gastrointestinal tract is functional
Gastrointestinal bleeding	
Ischemic colitis	
Pancreatitis/hyperamylasemia	NPO
	If severe, use parenteral nutrition; enteral nutrition may be tolerated
Embolic strokes	Dysphagia: use enteral nutrition if the patient is at risk for aspirating oral intake
Hallucinations/disorientation	

may be necessary, such as consistent carbohydrate diets for persons with diabetes. Oral intake will vary, ranging from good to extremely poor. Persons with extremely poor appetites may benefit from an unrestricted diet, use of liquid oral supplements, small meals with snacks, and a daily multivitamin supplement.

Patients who remain on ventilators after a few days or have impaired swallowing will need alternate routes of nutrition. If the gastrointestinal tract is functional, enteral nutrition is preferred; otherwise, parenteral nutrition will be necessary. The type of enteral product and concentration of the parenteral nutrition will depend on cardiac status, severity of impairment of other organs, and treatment of organ failure. These critically ill patients are also at risk for developing the refeeding syndrome.

When to initiate enteral nutrition in the cardiac surgical patient is a controversial issue. The potential for hemodynamic instability and the use of inotropes have led some to believe that enteral nutrition should not be utilized. However, one small study involving nine postoperative stable cardiac patients on dobutamine and/or norepinephrine, who were started on enteral nutrition the first day after surgery, found that tube feeding improved cardiac index and increased splanchic blood flow.[9] The patients received a polymeric product running at a continuous rate that provided 130% of measured energy expenditure. Blood glucose and insulin levels indicated that the tube feeding was being metabolized. There was no evidence of bowel ischemia.

In another study, the researchers initiated tube feeding in ventilated cardiac surgery patients within three days of surgery and found very few incidences of intolerance.[10] Vomiting occurred once in 19% of the patients, and it happened early during the study period. Twenty-five percent of the patients developed diarrhea, which was attributed to antibiotics. Aspiration occurred in 10% of the patients. Considering these studies, early enteral nutrition can be well tolerated in critically ill, hemodynamically stable cardiac surgery patients on inotropes.

Calorie and protein requirements are similar to those needed for patients undergoing major surgery;[11,12] refer to Table 31.1 for requirements. Calorie and protein requirements increase with severity of illness. Protein requirements may need to be adjusted for renal failure.

31.3 CARDIAC TRANSPLANT PATIENTS

The nutritional status and nutrition care of critically ill cardiac transplant candidates are identical to those of cardiac patients. Malnutrition should be treated aggressively, if possible, because persons who are malnourished preoperatively have a significantly higher mortality and morbidity rate than those who are well nourished.[13] Malnourished patients are at greater risk for postoperative infection, which will adversely influence survival.[14] Most transplant candidates will be in good nutritional status. One study found that 56% of transplant candidates were in good nutritional status, 25% were marginally compromised, and cardiac cachexia was found in 19% of the candidates.[4]

Postoperative nutrition care of cardiac transplant patients is similar to that of cardiac surgical patients. Patients are extubated within 24 to 48 hours of transplant, started on small amounts of clear liquids, and then advanced to a heart-healthy 3 to 4 g sodium diet with a mild fluid restriction, usually within five days of transplant.[15] Initially there may be some nausea, due to the loading doses of immunosuppressive medications, but this usually resolves within one or two days. Oral intake ranges from good to poor. Patients who are not eating well will benefit from unrestricted diets, liquid oral supplements, and a daily multivitamin supplement.[15]

The need for enteral or parenteral nutrition support in the postoperative period is rare. It will be necessary for patients who are unable to wean off mechanical ventilation within a few days of surgery and for those with neurological impairment or extreme anorexia. Most patients will have a functioning gastrointestinal tract, so enteral nutrition is preferred. The type of enteral product is dependent on the acute medical status of the patient; for example, if the patient has pulmonary edema, then a concentrated 2 cal/ml product should be prescribed.

Nutritional requirements reflect the hypermetabolism associated with surgery;[13,16,17] refer to Table 31.1 for requirements. Patients who develop infection will have greater requirements.

31.4 MECHANICAL DEVICES

There are many options for mechanical devices available for use in critically ill cardiac patients. The most commonly used device is the intra-aortic balloon pump (IABP), a short-term therapy usually not lasting more than a week. If the patient is not mechanically ventilated or receiving high-flow oxygen therapy, oral nutrition is preferred, using a heart-healthy, sodium- and fluid-restricted diet. However, it may be difficult for the patient to eat and drink while in a prone position, because the elevation of the head of the bed is limited to thirty degrees. For those who are mechanically ventilated, alternate routes of nutrition support will be needed if the patient is not extubated within a few days.

One study examined the energy expenditure of patients on IABP, and the results indicated that they were hypermetabolic.[18] Predicted resting energy expenditure, using the Harris–Benedict equation, was 1200 calories. Measured resting energy expenditure was 1600 calories on the second day of IABP and had increased to about 1800 calories on the third day.

Ventricular assist devices (VADs) are bridges to cardiac transplant that may be implanted when a transplant candidate becomes critically ill while waiting for a donor heart. Also, VADs may be used for a very critically ill cardiac patient who needs additional support while waiting for medical and surgical treatments to take effect. VADs take over the pumping action of either the left or right side of the heart while leaving the heart in place.[19] They are *internal* or *external*, depending on the location of the device in relation to the body.[19] Internal devices are much smaller than the external ones, thus promoting greater mobility. However, they may be too large for adults with small abdominal cavities.[19] Power is provided from an external source and funneled to the device through drive lines.[19] Complications from using VADs include bleeding during the immediate postoperative period, strokes and other neurological dysfunctions, thromboemboli, and infection.[19] About 25% of the patients will develop a "pump pocket" infection.[19] Some may also develop elevated panel reactive antibodies (PRA), indicating the presence of antihuman leukocyte antigen (HLA) antibodies.

Treatment for PRA is plasmapheresis; blood is removed from the patient to separate out the antibodies, fresh plasma or albumin is added to restore blood volume, and then the blood is returned to the patient.[20]

VADs can pose nutritional challenges. The internal devices can be noisy, sit on top of the stomach, and, depending on type, can weigh as much as 2.5 pounds. It is difficult to assess gastrointestinal function because the abdominal area is distended from the device and the pumping noise of the device masks bowel sounds.

Most patients on VADs will be able to resume oral intake within three days of implant. There is usually no need for diet and fluid restrictions because the devices depend on adequate blood volume to work properly. Restricting fluids may promote mechanical malfunctions. If complications occur, diet and fluids will need to be adjusted based on organ failure and its treatment to prevent further organ damage. For example, if the patient has acute renal failure and is on dialysis, the patient will need a diet appropriate for dialysis. Oral intake will vary; some patients will eat well and others will have poor appetites. Early satiety can occur due to the VADs' location in the abdominal cavity. Patients with early satiety will benefit from small, frequent meals with use of oral supplements until their appetites improve.

If the patient is unable to resume oral intake within a few days, alternate routes of nutrition support are needed. Enteral nutrition is preferred, but it is a challenge to place feeding tubes successfully. Because VADs are on top of the stomach, they may hinder placement below the stomach and may hide the feeding tube on abdominal radiography. Parenteral nutrition should be avoided, if possible, due to its potential to promote infection. These patients are already at risk for infection from the drive line sites. Selection of tube-feeding product depends on the acute medical condition. Sometimes, the patient may have been severely fluid overloaded at the time of VAD placement, so a concentrated, 2 cal/ml product is needed until fluid status improves. If there is no edema, a standard 1 cal/ml product should be administered. The nutrition support must take into account any organ failure and its treatment. For example, if the patient develops acute renal failure and is on dialysis, the tube-feeding product must be appropriate for a dialysis patient.

31.5 THORACIC PATIENTS

Thoracic surgical patients may spend less than 24 to 48 hours in the ICU postoperatively to wean off ventilators. All patients will resume oral intake after extubation, with the exception of those having upper gastrointestinal surgery. Persons with esophageal cancer and sometimes hiatal hernias may have feeding jejunostomies placed at the time of surgery so that enteral nutrition will be initiated within a few days of surgery.

This is a population characterized by lung or esophageal cancer, usually in the early stages prior to development of metastases. Some patients may have preoperative chemotherapy or radiation to shrink tumors to a resectable size. Consequently, preoperative nutritional status ranges from good to poor, with some patients having weight loss. Patients with esophageal cancer have the greatest risk of malnutrition, due to tumor obstruction of the gastrointestinal tract, but many will not have significant impairment of oral intake. It is not uncommon to have an obese patient undergoing esophagectomy.

Thoracic patients remain in the ICU only if they become critically ill. Two-thirds of postoperative problems, if they occur, are cardiopulmonary, ranging from arrhythmias to respiratory failure.[21] Postoperative respiratory failure is the major cause of mortality in this population.[21] Another complication is anastomotic leaks, which can have devastating consequences because they significantly increase the risk of sepsis and multiple organ system failure.[21] Other complications with nutritional implications include the development of esophageal fistulas and pneumonia.[21]

Generally, critically ill thoracic patients remain in the ICU because they require mechanical ventilation. Enteral nutrition should be initiated within a few days of surgery if the patient is unable to be weaned off the ventilator. Selection of tube-feeding product is dependent on the specific organ failure and its severity. Most patients with respiratory failure will do well with a standard 1 cal/ml product, but those with pulmonary edema will need a fluid-restricted product. If multiple system organ failure develops, the product needs to be appropriate for the organ failure. For example, a septic patient with acute renal failure and receiving dialysis will need a product appropriate for dialysis. Parenteral nutrition will be required for the patient with upper gastrointestinal surgery if the gastrointestinal tract is dysfunctional due to the development of esophageal fistulas, anastomotic leaks, wound dehiscence, or paralytic ileus.

Nutritional requirements are similar to those of other major surgeries. Those requirements will increase significantly if wound dehiscence, anastomotic leaks, or sepsis occurs.

31.6 LUNG TRANSPLANT PATIENTS

Lung transplant candidates should be in good nutritional status prior to transplant. Ideally, transplant candidates should be within 20% of ideal body weight.[22] Mortality rate significantly increases with cachexia.[22] Obesity hinders mobilization and restricts diaphragmatic function.[22] Consequently, some obese candidates will require weight reduction prior to transplant. Persons with cystic fibrosis who are underweight may need supplemental enteral nutrition to achieve and maintain desirable weight. Some cystic fibrosis patients may have percutaneous endoscopic gastrostomy (PEG) tubes implanted preoperatively to improve nutritional status. Persons likely to be malnourished are those with cystic fibrosis, emphysema, or bronchiectasis, whereas persons with pulmonary hypertension or pulmonary fibrosis tend to be well nourished.[23]

Most lung transplant candidates will never be ill enough to be admitted to an ICU. Requiring mechanical ventilation preoperatively is a risk factor for a survival rate of less than one year after transplant.[24] Consequently, critically ill patients most likely will not be listed for transplant.

Lung transplant surgery puts stress on all organs and promotes catabolism.[23] Immediate postoperative complications include reperfusion injury, resulting in pulmonary edema; acute rejection; and infection.[25] Early graft dysfunction occurs in 10 to 20% of the patients, causing respiratory failure, pulmonary hypertension, pulmonary edema, and right-sided heart failure.[25] Other complications include sepsis, bronchial dehiscence, hemorrhage, air embolism, and ischemic injury.[23]

Most lung transplant patients will be able to resume oral intake within 5 days of surgery. Usually, extubation occurs within the first 24 hours of surgery. Initiating oral intake is dependent not only on gastrointestinal function but also on respiratory status. It is not uncommon for patients to require several days of high-flow oxygen therapy after extubation, thus preventing resumption of oral intake. Once the patient no longer needs high-flow oxygen therapy, clear liquids can be initiated. The diet is advanced to one that is low in cholesterol, saturated fat, and total fat with a 3 to 4 g sodium restriction, due to the long-term side effects of immunosuppressive medications. Oral intake will vary and generally patients will eat well.

If the patient requires mechanical ventilation for more than a few days, enteral nutrition should be initiated. If pulmonary edema is present, the tube-feeding product should be a concentrated, 2 cal/ml product; otherwise, a standard 1 cal/ml product will be acceptable. There may be the rare patient with multiple organ failure that involves the gastrointestinal tract; parenteral nutrition will be required.

Cystic fibrosis patients need pancreatic enzyme replacement therapy during the immediate postoperative period. If the patient is NPO, these are administered 3 to 4 times daily as enteric-coated capsules through a nasogastric tube or an existing PEG tube. If the cystic fibrosis patient is receiving enteral nutrition through a small-bore nasoenteric tube in the postpyloric position, the replacement enzymes need to be in a powder form, such as crushed Viokase tablets, mixed with water, and then administered through the feeding tube 3 to 4 times daily. The amount of enzyme replacement is dependent on usual dose and tolerance to the tube feeding.

Nutritional requirements during the postoperative period are similar to those of other major surgeries;[23] see Table 31.1 for requirements. If infection is present, caloric needs will be elevated.

REFERENCES

1. Porth, C., Heart failure, in *Pathophysiology*, Lippincott Company, Philadelphia, 1982, pages 216–221.
2. Chicago Dietetic Association, The South Suburban Dietetic Association, and Dietitians of Canada, Congestive heart failure, in *Manual of Clinical Dietetics*, 6th ed., American Dietetic Association and Dietitians of Canada, Chicago, IL, 2000, pages 259–263.
3. Kirklin, J.K., Young, J.B., and McGiffin, D.C., Pathophysiology and clinical features of heart failure, in *Heart Transplantation*, Churchill-Livingstone, Philadelphia, 2002, pages 107–138.
4. Frazier, O.H., Van Buren, C.T., Poindexter, S.M., and Waldenberger, F., Nutritional management of the heart transplant recipient, *J. Heart Transplantation*, 4, 450, 1985.
5. Kirklin, J.K., Young, J.B., and McGiffin, D.C., Medical and nontransplant surgical therapy of heart failure, in *Heart Transplantation*, Churchill-Livingstone, Philadelphia, 2002, pages 139–197.
6. Mehta, S.M. and Pae, W.D., Complications of cardiac surgery, in *Cardiac Surgery in the Adult*, Edmunds, L.H., Ed., McGraw-Hill, New York, 1997, pages 369–402.
7. Bojar, R.M., Fluid management, renal and metabolic problems, in *Perioperative Care in Cardiac Surgery*, 3rd ed., Blackwell Science, Malden, MA, 1999, pages 337–369.
8. Utley, J.R., Leyland, S.A., and Edmunds, L.H., Preoperative evaluation, in *Cardiac Surgery in the Adult*, Edmunds, L.H., Ed., McGraw-Hill, New York, 1997, pages 145–164.
9. Revelly, J., Tappy, L., Berger, M., Gersbach, P., Cayeux, C., and Chiolero, R., Early metabolic and splanchic responses to enteral nutrition in postoperative cardiac surgery patients with circulatory compromise, *Intens. Care Med.*, 27, 540, 2001.
10. Kesek, D.R., Akerlind, L., and Karlsson, T., Early enteral nutrition in the cardiothoracic intensive care unit, *Clin. Nutr.*, 21, 303, 2002.
11. Chicago Dietetic Association, The South Suburban Dietetic Association, and Dietitians of Canada, Cardiac surgery, in *Manual of Clinical Dietetics*, 6th ed., American Dietetic Association and Dietitians of Canada, Chicago, IL, 2000, pages 255–258.
12. Chicago Dietetic Association, The South Suburban Dietetic Association, and Dietitians of Canada, Nutrition assessment of adults, in *Manual of Clinical Dietetics*, 6th ed., American Dietetic Association and Dietitians of Canada, Chicago, IL, 2000, pages 3–38.
13. ASPEN, Board of Directors and the Clinical Guidelines Task Force, Guidelines for the use of parenteral and enteral nutrition in adult and pediatric patients: solid organ transplants, *J. Parenter. Enteral Nutr.*, 26(suppl.), 74SA, 2002.
14. Hasse, J.M., Nutrition assessment and support of organ transplant recipients, *J. Parenter. Enteral Nutr.*, 25, 120, 2001.
15. Chicago Dietetic Association, The South Suburban Dietetic Association, and Dietitians of Canada, Heart transplant, in *Manual of Clinical Dietetics*, 6th ed., American Dietetic Association and Dietitians of Canada, Chicago, IL, 2000, pages 517–523.
16. Poindexter, S.M., Nutrition support in cardiac transplantation, *Topics Clin. Nutr.*, 7, 12, 1992.
17. Hasse, J.M., Recovery after organ transplantation in adults: the role of postoperative nutrition therapy, *Topics Clin. Nutr.*, 13, 15, 1998.
18. Paccagnella, A., Calo, M., Cipolotti, G., Manuali, A., Da Col U., Giacomin, A., and Simini, G., Total parenteral nutrition in patients with intra-aortic balloon counterpulsation, *Scand. J. Thor. Cardiovasc. Surg.*, 27, 35, 1993.
19. Kirklin, J.K., Young, J.B., McGiffin, D.C., Holmann, W.L., and Kormos, R.L., Mechanical support of the failing heart, in *Heart Transplantation*, Kirklin, J.K., Young, J.B., and McGiffin, D.C., Eds., Churchill-Livingstone, Philadelphia, 2002, pages 252–289.
20. Kirklin, J.K., Young, J.B., McGiffin, D.C., and George, J.F., Immunosuppressive modalities, in *Heart Transplantation*, Kirklin, J.K., Young, J.B., and McGiffin, D.C., Eds., Churchill-Livingstone, Philadelphia, 2002, pages 390–463.
21. Todd, T.R.J. and Ralph-Edwards, A.C., Perioperative management, in *Thoracic Surgery*, Pearson, F.J., Cooper, J.D., Deslauriers, J., Ginsberg, R.J., Hiebert, C.A., Patterson, G.A., and Urshel, H.C., Eds., Churchill-Livingstone, New York, 2002, pages 139–154.
22. Mohindra, V. and Doyle, R.L., Clinical evaluation of heart-lung and lung transplantation candidates, in *Heart and Lung Transplantation*, 2nd ed., Baumgartner, W.A., Kasper, E., Reitz, B.R., and Theodore, J., Eds., W.B. Saunders Company, Philadelphia, 2002, pages 64–73.

23. Chicago Dietetic Association, The South Suburban Dietetic Association, and Dietitians of Canada, Lung transplant, in *Manual of Clinical Dietetics*, 6th ed., American Dietetic Association and Dietitians of Canada, Chicago, IL, 2000 , pages 541–546.
24. Zuckerman, J.B. and Kotloff, R.M., Lung transplantation for cystic fibrosis, *Clin. Chest Med.*, 19, 535, 1998.
25. Moon, M.R., Barlow, C.W., and Robbins, R.C., Early postoperative care of lung and heart-lung transplant recipients, in *Heart and Lung Transplantation*, 2nd ed., Baumgartner, W.A., Kasper, E., Reitz, B.R., and Theodore, J., Eds., W.B. Saunders Company, Philadelphia, 2002, pages 225–232.

32 Traumatic Brain Injury and Stroke

L. Lee Jimenez
Sodexho Food Services

Frank Davis
Memorial Health University Medical Center

CONTENTS

32.1 TYPES OF BRAIN INSULTS

Traumatic brain injury (TBI) accounts for almost 40% of all trauma-related deaths, resulting in as many as 56,000 deaths per year in the U.S. (1). The financial impact is staggering, exceeding $75 to $100 billion annually, when one considers both direct medical expenses and loss of productivity (2). The majority of those injured are under the age of 35, which are often the most productive years (3). Common causes of death due to TBI are outlined in Figure 32.1. Above the age of 65, fatal neurological injury occurs most often from cerebrovascular accidents or strokes, with a death rate that is approximately triple that of TBI (4,5). In 80% of the cases, strokes are secondary to ischemia (too little blood flow, primarily embolic disease), with hemorrhage causing the other 20% (6). Demographically, males experience a higher incidence of strokes and African-Americans are significantly more likely to have a stroke than Caucasians (4).

In TBI, the initial insult (the actual blunt or penetrating injury) is often classified as the *primary injury* (7). Intracranial events that can occur after the initial injury are often referred to as the *secondary injury*. These events, which often occur while under the care of the medical team, can lead to an exacerbation of the initial insult. Secondary injury includes hypoxia, decreased perfusion (hypotension), elevated intracranial pressure (ICP), delayed bleeding or hematoma formation, cerebral edema, and seizures (7). It is estimated that 10 to 15% of patients with severe brain injury will succumb to medically and surgically intractable elevated ICP, which is associated with a mortality of 84 to 100% (8). Management of increased ICP may include mild hyperventilation, osmotic agents such as mannitol, hypertonic fluids to include 3% NaCl, the placement of intraventricular catheters

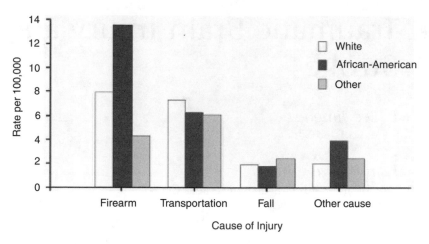

FIGURE 32.1 Traumatic brain injury–related death rates by cause and race, United States, 1994. Age adjusted to 1990 U.S. population.

TABLE 32.1
Glasgow Coma Scale

Eyes	Open	Spontaneous	4
		To sound	3
		To pain	2
		Never	1
Best verbal response		Orientated	5
		Confused conversation	4
		Inappropriate words	3
		Incomprehensible sounds	2
		None	1
Best motor response		Obeys commands	6
		Localize pain	5
		Flexion — withdrawal	4
		Flexion — abnormal	3
		Extension	2
		None	1
		TOTAL	3–15

Source: From G. Teasdale and B. Jennett, *Acta Neurochirurgica*, 34, 46, 1976. With permission.

to drain cerebrospinal fluid, optimizing cerebral perfusion pressure with intravascular volume expansion and vasopressor therapy, and drug therapy such as barbiturates (7).

The Glasgow Coma Score (GCS) (Table 32.1) utilizes postinjury observations to classify the severity of head injuries and predict outcome. Though initially intended to be used early in the hospital course, in general, the later that the GCS measurement is made, the more accurate its value as a prognostication tool in predicting long-term mortality and disability (1). Mild injuries (GCS 13 to 15) make up the majority of brain injuries and are not usually associated with long-term deficits. Patients with moderate head injury (GCS 8 to 12) constitute a heterogeneous population; up to 20% of these patients will progress to severe brain damage (7). The prognosis for severe brain injuries, as indicated by a GCS of < 8, is very poor. Of hospitalized patients admitted with brain injury, the ratio of mild to moderate to severe injury is 8:1:1 (1).

32.2 GOALS OF NUTRITION SUPPORT

As described comprehensively in Chapter 1, the response to stress is characterized by a significant increase in energy expenditure (EE) and nitrogen (N) losses. The obligatory mobilization of lean body mass (LBM) observed with brain injury is estimated to be up to 25 g N per day, or triple the normal turnover rate, which would cause a 70 kg man to lose 10% of LBM in a week (8). Minor changes in body composition are rarely of clinical significance, but losses of 10% or more LBM have been associated with increased morbidity (9). Although aggressive nutritional support should not be expected to prevent the loss of LBM that is characteristic of the hypercatabolic state (9), the attenuation of these losses is attainable with the adequate provision of energy and protein (10).

32.3 TIMING OF NUTRITION SUPPORT

A strategy for nutritional support in the patient with an acute brain injury should be developed as soon as the patient is stabilized and adequately resuscitated. The selected route of nutritional support should provide consistent nutrient delivery, which should commence as early as feasible into the hospital course particularly for patients with moderate to severe TBI (11). Early nutritional support, defined as initiation within 24 to 48 hours of ICU admission, has been demonstrated in a recent review of randomized, controlled trials to be associated with a trend toward less infectious morbidity and overall mortality in ICU patients (12). In stroke patients and patients with TBI, early nutrition support has been associated with enhanced immune function, decreased infections, reduced ICU and total hospital days, and improved neurological outcome (13–16).

32.4 ENTERAL VS. PARENTERAL

Although some early research demonstrated improved outcomes with parenteral nutrition (PN) compared to enteral nutrition (EN) (17), more current literature clearly shows an advantage of enteral feedings. As described in Chapter 12, EN has been associated with a significant decrease in infectious complications, compared with PN, in critically ill patients (12). In patients with brain injury, the American Society of Enteral and Parenteral Nutrition (ASPEN) recommends that EN be utilized in lieu of PN when the gastrointestinal tract is functional and EN is tolerated (11).

32.5 GASTRIC VS. SMALL BOWEL FEEDING

Delayed gastric emptying in patients with brain injury has been well documented and appears to correlate closely with severity of injury and elevation of ICP (18–20). The intolerance of feeding delivered into the stomach precludes consistent nutrient delivery and worsens the negative nitrogen balance (21). The importance of nutritional access that allows for consistent nutrient delivery is underscored by the observation that energy needs and nitrogen losses increase over time (22). Utilization of prokinetic agents (PKA) is associated with enhanced gastrointestinal transit in critically ill patients (23); however, when studied in patients with severe brain injuries, PKA did not significantly improve gastric emptying (24), nor did its addition facilitate a faster advancement to goal nutrition (25). A further concern is that lower esophageal sphincter (LES) tone is often impaired in the majority of patients with head injuries and strokes, which could potentially increase the risk of aspiration, particularly in patients with a low GCS who are unable to protect their airway due to a diminished gag reflex (26,27).

Another important factor in decreasing the risk of aspiration in critically ill patients is head positioning. The consensus statement from the North American Summit on Aspiration in the Critically Ill Patient includes a recommendation for elevating the head of the bed > 30 to 45 degrees in *all* patients receiving EN (28). There are data to support that this positioning may also be of benefit in lowering ICP in traumatic head injuries (29); however, in patients with ischemic stroke, a lower or flat head position may increase blood flow to ischemic brain tissue (30). In those patients for whom the head of bed cannot be elevated and who have other risk factors for aspiration, (i.e., impaired consciousness), it is recommended that EN be provided via a small bowel (SB) feeding tube distal to the ligament of Treitz (28).

Delivery of EN via SB access was associated with enhanced nutritional delivery, a more rapid advancement to goal regimen, and a decreased incidence of ventilator-associated pneumonia (VAP), when compared to gastric delivery in a recent meta-analysis (31). In patients with brain injury, SB feeding provides an improvement in nitrogen balance when compared to gastric feeding and total parenteral nutrition (TPN) (32). Enhanced neurological recovery and the ability to consistently deliver EN early in the hospital course have also been demonstrated when SB feeding is utilized (16,32). In patients maintained in a pharmacologically induced coma (GCS = 3) due to refractory elevated ICP, SB feeding has been shown to be an important adjunct in EN provision (33). Though the superior tolerance of SB feeding is suggested in the majority of studies of EN in brain injury, one study demonstrated that patients with TBI could be consistently fed early into the hospital course (day 3.6) via percutaneous endoscopic gastrostomy (PEG) with a low complication rate (4%) (34). When the gastric route is used, continuous feeding is more likely to be associated with a reduced incidence of feeding intolerance and a faster advancement to goal when compared to bolus delivery (25).

Historically, a limiting factor in the utilization of SB access has been the lack of success in reliably positioning nasoenteric access devices into the small bowel. With blind, bedside positioning, SB intubation rates vary widely, from 15 to 95% (35,36). The highest rates of success for blind SB intubation have been reported when a small number of clinicians are dedicated to providing this service (36,37). This program has been developed at our own institution with marked success over a relatively short period of time. Blind, bedside placement of SB feeding tubes is less than one-tenth the cost of endoscopically placed tubes (35). Because SB delivery is likely to be better tolerated than gastric EN in this population, the availability of SB access may be associated with a decrease in TPN usage, the daily cost of which is approximately 5 to 7 times the daily cost of enteral delivery (35). The potential to decrease the incidence of VAP by lowering the risk with SB feeding also has significant financial implications: it has been estimated that a facility loses up to $20,000 per case of VAP (1986 dollars) (38). Because nutritional support should minimize potential complications associated with the route of delivery, a recommendation of ASPEN is that SB tube placement initially be attempted by blind, directed, and/or spontaneous method and, if unsuccessful, fluoroscopy or endoscopy be utilized to obtain SB access (11).

Once patients begin to make the transition to the convalescence phase of their injury, plans for long-term enteral access should be initiated. To avoid nasal irritation and enhance patient comfort, long-term access should be considered when EN is anticipated for > 4 weeks (39). PEG is the most commonly used route for long-term enteral access. Impaired gastric emptying is frequently observed early in this population and may persist for up to 25 days after injury (20). In addition, comprised LES function and the decreased level of consciousness characteristic of patients with brain injury create a predisposition for aspiration (26). To that end, the Brain Trauma Foundation's Guidelines for the Management of Severe Head Injury recommend consideration of jejunal feeding via gastrojejunostomy to improve enteral feeding tolerance (8). Unfortunately, the effectiveness of the gastrojejunostomy is sometimes limited by the susceptibility of the jejunal extension for dislodgment, kinking, and occlusion. Other surgical options for jejunal access would include a laparoscopic or open jejunostomy tube, both of which require a trip to the operating room.

32.6 NUTRITIONAL ASSESSMENT

The well established variance of metabolic requirements in brain injury, reaching up to 250% above expected EE, has been paralleled to that of patients with 20 to 40% of their body surface area burned (22,40–42). Fine-tuning the nutrition care plan is essential, because the exogenous provision

TABLE 32.2
Factors that Influence Energy Requirements in Brain-Injured Patients

Factor	Effect on EE
Pharmacological Interventions	
Barbiturates (49–51)	↓ 28–40%
	(also ↓ N excretion)
Beta-blockers (52)	↓ 6%
Neuromuscular blocking agents (with morphine) (40,53)	↓ 20–42%
Physiological Observations	
Increased muscle activity (51)	↑ 42–91%
Pulmonary toilet, suctioning, turning, spontaneous activity, painful stimuli (40)	↑ 7–66%
Elevated body temperature (65)	↑ 10% per °C
Thermic effect of food (53)	↑10%

of nutrients that is timely and compatible with metabolic demands has been demonstrated to enhance neurological recovery and overall outcomes (16,43,44). Predictive formulas estimating nutritional needs have proved inadequate in this population (42,45); therefore, indirect calorimetry is the preferred method for estimating EE (11,45). A decrease in metabolic rate that is 24 to 30% less than basal rates has been observed in patients who progressed to brain death (46). If this deterioration appears imminent, hypocaloric feeding should be considered and TPN avoided in order to decrease the risk of hepatic steatosis, which could potentially affect the viability of successful organ donation (47).

The limited availability of indirect calorimetry impedes its routine usage at many facilities, but it is hoped that, with the advent of less cumbersome and more affordable calorimeters (48), this gold standard for calculating energy requirements will be more readily available and applicable for critically ill patients. When this measurement is not feasible, a comprehensive nutritional assessment should be as performed, with special attention to the effect of commonly used pharmacological agents. Barbiturates have been demonstrated to exert a beneficial effect on lowering ICP, partly by lowering metabolic demands and subsequently decreasing cerebral blood flow and volume (8). This class of drugs, as well as neuromuscular-blocking agents and beta-blockers, can cause clinically significant changes in energy and protein demands; therefore, consideration of these drugs should be an essential component of the nutritional assessment (see Table 32.2) (40,49–53). This is particularly important, because it has been suggested that the wide range of metabolic demands of brain-injured patients can be explained by the muscle tone resulting from the administration of these medications, rather than the actual injury, ICP, or level of consciousness (51).

Propofol is a commonly used sedative in an emulsion base of soybean oil in water that delivers 1.1 kcal/ml. These calories should be considered with the nutrition support regimen, adjusting as necessary to maintain consistent nutrient delivery without overfeeding (54). In patients receiving propofol, SB delivery should be considered for optimal tolerance, because impaired GI transit may be observed due to the generalized relaxing effect of the drug on visceral smooth muscle (28). Utilizing a low-fat, high-protein formula can minimize additional calories provided by fat in patients receiving EN. If the patient is receiving PN, care should be taken to reduce or even eliminate the lipid infusion so as to maintain a lipid infusion of less than 1 g/kg/d (54).

When indirect calorimetry is not available, a guideline for calculating energy requirements for nonparalyzed patients is 140% of estimated metabolic expenditure, such as that calculated by the Harris–Benedict or other predictive equation (see Chapter 6); for patients who are paralyzed, replacement should be aimed at 100% of predicted basal metabolic expenditure (8). If the general guideline of 20 to 35 kcal/kg is utilized, the low end of this range is appropriate for paralyzed patients, reserving the upper limit for nonparalyzed patients. For obese patients, weight may need to be adjusted to approximate LBM. Protein should be delivered at 1.5 to 2 g/kg (55), though it is important to recognize that positive nitrogen balance is likely not attainable in the postinjury phase of acute brain injury (22). Enteral or parenteral formulations containing 15 to 20% of total kcal as protein are recommended in order to help counteract the marked hypercatabolism (8).

There are little data available on the role of micronutrients in brain injury. Zinc supplementation has been associated with improved neurological recovery when provided early in the postinjury period (56), but more research is warranted.

32.7 MONITORING NUTRITION SUPPORT

In the past, fluid restriction was a common practice in patients with elevated ICP to help reduce ICP by decreasing total circulating volume. Today, however, most data suggest resuscitation to a normal intravascular volume, with the avoidance of hyponatremia and hypo-osmolarity. Isotonic fluid is usually recommended, with some recent data suggesting the use of hypertonic saline with inconclusive survival advantage (57).

Abnormal sodium levels are frequently observed in the brain-injured population. Hypernatremia and hyperosmolality due to diabetes insipidus (DI) may frequently develop in patients with severe cerebral disease or injury. DI are characterized by urinary output of more than 300 ml/h with a specific gravity < 1.005, along with a rising serum sodium (inappropriately dilute urine with rising serum sodium and osmolality). These patients often require the aggressive use of desmopressin acetate (DDAVP) via the intravenous (IV) or subcutaneous route. In cases of severe hypernatremia, one might consider replacing the excessive urine output with intravenous D5W.

Although not as common as the preceding complication, hyponatremia can also occur due to the syndrome of inappropriate antidiuretic hormone (SIADH) or cerebral salt wasting (CSW). The physiological response elicited by SIADH results in renal conservation of water and a dilutional hyponatremia that is treated with a water restriction. To facilitate a negative fluid balance, concentrated enteral or parenteral formulations (or both) should be provided.

In contrast to SIADH, the primary defect in CSW is due to the kidneys' inability to conserve salt, with resultant salt wasting and volume depletion. Once the presence of CSW is confirmed (dilute, high-volume urine, as opposed to concentrated, low-volume urine in SIADH), appropriate treatment consists of volume and salt replacement, which may be accomplished by IV normal or, rarely, hypertonic saline, and/or enteral salt provision (58). The prompt and accurate differentiating between these two causes of hyponatremia is of utmost importance; failure to do so can lead to an inappropriate hypovolemia, which can be fatal in this population.

The potential interaction of drugs with nutrients should be considered in every nutrition support regimen. Phenytoin, an anticonvulsant, is commonly prescribed to be administered on an empty stomach, causing interruption of continuous EN. Frequent disruption of EN delivery is a concern, because it is has been shown that critically ill patients receive nutrition that is significantly less than their nutritional requirements (59). To avoid routine EN interruptions, the IV route for phenytoin administration may be a better option.

Another drug frequently utilized in this population is mannitol, an osmotic diuretic, which has proved to be effective in controlling ICP. Especially when administered in large doses, mannitol has an increased risk of acute tubular necrosis and can also cause significant osmolarity disturbances (8).

Intensive glucose control, defined as between 80 and 110 mg/dl, has recently been identified as advantageous in critical care management (60); however, the optimal maximum glucose level has not yet been established. Hyperglycemia may be exacerbated by steroids, although the routine addition of steroids to reduce ICP and improve outcomes is no longer suggested (8).

The use of serum transport proteins as a measure of nutritional adequacy in times of injury has limitations, and it is essential to understand the hepatic reprioritization that occurs in response to stress for accurate interpretation (see Chapter 5). During the hypercatabolic response, hepatocytes down-regulate the production of transport proteins, with a concomitant increase the production of "survival" or acute-phase proteins, such as C-reactive protein (CRP) (61). Because significantly elevated CRP levels have been observed in brain-injured patients with mean values peaking at > 11 times the normal range (62), interpreting prealbumin as a reflection of nutritional adequacy should be done cautiously and in concert with CRP. For instance, if CRP is normal and prealbumin is low, the appropriateness of the current regimen should be reevaluated because, generally, in patients with a healthy, noncirrhotic liver (provided the majority [> 55%] of nutritional needs are being delivered), an increase in prealbumin of 4 to 5 mg/dl per week can be anticipated (61). Higher levels of prealbumin may be observed with the concurrent administration of steroids (63). It is useful to monitor serial prealbumin in conjunction with CRP to evaluate the degree of hypercatabolism and the adequacy of the nutrition support being provided (64).

The significantly increased nitrogen excretion in this population has led some authors to advocate nitrogen balance studies to assess nutritional adequacy in this population (22,40). In addition to being logistically difficult to obtain, these studies are influenced by a variety of factors, such as the level of calorie and nitrogen intake, insensible losses, presence of hematuria, and inadequate urine collection, making these values complicated to interpret. The practicality, cost, and the established correlation of prealbumin with nitrogen balance studies suggests that prealbumin, with the previously mentioned caveats about its interpretation, is a preferred parameter for monitoring the appropriateness of nutrition support (61,62).

32.8 CONCLUSION

Nutrition support in acute brain injury can pose significant challenges for the clinician. A summary of commonly encountered problems in brain-injured patients is provided in Table 32.3. As previously stated, nutrition support should be initiated as early as feasible in the hospital course for maximal therapeutic benefit. Because the route chosen for nutritional delivery should be that which allows for reliable and consistent nutrient delivery, SB access is strongly suggested, particularly in the acute phase of brain injury. Ongoing nutritional assessment and monitoring should be conducted that includes physical observations and the usage of medications that could significantly affect metabolic demands.

No longer is PN recommended for first-line nutritional support in this patient population (11). With the increasing availability of SB feeding tubes, the barriers that have plagued safe and reliable gastric feeding can be avoided, and patients can benefit from the numerous benefits of enteral nutrition.

32.9 CASE STUDY

32.9.1 CLINICAL PRESENTATION

J.D. is a 24-year-old male who arrives at the trauma center for work-up and treatment of injuries received in a motor vehicle accident in an outlying county. GCS was 6 on admission, and a CT scan of the head was obtained. The CT revealed a subarachnoid hemorrhage and small subdural hematoma, and the patient was immediately taken to the operating room for placement of a ventricular ICP monitor. With the exception of a broken rib revealed on chest x-ray, other diagnostic exams were unremarkable, and the patient, now intubated, was transferred to the ICU.

J.D. receives propofol at 15 ml/h and PCA at 3 mg/h. He has bouts of elevated ICP (normal values 0 to 15 mmHG) and is given mannitol for this, while serum osmolarity is monitored every 12 hours. A nasogastric (NG) tube is in place and has drained 350 ml over the first 24 hours. Prealbumin at admission was 22.5 mg/dl, and the team would like to start enteral feeds via the NG tube to maintain nutritional status.

TABLE 32.3

Potential Nutrition Related Complications in Patients with Acute Brain Injury

Complication	Possible Cause(s)	Suggested Response
Abdominal distention	Ileus	May require PN
	Hypoperfusion	If possible, low rate, semielemental
	Medications	formula for trophic benefits
Aspiration	Elevated ICP	Jejunal feeding
	Decreased LES tone	NG/OG tube for decompression if high
	Impaired gastric emptying	gastric residuals continue with jejunal
	Incompetent gag reflex	feeding
	Medications that delay gastric emptying	+/- Addition of PKA if jejunal feeding is not feasible
Diarrhea	Hyperosmotic (e.g., sorbitol-containing) medication elixirs or suspensions	Change medications to nonliquid or IV form
	Antibiotic therapy	Addition of probiotic
	Bowel program, prokinetic agents	Ensure that bowel program, prokinetic
	Infectious causes	agents have been discontinued
		Rule out infectious causes (e.g., *C. difficile*)
Elevated residuals	Delayed gastric emptying due to elevated ICP, brain injury	Jejunal feeding
	Medications (opioids, barbiturates)	Avoid bolus feeding
	Ventilator settings	Diligent glucose management
	Hyperglycemia	
Hyperglycemia	Injury to brain	Tight BG control with insulin infusion as
	Corticosteroid therapy	needed
	Overfeeding	Indirect calorimetry
Hypertriglyceridemia	Impending organ failure	Avoid prolonged propofol usage
	Overfeeding	Indirect calorimetry
	Propofol	
Negative nitrogen balance	Characteristic of brain injury	Ensure sufficient energy and protein
	Suboptimal energy or protein provision	administration
	Corticosteroid usage	Indirect calorimetry
		Follow CRP with prealbumin to help gauge catabolism

Question:

Would this patient be expected to tolerate gastric feeds?

Comment:

The low GCS score, use of narcotic analgesia and propofol, and elevated ICP are all factors that would predispose J.D. to gastric feeding intolerance (18–20,28). If at all possible, a postpyloric tube should be placed to allow early EN, which has been associated with improved outcomes in this population (14–16).

Question:

What is J.D.'s nutritional status upon admission?

Comment:

J.D. was eating regularly (3 meals/d) per spouse prior to his motor vehicle accident. He is 71 inches and 195 pounds (89 kg), and prealbumin was within normal limits. By all indications, it appears that J.D., like the majority of trauma patients, was well nourished at the time of injury. However, the obligatory mobilization of LBM that is characteristic of brain injury could cause him to lose a significant amount of LBM in a short amount of time (8). In view of this, nutritional support should start early and avoid frequent interruptions (11).

Question:

What type of enteral formula should be provided?

Comment:

A high-protein, low-fat formula should be delivered, considering the calories provided via the propofol drip, advancing the EN infusion to goal once the propofol is discontinued. It is a good idea to monitor serum triglycerides if the propofol is continued for a prolonged period of time (54).

Question:

How would J.D.'s nutritional needs be assessed?

Comment:

If the clinician is unable to obtain an indirect calorimetry study, the Harris–Benedict equation, with a factor of 1.4, would equate to 2833 kcal or ~32 kcal/kg. Using the upper range of kcal/kg (approximately 30 to 35 kcal/kg) would be appropriate for J.D. because he is not receiving neuromuscular-blocking agents. For protein needs, 1.5 to 2 g/kg would deliver 134 to 178 g/day, which can be accomplished with a high-protein formula.

Question:

It is now post trauma day #6, and J.D. has been receiving postpyloric feeding at goal for the last 4 days. A prealbumin is obtained and reveals a level of 11.3 mg/dl. How do you explain?

Comment:

The synthesis of prealbumin is immediately down-regulated after an injury due to the increased production of acute-phase proteins. Even with adequate exogenous provision of nutrients, the prealbumin will not increase if acute-phase proteins are elevated. CRP is a good marker of underlying inflammation, and its changes can be inversely correlated with non-acute-phase proteins, (e.g., prealbumin) (61). As long as the CRP is elevated, the prealbumin will often not increase significantly and thus is not an indicator to increase nutritional support. However, in the absence of liver dysfunction, if the CRP normalizes and the prealbumin fails to rise, one should consider measuring the adequacy of energy and protein delivery with indirect calorimetry and a nitrogen balance study.

Question:

It is now post trauma day #20, and though J.D. is demonstrating significant improvement, it appears that he will not be able to resume oral nutrition in the near future. What type of access would you recommend?

Comment:

Long-term enteral access should be provided when the need for access is expected to be more than 4 weeks (39). Though delayed gastric emptying has been observed up to 25 days after brain injury (20), this has not been the usual experience of these authors. Given the problems with long-term jejunal access (i.e., frequent kinking, occlusion, and even dislodgement), an initial step would to be to place a PEG tube. One can then initiate gastric feeding while monitoring gastric residuals and bowel function and watching closely for signs of aspiration. A convenience of the gastric route during the subacute and chronic phases is the ability to provide bolus feeding in most patients, avoiding the need for a continuous infusion pump, and making ambulation easier during physical therapy. If the patient fails the gastric route, then one must consider either a jejunal extension through the gastrostomy tube or a surgically placed jejunostomy tube.

REFERENCES

1. Krauss JF, McArthur DL. Epidemiologic aspects of brain injury. *Neurol. Clin.* 1996; 14: 435–450.
2. *Injury in America: A Continuing Public Health Problem.* National Academy Press, Washington, DC, 1985.
3. Brunner CS. Neurologic impairments. In: *Contemporary Nutrition Support Practice: A Clinical Guide.* Matarese LE, Gottschlich MM, Eds. W.B. Saunders, Philadelphia, 1998, 384–395.
4. National Center for Health Statistics. Accessed February 10, 2004: http://www.cdc.gov.
5. *Traumatic Brain Injury in the United States: A Report to Congress.* Accessed February 10, 2004: www. cdc.gov.
6. Pulsinelli WA. Cerebrovascular diseases: principles. In: *Cecil Textbook of Medicine.* Goldman L, Bennett JC, Eds. W.B. Saunders, Philadelphia, 2000, 2092–2099.
7. Vender JR, Cresci GA, Lee MR. Nutritional considerations in severe brain injury. In: *Nutritional Considerations in the Intensive Care Unit.* Shikora SA, Martindale RG, Schwaitzberg SD, Eds. Kendall/Hunt, Dubuque, IA, 2002, chap. 22.
8. Bullock R, Chestnut RM, Clifton G, et al. Guidelines for the management of severe head injury. *Brain Trauma Foundation* 1995; 14: 1–15.
9. Wilmore DW. Catabolic illness: strategies for enhancing recovery. *N. Engl. J. Med.* 1990; 325: 695–702.
10. Loder PB, Smith RC, Kee AJ, et al. What rate of infusion of intravenous nutrition solution is required to stimulate uptake of amino acids by peripheral tissues in depleted patients? *Ann. Surg.* 1990; 211: 360–368.
11. ASPEN Board of Directors and The Clinical Guidelines Task Force. Guidelines for the use of parenteral and enteral nutrition in adult and pediatric patients. *JPEN* 2002; 26 (Suppl): 15A–1385A.
12. Heyland DK, Dhaliwal R, Drover JW, et al. Canadian clinical practice guidelines for nutrition support in mechanically ventilated, critically ill adult patients. *JPEN* 2003; 27: 355–373.
13. Nyswonger GD, Helmchen RH. Early enteral nutrition and length of stay in stroke patients. *J. Neurosci. Nurs.* 1992; 24: 220–223.
14. Graham TW, Zadrozny DB, Harrington T. The benefits of early jejunal hyperalimentation in the head-injured patient. *Neurosurgery* 1989; 25: 729–735.
15. Sacks GS, Brown RO, Teague D, et al. Early nutrition support modifies immune function in patients sustaining severe head injury. *JPEN* 1995; 19: 387–392.
16. Taylor SJ, Fettes SB, Jewkes C, et al. Prospective, randomized, controlled trial to determine the effect of early enhanced enteral nutrition on clinical outcome in mechanically ventilated patients suffering head injury. *Crit. Care Med.* 1999; 27: 2525–2531.
17. Young B, Ott L, Twyman D, et al. The effect of nutritional support on outcome from severe head injury. *J. Neurosurg.* 1987; 67: 668–676.
18. Kao CH, ChangLai AP, Chieng PU, et al. Gastric emptying in head-injured patients. *Am. J. Gastro.* 1998; 93: 1108–1112.
19. Norton JA, Ott LG, McClain C, et al. Intolerance to enteral feeding in the brain-injured patient. *J. Neurosurg.* 1988; 68: 62–66.
20. Ott L, Young B, Phillips R, et al. Altered gastric emptying in the head-injured patient: relationship to feeding intolerance. *J. Neurosurg.* 1991; 74: 738–742.
21. Weekes E and Elia M. Observations on the patterns of 24-hour energy expenditure changes in body composition and gastric emptying in head-injured patients receiving nasogastric tube feeding. *JPEN* 1996; 20: 31–37.
22. Clifton GL, Robertson CS, Grossman RG, et al. The metabolic response to severe head injury. *J. Neurosurg.* 1984; 60: 687–696.
23. Booth CM, Heyland DK, Paterson WG. Gastrointestinal promotility drugs in the critical care setting: a systematic review of the evidence. *Crit. Care Med.* 2002; 30: 1429–1435.
24. Marino LV, Kiratu EM, French S, et al. To determine the effect of metoclopramide on gastric emptying in severe head injuries: a prospective, randomized, controlled trial. *Br. J. Neurosurg.* 2003; 17: 24–28.
25. Rhoney DH, Parker D, Formea CM, et al. Tolerability of bolus versus continuous gastric feeding in brain-injured patients. *Neurol. Res.* 2002; 24: 613–620.

26. Saxe JM, Ledgerwood AM, Lucas CE, et al. Lower esophageal sphincter dysfunction precludes safe gastric feeding after head injury. *J. Trauma* 1994; 27: 581–586.

27. Lucas CE, Yu P, Vlahos A, et al. Lower esophageal sphincter dysfunction often precludes safe gastric feeding in stroke patients. *Arch. Surg.* 1999; 134: 55–58.

28. McClave SA, DeMeo MT, DeLegge MH, et al. North American summit on aspiration in the critically ill patient: consensus statement. *JPEN* 2002; 26 (Suppl): S80–S85.

29. Winkelman C. Effect of backrest position on intracranial and cerebral perfusion pressures in traumatically brain-injured adults. *Am. J. Crit. Care* 2000, Nov 9 (6): 373–380.

30. Wojner AW, El-Mitwalli A, Alexandrov AV. Effect of head positioning on intracranial blood flow velocities in acute ischemic stroke: a pilot study. *Crit. Care Nurs. Q.* 2002; 24 (4): 57–66.

31. Heyland DK, Drover JW, Dhaliwal R, et al. Optimizing the benefits and minimizing the risks of enteral nutrition in the critically ill: role of small bowel feeding. *JPEN* 2002; 26 (Suppl): S51–S57.

32. Kirby DK, Clifton GL, Turner H, et al. Early enteral nutrition after brain injury by percutaneous endoscopic gastrojejunostomy. *JPEN* 1991; 15: 298–302.

33. Magnuson B, Hatton J, Williams S, et al. Tolerance and efficacy of enteral nutrition for neurosurgical patients in pentobarbital coma. *Nutr. Clin. Pract.* 1999; 14: 131–134.

34. Klodell CT, Carroll M, Carrillo EH, et al. Routine intragastric feeding following traumatic brain injury is safe and well tolerated. *Am. J. Surg.* 2000; 179: 168–171.

35. Ott L, Annis K, Hatton J, et al. Postpyloric enteral feeding costs for patients with severe head injury: blind placement, endoscopy, and PEG/J versus TPN. *J. Neurotrauma* 1999; 16: 233–242.

36. Cresci G, Martindale R. Bedside placement of small bowel feeding tubes in hospitalized patients: a new role for the dietitian. *Nutrition* 2003; 19: 843–846.

37. Taylor B, Schallom L. Bedside small bowel feeding tube placement in critically ill patients utilizing a nurse/dietitian team approach. *Nutr. Clin. Pract.* 2001; 16: 258–262.

38. Boyce JM, Potter-Bynoe G, Dziobek L, et al. Nosocomial pneumonia in Medicare patients: hospital costs and reimbursement patterns under the prospective payment system. *Arch. Int. Med.* 1991; 151: 1109–1114.

39. Cresci GA. Enteral access: the role of the nutrition support dietetics professional. *Support Line* 2002; 24: 12–18.

40. Clifton GL, Roberton CS, Choi SC. Assessment of nutritional requirements of head-injured patients. *J. Neurosurg.* 1986; 64: 895–901.

41. Bruder N, Dumong JC, Francois G. Evolution of energy expenditure and nitrogen excretion in severe head-injured patients. *Crit. Care Med.* 1991; 19: 43–48.

42. Moore R, Najarian MP, Konvolinka CW. Measured energy expenditure in severe head trauma. *J. Trauma* 1989; 29: 1633–1636 .

43. Young B, Ott L, Twyman D, et al. The effect of nutritional support on outcome from severe head injury. *J. Neurosurg.* 1987; 67: 668–676.

44. Graham TW, Zadrozny DB, Harrington T. The benefits of early jejunal hyperalimentation in the head-injured patient. *Neurosurgery* 1989; 25: 729–735.

45. Sunderland PM, Heilbrun MP. Estimating energy expenditure in traumatic brain injury: comparison of indirect calorimetry with predictive formulas. *Neurosurgery* 1992; 31: 246–253.

46. Bitzani M, Mutamis D, Nalbandi V, et al. Resting energy expenditure in brain death. *Int. Care Med.* 1999; 25: 970–976.

47. Lifelink, personal communication, 2003.

48. Nieman DC, Trone GA, Austin MD. A new handheld device for measuring resting metabolic rate and oxygen consumption. *JADA* 2003; 103: 588–592.

49. Fried RC, Dickerson RN, Guenter PA, et al. Barbiturate therapy reduces nitrogen excretion in acute head injury. *J. Trauma* 1989; 29: 1558–1564.

50. Dempsey DT, Guenter PA, Mullen JL, et al. Energy expenditure in acute trauma with and without barbiturate therapy. *Surg. Gynecol. Obstet.* 1985; 160: 128–134.

51. Fruin AH, Taylon C, Pettis MS. Calorie requirements in patients with severe head injuries. *Surg. Neurol.* 1986; 25: 25–28.

52. Chiolero RL, Breitenstein E, Thorin D, et al. Effects of propranolol on resting metabolic rate after severe head injury. *Crit. Care Med.* 1989; 17: 328–334.

53. McCall M, Jeejeebhoy K, Pencharz P, et al. Effect of neuromuscular blockage on energy expenditure in patients with severe head injury. *JPEN* 2003; 27: 27–35.

54. Roth MS, Martin AB, Katz JA. Nutritional implications of prolonged propofol use. *Am. J. Heath-Syst. Pharm.* 1997; 54: 694–695.

55. Varella L, Fastremski CA. Neurological impairment. In: *The Science and Practice of Nutrition Support.* Gottschlich MM, Ed. Kendall/Hunt, Dubuque, IA, 2001, chap 20.

56. Young B, Ott L, Kasarskis E, et al. Zinc supplementation is associated with improved neurologic recovery rate and visceral protein levels of patients with severe closed head injury. *J. Neurotrauma* 1996; 13(1): 25–34.

57. Shackford SR, Bourguignon PR, Wald SL, et al. Hypertonic saline resuscitation of patients with head injury: a prospective, randomized clinical trial. *J. Trauma* 1998; 44: 50–58.

58. Zafonte RD, Mann NR. Cerebral salt wasting syndrome in brain injury patients: a potential cause of hyponatremia. *Arch. Phys. Med. Rehab.* 1997; 78: 540–542.

59. McClave SA, Sexton LK, Spain DA, et al. Enteral tube feeding in the intensive care unit: factors impeding adequate delivery. *Crit. Care Med.* 1999; 27: 1252–1256.

60. Van den Berghe G, Wouter P, Weekers F, et al. Intensive insulin therapy in critically ill patients. *N. Engl. J. Med.* 2001; 345:1359–1367.

61. Spiekerman AM. Proteins used in nutritional assessment. *Clin. Lab. Med.* 1993; 13: 353–369.

62. Boosalis MG, Ott L, Levine AS, et al. Relationship of visceral proteins to nutritional status in chronic and acute stress. *Crit. Care Med.* 1989; 17: 741–747.

63. Oppenheimer JH, Werner SC. Effect of prednisone on thyroxine-binding proteins. *J. Clin. Endocrinol. Metab.* 1966; 26: 715–721.

64. Bernstein L, Bachman TE, Meguid M, et al. Measurement of visceral protein status in assessing protein and energy malnutrition: standard of care. *Nutrition* 1995; 11: 169–171.

65. Bruder N, Raynal M, Pellissier D, et al. Influence on body temperature, with or without sedation, on energy expenditure in severe head-injured patients. *Crit. Care Med.* 1998; 26: 568–557.

33 Acute Pancreatitis

Rémy F. Meier
Kantonsspital Liestal

Christoph Beglinger
University Hospital Basel

CONTENTS

33.1 INTRODUCTION

The clinical patterns of acute pancreatitis vary from mild disease to severe necrotizing pancreatitis with local and systemic complications. Classifying acute pancreatitis by the Atlanta criteria, (1) approximately 75% of the patients have a mild disease, with a mortality rate below 1% (2). Mortality increases to up to 20% if the disease progresses to severe necrotizing pancreatitis (3–6). These patients often develop nutritional deficiencies during the prolonged and complicated course of the disease. This can have fatal consequences, especially in patients already malnourished at the time of the initial attack (7).

For a long time, oral or enteral nutrition support was regarded as harmful, because stimulation of the exocrine pancreatic secretion was considered a risk for exacerbating autodigestive processes. These concerns formed the basis for the concept of placing patients on bowel rest; intravenous nutritional support was used to bypass the stimulatory effect of oral or enteral nutrition until the patient had recovered.

During the last decade, knowledge about the beneficial effects of enteral nutrition and better understanding of the disease have fundamentally changed this concept.

33.2 MALNUTRITION IN ACUTE PANCREATITIS

Malnutrition is a common problem in patients with pancreatitis. A coincidence of malnutrition in chronic alcoholics is present in 50 to 80%, and alcohol-induced pancreatitis is one of the major causes of the disease (7).

Protein-calorie malnutrition can also arise or worsen because of depletion of nutrients and the hypermetabolic state during acute pancreatitis.

Specific and nonspecific metabolic changes occur during acute pancreatitis. Pain and the inflammatory response triggered by the autodigestive processes, which are modulated by a variety of proinflammatory cytokines, can increase the basal metabolic rate. This can result in an increased energy consumption (8). The resting energy expenditure varies according to the severity and the length of the disease. If metabolic expenditure is measured daily by indirect calorimetry, the values show a wide range, according to the severity of acute pancreatitis. If these patients develop sepsis, 80% of them show an elevation in protein catabolism and an increased nutrient requirement (8,9). The negative nitrogen balance determines clinical outcome. Sitzmann et al. reported a tenfold increased mortality rate when the nitrogen balance was negative, compared to those patients with a positive balance (10). Whether negative nitrogen balance is the principle factor for outcome is not clear. The relationship between nitrogen balance and outcome may only reflect the relationship between nitrogen balance and severity of disease; none of the studies was stratified according to disease severity (11).

33.3 SPECIFIC SUBSTRATE METABOLISM IN ACUTE PANCREATITIS

33.3.1 CARBOHYDRATES

Glucose metabolism in acute pancreatitis is determined by an increase in energy demand. Endogenous gluconeogenesis is increased as a consequence of the metabolic response to the severe inflammatory process. Glucose is an important source of energy and can partially counteract the intrinsic gluconeogenesis from protein degradation. This can counteract, to a certain degree, the deleterious and unwanted effects of protein catabolism (12). Application of carbohydrates with concomitant restriction of lipids reduces the risk of hyperlipidemia, but hyperlipidemia cannot be completely avoided.

The maximum rate of glucose oxidation is approximately 4 mg/kg/min. The administration of glucose in excess can be harmful, and even wasteful, because of lipogenesis and glucose recycling. Furthermore, hyperglycemia and hypercapnia can occur. Hyperglycemia can lead to increased infections and metabolic complications. Glucose levels can also be increased because of the frequently impaired insulin secretion. Hyperglycemia following glucose infusion can only partly be corrected with exogenous insulin administration. There is little evidence that supplemental insulin is beneficial to patients. Monitoring blood glucose levels seems to be adequate.

Intravenous glucose administration does not stimulate exocrine pancreatic secretion (13–15). Enteral perfusion of glucose into the jejunum is only a weak stimulus for exocrine pancreatic secretion.

33.3.2 PROTEINS AND AMINO ACIDS

A negative nitrogen balance is often seen in severe acute pancreatitis. The protein losses must be minimized in these patients, and the increased protein turnover must be compensated. Deficiencies in certain amino acids may enhance pancreatic inflammation, leading to a potential vicious cycle (16). Intravenous administration of protein hydrolysates either inhibits exocrine pancreatic secretory responses or has no effect (13,17), but amino acids can stimulate gastric acid secretion, which in turn may stimulate the pancreatic secretory response through stimulatory mechanisms in the duodenum. Jejunal perfusion of elemental diets containing defined amounts of protein or amino acids is well tolerated and does not stimulate exocrine pancreatic secretion. In contrast, gastric and duodenal perfusions of proteins are potent stimulants of pancreatic secretory responses. Regardless of whether an elemental diet is ingested orally or infused into the duodenum or the jejunum, the elemental diet results in less stimulation than a standard diet infused at the same level (18–24). Elemental diets are regarded as the most beneficial diet for patients with acute pancreatitis, but clinical experience with infusing intact proteins in the jejunum has not shown major negative effects on outcome.

33.3.3 LIPIDS

Hyperlipidemia is a common observation in acute pancreatitis. Increases in cholesterol and free fatty acid serum concentrations have been reported. The mechanism of altered lipid metabolism is not entirely clear (altered lipid oxidation or lipid clearance?). Serum lipid concentrations return to normal ranges if the acute phase of acute pancreatitis is over and the patient is recovering. On the other hand, in some patients with hyperlipidemia, an increased risk of developing acute pancreatitis was reported. Hypertriglyceridemia ranging up to 80 to 100 mmol/l was seen in these patients, with hyperlipidemia preceding pancreatitis (25). In animals, infusion of high amounts of triglycerides induced pancreatitislike changes with a rise of free fatty acids in the serum. This process can enhance the formation of microthrombi and aggravate the disease by ischemic injury to the pancreatic tissue. Furthermore, in the injured pancreas, capillary permeability can increase, followed by a leakage of activated pancreatic enzymes (26,27). This in turn may promote local hydrolysis of triglycerides from chylomicrons, which can exhibit local toxicity toward capillary membranes, causing further damage to the pancreas.

Pancreatic exocrine secretion is not stimulated by intravenous lipids (18,28–32). However, four cases have been reported in the literature in which acute pancreatitis developed after intravenous infusion of fat emulsions (33–35). In these cases, serum triglycerides or other lipid levels were not well documented or reported. Furthermore, in these patients additional diseases and drug therapies could be involved in the development of the unwanted effect.

The stimulation of exocrine pancreatic secretion by enteral administration of lipids depends on the anatomic site of administration. Lipids perfused into the stomach and into the duodenum are powerful stimuli. If the same amount of lipid is given into the distal jejunum, only a minimal stimulation of exocrine pancreatic secretion occurs. Taking all these arguments together, there is no convincing evidence that would suggest a contraindication to the use of triglycerides or other fats in patients with acute pancreatitis, provided that these patients are monitored for hypertriglyceridemia.

33.4 NUTRITIONAL SUPPORT IN ACUTE PANCREATITIS

Specific nutritional support depends on the severity of the disease. It is therefore essential to define the patients at risk. The patient must be assessed at the time of admission and during the course of the disease. The most important patients are those developing severe necrotizing pancreatitis. Patients with mild to moderate pancreatitis usually recover within 7 to 10 days.

33.4.1 SEVERITY ASSESSMENT

Prediction of the progress of acute pancreatitis at the time of admission can be difficult, but an assessment of severity is necessary to plan nutritional interventions. Nutritional support ranges from no nutrition to full enteral or parenteral nutrition (or both), according to the development of the disease.

Several prognostic scoring systems, which include clinical, laboratory, and radiological criteria, are available (36–38). The Atlanta classification of severity defines severe acute pancreatitis on the

---

TABLE 33.1
Ranson's Criteria of Severity for Acute
Pancreatitis

Admission Criteria
Age > 55 years
White blood count > 16,000/mm³
Glucose > 200 mg/dl
Lactate dehydrogenase > 350 IU/l
Aspartamine transaminase > 250 U/l

Following Initial 48 Hours Criteria
Hematocrit decrease of > 10%
Blood urea nitrogen increase of 5 mg/dl
Calcium < 8 mg/dl
PaO_2 < 60 mg Hg
Base deficit > 4 mEq/l
Fluid sequestration > 6 l

Source: From Ranson JH, Rifkind KM, Roses DF, Fink SD,
Eng K, Spencer FC, *Surg. Gynecol. Obstet.* 1974; 139: 69–81.

---

basis of standard clinical manifestations: a score of 3 or more in the Ranson criteria (Table 33.1) or a score of 8 or more in the APACHE II criteria, and evidence of organ failure and intrapancreatic pathological findings (necrosis or interstitial pancreatitis) (1). This classification is helpful because it also allows comparison of different trials and methodologies.

The severity of acute pancreatitis based on imaging procedures is based on the Balthazar score, which predicts severity on CT appearance, including presence or absence of necrosis. Failure of pancreatic parenchyma to enhance during the arterial phase of intravenous contrast-enhanced CT indicates necrosis, which predicts a severe attack if more than 50% of the gland is affected (39). Other markers include measurement of concentrations of serum C-reactive protein (CRP) or urinary trypsinogen activation peptide (TAP); both are useful in clinical practice. CRP concentration has an independent prognostic value. A peak of more than 210 mg/l on day 2 through 4, or more than 120 mg/l at the end of the first week, is as predictive as multiple-factor scoring systems (40). Urinary TAP, which is released during activation of trypsinogen to trypsin, has been shown to predict accurately the severity of acute pancreatitis 24 hours after onset. Urinary TAP is suggested as a single marker for severity assessment (41), but it is not yet available as a routine test.

33.4.2 ROUTE OF NUTRIENT DELIVERY

Oral feeding is known to increase abdominal pain in patients with acute pancreatitis. Therefore, patients were either fasted or the nutrients were given by the parenteral route to put the pancreas "at rest."

Patients with mild to moderate acute pancreatitis can usually start with an oral diet within the first three days of onset if their pain is diminished and the pancreatic enzymes have a tendency to return to normal (42). The only available study reported that, in 21% of patients, pain relapses occurred during oral refeeding on day 1 or 2. Patients at risk were those with a serum lipase concentration three times higher than those of the upper limit and with a higher CT-Balthazar score (42).

33.4.2.1 Total Parenteral Nutrition or Enteral Nutrition

Traditionally, total parenteral nutrition (TPN) was used to avoid stimulation of the exocrine pancreatic secretory response. In mild to moderate pancreatitis, two prospective studies are available comparing TPN with a nasojejunal feeding regimen or no nutritional support (43,44); the studies showed no difference in outcome. However, TPN was more expensive or accompanied by an increase in catheter-related infections (43); furthermore, TPN was associated with a longer hospital stay (44). Finally, TPN was associated with more hyperglycemia and other metabolic disturbances. In recent years, it has become clear that these complications were often the consequence of overfeeding (45). Van den Berghe et al. showed, irrespective of the route of nutritional support, that the control of hyperglycemia with insulin reduced mortality in critically ill patients (46).

Several studies in patients with trauma, thermal injury, and major gastrointestinal surgery have shown a reduction in septic complication with enteral feeding (47,48). Enteral nutrition helps to maintain mucosal function and limits absorption of endotoxin and cytokines from the gut (49–51). In animals with induced pancreatitis, enteral nutrition prevented bacterial translocation (52); whether this is of clinical relevance in patients with acute pancreatitis is still unclear (53).

Recently, strategies have changed: nutritional management has shifted from parenteral to enteral feeding. Enteral feeding in acute pancreatitis may reduce catabolism and loss of lean body mass, modulate the acute-phase response, and preserve visceral protein metabolism, with the potential to down-regulate the splanchnic cytokine response (54). Furthermore, enteral nutrition has been shown to be safe and well tolerated. Several prospective, randomized clinical trials have been performed in the past few years comparing enteral with parenteral nutrition in patients with acute pancreatitis. In the first prospective study, by McClave et al., patients with mild to moderate acute pancreatitis were randomized either to total parenteral nutrition or to total enteral nutrition via a nasojejunal tube (43). Both groups received an isocaloric, isonitrogenous solution within 48 hours after admission to the hospital. The outcome in both groups revealed no statistical differences in infectious complications, length of ICU stay, length of hospital stay, or days to oral food intake. In the TPN group, a significantly higher glucose concentration in the first five days was found. The caloric goal was reached in 82% of the patients with enteral feeding, compared to 96% of patients with TPN (43).

A second prospective, randomized study compared either a nasojejunal tube feeding with a semielemental diet or TPN within 48 hours of admission in patients with severe necrotizing acute pancreatitis (55). Enteral feeding was well tolerated without adverse effects on the course of the disease, but patients who received enteral feeding experienced fewer septic complications and fewer total complications than those receiving parenteral nutrition. Furthermore, the costs of nutritional support were three times higher in the patients receiving TPN. This study showed that, in severe acute pancreatitis, enteral nutrition support was beneficial compared to patients with mild or moderate pancreatitis (43).

These findings are supported by two other studies. Windsor et al. compared parenteral nutrition with enteral nutrition in patients with acute pancreatitis of all levels of severity (54). This study demonstrated that enteral nutrition attenuates the acute-phase response in acute pancreatitis and improves disease severity and clinical outcome, despite the fact that the pancreatic injuries were virtually unchanged on CT scan. In the enteral feeding group, SIRS and sepsis were reduced, resulting in a beneficial clinical outcome (APACHE II score and C-reactive protein). In this study, unfortunately, only a few patients had severe pancreatitis, and the total amounts of nutrient received revealed marked differences between the enteral and the parenteral groups. Furthermore, these positive results of the Windsor study could not be confirmed by Powell et al. with respect to the inflammatory response in patients with prognostically severe acute pancreatitis (56).

Abou-Assi et al. selected 156 patients with acute pancreatitis during a 12-month period (57). During the first 48 hours, all patients were treated with IV fluid and analgesics. In this study, 87% of patients had mild, 10% had moderate, and 3% had severe disease. Those patients who improved were fed orally afterward. The nonresponders were randomized to receive nutrients either by a nasojejunal tube or by TPN. Seventy-five percent of the initially enrolled patients improved with the oral regimen and were discharged within 4 days. Fifty-four percent of the enteral group (n = 26) and 88% of the TPN group (n = 27) received inadequate energy intake. The patients in the enteral group were fed for a significantly shorter period (mean 6.7 days vs. 10.8 days [TPN]) and had significantly fewer metabolic and septic complications. Hyperglycemia requiring insulin therapy was significantly higher in the parenterally fed patients. Despite fewer complications in the enteral group, the mortality was similar in the two groups. The authors concluded that hypocaloric enteral feeding is safer and less expensive than parenteral feeding and bowel rest in patients with acute pancreatitis.

Enteral nutrition in severe acute pancreatitis is today performed by placing a jejunal feeding tube distally to the ligament of Treitz. The tubes are placed either with fluoroscopic help or by endoscopy. Normally, jejunal tubes are well tolerated without an exacerbation of pancreatitis-related symptoms (43,58–60). Rarely, proximal migration of the feeding tube and a subsequent pancreatic stimulation can aggravate acute pancreatitis (61). Severe ileus, preventing enteral feeding in the early stages of disease, can be a problem. Partial ileus is not a contraindication to enteral feeding, because these patients frequently tolerate continuous low-volume nasojejunal nutrients. In patients not tolerating nasoenteral feeding tubes, laparascopic jejunostomies are performed in some institutions. There are no convincing data to support this approach. Whether jejunal feeding is absolutely necessary is not completely clear. Minimizing stimulation of the exocrine pancreatic secretion would support the route of jejunal feeding. It is, however, controversial whether stimulation of pancreatic secretion is important for the outcome of the disease. Recently, a randomized study of nasogastric vs. nasojejunal feeding in severe acute pancreatitis was published (62). In this study, nasogastric feeding was safe; little difference was documented between the two methods with respect to pain, analgesic requirements, serum CRP concentrations, or clinical outcome (62).

33.4.3 NUTRIENT REQUIREMENTS

Patients with severe acute pancreatitis are hypermetabolic. They have a nonsuppressible gluconeogenesis, despite sufficient caloric intake, and increased ureagenesis and an accentuated net protein catabolism, which can go up to 40 g nitrogen/d. Glucose supply cannot completely inhibit intrinsic gluconeogenesis and the status of acute catabolism. The more severe acute pancreatitis is, the more excessive is hypermetabolism. Resting energy expenditure can be variable in these patients. Seventy-seven to 158% of the predicted energy expenditure is reported (9). If the disease is complicated by sepsis or multiorgan failure, the resting energy expenditure is significantly increased (9,63). In severe acute pancreatitis, the Harris–Benedict equation is not sensitive enough to estimate caloric expenditure. In these cases, indirect calorimetry is recommended to avoid over- or underfeeding.

For enteral or parenteral nutrition, ~25 to 35 kcal/kg BW/d are recommended. It is important to avoid overfeeding and hyperglycemia (57). Blood glucose concentrations should not exceed 10 mmol/l. Insulin treatment is recommended, but the doses should not be higher than 4 to 6 unit/h. The impaired glucose oxidation rate cannot be normalized by insulin administration. Normally, 3 to 6 g/kg BW/d of carbohydrates can be recommended.

The optimal goal of protein supply is between 1.2 and 1.5 g/kg BW/d. A high protein intake should be given only to patients with a severe negative nitrogen balance. Lower protein intake should be given to patients with renal or severe hepatic failure.

Fat can be safely given up to 2 g/kg BW/d, but blood triglyceride levels must be monitored carefully. Triglycerides should not be higher than 12 mmol/l.

The nutrient recommendations are easier to obtain with TPN than with enteral nutrition. Enteral solutions contain fixed amounts of the different nutrients. The enteral intake of the different nutrients can only be regulated by changing the application time. Today, 24-hour continuous jejunal feeding is most often used.

33.5 PRACTICAL APPROACH FOR NUTRITIONAL SUPPORT IN ACUTE PANCREATITIS

If nutritional support is indicated, early enteral nutrition by a jejunal tube is recommended as a first step. When side effects occur or the caloric goal cannot be reached, enteral nutrition should be combined with parenteral nutrition. Substantial experimental evidence exists that enteral feeding in severe acute pancreatitis can down-regulate the systemic inflammatory response and promote beneficial effects on GI functions. The impaired gut motility may facilitate the colonization of the intestine with pathogenic bacteria and may contribute to bacterial translocation of the intestinal wall, with subsequent superinfection of the pancreatic necrosis. For this reason, a low volume of an enteral solution continuously perfused to the jejunum is also recommended if TPN must be given in situations in which full enteral nutrition is not possible (e.g., prolonged paralytic ileus).

33.5.1 MILD TO MODERATE ACUTE PANCREATITIS

There is no evidence that aggressive nutritional support (enteral or parenteral) has a beneficial effect on clinical outcome in patients with mild to moderate acute pancreatitis. Early enteral nutrition support can be of importance in patients with preexisting severe malnutrition or in patients for whom early refeeding is delayed. Unfortunately, there are no clinical data available to support this.

The European guidelines recommend the following three steps of nutritional treatment in these patients (64). The initial management involves (2 to 5 days) fasting, analgesics, and IV fluid and electrolyte replacement. If pain is controlled and enzymes are regredient, a diet rich in carbohydrates and moderate in protein and in fat can be started. Normally, this patient can be discharged to home after 4 to 7 days, with a normal diet (Figure 33.1).

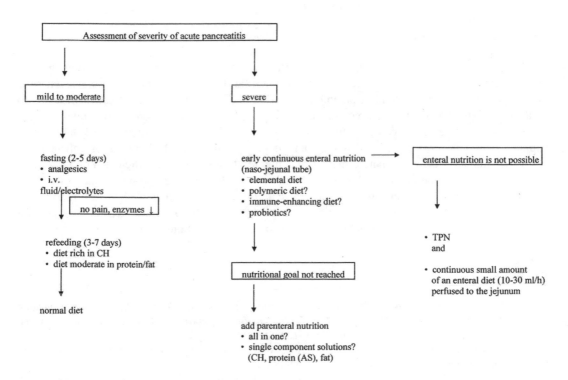

FIGURE 33.1 Nutritional support in acute pancreatitis.

33.5.2 Severe Pancreatitis

In patients with severe pancreatitis, who have complications or need surgery, early nutritional support (enteral or parenteral) is necessary to prevent the adverse effect of nutrient deprivation. Nutrient delivery (enteral or parenteral) should be determined by patient's tolerance.

The European guidelines recommend to start early, continuous enteral feeding by a jejunal tube as soon as clinical signs predict severe pancreatitis (64). Most often, an elemental diet is used, but standard enteral or immune-enhancing formulations are also given. At present, the optimal nutrient formulation is still unclear, due to the lack of controlled clinical trials.

Recently, two studies have been published with specific enteral formulations. Hallay et al., in a small study, reported a beneficial effect of a glutamine-rich, multifiber diet compared to a standard fiber diet on the recovery of IgG, IgM proteins, and on a shorter duration of the disease (51). A second study examined the efficacy of the enteral administration of the probiotic *Lactobacillus plantarum* in patients with severe acute pancreatitis (65). Twenty-two patients received live bacteria with oat fiber, and 23 patients received the same formulation with heat-killed bacteria. In the group with live bacteria, only one patient developed a septic pancreatic complication requiring surgery, compared to the control group with 7 patients ($p < 0.023$). These observations are exciting, but for the time being it is not possible to recommend this approach as a routine procedure. Larger trials are required to confirm these results.

If the enteral approach is insufficient, parenteral nutrition should be added. Usually, the combined nutritional support allows the patient to reach the nutritional goals.

In cases where TPN is given as first line, a continuously perfused small amount of an enteral diet (10 to 30 ml/h) perfused to the jejunum should be tried in parallel. The administration of fat in parenteral nutrition can be regarded as safe, if hypertriglyceridemia (< 12 mmol/l) is avoided (Figure 33.1).

33.6 CONCLUSION

Seventy-five to 80% of patients with acute pancreatitis have a mild to moderate disease and do not need specific nutritional support. Early oral refeeding can be started within a few days. There is no evidence that specific enteral or parenteral nutrition is of benefit in these patients. There are no data available to give a nutritional recommendation in patients with severe preexisting malnutrition.

Patients with severe disease, complications, or the need for surgery require early nutritional support. In patients with severe pancreatitis, an enteral jejunal approach should be established, but parenteral nutrition is an alternative method when enteral nutrition is insufficient. For the future, several factors must be clarified: the timing of nutritional therapy, the optimal feeding site (oral, gastric, jejunal, or TPN), and the optimal nutrient formulation (elemental diet, polymeric diet, immune-enhancing diet, or pre- and probiotics). Furthermore, in future studies a clear stratification of the patients according to their nutritional status on admission should be performed.

REFERENCES

1. Bradley EL and members of the Atlanta International Symposium. A clinically based classification system for acute pancreatitis: summary of the International Symposium on Acute Pancreatitis, Atlanta, GA, Sept. 11–13, 1992. *Arch. Surg.* 1993; 128: 586–590.
2. Winslet MC, Hall C, London NJM, Neoptolemos JP. Relationship of diagnostic serum amylase to aetiology and prognosis in acute pancreatitis. *Gut* 1992; 33: 982–986.
3. Bradley EL. Indications for surgery in necrotizing pancreatitis: a millennium review. *J. Pancreas* 2000; 1: 1–3.
4. Ashley SW, Perez A, Pierce EA, Brooks DC, Moore FD Jr., Whang EE, Banks PA, Zinner MJ. Necrotizing pancreatitis. *Ann. Surg.* 2001; 234: 572–580.

5. Buchler MW, Gloor B, Muller CA, Friess H, Seiler CA, Uhl W. Acute necrotizing pancreatitis: treatment strategy according to the status of infection. *Ann. Surg.* 2000; 232: 619–626.
6. Slavin J, Ghaneh P, Sutton R, Hartley M, Rowlands P, Garvey C, Hughes M, Neoptolemos J. Management of necrotizing pancreatitis. *World J. Gastroenterol.* 2001; 7: 476–481.
7. Robin AP, Campbell R, Palani CK, Liu K, Donahue PE, Nyhus LM. Total parenteral nutrition during acute pancreatitis: clinical experience with 156 patients. *World J. Surg.* 1990; 14: 572–579.
8. Shaw JH, Wolfe RR. Glucose, fatty acid, and urea kinetics in patients with severe pancreatitis: the response to substrate infusion and total parenteral nutrition. *Ann. Surg.* 1986; 204: 665–672.
9. Dickerson RN, Vehe KL, Mullen JL, Feurer ID. Resting energy expenditure in patients with pancreatitis. *Crit. Care Med.* 1991; 19: 484–490.
10. Sitzmann JV, Steinborn PA, Zinner MJ, Cameron JL. Total parenteral nutrition and alternate energy substrates in treatment of severe acute pancreatitis. *Surg. Gynecol. Obstet.* 1989; 168: 311–317.
11. Klein S, Kinney J, Jeejeebhoy K, Alpers D, Hellerstein M, Murray M, et al. Nutrition support in clinical practice: review of published data and recommendations for future research directions. National Institutes of Health, American Society for Parenteral and Enteral Nutrition, and American Society for Clinical Nutrition. *J. Parenter. Enteral Nutr.* 1997; 21: 133–156.
12. Alpers DH. Digestion and absorption of carbohydrates and protein. In: Johnson LR et al. (eds), *Physiology of the Gastrointestinal Tract* (2nd edition). Raven Press, New York, 1987, 1469–1487.
13. Niederau C, Sonnenberg A, Erckenbrecht J. Effects of intravenous infusion of amino acids, fat, or glucose on unstimulated pancreatic secretion in healthy humans. *Dig. Dis. Sci.* 1985; 30: 445–455.
14. Klein E, Shnebaum S, Ben-Ari G, Dreiling DA. Effects of total parenteral nutrition on exocrine pancreatic secretion. *Am. J. Gastroenterol.* 1983; 78: 31–33.
15. Lam WF, Masclee AA, de Boer SY, Souverijn JH, Larners CB. Effect of acute hyperglycemia on basal and cholecystokinin-stimulated exocrine pancreatic secretion in humans. *Life Sci.* 1997, 60: 2183–2190.
16. Silberman H, Dixon NP, Eisenberg D. The safety and efficacy of a lipid-based system of parenteral nutrition in acute pancreatitis. *Am. J. Gastroenterol.* 1982; 77: 494–497.
17. Variyam EP, Fuller RK, Brown FM, Quallich LG. Effect of parenteral amino acids on human pancreatic exocrine secretion. *Dig. Dis. Sci.* 1985; 30: 541–546.
18. Stabile BE, Debas HT. Intravenous versus intraduodenal amino acids, fats, and glucose as stimulants of pancreatic secretion. *Surg. Forum* 1981; 32: 224–226.
19. McArdle AH, Echave W, Brown RA, et al. Effect of elemental diet on pancreatic secretion. *Am. J. Surg.* 1974; 128: 690–694.
20. Guan D, Hideki O, Green GM. Rat pancreatic secretory response to intraduodenal infusion of elemental vs polymeric defined-formula diet. *J. Parenter. Enteral Nutr.* 1994; 18: 335–339.
21. Cassim MM, Allardyce DB. Pancreatic secretion in response to jejunal feeding of elemental diet. *Ann. Surg.* 1974; 180: 228–231.
22. Grant JP, Davey-McCrae J, Snyder PJ. Effect of enteral nutrition on human pancreatic secretions. *J. Parenter. Enteral Nutr.* 1987; 11: 302–304.
23. Vidon N, Hecketsweiler P, Butel J, et al. Effect of continuous jejunal perfusion of elemental and complex nutritional solutions on pancreatic enzyme secretion in human subjects. *Gut* 1978; 19: 194–198.
24. Ragins H, Levenson SM, Signer R, Stamford W, Seifter E. Intrajejunal administration of an elemental diet at neutral pH avoids pancreatic stimulation: studies in dog and man. *Am. J. Surg.* 1973; 126: 606–614.
25. Greenberger NJ. Pancreatitis and hyperlipidemia. *N. Engl. J. Med.* 1973; 289: 586–587.
26. Cameron JL, Capuzzi DM, Zuidema GD, Margolis S. Acute pancreatitis with hyperlipidemia: evidence for a persistent defect in lipid metabolism. *Am. J. Med.* 1974; 56: 482–487.
27. Farmer RG, Winkleman EL, Brown HB, Lewis LA. Hyperlipoproteinemia and pancreatitis. *Am. J. Med.* 1973; 54: 161–165.
28. Burns GP, Stein TA. Pancreatic enzyme secretion during intravenous fat infusion. *J. Parenter. Enteral Nutr.* 1987; 11: 60–62.
29. Fried GM, Ogden WD, Rhea A, Greeley G, Thompson JC. Pancreatic protein secretion and gastrointestinal hormone release in response to parenteral amino acids and lipid in dogs. *Surgery* 1982; 92: 902–905.

30. Konturek SJ, Tasler J, Cieszkowski M, et al. Intravenous amino acids and fat stimulate pancreatic secretion. *Am. J. Physiol.* 1979; 233: E678–E684.
31. Stabile BE, Borzatta M, Stubbs RS, Debas HT. Intravenous mixed amino acids and fats do not stimulate exocrine pancreatic secretion. *J. Physiol.* 1984; 246: G274–G280.
32. Edelmann K, Valenzuela JE. Effect of intravenous lipid on human pancreatic secretion. *Gastroenterology* 1983; 85: 1063–1068.
33. Buckspan R, Woltering E, Waterhouse G. Pancreatitis induced by intravenous infusion of a fat emulsion in an alcoholic patient. *South. Med. J.* 1984; 77: 251–252.
34. Lashner BA, Kirsner JB, Hanauer SB. Acute pancreatitis associated with high-concentration lipid emulsion during total parenteral nutrition therapy for Crohn's disease. *Gastroenterology* 1986; 90: 1039–1041.
35. Noseworthy J, Colodny AH, Eraklis AJ. Pancreatitis and intravenous fat: an association in patients with inflammatory bowel disease. *J. Pediatr. Surg.* 1983; 18: 269–272.
36. Blamey SL, Imrie CW, O'Neill J, Gilmour WH, Carter DC. Prognostic factors in acute pancreatitis. *Gut* 1984; 25: 1340–1346.
37. Knaus WA, Draper EA, Wagner DP, Zimmermann JE. APACHE II: a severity of disease classification system. *Crit. Care Med.* 1985; 13: 819–829.
38. Ranson JH, Rifkind KM, Roses DF, Fink SD, Eng K, Spencer FC. Prognostic signs and the role of operative management in acute pancreatitis. *Surg. Gynecol. Obstet.* 1974; 139: 69–81.
39. Balthazar EJ, Robinson DL, Megibow AJ, Ranson JH. Acute pancreatitis: value of CT in establishing prognosis. *Radiology* 1990; 174: 331–336.
40. Wilson C, Heads A, Shenkin A, Imrie CW. C-reactive protein, antiproteases and complement factors as objective markers of severity in acute pancreatitis. *Br. J. Surg.* 1989; 76: 177–181.
41. Neoptolemos JP, Kemppainen EA, Meyer JM, et al. Early prediction of severity in acute pancreatitis by urinary trypsinogen activation peptide: a multicentre study. *Lancet* 2000; 355: 1955–1960.
42. Levy P, Heresbach D, Pariente EA, Boruchowicz A, Delcenserie R, Millat B, et al. Frequency and risk factors of recurrent pain during refeeding in patients with acute pancreatitis: a multivariate multicentre prospective study of 116 patients. *Gut* 1997; 40: 262–266.
43. McClave SA, Greene LM, Snider HL, Makk LJ, Cheadle WG, Owens NA, et al. Comparison of the safety of early enteral vs parenteral nutrition in mild acute pancreatitis. *J. Parenter. Enteral Nutr.* 1997; 21: 14–20.
44. Sax HC, Warner BW, Talamini MA. Early total parenteral nutrition in acute pancreatitis: lack of beneficial effects. *Am. J. Surg.* 1987; 153: 117–124.
45. Nordenstrom J, Thorne A. Benefits and complications of parenteral nutritional support. *Eur. J. Clin. Nutr.* 1994; 48: 531–537.
46. Van den Berghe G, Wouters P, Weekers F, et al. Intensive insulin therapy in critically ill patients. *N. Engl. J. Med.* 2001; 345: 1359–1367.
47. Trice S, Melnik G, Page CP. Complications and costs of early postoperative parenteral versus enteral nutrition in trauma patients. *Nutr. Clin. Pract.* 1997; 12: 114–119.
48. Heyland DK, Novak F, Drover JW, Jain M, Su X, Suchner U. Should immunonutrition become routine in critically ill patients? A systematic review of the evidence. *JAMA* 2001; 286: 944–953.
49. Buchman AL, Moukarzel AA, Bhuta S, et al. Parenteral nutrition is associated with intestinal morphologic and functional changes in humans. *J. Parenter. Enteral Nutr.* 1995; 19: 453–460.
50. Lange JF, van Gool J, Tytgat GN. The protective effect of a reduction in intestinal flora on mortality of acute haemorrhagic pancreatitis in the rat. *Hepatogastroenterology* 1987; 34: 28–30.
51. Hallay J, Kovács G, Szatmári K, Bakó, Szentkereszty ZS, Lakos G, Sipka S, Sápy P. Early jejunal nutrition and changes in the immunological parameters of patients with acute pancreatitis. *Hepato-Gastroenterology* 2001; 48: 1488–1492.
52. Kotani J, Usami M, Nomura H, Iso A, Kasahara H, Kuroda Y, Oyanagi H, Saitoh Y. Enteral nutrition prevents bacterial translocation but does not improve survival during acute pancreatitis. *Arch. Surg.* 1999; 134: 287–292.
53. MacFie J. Enteral versus parenteral nutrition: the significance of bacterial translocation and gut-barrier function. *Nutrition* 2000; 16: 606–611.

54. Windsor AC, Kanwar S, Li AG, Barnes E, Guthrie JA, Spark JI, et al. Compared with parenteral nutrition, enteral feeding attenuates the acute phase response and improves disease severity in acute pancreatitis. *Gut* 1998; 42: 431–435.

55. Kalfarentzos F, Kehagias J, Mead N, Kokkinis K, Gogos CA. Enteral nutrition is superior to parenteral nutrition in severe acute pancreatitis: results of a randomized prospective trial. *Br. J. Surg.* 1997; 84: 1665–1669.

56. Powell JJ, Murchison JT, Fearon KCH, Ross JA, Siriwardena AK. Randomized controlled trial of the effect of early enteral nutrition on markers of the inflammatory response in predicted severe acute pancreatitis. *Br. J. Surg.* 2000; 87: 1375–1381.

57. Abou-Assi S, Craig K, O'Keefe SJD. Hypocaloric jejunal feeding is better than total parenteral nutrition in acute pancreatitis: results of a randomized comparative study. *Am. J. Gastroenterol.* 2002; 97: 2255–2262.

58. Cravo M, Camilo ME, Marques A, Pinto Correia J. Early tube feeding in acute pancreatitis: a prospective study. *Clin. Nutr.* 1989; Suppl. 8: 14(A).

59. Kudsk KA, Campbell SM, O'Brien T, Fuller R. Postoperative jejunal feedings following complicated pancreatitis. *Nutr. Clin. Pract.* 1990; 5: 14–17.

60. Nakad A, Piessevaux H, Marot JC, Hoang P, Geubel A, Van Steenbergen W, Reynaert M. Is early enteral nutrition in acute pancreatitis dangerous? About 20 patients fed by an endoscopically placed nasogastrojejunal tube. *Pancreas* 1998; 17: 187–193.

61. Scolapio JS, Malhi-Chowla N, Ukleja A. Nutrition supplementation in patients with acute and chronic pancreatitis. *Gastroentrol. Clin. North Am.* 1999; 28: 695–707.

62. Eatock FC, Brombacher GD, Steven A, Imrie CW, McKay CJ, Carter R. Nasogastric feeding in severe acute pancreatitis may be practical and safe. *Int. J. Pancreatol.* 2000; 28: 23–29.

63. Bouffard YH, Delafosse BX, Annat GJ, Viale JP, Bertrand OM, Motin JP. Energy expenditure during severe acute pancreatitis. *J. Parenter. Enteral Nutr.* 1989; 13: 26–29.

64. Meier R, Beglinger C, Layer P, Gullo L, Keim V, Laugier R, Friess H, Schweitzer M, MacFie J. ESPEN guidelines on nutrition in acute pancreatitis. *Clin. Nutr.* 2002; 21: 173–183.

65. Olah A, Belagyi T, Issekutz A, et al. Randomized clinical trial of specific lactobacillus and fibre supplement to early enteral nutrition in patients with acute pancreatitis. *Br. J. Surg.* 2002; 89: 1103–1107.

34 Nutritional Support of the General Surgical ICU Patient

Kenneth A. Kudsk
University of Wisconsin — Madison

CONTENTS

34.1 INTRODUCTION

Planning for nutritional support of the critically ill patient begins during the initial interaction between physician and patient. Although many ICU patients present in a hypermetabolic state due to critical illness where prolonged recovery is expected, there is a definite group of patients whose critical illness results from complications of surgical therapy. In this group, early identification of the high-risk patient may lead to preemptive preoperative nutritional support, where specific intra-operative procedures (such as GI tract cannulation) can reduce postoperative complications and preclude long ICU stays. Thus, treatment of critical illness *and* prevention of critical illness are appropriate parts of an aggressive nutrition approach.

Well nourished patients or patients with mild malnutrition with oral intake delayed for only 4 to 5 days following surgery require no specialized nutritional support. Malnourished patients with severely compromised nutritional status have compromised lean tissue mass and impaired ability to heal at the onset. When critical illness develops in patients with marginal nutritional status, retention of sodium water, further loss of lean body mass due to immobilization and hypermetabolism, and the development of organ or multiple organ dysfunction increases susceptibility to infectious complications and healing problems. These factors increase ICU and hospital stay, as well as mortality.

34.2 PRE-EXISTING NUTRITIONAL STATE: OPPORTUNITY FOR PREVENTIVE NUTRITIONAL THERAPY

Every surgical procedure carries some risk of postoperative complications. This risk correlates with the magnitude and complexity of individual procedures.[1] In elective general surgery, particularly high-risk operations include esophagectomy, gastrectomy, operations upon the pancreas and duodenum, and major hepatobiliary procedures. Major colorectal procedures, especially abdomino-perineal resections, have a higher complication rate than simple colectomies. Clinical evidence demonstrates that preoperative nutrition in patients with significant preexisting nutrition deficits reduces the risk of complications and directly impacts critical care.[2,3] The VA Cooperative Study clearly showed that intravenous nutritional support increases complications in well nourished or mildly malnourished patients, a population probably not at risk of nutrition-related complications.[2] However, the intervention significantly improves healing (reduced wound dehiscence, anastomotic failures, etc.) and exerts a beneficial effect on infectious complications when used preoperatively for 7 to 14 days in severely malnourished patients. In another VA study of surgical risk, serum albumin was the single best predictor of complication risk in patients undergoing surgical procedures.[4] This risk is related to the type of surgical procedure, because there is a linear increase in complications in patients undergoing elective GI surgery as preoperative albumin decreases from normal level to levels below 2.0 g/dl.[1] Patients undergoing esophagectomy appear at risk if albumin drops below 3.75 g/dl. Complications increase in patients undergoing gastrectomy or pancreatic surgery when preoperative albumin levels drop below 3.25 g/dl. Patients undergoing elective colectomy have little increased risk unless preoperative albumin levels drop below 2.5 g/dl. Therefore, albumin can be used as a simple marker for preoperative nutritional status in nonhypermetabolic general surgical patients.

Simple clues of preexisting malnutrition can also be obtained through detailed nutritional history. Involuntary weight loss of 20% over 2 to 6 months or 10% over 1 month closely associates with increased postoperative complications. Thus, calculation of the percent of body weight loss or the percent of usual body weight can guide the clinician in assessing nutritional risk. Other clues include symptomatic Crohn's disease with progressive weight loss, a history of alcoholism or drug abuse, or chronic malabsorption symptoms. With these warnings and evidence of a deteriorating nutritional state, 7 to 10 days of preoperative enteral or parenteral feeding can reduce critical illness by avoiding complications. In addition, the history can guide the clinicians to gain access to the gastrointestinal tract to allow direct small bowel feeding in the postoperative period. Most intestinal surgery results in gastroparesis or an atonic colon but leaves the small intestine capable of absorbing nutrients. Placement of a tube into the jejunum permits the opportunity to feed enterally and precludes the need for intravenous nutrition and its attendant complications. There is significant evidence that enteral delivery of nutrients significantly reduces infectious complications that would develop in unfed or parenterally fed patients.[5,6] Whether or not enteral access is obtained, nutritional support should be instituted in the early postoperative phase of patients at high risk of complications to obviate progressive starvation-induced malnutrition, rather than waiting until complications develop.

34.3 RESPONSE TO STRESS AND INJURY IN CRITICAL ILLNESS

The hypermetabolism in critical illness is related to increased levels of the counterregulatory hormones epinephrine, norepinephrine, and cortisol, which blunt pancreatic secretion of insulin release, reduce tissue responsiveness to insulin, and accelerate proteolysis, gluconeogenesis, and the acute-phase protein response.[7] IL-6 stimulates hepatic production of acute-phase proteins, such as C-reactive protein and alpha1-acid glycoprotein, and inhibits production of constitutive proteins, such as albumin and prealbumin (transythyretin).[8] As a result, albumin is not a marker of nutritional status. Under these conditions, measurements of C-reactive protein and prealbumin probably best reflect resolution of the inflammatory state (decreasing CRP levels) and response to nutritional therapy (increasing serum prealbumin).

This metabolic response also inhibits starvation adaptation and ketone body production; as a result, gluconeogenesis is the primary energy source. Because glucose stores are depleted within 18 hours of fasting, glucose production becomes dependent on proteolysis as a carbon source, which accelerates lean tissue deterioration. Although specialized nutrition support can provide metabolic substrate, the important issue is to control the metabolic response through debridement of necrotic tissue, drainage of abscesses, prevention or treatment of infection, and use of other medical and surgical therapies to control factors that otherwise continue to drive the hypermetabolism. Control of this response is a paramount consideration in the overall nutritional support of critically ill patients.

Other predictive tools have been studied and determine nutritional rush in surgical patients preoperatively. These include the Prognostic Nutritional Index, which correlates with risk in the equation:[9]

$$PNI\ (\%) = 158 - 16.6\ (ALB) - 0.78\ (TSF) - 0.20\ (TFN) - 5.8\ (DH)$$

In this equation, PNI is the risk of complication, ALB is serum albumin in g/dl, TSF is triceps skin fold thickness in mm, TFN is serum transferrin in mg/dl, and DH is delayed hypersensitivity reactions to one of three recall actions. Because DH is not commonly used today, this score has been simplified by replacing with a lymphocyte score of 0 to 2, where 0 is less than 1000 total lymphocytes per mm^3, 1 is 1000 to 2000 total lymphocytes per mm^3, and 2 is more than 2000 lymphocytes per mm^3. The higher the PNI, the greater the risk of complications. In this equation, albumin is the primary factor in the equation. Finally, subjectively global assessment evaluates organ status by determining changes in organ function, body composition, and the restriction of nutrient intake in the disease process.[10] There appears to be close inter observer agreement using this technique.

Unfortunately, no gold standard exists to quantify nutritional status. Malnutrition is a continuum, and significant preexisting malnutrition is just as important in the development of complications as the operative procedure, the gravity of illness, and the degree of hypermetabolism induced by the disease process.

34.4 NUTRIENT REQUIREMENTS

34.4.1 ENERGY

The Harris–Benedict equation uses gender, height, weight, and age to determine basal energy expenditure (BEE).[11]

In males:

$$BEE = 66 + (13.8 \times weight\ in\ kg) + (5 \times height\ in\ cm) - (6.8 \times age)$$

In females:

$$BEE = 655 + (9.6 \times weight\ in\ kg) + (1.7 \times height\ in\ cm) - (4.7 \times age)$$

Although these values were previously increased by stress factors of 1.5 to 2 and activity factors, recent measurements with indirect calorimetry show that these corrections lead to overestimates of energy expenditure.[12] At most, the correct estimate is 15% greater than the BEE. Current recommendations for ICU patients are 25 (to 30) total kcal/kg/d. With this value, the formula meets the energy requirements with overfeeding in less than 20%.[13] In cases of significant fluid overload from resuscitation, estimated normal body weight should be obtained by history from the family (or patient); in obese patients, an adjusted body weight of 10 to 25% over the ideal body weight should be used in calculations.

Metabolic carts measure CO_2 production and oxygen consumption to assess more accurately the specific nutrient requirements via the Weir Equation.[14] Accurate data, however, mandate dedicated personnel with very well defined protocols, which usually are not instituted. There are also significant problems in patients with a high FIO_2 (> 0.6), air leaks from chest tubes, high levels of PEEP, or leaks at tracheostomies. Therefore, the technique is most unreliable in patients who need it most. Indirect calorimetry is not recommended for routine patient management but can be valuable in institutions with the appropriate resources to support the carts.

34.4.2 PROTEIN REQUIREMENTS

With no renal dysfunction, the recommended range of protein in stressed and critically ill patients is 1.5 (to 2) g/kg/d. These numbers are used with enteral or parenteral feeding. With this dose of protein, BUN levels remain within normal levels and rarely rise above 40 mg/dl. As stress resolves, protein requirements can be decreased toward 1 g/kg/d. Burn patients are typically administered 2 to 2.5 g/kg/d due to excessive urinary nitrogen and wound protein losses. In the critically ill patient population, administration of greater amounts of protein than recommended offer little clinically but are capable of raising the BUN to high limits and elevating the BUN-to-creatinine ratio. There is no evidence that formulas enriched with branched-chain amino acids in stress or essential amino acid formulations in acute renal failure provide additional benefits over standard amino acid or protein formulas. Some nitrogen-rich specialty enteral diets are enriched with arginine, glutamine, or both. Typically, BUN levels will climb but rarely to greater than 60 mg/dl unless renal function is compromised.

34.4.3 GLUCOSE AND FAT REQUIREMENTS

A maximum of 4 to 5 mg/kg/min (approximate 7.2 g/kg/d) of glucose can be oxidized.[15] Blood glucose should be maintained well below 200 mg/dl because there is evidence of increased infectious complications with elevated blood glucose. Recently, work promotes aggressive insulin infusion to keep blood glucose between 80 and 120 mg/dl in critically ill patients.[16] A significant reduction in mortality was noted but, interestingly enough, only in thoracic and cardiac surgery patients, with no obvious benefit in the subpopulations of patients undergoing abdominal, vascular, or other general surgical procedures. No medical ICU patients were studied. Administration of glucose should meet approximately 60 to 70% of the total nonprotein caloric requirements with the remaining met by fat.

Lipid infusion with TPN should be given to provide approximately 1 g/kg/d, with a maximum dose of 2.5 g/kg/d. In most enteral formulas, the calorie-to-nitrogen ratio and fat composition are predetermined and are well below these levels. With IV feeding, a higher percentage of fat administration may better control glucose levels in patients with diabetes or those receiving corticosteroids, but it also may induce hyperlipidemia, cholestasis, and perhaps immunosuppressive effects. If triglyceride levels climb above 300 mg/dl, lipid should be reduced or withheld. There is no evidence that IV lipid aggravates acute pancreatitis that is not hyperlipidemia induced.

34.4.4 TIMING OF NUTRITIONAL SUPPORT

Severely malnourished patients at high risk of postoperative complications may benefit from 7 to 10 days of preoperative nutrition. Such patients include those with hypoalbuminemia (unrelated to stress), involuntary weight loss > 20% over 3 to 5 months or 10% acute weight loss over 1 month. In the VA Cooperative Study, 395 malnourished patients requiring laparotomy or noncardiac thoracotomy were randomized to preoperative for 7 to 15 days or an ad lib diet.[2] Preoperative parenteral feeding significantly reduced incidence of noninfectious complications in the severely malnourished group, with no increase in infectious complications. Similar studies with enteral feeding show similar results.[17,18] There is no evidence that specialized preoperative nutrition provides benefit to well nourished or mildly malnourished patients.[19] One should proceed with surgery, obtain enteral access as indicated, and institute early postoperative enteral nutrition. For patients in whom enteral access cannot be obtained and are unlikely to resume a diet in 4 to 5 days, it seems rational to institute intravenous nutrition to prevent subsequent starvation-induced progressive malnutrition. If the patient is expected to start a diet and advance within 5 to 7 days of surgery, no parenteral nutrition is indicated. Braga and colleagues presented data showing that 5 days of preoperative feeding of well nourished patients undergoing surgery with an immune-enhancing oral supplement benefited compared to patients who received no such supplementation.[17] This suggests a pharmacologic effect of specialty nutrients in well nourished patients. In another study, the same authors documented that an immune-enhancing diet given preoperatively for 7 days and continued postoperatively led to significantly reduced complications, compared to patients administered postoperative parenteral nutrition or standard enteral feedings in the postoperative period.[18]

34.4.5 ROUTE OF NUTRITION

There is substantial evidence that enteral delivery of nutrients improves immunologic defenses and clinical outcome, compared to parenteral feeding.[5,6,20–22] As a result, enteral feeding is a preferred mode when possible. Contraindications to enteral feeding include profound abdominal distension, intestinal obstruction, potential bowel ischemia, short gut, multiple enterocutaneous fistulas, gastrointestinal hemorrhage that might require subsequent surgery, severe small bowel mucosal disease, and multiple anastomosis or stricturoplasties. Under these conditions, parenteral feedings should be instituted to avoid progressive starvation-induced malnutrition. After almost all major GI surgery, however, atony of the GI tract ileus precludes successful intragastric feeding. Fortunately, this ileus persists only in the colon and stomach. When direct small bowel access is obtained, early enteral feeding can usually be administered within 24 hours of surgery. Although it has been recommended that enteral feeding be instituted in the very early postoperative period, it is our policy to start feedings on the first postoperative day after resuscitation is complete, patients are hemodynamically stable, and there is good splanchnic perfusion. Bowel sounds are not necessary to institute feedings, but the patient should be observed for signs of intolerance, such as significant new tachycardia, onset of abdominal distention, cramping, or reflux of tube feedings into the NG tube after initiation of small bowel feeding. Tube feedings can be increased every 8 to 24 hours. Most patients are alert enough to describe abdominal cramping. If this is persistent, the rate should not be advanced; if cramping is severe, slow to a more tolerable rate.

Many patients in whom celiotomy was not performed or enteral access not obtained will still tolerate intragastric feeding after 3 to 4 days. The NG tube can be clamped and residuals checked every 4 hours. If residuals are low (less than 200 cc) feedings can be attempted at 50 ml/h and residuals measured every 4 hours. If residuals remain low at less than 200 ml, tube feedings can be advanced by 25 to 50 ml each 12 hours to goal rate. The head of the bed should be elevated 30 degrees or more, because the GE junction is the most dependent area of the stomach and feedings will pool at this area in the supine patient. If tube feedings are tolerated with the NG feeding, the tube should be removed and replaced by a small-bore tube to minimize reflux.

Gastrointestinal agents can be given if residuals remain high.[23,24] If the gastroparesis persists, access into the third or fourth portion of the duodenum and beyond the ligament of Treitz can be obtained in several ways. Success reaches 90% with blind advancement of the nasojejunal tube by experienced clinicians.[25] Radiological advancement of the tube under fluoroscopy and, in some circumstances, upper endoscopy can be used. It is usually possible to advance the tube into the distal duodenum or small intestine in most patients. Institutional resources should dictate the method used for this access.

Several methods are available to gain access for small bowel feeding at celiotomy. A small-bore tube can be advanced through the nose or mouth and guided by the surgeon beyond the ligament of Treitz. These tubes require commitment of the nursing staff to avoid dislodgement during patient movement or by agitated patients. Nasoenteric tubes also tend to flip back into the stomach. Direct small bowel tube access with a 5 or 7 Fr needle catheter jejunostomy (NCJ) or larger-bore 14, 16, or 18 Fr catheter is more reliable. Five or 7 Fr NCJ should be used when access is required for 3 to 4 weeks and not longer. Larger-bore tubes are best for patients who need long-term access such as those patients expected to go to nursing homes or have prolonged in-hospital recovery. The advantage of large-bore tubes is they can be exchanged after the tract is formed in 6 to 8 days. Once NCJs are lost, they cannot be replaced. Five Fr NCJs tolerate defined formula diets or commercially prepared fiber-containing diets but clog with immune-enhancing diets or if protein is added to commercial diets. Seven Fr NCJs tolerate either of these diets. With either a 5 or a 7 Fr catheter, medications should not be given via the NCJ, even in the elixir form, because they coagulate tube feedings, causing early tube loss.[26] NCJ obstruction within 24 to 48 hours of insertion is usually due to a kink at the fascia and can be corrected by withdrawing the catheter while flushing. The catheter immediately flows, and the tube can be withdrawn to cut off the kink and reattach the connector. A final technique for decompressing the stomach and feeding the small bowel is a transgastric jejunostomy. These tubes are advanced through a suture in the stomach and held in place by an intragastric balloon. Some tubes come with stylets or channels that allow the tube to advance through the pylorus and into the small intestine.[27] The jejunal limb for feeding is small in diameter, and the catheter should be treated similarly to a 5 Fr NCJ tube, precluding use of immune-enhancing diets, medications, and the addition of protein to enteral formulas.

Technical considerations are important in construction of a jejunostomy. An insertion site in the small bowel should have a long mesentery and adequate length beyond the ligament of Treitz to preclude tethering and dislodgement if the patient develops distension. Second, a Witzel tunnel should be created for approximately 3 to 5 cm to preclude dislodgement into the peritoneal cavity. This segment should be sutured to the anterior abdominal wall with 3 to 4 sutures just lateral to the rectus sheath to eliminate the chance of torsion or volvulus at the attachment site and minimize the opportunity for small bowel to lineate over the site. The external portion of the catheter should be short to reduce dislodgement of the catheter by patients. No communication should exist between the tube and peritoneal cavity.

34.5 CHOOSING THE ENTERAL FORMULA

The degree of hypermetabolism and severity of stress determine the type of formula. Whether intragastric or small bowel feedings are used, complex formulas with intact proteins, carbohydrates, and fat can be used without significant absorptive problems. Chemically defined diets are used primarily in patients with existing mucosal disease or significant absorptive disorders. Most formulas with calorie-to-nitrogen ratios of 100:1 to 151:1 are appropriate. Fiber-containing diets are well tolerated. An advantage is that the fiber is metabolized by bacteria to short-chain fatty acids, which serve as an energy substitute for colonocytes for water absorption.[28]

In severe stress, specific substitutes may be beneficial in supporting the metabolic and immunologic functions. Immune-enhancing diets (IEDs) contain various combinations of omega-3 fatty acids, glutamine, branched-chain amino acids, and arginine. In trauma, the formulas are effective in the most severely injured patients but are probably not necessary in less severely injured patients.[6] Patients with severe chest, intra-abdominal, musculoskeletal, or head injuries who are intubated and required significant resuscitation probably will benefit from these diets. These patients will typically have an injury severity score of greater than 18 to 20 or multiple intra-abdominal injuries involving the pancreas, duodenum, liver, or colon.[5,6,29] There is evidence that preoperative feeding in general surgical malnourished patients and continuation of these diets postoperatively reduces infectious complications following major gastrointestinal surgery. Most of the studied populations have had surgical resection for malignancies, but it is likely that the magnitude of surgery, rather than malignancy, is the important issue.

These formulas, however, should not be the routine enteral feeding product but should be limited for use in patients at greatest risk of nutrition-related complications. Recent recommendation for use of IEDs include moderate to severely malnourished patients undergoing elective esophageal, gastric, or pancreatic surgery or major hepatobiliary surgery, with the most likely benefit being observed in the more severely malnourished patients.[29] These formulas may not be as beneficial in patients undergoing colon or rectal surgery unless severe malnutrition exists. However, recent work by Braga studying patients undergoing elective surgery for colorectal carcinoma noted a reduction in infectious complications in patients receiving those diets preoperatively for 7 days.[30] Populations who *may* benefit from these specialty diets but for whom data are still lacking are those undergoing major vascular reconstruction with known pulmonary disease, those with preexisting malnutrition undergoing major head and neck surgery, patients with third-degree burns > 30%, or ventilator-dependent, nonseptic medical and surgical patients. One subpopulation of patients may be at an increased risk with these supplemented diets.[29] One study showed that elderly males septic with pneumonia had increased mortality. A second, recently published study demonstrated an increase in mortality in patients who were septic from other causes.[31] Thus, until further data clarify this issue, IEDs are not recommended in patients with established or impending sepsis.

34.6 COMPLICATIONS OF ENTERAL FEEDING

Aspiration, abdominal distension, intestinal intolerance, and diarrhea are the most common complications of enteral feeding.[32,33] These issues are discussed in detail in Chapter 19.

34.7 PARENTERAL FEEDING

If enteral feeding is not possible, the concentrated parenteral formula must be administered through a central line for dilution by the rapid blood flow. In critically ill general surgery patients, peripheral nutrition is rarely used. Generally, 1.5 to 2.5 l are administered per day, containing 1.5 g of protein and 25 kcal/kg through a dedicated central venous port. Peripheral nutrition is undesirable, because there is no evidence that formulas which fail to approximate energy needs will significantly improve outcome. In addition, the high fat content typically used impairs reticuloendothelial function. With central parenteral nutrition, the macronutrient substrates carbohydrate, protein, and fat can be combined in one container as a three-in-one formula or total nutrient admixture (TNA). Continuous infusion of lipid improves utilization and may diminish immune suppression. Addition of insulin can maintain blood glucose in stressed patients. Recent data suggest that glucose control at levels of 80 to 120 mg/dl with insulin improves clinical outcome.[16] The benefit of this restricted glucose range occurred primarily in postcardiac surgery and not in general surgical patients. In the United States, all lipid emulsions come from vegetable oils, which are rich in omega-3 fatty acids. Omega-3 fatty acids are metabolized to prostaglandins and leukotrienes of the 2 and 4 series, which are immunosuppressive and proinflammatory. Structured lipids, with medium- and long-chain glyceride combinations, are available outside the United States and may obviate this complication. Lipid in parenteral feeding should be reduced if propofol is used for sedation because of propofol's high lipid content.

Critically ill patients should receive daily multivitamins containing folic acid and vitamins B1, B6, C, and K. Vitamin K can be administered in a daily dose of 0.5 to 1 mg or a weekly dose of 5 to 10 mg. It is probably advisable to supplement TPN with thiamin (25 to 50 mg/d) in patients with a history of alcohol abuse. Standard solutions containing selenium, chromium, copper, magnesium, and zinc should also be added. Zinc (an additional 5 to 10 mg/d) should be supplemented in patients with ongoing small bowel or pancreatic fistulas. Hepatic cholestasis mandates that copper and magnesium be withheld due to impaired biliary excretion. Manganese has caused neurological damage in patients with chronic liver or cholestasis, due to deposition in the basal ganglion. In these patients, 5 mg of zinc, 60 μg of selenium, and 12 μg of chromium should be added individually.

34.7.1 COMPLICATIONS OF PARENTERAL FEEDING

Daily measurements of sodium, potassium, calcium, phosphorus, magnesium, bicarbonate, chloride, and glucose should be obtained for several days after institution of parenteral feeding. Serum glucose should be checked with fingerstick glucoses several times daily. Hyperglycemia can be treated by decreasing glucose administration or by adding insulin to the TNA solution. A separate insulin infusion may be useful in some circumstances to control glucose levels. Administration of TNA can cause dramatic intracellular shifts of potassium, phosphorus, and magnesium, particularly in patients with preexisting malnutrition or those who receive diuretics with hypolipemia. In particular, potassium levels below 3.2 meq require treatment prior to institution of TNA. A similar approach should be used for magnesium and phosphate.[34] For patients with mild hypophosphatemia (2.4 to 3 meq/dl), 0.16 mmol/kg of phosphate (as the potassium or sodium salt) should be administered. For moderate hypophosphatemia of 1.6 to 2.3 meq/dl, 0.32 mmol/kg and, for severe hypophosphatemia (less than 1.6 meq/dl), 0.64 mmol/kg of phosphate should be administered. Phosphate administered as the potassium salt contains 2 mmol for every 3 meq of potassium. The sodium salt contains 3 mmol phosphate for 4 meq of sodium. Phosphate should be administered over 4 to 6 hours for mild and moderate hypophosphatemia and over 8 to 12 hours for severe hypophosphatemia. In more aggressive situations, up to 7.5 mmol of phosphate per hour (45 mmol in a 24-hour period) have been administered safely. Dosing of the phosphate for moderate to severe hypophosphatemia should be completed prior to instituting parenteral feeding.

Hypomagnesemic patients should receive magnesium sulfate over 12 to 24 hours, because more rapid infusion results in urinary excretion.[35] For a serum magnesium of 1.6 to 1.8 meq/dl, 0.5 meq (0.05 g/kg) should be infused over 12 hours. For patients with magnesium levels less than 1.5, the infusion should be given over 24 hours. For serum magnesium of 1 to 1.5 meq/dl, 0.1 g/kg or 1.0 meq/kg is indirect, while 0.15 g/kg or 1.5 meq/kg is recommended for severe hypophosphatemia. One gram of magnesium sulfate contains 8 meq of magnesium. Actual body weight is used for calculations unless greater than 130% of ideal body weight. If greater than 130%, ideal body weight should be used for dose calculation. Patients with extremely low magnesium serum concentrations (less than 1 mg/dl) or symptomatic patients sustaining tetany or seizures should receive 1 to 2 g of magnesium sulfate over 10 minutes, followed by an infusion over 12 to 24 hours, depending upon the preceding dose. It takes 36 to 48 hours for magnesium to be distributed to all tissues, and the levels should be reassessed at that time.

Critically ill patients should receive approximately 30 mmol/d of phosphorus via parenteral feeding and 15 to 30 meq of magnesium. Electrolytes should be monitored daily for 5 to 7 days and, once stabilized, can be reduced to twice a week. Usually, however, ICU patients have electrolytes checked daily.

34.8 MONITORING

Outcome goals should be established for enteral and parenteral feeding. Although the goal is maintenance of lean body mass, complete maintenance is impossible in stressed, critically ill, immobilized patients. Nitrogen balance can be determined on a weekly basis by calculating the difference between nitrogen intake and urinary nitrogen output over a 24-hour period. It is rarely possible to obtain positive nitrogen balance in immobilized patients until disuse atrophy has occurred over the first 2 to 3 weeks. Ideally, a nitrogen balance of −2 to 0 g/d is reasonable in the critical care setting. Plasma protein concentration can be used to indicate nutrition support efficacy. Although albumin concentrates drop precipitously during critical illness due to dilution, a long half-life ($T^1/_2$ 21 d), an increase in permeability and IL-6, other proteins with shorter half-lives, such as prealbumin (transthyretin: $T^1/_2$ 2 d) and transferrin ($T^1/_2$ 7 d), can be monitored weekly. Similarly, weekly C-reactive protein (CRP) evaluation provides a measure of acute-phase protein response due to IL-6 levels. An elevated CRP with depressed prealbumin reflects the systemic response to inflammation. A low prealbumin with a low CRP is more indicative of suboptimal protein or energy administration (unless the patient is on high-dose steroids). Other, more subjective methods of assessment should be used, such as the development of granulation tissue in a healing wound or decreasing fistula output, which reflect positive response to nutrition therapy. Using a combination of clinical and objective laboratory tests, the clinician can prevent complications and optimize delivery of nutritional support in the critically ill general surgical patients.

34.9 SUMMARY

Nutrition support is an integral part of ICU care in general surgical patients. Those likely to develop complications can often be identified preoperatively through a complete history and physical and the addition of simple laboratory tests. Ideally, nutrition can be provided preoperatively to high-risk patients and enteral access obtained to allow a higher success rate with gastrointestinal feeding. When the GI tract cannot be used, parenteral feeding allows delivery of adequate macro- and micronutrients to the ICU patient.

REFERENCES

1. Kudsk, K.A., et al., Preoperative albumin and surgical site identify surgical risk for major postoperative complications, *JPEN,* 27, 1, 2003.
2. The Veterans Affairs Total Parenteral Nutrition Cooperative Study Group, Perioperative total parenteral nutrition in surgical patients, *NEJM,* 325, 525, 1991.
3. Braga, M. et al., Nutritional approach in malnourished surgical patients, *Arch. Surg.,* 137, 174, 2002.
4. Daley, J. et al., Risk adjustments of the postoperative morbidity rate for the comparative assessment of the quality of surgical care: results of the National Veterans Affairs Surgical Risk Study, *J. Am. Coll. Surg.,* 185, 328, 1997.
5. Kudsk, K.A. et al., Enteral versus parenteral feeding: effects on septic morbidity after blunt and penetrating abdominal trauma, *Ann. Surg.,* 215, 503, 1992.
6. Moore, F.A., Moore, E.E., and Jones, T.N., Benefits of immediate jejunostomy feeding after major abdominal trauma: a prospective randomized study, *J. Trauma,* 26, 874, 1986.
7. McClave, S.A. and Snider, H.L., Understanding the metabolic response to critical illness: factors that cause patients to deviate from the expected pattern of hypermetabolism, *New Horizons,* 2, 139, 1994.
8. Ohzato, H. et al., Interleukin-6 as a new indicator of inflammatory status: detection of serum levels of interleukin-6 and C-reactive protein after surgery, *Surgery,* 111, 201, 1992.
9. Buzby, G.P. et al., Prognostic nutritional index in GI surgery, *Am. J. Surg.,* 139, 160, 1980.
10. Pablo, A.M., Izaga, M.A., and Alday, L.A., Assessment of nutritional status on hospital admission: nutritional scores. *Nutrition,* 57, 824, 2003.
11. Kudsk, K.A., Sacks, G.S., and Brown, R.O., Nutritional support. In *Trauma,* 5th edition, Mattox, K.L., Feliciano, D.V., and Moore, E.E., Eds. McGraw-Hill, New York, 2004, Chapter 61.
12. Hunter, D.C. et al., Resting energy expenditure in the critically ill: estimations versus measurement, *Br. J. Surg.,* 75, 875, 1988.
13. Hwang, T.L., Hwang, S.L., and Chen, M.F., The use of indirect colorimetry in critically ill patients: relationship with measured energy expenditure to injury severity score, a septic severity score, and Apache II score, *J. Trauma,* 34, 247, 1993.
14. Campbell, S.M. and Kudsk K.A., "High tech" metabolic measurements: useful in daily clinical practice? *JPEN,* 12, 610, 1988.
15. Wolfe, R., Allsop, J., and Burke, J., Glucose metabolism in man: responses to intravenous glucose infusion, *Metabolism,* 28, 210, 1979.

16. Van den Berghe, G. et al., Intensive insulin therapy in critically ill patients, *N. Engl. J. Med.*, 345, 1359, 2001.

17. Gianotti, L. et al., A randomized controlled trial of preoperative oral supplementation with a specialized diet in patients with gastrointestinal cancer, *Gastroenterology*, 122, 1763, 2002.

18. Braga, M. et al., Preoperative oral arginine and n-3 fatty acid supplementation improves the immunometabolic host response and outcome after colorectal resection for cancer, *Surgery*, 132, 805, 2002.

19. Heslin, M.J. et al., A prospective, randomized trial of early enteral feeding after resection of upper gastrointestinal malignancy, *Ann. Surg.*, 226, 567, 1997.

20. Moore, F.A. et al., TEN vs. TPN following major abdominal trauma: reduced septic morbidity, *J. Trauma,* 29, 916, 1989.

21. Moore, F.A. et al., Early enteral feeding, compared with parenteral, reduces postoperative septic complications: the results of a meta-analysis, *Ann. Surg.*, 216, 172, 1992.

22. Kudsk, K.A., Minard, G., Croce, M.A., Brown, R.O., Lowrey, T.S., Pritchard, E., Dickerson, R.N., and Fabian, T.C., A randomized trial of isonitrogenous enteral diets following severe trauma: an immune-enhancing diet (IED) reduces septic complications, *Ann. Surg.*, 224, 531, 1996.

23. Dive, A. et al., Effect of erythromycin on gastric motility in mechanically ventilated critically ill patients: a double-blind, randomized, placebo-controlled study, *Crit. Care Med.*, 23, 1356, 1995.

24. MacLaren, R. et al., Sequential single doses of cisapride, erythromycin, and metoclopramide in critically ill patients intolerant to enteral nutrition: a randomized, placebo-controlled, crossover study, *Crit. Care Med.*, 28, 438, 2000.

25. Zaloga, G.P., Bedside method for placing small bowel feeding tubes in critically ill patients: a prospective study, *Chest,* 100, 1643, 1991.

26. Cutie, A.J., Altman, E., and Lenkel, L., Compatibility of enteral products with commonly employed drug additives, *JPEN*, 7, 186, 1983.

27. Winkler, M.J., Korunda, M.J., Garmhausen, L., and Kudsk, K.A., Jejunal cannulation via Stamm gastrostomy: an improved technique for feeding jejunostomy at laparotomy. *Surg. Rounds*, 18, 469, 1995.

28. Spapen, H. et al., Soluble fiber reduces the incidence of diarrhea in septic patients receiving total enteral nutrition: a prospective, double-blind, randomized, and controlled trial, *Clin. Nutr.*, 20, 301, 2001.

29. Proceedings from summit on immune-enhancing enteral therapy, *JPEN*, 25, S1, 2001.

30. Braga, M. et al., Preoperative oral arginine and n-3 fatty acid supplementation improves the immunometabolic host response and outcome after colorectal resection for cancer, *Surgery,* 132, 805, 2002.

31. Bertolini, G. et al., Early enteral immunonutrition in patients with severe sepsis: results of an interim analysis of a randomized multicentre clinic trial, *Intens. Care Med.*, 29, 834, 2003.

32. Jones, T.N. et al., Gastrointestinal symptoms attributed to jejunostomy feeding after major abdominal trauma: a critical analysis, *Crit. Care Med.*, 17, 1146, 1989.

33. Edes, T.E., Walk, B.E., and Austin, J.L., Diarrhea in tube-fed patients: feeding formula not necessarily the cause, *Am. J. Med.*, 88, 91, 1990.

34. Clark, C.L. et al., Treatment of hypophosphatemia in patients receiving specialized nutrition support using a graduated dosing scheme: results from a prospective trial, *Crit. Care Med.,* 23, 1504, 1995.

35. Topf, J.M. and Murray, P.T., Hypomagnesemia and hypermagnesemia, *Rev. Endocr. Metab. Disorder,* 4, 195, 2003.

Section VII

General Systemic Failures

35 Systemic Inflammatory Response and Sepsis: A Multidisciplinary Approach to the Nutritional Considerations

Mark H. Oltermann
Texas Tech Medical Center — Amarillo

CONTENTS

35.1 INTRODUCTION

The nutritional care of intensive care unit (ICU) patients who are septic can be very challenging. There is no Grade A recommendation on how best to feed them (see Table 35.1 for grading definitions) (1). There is debate as to whether they should be fed at all (2,3). The stakes are high. There are over 750,000 U.S. cases annually, with over 200,000 deaths (mortality rate of 28.6%).

TABLE 35.1
Grading System

Grading of Recommendations
   Grade A. Supported by at least two Level I studies
   Grade B. Supported by at least one Level I study
   Grade C. Supported by Level II investigations
   Grade D. Supported by Level III investigations
   Grade E. Level IV or V evidence only
Grading of Evidence
   Level I. Large, prospective, randomized trials with little risk of false positive or false negative error
   Level II. Small randomized trials with higher risks of false positives or false negatives
   Level III. Nonrandomized trials with contemporaneous controls
   Level IV. Nonrandomized trials with historical controls
   Level V. Case series or expert opinion

Source: Adapted from Sackett DL, *Chest* 1989, 95, 2S–4S.

The average cost per case is over \$22,000, with an annual national burden of over \$16 billion (4). It would make some sense that avoiding malnutrition by aggressive feeding programs would improve outcomes, but definitive literature is lacking. It is best to start with some definitions prior to reviewing pertinent literature and, hopefully, come to some solid recommendations. For the purposes of this chapter, no attempt will specifically be made to separate "medical" from "surgical" sepsis. Both need aggressive approaches to source control.

35.2 DEFINITIONS

Nutritional manipulation is defined as forced feeding of an enteral nutrition via an enteral feeding tube, parenteral nutrition, intravenously or a combination thereof. This term does not include oral supplements or special diets that are expected to be taken spontaneously by mouth. The systemic inflammatory response syndrome (SIRS) is the host's nonspecific cascade of inflammatory events that occur in response to some type of insult (infection, trauma, burns, pancreatitis, or major surgery). For literature purposes, SIRS is defined by at least two of the following manifestations:

- Temperature > 38°C or < 36°C
- Heart rate > 90 beats/min
- Respiratory rate > 20 breaths/min, or a $PaCO_2$ < 32 mmHg
- WBC count > 12,000 cells/mm^3, < 4,000 cells/mm^3, or > 10% immature forms

These criteria are nonspecific. An athlete just finishing a race would meet SIRS criteria. To be more specific, the insult should be the initiator of the manifestations. It is important to note, however, that the manifestations themselves are felt to be caused by the host response to the insult via hormones, cytokines, and inflammatory cells. *Sepsis* is defined as SIRS that is due to infection (the invasion of normally sterile tissues by microorganisms, their products, or both). *Severe sepsis* is defined as sepsis with at least one SIRS-induced organ dysfunction. *Septic shock* is severe sepsis that requires medical support of blood pressure in spite of the patient receiving "adequate" volume resuscitation. If more than one organ is dysfunctional, the term *multiple organ dysfunction syndrome* (MODS) is used; if organs are failing, the patient is said to have *multiple organ failure syndrome* (MOFS). MOFS is the leading cause of death in noncoronary ICUs today. The definition of dysfunctional organs has varied from author to author in the past (5,6,7), but can generally be summarized as in Table 35.2.

TABLE 35.2
Organ Failure Definitions

Respiratory: Acute lung injury (ALI) or adult respiratory distress syndrome (ARDS). ALI requires bilateral lung infiltrates, no evidence of heart failure, and PaO_2/FIO_2 ratio of less than 300 mm Hg. ARDS is just more severe, with a PaO_2/FIO_2 ratio of less than 250 mm Hg.

Renal: Oliguria in spite of "adequate" volume replacement, or an acute rise in serum creatinine.

Central nervous system: Altered mental status, or a Glascow coma score of < 15.

Hepatic: Jaundice, or an acute rise in liver enzymes.

Cardiovascular: Hypotension in spite of "adequate" fluids, or evidence of an acute dilated cardiomyopathy.

Gastrointestinal: Stress ulcer bleeding.

Hematologic: Low platelet count, or an increase in protime (PT), partial thromboplastin time (PTT), or an increase in D-dimer levels not explained by other diseases.

Systemic: Lactic acid levels greater than two times normal.

As noted earlier, sepsis is only one cause of SIRS (although probably the most common cause). But it is the SIRS itself that appears to cause the organ dysfunction, not the infection *per se*. What is not known is whether the SIRS produced by infection is different from the SIRS from another source. More specifically, does the nutritional manipulation of the septic patient need to be different from that of the nonseptic SIRS patient?

35.3 NONNUTRITIONAL CARE OF THE SEPTIC PATIENT

Before reviewing the nutritional literature, it is imperative to review the care of septic patients in general, as well as other literature related to the care of ICU patients. It is important to understand what the drivers of mortality are for septic patients. Many of these ICU articles have reached the journals subsequent to the controversial nutritional literature. Nutritional studies tend to have small numbers; these studies' outcomes could easily be influenced by noncompliance in areas of care that have clearly been shown to improve survival.

35.3.1 RESUSCITATION

The first steps in the management of a septic patient are the same as in all critically ill patients: airway, respiration, and organ perfusion. A recent article by Rivers et al. (8) randomized septic patients presenting to the emergency department (ED) with hypotension or lactic acidosis to either "standard" care or at least 6 hours of "goal-directed therapy." The early goal-directed therapy (EGDT) involved protocols that directed more aggressive fluids, inotropic support (dobutamine), and red blood cell transfusions during this first six hours. The ICU physicians ultimately caring for the patients after six hours were unaware of the patient assignments. Mortality was significantly reduced with EGDT from 46.5 to 30.5%. This equates to one life saved for every 7 patients treated with EGDT (number needed to treat [NNT] = 7). The best endpoints of resuscitation after the first 6 hours are issues of ongoing debate in critical care circles, and no definitive answers can be given at this time.

35.3.2 SOURCE CONTROL

Although not based on prospective randomized trials, it has been known anecdotally for many years that *in patients with severe sepsis* (at least one SIRS-induced organ dysfunction), delay in removal of an easily reversible source of infection (collection of pus, dead colon, or infected foreign body) leads to an increase in mortality (9). Every hour that there is ongoing stimulation of the inflammatory cascade increases the likelihood that the patient will progress to MODS and MOFS.

35.3.3 ANTIMICROBIALS

The data to document increases in mortality with inadequate antibiotics are not randomized but are nonetheless profound. Kollef et al. showed a fourfold increase in mortality (12.2 to 52.1%) for ICU patients receiving inadequate antibiotics (10). In ICU patients specifically noted to have bloodstream infection, Ibrahim documented that mortality increased from 28.4 to 61.9% (11). These two studies together equate to an approximate NNT of 3 and demonstrates the critical importance of proper antibiotic choices.

35.3.4 VENTILATOR MANAGEMENT

Most septic patients for whom nutritional manipulation is considered are on a ventilator. Recent data have shown that the type of ventilator strategy utilized influences mortality rates. The ARDS Network documented a lowered mortality rate from 39.8 to 31% (NNT = 11) by utilizing a lower tidal volume "lung protective strategy" in patients with ALI/ARDS (12). Although this was not specifically a sepsis study, many of the patients had sepsis as their initiating event. Nutrition studies done today that utilize mostly intubated patients would need to specify ventilator strategy utilized to ensure comparable patients in both experimental and control arms.

35.3.5 MANIPULATION OF THE COAGULATION CASCADE

During sepsis, it has been demonstrated that there is overlap between the inflammatory and coagulation cascades. In February, 2001, the results of a multicenter trial were published, showing efficacy of activated protein C (drotrecogin alfa: Xigris®) for patients with severe sepsis (13). Mortality was reduced from 30.8 to 24.7% (NNT = 16). This agent was eventually FDA approved for a sicker population of patients with an APACHE II score > 25. This subgroup showed greater efficacy, with a lowering of mortality from 43.7 to 30.9% (NNT = 8). Patients not eligible for activated protein C may still benefit from coagulation manipulation. In the retrospective analysis of the two recent large sepsis trials (activated protein C and antithrombin III), it was noted in the placebo arms that those patients who received deep venous thrombosis prophylaxis doses of subcutaneous heparinoid products, compared to those who did not, had a lowered mortality rate of 42 to 32.8% (NNT = 11) (14). These results were unrelated to pulmonary embolism. Although this is retrospective analysis of prospective data and not randomized, it remains very intriguing.

35.3.6 CORTICOSTEROIDS

Early trials of high-dose steroids in sepsis patients have been negative. However, there are new data for more physiologic doses of steroids in this patient population. Annane et al. showed improved survival in severe septic shock patients who were defined as "steroid responsive" based on a cosyntropin stimulation test (15). Mortality was reduced from 63 to 53% (NNT = 10). Marik and Zaloga suggest that a random cortisol level of < 25 μg/dl in a septic shock patient is an adequate threshold to treat (16).

35.3.7 AGGRESSIVE SERUM GLUCOSE CONTROL

Van den Berghe randomized postoperative surgical patients to an aggressive serum glucose control protocol vs. a more liberal protocol (17). Although this was not specifically a sepsis study, the greatest reduction in mortality involved deaths due to MOFS with a proven septic focus. In patients sick enough to remain in an ICU for > 5 days, mortality was reduced from 20.2 to 10.6% (NNT = 10). Interestingly, aggressive glucose control also significantly reduced acute renal failure requiring dialysis, the number of red blood cell transfusions, and critical illness polyneuropathy.

35.3.8 Multidisciplinary, Intensivist-Led ICU Team

Without even a discussion of nutrition, areas have been addressed that significantly influence mortality of the septic patient. It is logical that full-time ICU physicians familiar with the critical care literature and leading a multidisciplinary team of nurses, therapists, dietitians, and pharmacists would improve outcomes. In a review article by Young and Birkmeyer, relative reductions in mortality rates for intensivist-model ICUs ranged from 15 to 60% (18). Conservative estimates were that over 50,000 lives could be saved per year in the U.S. if intensivists were fully implemented. Although the studies were not prospectively randomized, there was enough evidence for the Leapfrog Group to make intensivists part of its hospital safety initiative (19).

35.4 GOALS OF NUTRITION

The ultimate goal of nutritional manipulation of the patient is to improve morbidity and mortality. Mortality is fairly objective, although the timing that correlates best with efficacy (ICU mortality, hospital mortality, 28-day mortality, or 6-month mortality) is still debated. Assuming that the intensivist-led team has fully addressed all of the previous issues in a timely fashion, does nutrition play a role? The absolute answer is unclear but ranges from a possible worse survival all the way to a reduction in mortality from 32.2 to 19.1% (2,20,21). Morbidity is harder to keep objective. ICU days, ventilator days, and hospital length of stay are influenced by many other issues besides patient improvement. Early mortality influences numbers of patients who do not develop morbidity complications. Nosocomial infections, especially pneumonia, lack gold-standard definitions. Other commonly cited goals of nutrition may not correlate well with improved morbidity and mortality. Weight gain may be limited to fat and water. Nitrogen balance studies are prone to error and primarily become positive when the patient can physically exercise more (restore skeletal muscle). No studies have been done that *titrated* nutrition to any of these intermediary endpoints and compared complication rates.

35.5 NUTRITIONAL MANIPULATION VS. NOTHING BY MOUTH (NPO)

Unless research subjects' rights are abandoned, it is unlikely we will ever have a truly prospective randomized placebo (daily tray brought into room) controlled nutrition trial in any ICU. Some feel it is unethical to force-feed any patient without such data. Therefore, we must extrapolate from data we do have, realizing the inherent shortcomings of that decision.

The mortality rate of severe sepsis (at least one organ dysfunction) is usually cited at 20%. If respiratory is the failing organ system, mortality increases to at least 30% (ARDS Network data). The risk of nutritional manipulation (complications of tubes, lines, and metabolic derangements) is around 5 to 10%. It would appear, then, that nutritional manipulation in these patients would have a favorable risk–benefit ratio. SIRS-induced respiratory failure patients are also likely to be NPO for > 5 days and therefore are at risk for starvation-related morbidity (nosocomial infections, delayed wound healing, pressure ulcers, and prolonged rehabilitation from massive lean body mass losses). It would seem that this subgroup of patients would benefit from nutrition.

There are two studies worth mentioning, but neither was specifically in septic patients. The first, by Rapp et al., attempted to randomize severe head injury patients to total parenteral nutrition (TPN) vs. enteral nutrition (22). This older article, published in 1983, documented improved survival in the TPN subgroup. As it turned out, the gastric-fed enteral arm took an average of 10 to 14 days to reach goal rate, so in many ways, this was a study of TPN vs. NPO. The improved survival was related to a decrease in subsequent septic complications. The other article, by Kudsk et al., randomized severe trauma patients to receive a standard enteral formula (n = 18) or a study formula (n = 17) (23). Patients who met the same entrance criteria but were not randomized because of lack of enteral access (n = 19) served as a "contemporaneous" control. Although not prospectively randomized to the control arm, they still provide insight to the natural history of this illness with little nutritional manipulation (only 2 of 19 control patients received any nutrition prior to a complication). The control patients indeed had the worse outcomes, with higher septic complications, longer hospital stays, and higher costs. Based on these two imperfect studies, it is concluded that severe SIRS patients will benefit from nutritional manipulation because of their high risk for nutrition-related complications. It is unlikely that further randomized research will be done in this area.

35.6 TIMING OF NUTRITION INTERVENTION

There are two different issues related to timing of nutrition in high-risk patients. The first is that severe hypermetabolic patients will not reach the anabolic phase of their illness for many weeks, so the sooner nutrition is started, the less lean body mass will be lost. During the hypermetabolic phase, overfeeding one day cannot make up for underfeeding previous days. Although it may not be cause and effect, most complications occur in patients who are in negative nitrogen balance (24). Second, although Cerra et al. documented that "late" enteral nutrition (started at least 3 days after start of hypermetabolism) compared to TPN did not influence the development of MOFS (25), there is enthusiasm that early enteral nutrition (started within 24 hours of ICU admission) can favorably influence the inflammatory cascade (26). However, a more recent study by Ibrahim et al. reported worse outcomes in mechanically ventilated patients fed early vs. late (after 5 days) (27).

35.7 ENTERAL VS. PARENTERAL

Chapter 12 provides greater detail into the benefits of enteral over parenteral nutrition and when to consider combination therapies. Even the most expensive enteral product is less expensive than TPN and is thought to have fewer complications. TPN does not have the opportunity to influence favorably gastrointestinal blood flow or the inflammatory cascade, as enteral nutrition may. It is easier to overfeed patients utilizing TPN. Parenteral fat solutions in the U.S. are very rich in the ω-6 fatty acids. High doses of the ω-6 fats can induce more proinflammatory cytokines. Most studies document an increase in infectious complications with TPN vs. enteral (28,29). However, a recent study of an immune enteral formula compared to TPN in septic patients appeared to show improved survival in the TPN subgroup (30). This article will be discussed in more detail later.

35.8 GASTRIC VS. POSTPYLORIC

Gastric feedings are typically given through a large-bore nasogastric tube. Postpyloric tubes are smaller and softer and reduce the incidence of regurgitation and micro aspiration (31). They are also more likely to reach goal rate in a timely fashion. Because up to 75% of patients enrolled in enteral nutrition trials do not get a "therapeutic dose" of enteral nutrition, more reliable and rapid postpyloric access should be sought. Various options exist (see Chapter 15); local protocols should be developed to ensure small bowel feedings. It is of note that the Ibrahim trial that documented worse outcomes of early vs. late enteral feeding in ventilated patients was with the use of gastric access (27). There was a higher rate of ventilator-associated pneumonia in gastric-fed patients.

35.9 NUTRIENT PROVISION

35.9.1 TOTAL ENERGY REQUIREMENTS

The optimum total caloric load for severe sepsis patients remains unstudied. General recommendations typically range from a low of 25 kcal/kg/d of ideal body weight (IBW) to as much as 35 or more kcal/kg/d of usual weight (with a correction factor for obese patients). This could be a doubling of caloric recommendations. There is growing evidence that overfeeding is harmful, leading to hyperglycemia and prolonged ventilator time. Some have even promoted "permissive underfeeding" as a strategy to improve outcomes (32). As patients progress along the SIRS/MODS/MOFS pathway, their cells are unable to take up glucose. Therefore, contrary to typical recommendations, as patients get sicker, they probably should be fed fewer total calories, not more. A goal of 25 total kcal/kg/d IBW should be adequate for most ICU patients. Higher loads should be reserved for patients not clinically responding to nutrition and objective evidence of higher metabolic needs (indirect calorimetry). "Not clinically responding" should have objective definitions, such as patients remaining in negative nitrogen balance in spite of improvement in inflammatory markers. Ideal body weight should be used because it is more representative of lean body mass.

35.9.2 MACRONUTRIENT MAKEUP

Nitrogen balance in hypermetabolic patients is more likely to respond to protein loading than it is to caloric loading. Therefore, the first decision relates to protein needs. Most recommend 1.5 gm/kg/d. When dealing with IBW, this number comes closer to 2.0 gm/kg/d. Protein calories should be subtracted from total to get nonprotein calories. The next decision is what percent of nonprotein calories should be carbohydrate vs. fat. The typical recommendation of 15 to 30% of total calories as fat (correlating to approximately 20 to 40% of nonprotein calories) appears too wide. There is a trend toward high-fat diets in diabetics (to facilitate glucose control) and in patients on ventilators (to aid in weaning). These diets are not physiologic and have not been vigorously studied to show improvements in meaningful outcomes. In fact, many believe that high-fat diets, especially those high in the ω-6 variety found in Intralipid, may be harmful and stimulate proinflammatory cytokines (33). Battistella et al. showed that trauma patients given TPN that included IV fat (25% of total calories) had higher infection rates and longer lengths of stay than those given no lipids for the first ten days (34). From the ventilator standpoint, there is no advantage to altering fat–carbohydrate ratios, as long as the patient is not overfed (35). In the Battistella article, the lipid patients actually had longer ventilator times. The data for enteral products that may have a mixture of fat types (ω-6, ω-3, medium-chain triglycerides, fish oils) are more complex and need more study. Therefore, for TPN patients, consider withholding IV fats completely for the first 10 days (in well nourished patients) or giving low doses (5 to 10% of nonprotein calories). Remember that IV propofol has become a very common sedative in ICUs today. The carrier solution is a 10% lipid solution, a rich source of ω-6 fat. These calories need to be taken into account from the dietary standpoint. Propofol's prolonged use (> 48 h) in high doses (> 20 ml/h) should be discouraged in SIRS patients.

35.9.3 SPECIFIC ENTERAL FORMULAS

One of the greatest controversies today in critical care nutrition involves the area of specialty immune enteral formulas, particularly in the septic patient. Based on bench and animal research, many commercial companies have formulated products with a variety of additives purported to help the SIRS/MODS/MOFS patient. Most of the additives have not been studied individually in ICU patients; therefore, one criticism is that there is no way to determine whether these are synergistic or antagonistic in final formulation. These are the immune-enhancing or immune-modulating formulas. They usually contain one or more of the following: arginine, ω-3 fatty acids, ribonucleic acids, and glutamine. Many articles show improvement in morbidity but only in patient subsets. Only one article has shown improvement in survival but has been criticized for "less rigorous" methodologies (21). Two of the largest studies have high "drop-out" rates based on the inability to get an adequate dose of formula (36,37). It is unprecedented to have 75% of patients enrolled in a trial not receive therapeutic amounts of "drug." How reliable is an intent-to-treat analysis in this scenario? Does a meta-analysis make it more accurate?

The meta-analysis by Heyland et al. of 2001 reviews the published and some unpublished data to that point (20). This was a strict intent-to-treat analysis and was the first to raise the question of whether immunonutrition may actually be harmful in certain subsets of ICU patients. As this argument has been debated since 2001, it seems to have capsulated to the septic patient who is at highest risk for harm, with the arginine content of the formula deemed the culprit. Septic patients are often the most inflamed, and giving an immune stimulant could be harmful. It is possible that the SIRS of sepsis is different from nonsepsis SIRS (trauma, major surgery). The immune literature is much stronger in acute trauma and elective major surgery. This is an enticing theory, although it remains just that: a theory.

The trend for the increase in mortality in the Heyland meta-analysis in critically ill patients (not just sepsis) is driven by three articles, and one is unpublished at the time of the writing of this text (Ross product). In the Ross study, presented at the Society of Critical Care Medicine Congress in 2003, there were significantly more deaths reported in the experimental formula (20/87, 23%) than with the control formula (8/83, 9.6%, p = 0.03). The excess deaths were mostly found in septic patients (pneumonia at baseline). Ten of 26 pneumonia patients receiving the experimental formula died (38.5%), whereas no pneumonia patients died in the control group (0/9, 0%). This appears very dramatic but is hard to discuss without published data as to whether severity of illness was the same and whether other "drivers" of mortality were equally applied. In addition, the arginine content of the Ross product (5 g/1000 kcal) is much lower than other immune formulas (about 12 g/1000 kcal).

In the trial by Bower et al., there were more deaths in the experimental formula group (24/153, 15.7%) than in the control (12/143, 8.4%) (36). This is nearly statistically significant, with a p value of 0.055, which went unreported in the original study. The mortality was mostly seen in the septic subgroup. Eleven of 44 septic patients receiving experimental formula died (25%), whereas only 4 of 45 (8.9%) control formula patients died. Again, this seems fairly dramatic. However, most of this difference is driven by the septic patients who were "unsuccessfully fed." It is difficult to imagine how supplemental arginine is contributing to mortality when the difference is primarily seen in those that do not get much formula. In fact, all of the mortality difference in the Bower study is being driven by the "unsuccessfully fed" subgroup (see Table 35.3).

In the Atkinson study, the third article to contribute significantly to the mortality data of the Heyland meta-analysis, there was a much higher overall mortality rate (46%) than was predicted based on APACHE II scores, and slightly higher in the experimental formula group (48% experimental, 44% control, not significant) (37). Approximately 20% of the patients in the study were septic, but the study design did not allow endpoint separation based on sepsis or SIRS. The

TABLE 35.3
Mortality Rates

Feeding Subgroup	Experimental Mortality	Control Mortality
79 unsuccessfully fed	13/47 27.7%	3/32 9.4%
200 successfully fed	10/100 10%	7/100 7%
20 unsuccessfully fed septic patients	5/15 33%	0/5 0%

remarkable aspect of this study was that over 50% of the patients enrolled were either unstable transfers from the wards or emergency transfers from other hospitals. In light of the fact that timely resuscitation (EGDT) has one of the most profound influences on mortality, it is hard to determine whether nutrition is actually being studied as an independent variable in mortality determination.

There are three other articles worth mentioning at this time on the debate of feeding the septic patient. The first is by Galban et al. and was included in the Heyland meta-analysis (21). However, this study did not carry as much weight because it was not felt to be as "rigorous." The trial only looked at ICU mortality and was not blinded. It also dropped some randomized patients and did not have a strict definition of sepsis. Nevertheless, the mortality rate was significantly lower (p = 0.05) in the experimental formula (17/89, 19.1%) than in the control formula (28/87, 32.2%). And, most pertinent to this discussion, it was a study specifically done in septic patients (pneumonia being the most common source) and utilized a formula high in arginine (12.5 g/1000 kcal free arginine). One other criticism of this article was that the improvement in survival was "only significant" in the least sick patients (APACHE II scores of 10 to 15) (38). In reality, there was improved survival in those with scores > 15, but did not reach statistical significance because of smaller numbers of patients.

The second article is by Gadek et al. and was not included in the Heyland meta-analysis (39). It specifically looked at ARDS patients, approximately half originating from sepsis. The experimental diet in this study is different from that utilized in the Bower, Atkinson, and Galban studies. It is a high-lipid formula (55.2% of total calories) but contains a wide variety of oils (not just the ω-6 variety), including ω-3 fatty acids. It also does not contain added arginine. Favorable outcomes that reached statistical significance included days of ventilatory support, ICU length of stay, and a decrease in the number of new organs failing. There was only a trend toward lower mortality. The only concern with this article is that the control formula also contains 55.2% of total calories as lipid, but essentially all of the ω-6 variety. Are the patients doing better only because of *worse* outcomes in the control formula?

The third article, recently published by Bertolini et al., randomized ICU patients to an immune enteral formula or TPN (30). Because of the concern in septic patients brought out by the Heyland meta-analysis, the septic subgroup was looked at separately, associated with the planned interim analysis after a total of 237 patients were enrolled. The authors did indeed find a significant increase in mortality in the septic patients given the enteral formula vs. TPN. However, there were only 39 septic patients of the total enrolled, and the experimental formula (different from that used by Bower et al.) was actually low in added arginine (5 g/1000 kcal) and high in ω-6 fatty acids. In addition, similar to the Atkinson study, over 50% of the septic patients came to the ICU from a hospital ward, making the standardization of aggressive resuscitation unclear.

How then do we summarize the immunonutrition literature? Recommendations vary, from a moratorium for septic patients because the formulas only shorten lengths of stay by increasing mortality (Heyland meta-analysis), all the way to improving survival by an absolute amount of 13.1% (Galban article). This correlates to one life saved for every 8 patients treated with an immune enteral formula. Current theory suggests that if the immune products do worsen survival, the high arginine content may be the culprit by causing an increase in nitric oxide production, to the patient's detriment. Nitric oxide may cause inappropriate vasodilatation. Concerns with the arginine hypothesis are as follows:

- The Heyland meta-analysis admits that "we found a higher (trend in) mortality in patients receiving immunonutrition in the subgroup of studies using formulas *other than those of high arginine content*" (20).
- There is some arginine present in all whole-protein formulas. Why is mortality higher in those patients only getting small doses of experimental formula (the "unsuccessfully fed" subgroup of the Bower trial), if it is due to high arginine content?

- A recent article by Argaman in septic pediatric patients (6 to 16 years old) reports an increase in arginine oxidation to both nitric oxide and urea, leading to negative arginine balance, suggesting that arginine is "conditionally essential" during sepsis (40).
- Recent experimental data suggest that the production of nitric oxide during sepsis may limit inappropriate vasoconstriction, inhibit leukocyte adhesion, and inhibit activation of nuclear transcription factor kappa B (NF-κB), which increases cytokine production (41). All of these would be favorable in severe sepsis.
- The phase III placebo controlled trial of a nitric oxide synthase inhibitor in septic patients was actually stopped early because of an increase in mortality in those patients receiving the experimental drug (42).

35.10 CONCLUSION

What recommendations can be made at this time for the nutritional management of the SIRS patient, with severe sepsis representing the most lethal form? Assuming nutritional manipulation does play a positive role in the survival of these patients, it can easily be overshadowed by noncompliance in the eight other areas already shown to have an independent role in mortality. This point cannot be overemphasized. The recommendations that follow are based on the current state of the nutritional literature for SIRS and severe sepsis.

Once the patient is well resuscitated (or in the operating room), enteral access should be obtained, preferably postpylorically. Low-dose (10 to 20% of needs) enteral nutrition should be begun early (within 24 hours of ICU admission), as long as the patient is not on high-dose vasopressor agents. Strive for conservative advancement in rate toward total caloric goal. Avoid high-fat diets, especially those of primarily the ω-6 variety. Avoid long-term (> 48 h) intravenous propofol for sedation. Consider supplemental TPN for those patients who tolerate enteral feedings poorly, remain on high-dose pressors, or start off significantly malnourished. The decision as whether to utilize an immune-modulating formula remains controversial. There is no gold standard enteral formula that has been studied vs. placebo in septic patients. There is the concern for a possible increase in mortality based on a formula's arginine content. Yet, at the same time, there is the Galban article, the only prospective randomized nutrition article ever to show an improvement in survival, and it is specifically in septic patients receiving a high-arginine formula. The potential survival benefit (NNT = 8) for the septic patient would save thousands of lives per year and may be as powerful as activated protein C, a drug currently costing over $7000 per patient. Therefore, until further studies are done, this decision will have to be made at the local hospital level by a multidisciplinary, intensivist-led team well versed in the total care of the septic patient. This would represent a Grade B recommendation (based on only one article). Objective protocols should be developed that specify which patients qualify, how to advance, when to stop, and when to switch. The choice of immune product should be made based on literature review; given the concern about an increase in mortality, all immune formulas cannot be looked upon as generically equivalent. In other words, nutrition decisions should be made like any other medical decision in medicine today. Gone are the days that it could be assumed that nutrition "makes no difference."

35.11 CASE STUDY

M.O. was a 25-year-old white male admitted to the hospital with nausea, vomiting, and shortness of breath. He had a history of quadriplegia secondary to a motor vehicle accident 5 years before. He was wheelchair bound but could move his left thumb and breathed without the use of artificial ventilation. The patient was six feet tall, with a usual weight of approximately 60 kg (IBW closer to 80 kg). He had been admitted before on at least two other occasions with abdominal distension that resolved with nasogastric suction and bowel rest. On this admission, he was felt to have aspiration pneumonia and was placed on antibiotics.

Thirty-six hours into his admission, he had a respiratory arrest and severe hypotension. Evaluation at that time showed a dilated colon consistent with volvulus. He was resuscitated and taken to the operating room, where a distended necrotic colon was removed and a colostomy placed. A nasojejunal feeding tube was manipulated into place while the abdomen was open.

Postoperatively, M.O. was in septic shock, requiring vasopressor agents and ventilation utilizing a lung-protective strategy. Serum cortisol level was greater than 25 μg/dl, so he was not started on steroids. Activated protein C was considered but not given because of his rapid improvement in organ dysfunction. He was, however, started on heparinoid products for deep venous thrombosis prophylaxis. TPN was started on postop day 1 because of M.O.'s marginal baseline nutritional status and, by this time, it had been 5 days since he had received a normal diet. Low doses of an immune-modulating formula (10 cc/h) were started down the feeding tube when the patient's vasopressors were at lower doses (within 24 hours of his operation). Glucose levels were kept normal utilizing an insulin drip. A metabolic cart was done to assess energy requirements, because it was felt that typical equations may not accurately predict M.O.'s needs because he was a chronic quadriplegic. Overfeeding may have increased carbon dioxide production and made it difficult to wean him from the ventilator. His measured resting energy expenditure (REE) was 1310 kcal/d, with a predicted energy expenditure of 1670 kcal/d. Goal rate was his measured REE, because he was only 78% of predicted. Over the next four days, the patient's enteral nutrition was gradually advanced and the TPN weaned. He was extubated on postop day number 4 and transferred out of ICU on postop day 6.

REFERENCES

1. Sackett DL: Rules of evidence and clinical recommendations on the use of antithrombotic agents. *Chest* 1989; 95: 2S–4S.
2. Koretz RL: Nutritional supplementation in the ICU: how critical is nutrition for the critically ill? *Am. J. Respir. Crit. Care Med.* 1995; 151: 570–573.
3. Marino PL and Finnegan MJ: Nutrition support is not beneficial and can be harmful in critically ill patients. *Crit. Care Clinics* 1996; 12 (3): 667–676.
4. Angus DC, Linde-Zwirble WT, Lidicker J, et al.: Epidemiology of severe sepsis in the United States: analysis of incidence, outcome, and associated costs of care. *Crit. Care Med.* 2001; 29 (7): 1303–1310.
5. Fry DE, Pearlstein L, Fulton RL, et al.: Multiple system organ failure: the role of uncontrolled infection. *Arch. Surg.* 1980; 115: 136–140.
6. Marshall JC, Cook DJ, Christou NV, et al.: Multiple organ dysfunction score: a reliable descriptor of a complex clinical outcome. *Crit. Care Med.* 1995; 23: 1638–1652.
7. Vincent JL, Moreno R, Takala J, et al.: The sepsis-related organ failure assessment (SOFA) score to describe organ dysfunction/failure. *Int. Care Med.* 1996; 22: 707–710.
8. Rivers E, Nguyen B, Havstad S, et al.: Early goal-directed therapy in the treatment of severe sepsis and septic shock. *N. Engl. J. Med.* 2001; 345: 1368–1377.
9. Jimenez MF and Marshall JC: Source control in the management of sepsis. *Int. Care Med.* 2001; 27: S49–S62.
10. Kollef MH, Sherman G, Ward S, et al.: Inadequate antimicrobial treatment of infections: a risk factor for hospital mortality among critically ill patients. *Chest* 1999; 115 (2): 462–474.
11. Ibrahim EH, Sherman G, Ward S, et al.: The influence of inadequate antimicrobial treatment of bloodstream infections on patient outcomes in the ICU setting. *Chest* 2000; 118: 146–155.
12. The Acute Respiratory Distress Syndrome Network. Ventilation with lower tidal volumes as compared with traditional tidal volumes for acute lung injury and the acute respiratory distress syndrome. *N. Engl. J. Med.* 2000; 342: 1301–1308.
13. Bernard GR, Vincent JL, Laterre PF, et al.: Efficacy and safety of recombinant human activated protein C for severe sepsis. *N. Engl. J. Med.* 2001; 344: 699–709.

14. Davidson BL, Geerts WH, and Lensing AWA: Low-dose heparin for severe sepsis. (Letter to editor.) *N. Engl. J. Med.* 2002; 347 (13): 1036–1037.

15. Annane D, Sebille V, Charpentier C, et al.: Effect of treatment with low doses of hydrocortisone and fludrocortisone on mortality in patients with septic shock. *JAMA* 2002; 288: 862–871.

16. Marik PE and Zaloga GP: Adrenal insufficiency during septic shock. *Crit. Care Med.* 2003; 31: 141–145.

17. van den Berghe G, Wouters P, Weekers F, et al.: Intensive insulin therapy in the critically ill patient. *N. Engl. J. Med.* 2001; 345: 1359–1367.

18. Young MP and Birkmeyer JD: Potential reduction in mortality rates using an intensivist model to manage intensive care units. *Effective Clin. Pract.* 2000; 3 (6): 284–289.

19. Milstein A, Galvin RS, Delbanco SF, et al.: Improving the safety of health care: the Leapfrog initiative. The Leapfrog Group. *Effective Clin. Pract.* 2000; 5: 313–316.

20. Heyland DK, Novak F, Drover JW, et al.: Should immunonutrition become routine in critically ill patients? A systematic review of the evidence. *JAMA* 2001; 286 (8): 944–953.

21. Galban C, Montejo JC, Mesejo A, et al.: An immune-enhancing enteral diet reduces mortality rate and episodes of bacteremia in septic intensive care unit patients. *Crit. Care Med.* 2000; 28: 643–648.

22. Rapp RP et al.: The favorable effect of early parenteral feeding on the survival in head-injured patients. *J. Neurosurg.* 1983; 58: 906–912.

23. Kudsk KA, Minard G, Croce MA, et al.: A randomized trial of isonitrogenous enteral diets after severe trauma: an immune-enhancing diet reduces septic complications. *Ann. Surg.* 1996; 224 (4): 531–543.

24. Church JM and Hill GL: Assessing the efficacy of intravenous nutrition in general surgical patients: dynamic nutritional assessment with plasma proteins. *JPEN* 1987; 11 (2): 135–139.

25. Cerra FB et al.: Enteral nutrition does not prevent multiple organ failure syndrome (MOFS) after sepsis. *Surgery* 1988; 104 (4): 727–733.

26. Lowry SF: The route of feeding influences injury responses. *J. Trauma* 1990; 30 (12): S10–S15.

27. Ibrahim EH, Mehringer L, Prentice D, et al.: Early versus late enteral feeding of mechanically ventilated patients: results of a clinical trial. *JPEN* 2002; 26 (3): 174–181.

28. Moore FA, Moore EE, Jones TN, et al.: TEN versus TPN following major abdominal trauma: reduced septic morbidity. *J. Trauma* 1989; 29 (7): 916–923.

29. The Veterans Affairs Total Parenteral Nutrition Cooperative Study Group. Perioperative total parenteral nutrition in surgical patients. *N. Engl. J. Med.* 1991; 325 (8): 525–532.

30. Bertolini G, Iapichino G, Radrizzani D, et al.: Early enteral immunonutrition in patients with severe sepsis: results of an interim analysis of a randomized multicentre clinical trial. *Int. Care Med.* 2003; 29: 834–840.

31. Heyland DK, Drover JW, MacDonald S, et al.: Effects of postpyloric feeding on gastroesophageal regurgitation and pulmonary microaspiration: results of a randomized controlled trial. *Crit. Care Med.* 2001; 29 (8): 1495–1501.

32. Zaloga GP and Roberts P: Permissive underfeeding. *New Horizons* 1994; 2 (2): 257–263.

33. Suchner U, Katz DP, Fürst P, et al.: Effects of intravenous fat emulsions on lung function in patients with acute respiratory distress syndrome or sepsis. *Crit. Care Med.* 2001; 29 (8): 1569–1574.

34. Battistella FD, Widergren JT, Anderson JT, et al.: A prospective, randomized trial of intravenous fat emulsion administration in trauma victims requiring total parenteral nutrition. *J. Trauma* 1997; 43 (1): 52–60.

35. Talpers SS, Romberger DJ, Bunce SB, et al.: Nutritionally associated increased carbon dioxide production: excess total calories vs high proportion of carbohydrate calories. *Chest* 1992; 102 (2): 551–555.

36. Bower RH, Cerra FB, Bershadsky B, et al.: Early enteral administration of a formula (Impact®) supplemented with arginine, nucleotides, and fish oil in intensive care unit patients: results of a multicenter, prospective, randomized, clinical trial. *Crit. Care Med.* 1995; 23 (3): 436–449.

37. Atkinson S, Sieffert E, Bihari D, et al.: A prospective, randomized, double-blind, controlled clinical trial of enteral immunonutrition in the critically ill. *Crit. Care Med.* 1998; 26 (7): 1164–1172.

38. Heyland DK: Immunonutrition in the critically ill patient: putting the cart before the horse? *Nutr. Clin. Pract.* 2002; 17 (5): 267–272.

39. Gadek JE, DeMichele SJ, Karlstad MD, et al.: Effect of enteral feeding with eicosapentaenoic acid, γ-linolenic acid, and antioxidants in patients with acute respiratory distress syndrome. *Crit. Care Med.* 1999; 27 (8): 1409–1420.

40. Argaman Z, Young VR, Noviski N, et al.: Arginine and nitric oxide metabolism in critically ill septic pediatric patients. *Crit. Care Med.* 2003; 31 (2): 591–597.

41. Marik PE: Cardiovascular dysfunction of sepsis: a nitric oxide and L-arginine-deficient state? *Crit. Care Med.* 2003; 31 (2): 591–597.

42. López A, Lorente JA, Steingrub J, et al.: Multiple-center, randomized, placebo-controlled, double-blind study of the nitric oxide synthase inhibitor 546C88: effect on survival in patients with septic shock. *Crit. Care Med.* 2004; 32 (1): 21–30.

36 Nutrition Support in Patients with Cancer and Immunodeficiency

Vanessa Fuchs
Mexico's General Hospital

Jose L. Sandoval
Mexico's National Institute of Respiratory Diseases

CONTENTS

36.1 CANCER

Patients with cancer are frequently malnourished because of direct or indirect effects of tumor, surgery, radiation therapy, or chemotherapy, in addition to psychological factors. Malnutrition reduces quality of life, decreases performance status, and increases morbidity and mortality. Malnutrition adversely affects tissue function and repair and humoral and cellular immunity. It is not surprising that a significant proportion of patients with cancer end up being critically ill because of these factors (1). Malnutrition experienced by patients with cancer can be related to the patient's nutritional status before the development of cancer, the tumor itself, and cancer therapy. Aggressive treatment may increase the degree of malnutrition. The combination of the effects of therapy along with progressive malnutrition may be a frequent cause of death (2).

TABLE 36.1
Cytokine Effects on Protein and Lipid Metabolism in Cancer Cachexia

	Protein	Carbohydrate	Lipid
TNF-α	Increased muscle proteolysis	Increased glycogenolysis	Decreased lipogenesis
	Increased protein oxidation	Decreased glycogen synthesis	Decreased LPL in fat tissue
	Increased hepatic protein	Increased gluconeogenesis	
	synthesis	Increased glucose clearance	
		Increased lactate production	
IL-1	Increased hepatic protein	Increased gluconeogenesis	Increased lipolysis
	synthesis	Increased glucose clearance	Decreased LPL synthesis
			Increased fatty acid synthesis
IL-6	Increased hepatic protein		Increased lipolysis
	synthesis		Increased fatty acid synthesis
IFN-α			Decreased lipogenesis
			Increased lipolysis
			Decreased LPL activity

Patients with cancer tend to be immunosuppressed, not only because of their illness but also due to the necessary treatments. The use of intensive nutritional support for some patients with cancer may promote weight gain and positive nitrogen balance, increase tolerance of cancer therapy, and improve immune response. The benefits of nutrition support in patients with cancer may outweigh concerns about nutrition effects on tumor growth. The choice of nutritional support is dependent on the availability of and access to a functional gastrointestinal (GI) tract, patient comfort and compliance, drug toxicity, and site of radiation therapy (2).

The value of nutrition support in critically ill patients with cancer and bone marrow transplantation is to provide exogenous substrates to meet protein and energy requirements, thereby protecting vital visceral organs and attenuating catabolic responses. Although improved clinical outcomes as a result of nutritional support have been inadequately studied, it seems logical that nutrition-related morbidity and mortality can be prevented or ameliorated by appropriate and timely interventions (1,3).

36.1.1 Metabolic Changes in Critically Ill Patients with Cancer

Nutritional problems associated with malignancy are important, ranging from localized effects induced by a tumor on the organ involved or adjacent structures to systemic effects caused by metastasis or humoral factors produced by these tumor cells. The critically ill cancer patient characteristically exhibits significant glucose intolerance, increased fat depletion, and protein turnover. The malnourished patient with cancer is also unable to conserve energy because of inefficient metabolism.

Several mediators are responsible for metabolic changes in patients with cancer. Mediators such as hormones, cytokines, and growth factors are responsible for the nutritional derangements in cancer cachexia (see Table 36.1). Components associated with daily energy expenditure include basal metabolic rate, the thermal effect of exercise, and the thermogenic effect of food intake. In critically ill patients, stress and illness are additional factors that increase energy expenditure (1). There is usually a negative energy balance, which results from a decrease in energy intake, due to anorexia, hypophagia, or both, and an energy expenditure that sometimes increases in absolute value and always fails to adapt to the condition of semistarvation. The rise in energy expenditure is usually slight (100 to 300 kcal/d) but, if not compensated by increased intake, can cause a loss of body fat of 0.5 to 1 kg or 1 to 2.3 kg of muscle mass per month (see Table 36.2) (4).

TABLE 36.2
Metabolic Abnormalities in the Cancer Patient

Carbohydrate
Increased gluconeogenesis from amino acids, lactate, and glycerol
Increased glucose disappearance and recycling
Insulin resistance

Lipid
Increased lipolysis
Increased glycerol and fatty acid turnover
Lipid oxidation noninhibited by glucose
Decreased lipogenesis
Decreased lipoprotein lipase activity
Nonconstant increase in plasma levels of NEFA
Nonconstant increase in plasma levels of lipid

Protein
Increased muscle protein catabolism
Increased whole-body protein turnover
Increased liver protein synthesis
Decreased muscle protein synthesis

36.1.2 NUTRITIONAL MANAGEMENT

Attainable goals of nutrition support in the critically ill patient include the minimization of starvation effects with regard to energy and substrates, the prevention of specific nutrient deficiencies, and the support of acute inflammatory response until resolution of hypermetabolic response and healing takes place. Calories sufficient to meet the energy needs of patients should be achieved.

Indirect calorimetry is the standard to allow precise measurements of the daily caloric expenditure in the clinical setting. If this is not available, predictive equations are typically utilized (see Chapter 6).

Carbohydrates remain the primary source of calories in hypermetabolic patients and constitute 60% of nonprotein calories. Exogenous insulin administration tends to be ineffective, increasing cellular uptake in septic patients because of inhibited glucose oxidation.

Protein demands are markedly increased in critically ill patients. The high catabolic rate is refractory to protein or glucose infusion, but protein synthesis is responsive to amino acid infusions, making nitrogen balance possible. Protein requirements in septic or injured patients range from 1.2 to 2 g/kg/d. The recommended nonprotein calorie–nitrogen ratio is usually 150:1, but highly stressed patients require a lower ratio of 80:1 to 100:1 (1).

Fluids and electrolytes should be supplied to maintain adequate urine output and normal serum electrolyte levels. Vitamins and trace elements must be provided according to the recommended dietary allowance (RDA). Regular monitoring of laboratory profile, including electrolytes, liver function, and lipid panel, can ensure adequate nutritional supplementation and prevent unwanted complications (1,2).

The timing of nutrition support is determined by the priorities in the care of critically ill patient. Nutrition intervention is appropriate in the catabolic phase when hemodynamic stability is attained. The transitions from one phase to another phase of convalescence require nutrition support, especially in the phase soon after recovery from the shock state.

36.1.3 ENTERAL VS. PARENTERAL NUTRITION

The general consideration is that if the gut works, use it. The enteral route is preferred for the provision of nutritional support in the critically ill patient. The enteral route has several advantages over parenteral nutrition:

- Easy administration
- Good tolerance
- Promotion of mucosal growth and development
- Assistance in maintaining the barrier function of the GI tract

Limitations of enteral feeding are the risk for aspiration and its contraindication in patients with ileus, especially postoperative ileus. In an article published by Kirby et al., the authors discuss the many advantages and changes that have occurred in the nutritional management of critically ill patients, patients with GI diseases, and patients with selected cancers. Mechanical obstruction is the only contraindication to enteral nutrition, according to the authors (5).

In patients without oral or enteral nutrition support, total parenteral nutrition (TPN) is an important alternative.

36.2 NUTRITION IN AIDS PATIENTS

Nutritional problems have been a part of the clinical aspects of AIDS. The origin of nutritional abnormalities in AIDS patients is multifactorial. The complex mechanisms that cause malnutrition include disorders of metabolism, hypercatabolism, effects on the alimentary tract, and drug–nutrient interaction. Other, complementary causes of malnutrition in HIV/AIDS patients include psychological, social, and economic factors (6).

Two main paradigms should be considered: cachexia and starvation (7). The pathophysiologic hallmark of cachexia is a disproportionate loss of lean body mass (LBM), which comprises the body cell mass (CM) and connective tissues, over the losses of body fat mass (FM), with relative preservation of the extracellular body water (BW). These changes result from an increase in metabolic rate, with catabolism predominating over anabolism. This catabolic state is triggered by events that result in production and release of cytokines; the involved cytokines include interleukin 1 (IL-1), IL-6, tumor necrosis factor (TNF), and interferon alpha (IFN-α) (8). In contrast, starvation results from voluntary or involuntary reduction in food intake or assimilation due to factors in a real way external to the tissues, such as dieting, poverty, famine, or malabsorption.

36.2.1 METABOLIC AND NUTRITIONAL CONSEQUENCES OF HIV INFECTION

Since HIV infection was recognized, wasting (defined as > 5% loss of body weight or BMI < 20.5 kg/m^2) has been a major clinical problem associated with both mortality and morbidity. The importance of wasting as a poor prognostic indicator was formally recognized adoption of unexpected weight loss as an AIDS-defining illness, the *AIDS wasting syndrome*. Wasting arises from a variety of causes, not least altered energy intake, but one of the most marked features of HIV is its ability to generate profound metabolic alterations even in the absence of clinically apparent disease (9).

36.2.1.1 Intestinal Abnormalities

Acute and chronic diarrhea and weight loss have become a part of the clinical diagnosis of AIDS in HIV-infected patients. A variety of causes have been defined; however, in many patients the cause still remains uncertain. Mucosal changes unassociated with documental infection have been called *HIV enteropathy* (10).

Malabsorption should be considered if intake meets the requirement but stabilization or recovery of weight is not achieved.

36.2.1.2 Malnutrition

36.2.1.2.1   Protein-Energy Malnutrition

Given the prominent wasting in AIDS, it is natural that an analogy would be made to protein-energy malnutrition (PEM) as it exists in non-HIV patients. Evidence for PEM in AIDS includes the changes in LBM and decreases in circulating levels of export proteins (e.g., serum albumin, prealbumin, and retinal binding protein) in the presence of progressive weight loss (11).

36.2.1.3 Micronutrient Deficiencies

The acute-phase response to infection, stress, and inflammation results in rapid shifts of micro-nutrients from plasma to tissues with sequestration in an intracellular compartment. This is certainly the case of iron, zinc, and vitamin A (12).

Vitamin levels have been measured in patients with various stages of HIV infections. A particularly compelling issue has been the possibility that vitamin B12 or folate deficiencies might underlie some of the cognitive changes that occur in AIDS (13). Vitamin B6 (pyridoxine) deficiency is common in CDC stage III HIV patients.

Megadoses of vitamins and trace elements are used frequently by HIV-infected individuals, but positive results have mainly come from studies in rural areas of Africa, where RDA was brought up to 100% and not exceeded (9).

The CDC define the AIDS wasting syndrome as profound involuntary weight loss greater than 10% of baseline body weight, plus either chronic diarrhea (at least two stools per day for > 30 days) or chronic weakness and documented fever for > 30 days (intermittent or constant in the absence of concurrent illness) or condition other than HIV infection that could explain the findings, for example, cancer, tuberculosis, cryptosporidiosis, or other specific enteritis (7).

Body weight, however, was demonstrated to be a poor indicator of malnutrition. Besides AIDS, wasting is correlated with reduced survival in other diseases.

36.2.2 Nutritional Intervention

The major goal in HIV-infected patients is the maintenance of lean body mass. Nutrition support should be focused on optimal nutrition but also on quality of life. Recommendations for nutrition interventions are shown in Table 36.3 (9).

An individual infected with HIV should be treated as a chronically infected patient. This means that optimum nutrition should be provided and given, ensuring also that malabsorption is not a problem.

Optimum nutrition is described as follows:

- 30 to 35 kcal/kg actual body weight
- 1.5 to 1.7 g protein/kg actual body weight

Micronutrient requirement should meet 100 to 150% RDA, not less, with special attention to the antioxidants. If malabsorption is present, the micronutrient status should be evaluated and, if necessary, supplemented orally.

In overweight patients, the provision of protein should meet this recommendation, but energy intake should be adapted to the desired weight of the patient. Especially in patients with lipodystrophy, adequate protein intake should be ensured (9).

Because nutritional therapy has clearly been shown to have a beneficial effect on the clinical course of immunologic status of critically ill patients, one must not disregard the potential positive

TABLE 36.3
Stepwise Approach to Optimal Nutrition Support for HIV Patients

Oral Diet

Oral nutrition *ad lib* without intervention if weight and condition remain stable. Goal is 30 to 35 kcal and 1.0 to 1.7 g
  protein/kg.

Oral Supplement

Nutritional counseling by dietitian with oral supplementation in case of malnutrition defined by weight loss of 10% in 6
  months (this could increase energy intake in about 50% of malnourished HIV-infected patients).

Enteral Nutrition

Enteral nutrition with polymeric formula meeting the criteria of optimal nutrition in case the patient is not able to meet
  these criteria orally or with supplements.
In case of diarrhea, oligomeric formula should be used to influence malabsorption.
The supplementation of sodium to the formula to an amount of 2400 mg/l could also influence the absorption of fluids.
Soluble fibers could be tested to influence diarrhea, but negative side effects should be considered.

Parenteral Nutrition

TPN should be considered if enteral route is not available to provide body with fluids and nutrients.
Most AIDS patients using TPN suffer from severe GI infections, such as crypto- or micropordiosis, in which fecal fat and
  protein loss is over 20%.
In cases of nontreatable infection, home TPN can be considered.
If the patient has frequent diarrhea, it is important to monitor electrolytes and adjust doses via IV.

benefits of nutritional therapy in the treatment of malnourished HIV/AIDS patients. As a result of
the escalating cost of treatment and the predicting increase AIDS incidence, HIV/AIDS nutritional
therapy regimens must be simple to administer and cost effective (14).

Before one initiates therapy, some authors advise interviewing each patient, performing a
complete physical examination, conducting a nutritional assessment, evaluating gut function, and
calculating daily caloric and protein requirements. The selection of oral, enteral, or parenteral diets
is crucial in the successful management of these patients (14).

Specific oral nutritional supplements have also been postulated to have beneficial effects on
HIV and the wasting syndrome. Individuals with higher levels of niacin and vitamins B1, B2, and
B6 have a survival advantage.

Antiretroviral therapy and the introduction of the protease inhibitors pose nutritional challenges
(15). All of the protease inhibitors and a few of the nucleoside reverse transcriptase inhibitors have
dietary requirements that facilitate absorption and subsequent pharmacologic action. Because most
patients report many symptoms, including gastrointestinal disturbances, stomach pain, fatigue, and
nausea (which are probably disease related but may be exacerbated by the drugs themselves), it is
important to provide adequate dietary counseling to avoid frustration, depression, and poor adherence to the prescribed regimen (16).

Enteral feeding may be useful if the absorptive function of the GI tract remains intact. An
elemental diet containing small peptides, branched-chain amino acids, or medium-chain triglycerides may be well tolerated if GI tract function is only partially intact. Low residue, lactose-free
preparations may limit the amount of diarrhea resulting from enteral feedings.

Enteral feeding by percutaneous endoscopic gastrostomy (PEG) tubes has been studied prospectively (17). Amino acids were supplied as small peptides, and 40% of the lipid was in the form
of medium-chain triglycerides. Although weight gain did not reach statistical significance, there
was a significant increase in body cell mass, fat content, and serum albumin concentrations.

Administration of TPN has been studied in a few small, uncontrolled series of AIDS patients
in attempts to facilitate weight gain and replete body cell mass. A retrospective study aimed to

assess the use of TPN in 22 patients with more than 10% loss of body weight showed that only 68% of the patients (n = 15) gained weight and only 40% of the patients returned to their previous activities (18). In another study, Kotler and colleagues demonstrated weight gain in 12 patients with AIDS receiving intravenous TPN (19).

An article demonstrated that TPN had a variable effect on body composition, with repletion occurring in patients with eating disorders or malabsorption syndromes and progressive depletion occurring in patients with serious systemic infections. Enteral nutrition can also replete body mass in AIDS patients without severe malabsorption (17).

Some authors suggest considering combining both enteral and parenteral support with metabolic support in the acute phase of illness and between bouts of infections to facilitate patient care and to restore lean tissue (20).

Because all HIV/AIDS patients differ in their nutritional requirements, diet tolerance, and degree of intestinal dysfunction, there is no single nutritional therapy regimen that can be utilized in the treatment of all these patients. It is recommended to individualize oral diets combined with food supplements and enteral and parenteral diets in the treatment of HIV/AIDS patients (14).

36.3 NUTRITION IN BONE MARROW AND STEM CELL TRANSPLANTATION

The earliest report of therapeutic marrow infusion dates to 1939, when a patient received intravenous marrow from his brother to treat aplastic anemia (21). The diseases treated by bone marrow transplantation are hematologic malignancies, solid tumors, and other pathologic conditions. These include acute myelogenous leukemia, chronic myelogenous leukemia, acute lymphocytic leukemia, myeloproliferative disorders, multiple myeloma, non-Hodgkin's lymphoma, and Hodgkin's disease. Solid tumors treated include breast cancer, testicular cancer, ovarian cancer, glioma, neuroblastoma, small-cell lung cancer, and non-small-cell lung cancer. Other pathological conditions treated include severe aplastic anemia, B-thalasemia, severe combined immunodeficiency, autoimmune diseases and some hereditary metabolic disorders (22).

At present, two types of bone marrow transplantation (BMT) can be performed:

* Allogenic (allo-BMT) — Transfers marrow from a donor to a recipient
* Autologous BMT (a-BMT) — Uses the patient's own marrow

The stem or progenitor cell transplant consists of autologous or allogenic infusion of hemopoietic cells collected from peripheral blood. The cells are collected after administration of hemopoietic growth factors, may or may not be associated with chemotherapy.

Irrespective of the type of BMT, conditioning regimens have tremendous and deleterious consequences on the anatomical and functional integrity of the gastrointestinal tract; the duration of profound neutropenia produces mucositis. Allo-BMT patients receive conditioning regimens combining high-dose chemotherapy with total-body irradiation to induce profound immunodepression. Total-body irradiation is extremely toxic, inducing severe and prolonged mucositis.

Within 7 to 10 days after chemotherapy or chemoradiotherapy, patients almost invariably develop oroesophageal mucositis and gastrointestinal toxicity. Both conditions may result in decreased oral intake, nausea, vomiting, diarrhea, decreased nutrient absorption, and loss of nutrients from the gut, especially amino acids, secondary to altered transmembrane transport of nutrients.

Bone marrow transplantation has evolved as a treatment option for patients with end-stage disease and those at high risk for relapse. The consequences of BMT that affect a patient's nutritional status include nausea, vomiting, mucositis, diarrhea, hepatic veno-occlusive disease (VOD), and graft-vs.-host disease (GvHD) (1).

Malnutrition is frequent in patients with solid tumors; impaired nutritional status before transplantation is a negative prognostic factor for outcome after BMT (22). Weight gain is an unreliable indicator of nutritional status but is significant in considering hepatic VOD, especially in the presence of jaundice and an abnormal liver profile. Metabolic abnormalities include increased protein catabolism, hyperglycemia, increased serum cholesterol and triglycerides, and deficiencies in vitamins (K, B12, thiamin, E, beta-carotene) and electrolytes and minerals (magnesium, zinc, selenium, copper). In recent years, indications for TPN have decreased in favor of enteral nutrition. However, TPN is still largely used in BMT, mainly because of the gastrointestinal sequelae associated with BMT; making placement of nasoenteric tubes poorly tolerated by BMT patients. Moreover, virtually all patients undergoing BMT have a central venous catheter placed through which TPN can be safely administered.

Although it was shown that energy expenditure may differ between a-BMT and allo-BMT patients, consensus exists that energy requirements in BMT recipients may reach 130 to 150% of predicted basal energy expenditure (23). Therefore, 30 to 35 kcal/kg body weight/d is usually recommended. Lipids may be safely administered, providing 30 to 40% of nonprotein energy. Protein needs are also elevated and generally satisfied by provision of 1.4 to 1.5 g/kg body weight/d of a standard amino acid solution. TPN was not strictly "total," because patients were allowed oral food intake.

Muscaritoli et al. report that TPN should be initiated on day 1 after allo-BMT and continue for 15 to 21 days according to the intensity and duration of mucositis; oral intake is not allowed during the TPN period to minimize the risk of gut contamination from food and diarrhea. TPN is not routinely administered to a-BMT patients unless complications occur, such as prolonged mucositis (24). Artificial nutrition has rapidly moved from simple supportive care to adjunctive therapy, because of the potential nutritional benefits of a specialized nutritional intervention, such as improvement of tolerance to chemoradiotherapy, prevention or reduction of mucositis, reduction of septic complications, maintenance of immunocompetence, and modulation of biological responses.

The possibility that the administration of specific nutritional substrates, such as lipids and glutamine, during the delicate phase of aplasia and bone marrow reconstitution, may influence outcome is an intriguing topic deserving further investigation in larger, controlled clinical trials.

36.3.1 GLUTAMINE

The rationale for administering glutamine-supplemented nutrition to BMT patients was initially based on the concept that glutamine is the primary fuel for enterocytes and for gut-associated lymphoid tissue and that its administration enterally or parenterally could prevent or mitigate treatment-induced gastrointestinal toxicity (24).

Glutamine administration after BMT was indeed shown to exert positive effects on nitrogen balance, incidence of infectious complications, lymphocyte counts (25), survival duration of hospital stay, and need for TPN (26).

Nutritional support is considered an integral part of the supportive care of BMT patients. TPN still represents the main tool for providing nutritional support to patients undergoing BMT, despite several attempts currently being made at different institutions to feed these patients enterally. The aim of TPN after BMT is to prevent secondary gastrointestinal toxicity and metabolic alterations induced by aggressive conditioning regimens. TPN appears to allow easy modulation of amount of fluid, electrolytes, and micronutrients provided, which may be necessary considering the complexity and severity of the clinical conditions possible in the post-BMT period. The timing of nutritional support may also be critical in determining the short-term outcome of BMT patients, although controlled data are lacking (24).

36.4 CASE STUDY

The patient is a 43-year-old female with gastric cancer. Four months ago, she began experiencing nausea, vomiting, and early satiety; she was taken to the hospital, where they ordered a CAT scan, in which a tumor was found. She was sent to the OR for a subtotal gastrectomy with a gastrojenunostomy and a palliative jejunostomy.

36.4.1 Clinical History

Mother deceased because of gastric cancer.
Father deceased because of hypertension complications
Two weeks after surgery, she was transferred to a large tertiary hospital because of a fistula. A catheter for TPN was placed. Two days later, the patient entered the OR again for fistula closure, and then was admitted to the ICU. She continued with TPN (1500 kcal, 1.6 gm/kg body wt) 75 g protein, 300 g CHO, 20 g lipid, plus additional electrolytes, micronutrients vitamins.

- Actual weight: 45 kg
- Height: 1.55 m
- Glucose: 118 mg/dl
- Blood urea nitrogen (BUN): 56 mg/dl
- Creatinine (Creat): 0.78 mg/dl
- Total protein (PT): 5.9 g/dl
- Albumin (Alb): 2.14 g/dl
- Globulin (Glob): 3.76 g/dl
- Total bilirubin (BT): 0.78 mg/dl
- Direct bilirubin (BD): 0.34 mg/dl
- Indirect bilirubin (BI): 0.44 mg/dl

36.4.2 Comments

The incidence of gastrojejunal or duodenal stump fistulas following subtotal gastrectomy or total gastrectomy has been reported to be 1 to 2% (27), approximately one-quarter of which originated from gastrojejunostomy. Suture line failure accounted for 82% of all gastroduodenal fistulas. The causes of fistulas arising from the gastrojejunostomy may be related to the suture line containing tumor, ischemia of the gastric stump due to high ligation of the gastric artery and vasa brevia, stomal obstruction, and pancreatitis or tension on the suture line.

In all clinical situations, if the gut is functional, then it should be used as the route for feeding. This is not a case or indication for parenteral nutrition. Once the fistula has developed, parenteral nutrition should be used as soon as possible. Serum albumin level is one of the best predictors of malnutrition, because it provides the clinician with an index of visceral and somatic protein stores in most medical illnesses. Exceptions include anorexia nervosa, severe edema, fluid overload, and congenital analbuminemia. Serum albumin (21-day half-life) is a marker of initial nutritional status; serum transferrin (7-day half-life) responds more rapidly to nutritional support.

The route of parenteral nutrition should be secondary to the principle of meeting the individual patient's calorie and protein goals. Peripheral parenteral nutrition can be used in patients who can tolerate high fluid volumes daily (3 l) necessary to obtain adequate calorie administration or as a supplement in patients in the early phase of enteral nutrition. Peripheral vein nutrition is limited by phlebitis caused by the high osmolality of the feeding solution. Traditional aseptic technique is required for placement of central venous catheters. The subclavian vein is the most commonly used site, followed by the internal jugular vein. Central catheters can also lead to thrombosis as a result of improper placement in the subclavian vein. Heparin (1000 units/l) or hydrocortisone (5 mg/l) added to the TPN solution can reduce the occurrence of thrombophlebitis.

REFERENCES

1. Wong P, Enriquez A, Barrera R. Nutrition support in critically ill patients with cancer. *Oncol. Crit. Care* 17(3): 743–767, 2001.
2. Robuck JT, Fleetwood JB. Nutritional support of the patient with cancer. *Focus Crit. Care* Apr. 19(2): 129-30,132-4, 136-8, 1992
3. Klein S, Kinney J, Jeejeeboy K, et al. Nutritional support in clinical practice: review of published data and recommendation for future research directions. *Am. J. Clin. Nutr.* 66: 683–706, 1997.
4. Bozzetti F. Nutritional support in cancer. In: Allison S, Fürst P, et al. *Basics in Clinical Nutrition,* 2nd ed. Galén, Czech Republic, 2000, 239–242.
5. Kirby DF, Teran JC. Enteral feeding in gastrointestinal diseases and cancer. *Gastrointestinal. Endosc. Clin. N. Am.* 1998 Jul. 8(3) :623–643.
6. Fajardo A, Lara C. Intervención nutricional en VIH/SIDA, una guía práctica para su intervención y seguimiento. *Gac. Méd. Mex.* 137(5): 489–500, 2001.
7. Kotler DP. The wasting report 1996, 11th International Conference on AIDS, Vancouver, BC.
8. Kalinkovich A, et al. Elevated serum levels of TNF receptors (s TNF-R) in patients with HIV infection. *Clin. Exp. Immunol.* 89: 351–355, 1992.
9. Jonkers CF, Sauerwein HP. Nutrition support in AIDS. In: Allison S, Fürst P, et al. *Basics in Clinical Nutrition,* 2nd ed. Galén, Czech Republic 2000, 247–250.
10. Ramratnam B, et al. A practical approach to managing diarrhea in the HIV-infected person. *AIDS Reader* 7(6): 190–196, 1997.
11. Kotler DP, et al. Wasting syndrome: nutritional support in HIV infection. *AIDS Res. Hum. Retroviruses* 10: 931–934, 1994.
12. McNally Kruse, L. Nutritional assessment and management for patients with HIV disease. *AIDS Reader* 8(3): 121–130, 1998.
13. Coodley GO, et al. Micronutrient concentrations in the HIV wasting syndrome. *AIDS* 7(12): 1595–6000, 1993.
14. Hickey MS, Weaver KE. Nutritional management of patients with ARC or AIDS. *Gastroenetrol. Clin. N. Am.* 17(3): 545–561, 1988.
15. Schwenk A. HIV infection and malnutrition. *Curr. Opin. Clin. Metab. Care* 1: 375–380, 1998.
16. Shevitz AH and Knox TA. Nutrition in the era of highly active antiretroviral therapy. *CID* 323 (15 June): 1769–1775, 2001.
17. Kotler DP, et al. Nutritional effects and support in the patients with AIDS. *J. Nutr.* 122: 723–727, 1992.
18. Singer P, et al. Clinical and immunologic effects of lipid-based parenteral nutrition in AIDS. *J. Parenter. Enteral Nutr.* 16: 165–167, 1992.
19. Kotler DP, et al. Effect of home TPN on body composition in patients with AIDS. *J. Parenter. Enteral Nutr.* 14: 454–458, 1990.
20. Tuttle-Newhall JE, Veerabaugu MP. Nutrition and metabolic management of AIDS during acute illness. *Nutrition* 9(3): 240–244, 1993.
21. Osgood EE, Riddle MC, Matthews TJ. Aplastic anemia treated with daily transfusion and intravenous marrow. *Ann. Intern. Med.* 13: 357–367, 1939.
22. Schulte C, Reinhardt W, Beelen D, Mann K, Schaefer U. Low T3-syndrome and nutritional status as prognostic factors in patients undergoing bone marrow transplantation. *Bone Marrow Transplant* 22: 1171–1178, 1998.
23. Chamouard Cogoluenhes V, Chambrier C, Michallet M, et al. Energy expenditure during allogeneic and autologous bone marrow transplantation. *Clin. Nutr.* 17: 253–257, 1998.
24. Muscaritoli M, Grieco G, Capria S, Iori AP, Rossi Fanelli F. Nutritional and metabolic support in patients undergoing bone marrow transplantation. *Am. J. Clin. Nutr.* 75: 183–190, 2002.
25. Piccirillo N, De Matteis S, et al. Glutamine-enriched parenteral nutrition after analogous peripheral blood stem cell transplantation: effects on immune reconstitution and mucositis. *Haematologica* 88(2): 192–200, 2003.
26. Ziegler TR, Young LS, Benfell K, et al. Clinical and metabolic efficacy of glutamine supplemented parenteral nutrition after bone marrow transplantation: a randomized double-blind, controlled study. *Ann. Int. Med.* 116: 821–828, 1992.
27. Schwartz S, Shiers T, Cowles W, *Principles of Surgery,* 5th ed. McGraw-Hill, New York, 479, 1991.

37 Endocrine Disorders in the Critically Ill Patient

Nicole M. Daignault and Daniel P. Griffith
Emory University Hospital

Concepcion Fernandez-Estivariz and
Thomas R. Ziegler
Emory University School of Medicine

CONTENTS

37.1 INTRODUCTION

Critical illness following major trauma, sepsis/infection, burns, or other severe inflammatory process induces complex hormonal alterations, with subsequent impact on endocrine, metabolic, nutritional, and immunological functions. The gravity of related endocrine responses may vary according to such factors as the magnitude and duration of catabolic stress, baseline nutritional status, age, and various pharmacological agents. The primary alterations with endocrine processes observed during periods of acute stress include, but are not limited to:

- Activation of the hypothalamic–pituitary–adrenocortical (HPA) system
- Increased counterregulatory hormone secretion by the pancreas, pituitary, and adrenal glands (i.e., growth hormone, cortisol, catecholamines, and glucagons)
- Stimulation of cytokine release by immune cells and other cell types (interleukins [IL-1, IL-6], tumor necrosis factor [TNF])
- Alterations with thyroid hormone metabolism and release
- Diminished gonadal steroid secretion
- Reductions in insulinlike growth factor-1 (IGF-1) and IGF binding protein-3 levels
- Resistance of peripheral tissue to anabolic hormones (i.e., insulin, growth hormone [GH], and IGF-1)

The cytokine- and counterregulatory hormone–induced acceleration of protein breakdown and the diminished secretion and tissue sensitivity to endogenous anabolic agents are major contributing factors to the protein-catabolic response observed during periods of acute illness.[1] The purpose of this chapter is to discuss the potential endocrine and metabolic alterations that may result from tissue injury or stress and the principal endogenous mediators involved. A more thorough examination of the metabolic manifestations of critical illness is made elsewhere.[2–4]

37.2 COUNTERREGULATORY HORMONAL RESPONSES AND FUEL METABOLISM IN CRITICAL ILLNESS

The metabolic response to critical illness or injury serves to increase the availability of critical macronutrient substrates necessary for survival (amino acids, glucose, free fatty acids [FFAs]), control the immune response, and alter anabolic and reproductive functions.[5,6] A sympathoadrenal release of glucagon, cortisol, catecholamines, and GH is induced by the stress response.[6] Such activity is stimulated by factors including hemorrhage, volume depletion, alterations in body temperature, acid–base alterations, oxygen and nutrient substrate availability, pain or other emotional stressors, infection, and trauma-induced inflammation or tissue damage. Hormonally induced alterations in response to critical illness may contribute to various physical indices of patient morbidity, including muscle atrophy, infection, gastrointestinal deterioration, and tissue injury.[2,3,5,6]

The various phases following tissue injury or stress are best exemplified following trauma, in which a clearly defined initiation point is evident. The ebb (early) phase is the initial metabolic response that occurs within the first 24 to 36 hours following injury. This period is characterized by profound volume depletion, reduced cardiac output, and subsequent alterations in tissue perfusion. Oxygen consumption and metabolic rate are reduced, and there may also be a simultaneous reduction in body temperature. Nitrogen loss due to protein catabolism is minor at this time. The increased rates of lipolysis and gluconeogenesis allow for a high production of FFAs and endogenous glucose to serve as primary fuel sources for vital organs, including cardiac muscle and brain. This phase is also characterized by increased serum counterregulatory hormone levels concomitant with lower insulin levels.[2–4,6]

Following the acute resuscitation period, if full recovery does not arise, the patient may make a transition to a more chronic stage ("flow phase"), which may be prolonged for several days to weeks, depending on the severity of illness and the response to clinical interventions.[7] This period is marked by increases in metabolic rate, catabolism, oxygen consumption, cardiac output, and possibly fever.[7] Rates of protein synthesis are accelerated, secondary to enhanced production of acute-phase proteins by the liver.[7] However, protein degradation surpasses the synthetic capacity, leading to a net negative nitrogen balance and erosion of lean body mass.[1,8] The degree of nitrogen loss in the critically ill patient is directly proportional to the level of physiological stress, regardless of nutritional support interventions.[2,3]

Although the mechanisms for the phenomenon of ICU wasting are incompletely understood, the counterregulatory hormones, in concert with proinflammatory cytokines, appear to play a major role.[1,3,4,9] Research has shown the release of catecholamines by the adrenal glands to play a central role in the maintenance of homeostasis after various insults.[4] Investigations with denervated heart preparations have provided evidence to support the ability of catecholamines to induce tachycardia in response to such stressors as cold, pain, oxygen deprivation, or muscle stimulations.[4] Others have demonstrated the importance of neural pathways in the initiation of the stress response. Studies have found a reduction in adrenal steroid production in animals that sustained burn injuries in denervated limbs, following medulla oblongata transection or transection of the spinal cord proximal to the site of injury.[4] However, obstruction of neural pathways during the flow phase of critical illness was not shown to alter whole-body thermogenesis.[4] Thus, neural pathways appear to play a role in the initiation of the stress response, rather than its perseverance.

Proinflammatory cytokines secreted primarily by immune cells have been identified as important agents in cell-to-cell communication and regulation of the metabolic response to injury.[1,4] Studies have demonstrated the requirement for IL-1, TNF-α, and IL-6 for induction of the majority of stress-induced metabolic alterations.[1,4] Evidence suggests a similar stress response occurs with TNF-α or endotoxin infusion in cancer patients and healthy subjects, respectively.[2] Fever and elevations in plasma concentrations of stress-related hormones and acute-phase proteins were observed in both instances.[4] Likewise, when TNF-α was administered to healthy subjects, findings consistent with the stress response, including plasma FFA and glycerol levels, hyperglycemia, and increased thermogenesis, were observed.[3,4]

Cytokines work indirectly and in conjunction with other mediators to elicit cellular responses.[9,10] TNF-α-induced alterations in glucagon release have been shown to be the responsible factor for the stimulation of glucose production during critical illness, rather than the TNF-α itself.[10] Moreover, the influence of TNF-α on protein metabolism may be driven by its impact on glucocorticoid release, and the thermogenic response of IL-1 is thought to be mediated by corticotrophin-releasing factor (CRF) or arginine vasopressin secretion.[4] Cytokine production and activity are regulated by the interaction between cytokine and endocrine systems. Hence, both proinflammatory and anti-inflammatory cytokine productions have been shown to be suppressed by glucocorticoids.[1,4]

An additive effect of combined glucagon, hydrocortisone, and epinephrine infusions in healthy subjects to enhance nitrogen loss, insulin resistance, glucose intolerance, leukocytosis, and metabolic rate has been demonstrated.[3,10,11] Likewise, mechanisms that may precipitate catabolism, including malnutrition, acid–base disturbances, and disuse muscle atrophy may be interrelated with hormonal and cytokine signals.[3] Not only does the accelerated release of amino acids from skeletal muscle during this period, of which approximately 70% are composed of glutamine and alanine, serve as important substrates for gluconeogenesis, but glutamine also acts as a primary fuel source for the gut mucosa and immune cells.[3]

The flow phase of critical illness is characterized by marked alterations in carbohydrate, protein, and lipid metabolism. Rates of gluconeogenesis and glycogenolysis, particularly by the liver, and glucose uptake by the tissues, particularly the reticuloendothelial system, wounds, and gastrointestinal and immune cells are increased.[11,12] Accelerated rates of glycolysis in peripheral tissues and a possible suppression of pyruvate dehydrogenase activity lead to higher lactate levels at this time.[11] Glycerol release by adipocytes is increased due to counterregulatory hormone–induced activation of lipolysis.[11] The increased levels of lactate, glycerol, and alanine, derived by activated muscle proteolysis, all serve as important fuel substrates for gluconeogenesis.[11] Stimulated rates of endogenous glucose production persist in the setting of hyperinsulinemia and hyperglycemia.[7,10,11] Insulin resistance observed during critical illness is believed to be largely due to the combined effects of the counterregulatory hormones (cortisol, norepinephrine, epinephrine, and glucagon) and cytokines, primarily IL-6 and TNF-α.[1,10,11] Clinical observations and data in animal models have shown reduced glycogenolysis and gluconeogenesis rates during periods of prolonged endotoxemia or septic shock.[10,11] Glucose uptake by macrophages remains accelerated; therefore, hypoglycemia may ensue if sufficient exogenous glucose administration is not provided. Thus, the cumulative metabolic alterations observed during this phase of critical illness serve to provide critical substrates for anabolism, synthesis of acute-phase proteins (i.e., C-reactive protein, alpha-macroglobulin, immunoglobulin), and host defense.[2,3]

37.3 CENTRAL AND PERIPHERAL ENDOCRINE RESPONSE PATTERNS DURING CRITICAL ILLNESS

The central and peripheral hormonal response patterns observed during critical illness vary depending on the course of illness. In the initial days following onset of major illness, secretions of the hypothalamus and anterior pituitary gland are generally increased, resulting in higher serum concentrations of corticotropin-releasing hormone (CRH), arginine vasopressin (AVP), adrenocorticotropin (ACTH), prolactin (PRL), leutinizing hormone (LH), and GH (Table 37.1). In contrast, decreased circulating thyroid-stimulating hormone (TSH) concentrations are common during this phase, probably due in part to augmented endogenous cortisol and dopamine secretion or their exogenous administration in individual patients.[6] More prolonged or chronic catabolic states are characterized by suppression in the anterior pituitary activity and hormone release and/or abnormalities in the normal diurnal rhythm of anterior pituitary hormones. Serum concentrations are

TABLE 37.1
Endocrine Response Patterns in Acute and Prolonged Critical Illness

	Acute (Initial 7–10 Days)	Prolonged (> 10 Days)
CRH	↑↑	NL to ↓
ACTH	↑↑	NL to ↓
TSH	NL to ↓	↓ to NL or ↑
PRL	↑	NL
AVP	↑	↑
LH	↑	NL to ↓
GH	↑	
Cortisol	↑↑	↑
Adrenal androgens	↓	↓
Aldosterone	↑	NL to ↓
Glucagon	↑↑	↑
Insulin	NL to ↓	↑
Catecholamines	↑↑	↑
Triiodothyronine (total)	↓↓	↓
Thyroxine (total)	NL to ↑	NL
IGF-1	↓	↓
IGFBP-3	↓	↓
IGFBP-3 protease activity	↑	NL to ↑
Testosterone	↓	↓

Note: Responses vary as a function of nature, timing, and severity of illness; underlying nutritional status; medications; and other factors. Alterations in pituitary hormone pulse amplitude and/or pulse number also may occur (e.g., GH, TSH). For abbreviations see text.

↑ = increased blood levels; ↓ = decreased blood levels; NL = generally normal blood levels.

variable but often remain increased during the recovery period, and AVP levels may remain elevated throughout the entire course of illness (Table 37.1).[2,3]

During the recovery period, there is a restoration of the sensitivity of the anterior pituitary gland to feedback control. The hormonal alterations observed in the critically ill patient may also be related to trauma- or illness-induced damage to the hypothalamus, hypophysis, or target organs.[2,3]

37.4 HYPOTHALAMIC–PITUITARY–ADRENAL (HPA) AXIS

37.4.1 CORTISOL

Cortisol is the primary corticosteroid released by the adrenal cortex.[12] The physiological stress response is characterized by a loss of the normal diurnal rhythm of ACTH and adrenal cortisol secretion, leading to elevated concentrations of CRH, ACTH, and serum cortisol.[3,8,14,15] There is a reduction in the ACTH response to CRH. The HPA axis is stimulated by neural hormonal pathways, which may be activated by cytokine mediators, neural and nociceptive input from the injury site, or baroreceptor stimulation induced by volume contraction.[2,14] Hypothalamic and pituitary hormone secretion may be induced by cytokines released during the inflammatory process, including IL-1, IL-6, and TNF-α.[2,10,13,14] These mediators may have an individual or a combined impact on HPA axis stimulation.[2,13,14]

During the acute phase of the stress response, increased CRH and ACTH release is thought to be responsible for elevations in cortisol levels.[14,16] In the prolonged or chronic phase of critical illness, cortisol levels remain increased, despite lower ACTH concentrations.[13–16] Thus, the stimulation of cortisol release may be due to impaired clearance or via an alternative pathway,[13,15] such as one involving endothelin.[5,15] The hypersecretion of cortisol has been speculated to have a protective role in the prevention of a possible overresponse in the inflammatory cascade of the host.[16] The stimulation of the HPA axis appears to be an adaptive response to illness or injury and may help to maintain homeostasis.[14] Likewise, alterations in carbohydrate and protein metabolism induced by hypercortisolism provide immediate fuel sources for the host.[15,16] However, the benefit of augmented cortisol secretion may be overshadowed by its ability to induce hyperglycemia and protein breakdown, impair wound healing, and suppress the immune response. Subnormal plasma cortisol levels are also directly correlated with morbidity and mortality in the critically ill patient.[5,13,14,16] In contrast to the increase of cortisol release, critical illness is associated with a dissociated, reduced production of the adrenal androgens dehydroepiandrosterone (DHEA) and DHEA sulfate by the adrenal glands (Table 37.1).[1–2] Blood androstenedione concentrations are decreased in burn patients but elevated in critically ill nonburn patients, depending on the degree of injury. Dehydro-epiandrosterone and DHEA sulfate concentrations are consistently decreased after severe illnesses or burns, whereas the DHEA response to ACTH administration is blunted.[1–2]

37.4.2 RENIN–ANGIOTENSIN ALDOSTERONE AXIS

A significant decrease in plasma aldosterone levels has been documented in critically ill subjects, associated with increased risk for mortality.[2,15] These patients were found to be persistently hypotensive, with normal serum potassium levels, increased plasma renin activity cortisol responses, and increased levels of 18-hydroxycorticosterone, the precursor to aldosterone.[2] Only a fraction of the subjects responded to ACTH or angiotensin II administration, indicating a possible impairment in zona glomerulosa function.[2] The observed hypoaldosteronism was determined to be correlated with other factors, including the administration of pharmacological agents such as dopamine, angiotensin-converting enzyme activity, or impairments in aldosterone clearance.[2] Reductions in serum aldosterone concentrations in the setting of an activated renin–angiotensin axis may indicate alterations in the metabolic pathway of pregnenolone from mineralocorticoid and adrenal androgen production to glucocorticoid synthesis, in catabolic conditions.[15]

37.4.3 Prolactin

Evidence suggests that PRL plays an important role in immunoregulation. T and B lymphocytes are equipped with prolactin receptors, and T-cells depend on prolactin for maintenance of immunocompetence.[16] Likewise, animal data demonstrate impaired immune system activity and increased mortality in response to nonlethal bacterial exposure following blockage of prolactin release.[17] Circulating prolactin levels are known to be increased during the acute period of critical illness;[5] however, these are normal to suppressed during the prolonged conditions of stress.[5,15,16] This alteration may play a role in the compromised immune function of the chronically stressed patient.[15,16]

37.4.4 Thyroid Hormone Axis

Secretion of the prohormone T4 by the thyroid gland is stimulated by TSH.[5,15] T4 is subsequently peripherally deiodinated and converted to the active form of T3 or the inactive metabolite, reverse T3.[5,15] Serum T3 concentrations have been shown to decrease within hours after onset of acute illness or stress.[15] Serum T4 levels may be normal or elevated, and reverse T3 levels are increased at this time.[5,15,16] The possible etiologies of this phenomenon of low thyroid syndrome are decreased T3 production due to altered T4 to T3 conversion,[15] augmented T4 and T3 turnover, and decreased T3 secretion.[5,16] The action of cytokines, including TNF, IL-1, and IL-6, may also be possible mediators.[6,15] Dopamine infusion during critical illness has been determined to contribute to reduced T3 levels via a direct suppression of TSH release and its potential impact on thyroid hormone turnover.[15] Likewise, glucocorticoids and somatastatin may inhibit TSH release by the pituitary, and glucocorticoids prevent normal T3 conversion from its precursor.[5,15,16]

T3 plays a vital role in fuel metabolism and protein synthesis and may regulate GH release and activity. Elevated levels of thyroid hormones may promote protein breakdown; therefore, low thyroid syndrome may indicate a protective response to inhibit the catabolic state classically observed during critical illness.[15,16] Although a higher incidence of mortality has been linked to decreased tissue levels of thyroid hormone in critically ill patients and very low TSH levels are a biomarker for poor ICU outcomes,[15] no benefit from T4 or T3 supplementation in this patient population has been identified.[15,16] Reduced T3 levels may also be associated with other conditions or states present during prolonged or chronic stress conditions, including altered mental status, fatigue, depression, impaired gallbladder or gastrointestinal function, pleural and pericardial effusion, hypernatremia, hypertriglyceridemia, and normocytic, normochromic anemia.[16]

37.4.5 Pituitary–Gonadal Axis

Testosterone is the most prevalent anabolic steroid produced in the body.[16] It is released in a pulsatile method by the pituitary gonadotropes.[16] Testosterone levels have been determined to correlate directly with nitrogen balance.[16] Evidence indicates reductions in testosterone levels in response to various stress conditions, including malnutrition, trauma, burns, chronic critical illness, opioids, and other psychological or physical stressors.[15–17] Impairment of Leydig cell function may be induced by acute stress conditions, thus leading to low testosterone concentrations with a simultaneous rise in LH levels and normal levels of follicle-stimulating hormone (FSH) and inhibin.[15,16] Reduced LH and FSH concentrations have been established in critically ill postmenopausal women, which has been shown to be directly related directly to clinical outcome.[16] Likewise, an association between decreased androgen synthesis and reduced LH pulsatile secretions and increased pulsatile frequency has been demonstrated in critically ill men.[15,16] This may indicate a compensatory mechanism of heightened LH secretion in response to stress-induced hypotestosteronemia.[16] However, this appears to be blocked at the pituitary level. The hypogonagotropic, hypogonadism state of prolonged critical illness was found by Van den Berghe et al. to be only somewhat combated by gonadotropin-releasing hormone (GnRH) pulsatile administration.[18] This lends support to the hypothesis that this phenomenon occurs at a combined hypothalamic, pituitary, and gonadal level.[18] The inhibition on LH secretion may be exacerbated by dopamine and opioid infusion.[15,16] The extent of testosterone reduction is strongly correlated with the magnitude of the stress response.[16] Moreover, normal gonadal function may not resume for weeks to months after recovery from illness or insult, thereby further prolonging the protein catabolic period.[2,3] The clinical efficacy of testosterone supplementation in critically ill patients has been investigated. Marginal improvements in nitrogen balance have been identified, but little information on clinical outcomes is available with use of this agent in ICU patients.[2,3]

The potential role for the administration of testosterone derivatives (i.e., oxandrolone) in catabolic states has also been evaluated in the literature. Oxandrolone has been shown to aid in wound healing, promote nitrogen retention, improve lean body mass (LBM) and body weight gain, and to facilitate the restoration of physical function in burn patients, regardless of age.[19–23] The mechanism for action has been associated with oxandrolone-induced alterations in gene expression for structural proteins and proteins involved in the regulation of protein synthesis.[23] The availability for the oral administration of oxandrolone and its limited androgenic side effects offer further advantages for its use in the clinical setting. Additional, well designed clinical trials to ascertain better the efficacy of oxandrolone supplementation in the critically ill patient are indicated.

37.4.6 Growth Hormone–Insulinlike Growth Factor Axis

Growth hormone (GH) is produced and released from the anterior pituitary somatotrope.[15] Its synthesis is stimulated by hypothalamic growth hormone–releasing hormone and suppressed by somatostatin.[6,12,13] GH may function as an anabolic agent directly, via a binding to its respective receptor, or indirectly, via activation of IGF-1 synthesis.[1,11,14,15] It is secreted in an episodic and pulsatile fashion.[12,15,16] GH secretion is increased and serum concentrations are elevated after acute onset of illness.[5,10,15] However, insulinlike growth factor (IGF-1) and IGF-2 levels are reduced at this time.[6] This phenomenon may be at least partially attributed to GH resistance, which may be induced by impairments in receptor function and activity.[12,15,16] Studies have also shown a blunted IGF-1 response after exogenous GH administration in septic vs. healthy subjects.[12] This confirms that GH fails to induce an equivalent response on IGF-1 synthesis during periods of acute stress.[6,12]

There is evidence to suggest that injury or the various mediators of the inflammatory response may also lead to lower circulating IGF-1 levels. IGF-1 synthesis may be acutely inhibited within hours after the onset of the stress response, and this suppression may be sustained for weeks in conditions of prolonged stress. The primary etiology for the down-regulation of IGF-1 appears to be due to reduced hepatic synthesis and release; however, alterations in the IGF-1 transcription and translation also appear to play a role.[1,6,12]

Variation in nutritional intake and nutrient composition also influences IGF-1 production and release. Inadequate caloric or protein intake may lead to reductions in hepatic IGF-1 mRNA and circulating IGF-1 concentrations. In addition, alterations in lipid composition have been found to influence IGF-1 levels. Endogenous supplementation of omega-3 fatty acids in burn patients has been shown to lead to higher IGF-1 concentrations, compared to standard lipids.[12] Likewise, a more rapid rate of IGF-1 recovery following injury has been demonstrated in animals that were fed via the enteral route vs. those who received an isocaloric, isonitrogenous parenteral nutrition regimen.[12]

Alterations in circulating IGF-1 and IGF-2 levels may be partially related to reductions in IGF binding protein levels. Under normal conditions, IGFs circulate as a large complex bound to IGFBP-3 and an acid-labile subunit (ALS).[12] This acts to improve the half-life and to provide an available source of IGF.[12] During states of catabolic stress, elevated IGFBP-3 protease secretion promotes the dissociation of this complex, and decreased IGFBP-3 and ALS levels prevent further binding.[6,15] Hence, the IGF half-life is decreased. There is a simultaneous augmentation of IGFBP-1 levels, possibly due to the elevation in serum cortisol and glucagon concentrations and a reduction in insulin secretion during the acute phase of illness. Elevated serum IGFBP-1 concentrations have been associated with a higher risk for mortality in ICU patients and have been shown to be resistant to aggressive insulin therapy.[24,25] The subsequent increased formation of an IGF-1 to IGFBP-1 complex aids in the removal of circulating IGF-1 levels. Cytokines, including TNF-α and IL-1, have been found to suppress IGF, promote GH resistance in animal models, and increase IGFBP-1 concentrations in prolonged states of critical illness.[6,12,15] Likewise, elevated catecholamine levels have been shown to increase IGFBP-1 levels in humans and to activate hepatic IGFBP-1 production in animals.[12] Prolonged dopamine administration may lead to a further decrease in IGF-1 concentrations.[16] Exogenous and endogenous glucocorticoids and somatostatin may also contribute to GH suppression in critical illness.[16] Prolonged periods of reduced GH concentrations during catabolic illness may negatively affect wound healing and the recovery process and contribute to mucosal and muscle atrophy.[16]

In prolonged critical illness, reduced pulsatile amplitude and more disorderly release of GH lead to intermittently decreased circulating GH concentrations. IGF-1 and IGFBP-3 levels are simultaneously decreased at this time.[6,15] Reductions in IGFBP-3 concentrations may be due to enhanced clearance or impaired synthesis. Studies in burn patients have identified increased IGFBP-3 proteolysis, and omega-3 fatty acid supplementation was shown to attenuate this response.[12] Gender differences in the GH–IGF-1 axis during prolonged critical illness have been identified, with men demonstrating less pulsatility and regularity in GH release.[5,15,26] Supplementation with GH secretagogues has been shown to enhance GH secretion and IGF-1, IGFBP-3, and ALS concentrations. Thus, the etiology of IGF-1 suppression in prolonged critical illness may be at the hypothalamic level, as opposed to the GH resistance observed during the acute state.

Researchers have investigated the efficacy of exogenous recombinant GH, recombinant IGF-1, or IGF-1–IGFBP-3 complex administration in reversing the marked catabolic response observed during severe illness.[1] Moderate improvements in protein anabolism and ureagenesis have been observed in response to GH supplementation.[5,27,28] Other data suggest a possible role of recombinant GH administration in improving antioxidant defenses and proinflammatory response, based on observed alterations in glutamine and TNF-α levels.[29] IGF-1 administration has been shown to have less of an effect, even in the setting of low IGF-1 concentrations.

On the contrary, significant increases in mortality in response to recombinant GH supplementation in critically ill patients have been demonstrated.[31] This may be induced by potential physiological alterations associated with GH, including hyperglycemia and increased splanchnic oxygen consumption in combination with increased blood flow to the skeletal muscles.[15] Hence, alterations in oxygen delivery may facilitate hypoxic-induced injury to the tissues, including the gastrointestinal tract and liver, in the already hemodynamically compromised patient. Moreover, the administration of GH or other anabolic agents may alter the circulation of glutamine and other important amino acids utilized by peripheral tissues, in response to inhibition of the normal catabolic process. This may provide evidence to support a possible protective role of skeletal muscle breakdown during critical illness. Additionally, the negative findings by some may be partially related to the timing of GH administration. Hence, outcome of patients who received GH prior to the onset of the systemic inflammatory response may have been adversely influenced by GH-induced stimulation of proinflammatory cytokine release.[6,30,31] These or other factors may be responsible for the results of a recent randomized and blinded study demonstrating significantly increased rates of mortality and multiple organ failure with high-dose recombinant GH administered during the acute post-ICU admission phase.[44]

37.4.7 MYOSTATIN

Synthesis of members of the transforming growth factor (TGF) family has been shown to be stimulated by cytokines secreted during the catabolic response to stress. Myostatin, a member of the TGF-α family, is known to be a negative regulator of LBM. Animal data indicate that the absence of myostatin leads to higher muscle mass. Likewise, elevations in myostatin levels have been identified in catabolic conditions, such as AIDS wasting, burns, and disuse atrophy. However, endotoxin injection or induction of hypermetabolic peritonitis was not shown to elicit a stimulatory response on myostatin levels. The increase in myostatin concentrations observed in burn patients may be due to a sustained rise in glucocorticoids that is unlike that observed during the other stress conditions examined. This may be supported by findings showing that dexamethasone administration has been shown to increase myostatin mRNA levels.[12]

37.5 HYPERGLYCEMIA AND INSULIN RESISTANCE DURING THE STRESS RESPONSE

Hyperglycemia and insulin resistance are commonly observed in critically ill patients, regardless of a preexisting history of diabetes. Alterations in glucose metabolism appear to be induced by counterregulatory hormone and cytokine secretions.[11,32] The subsequent metabolic milieu leads to activated glycolysis and hepatic gluconeogenesis, despite concomitant hyperglycemia and hyperinsulinemia.[11,32] Decreased sensitivity of insulin-dependent glucose uptake in the liver, skeletal muscle, and heart occurs in serious illness. However, glucose uptake by tissues not dependent on insulin, including the brain, red blood cells, and wounds, is enhanced.[10,11]

In the past, critical care practitioners generally attempted to achieve serum glucose concentrations of less than 200 mg/dl, given the hyperglycemic metabolic response to stress. However, recent findings in critically ill subjects and a wealth of evidence in other medical–surgical conditions support the efficacy of more aggressive blood glucose control in improvement of clinical outcome.[32–42] In a recent landmark trial, Van den Berghe and colleagues investigated the hypothesis that moderate hyperglycemia, defined as levels between 110 and 200 mg/dl, in critically ill subjects compromised clinical outcome, regardless of diabetic status.[33] In a prospective, randomized, controlled trial, they examined variances in morbidity and mortality in 1548 surgical ICU patients from a single institution in response to aggressive (blood glucose less than 110 mg/dl) or moderate (blood glucose 110 to 200 mg/dl) glycemic control.[33] They demonstrated a significant reduction in overall ICU mortality (8 to 4.6%, and 20.2 to 10.6% among patients with > 5-day ICU course) and a decreased prevalence of other morbidity indices, including nosocomial infections, acute renal failure requiring hemodialysis or hemofiltration, critical illness polyneurapathy, and transfusion requirements in response to intensive insulin therapy. A trend toward decreased ventilator and ICU days was also observed.[33]

In a follow-up analysis of their data, these investigators determined that the protective effects of intensive insulin treatment were attributed to the metabolic management of normoglycemia, rather than directly related to the insulin infusion itself.[43] The known anti-inflammatory actions of insulin may partially explain its beneficial effects on morbidity and mortality.[40,41] Hyperglycemia-induced alterations in white blood cell (WBC) function, including impaired granulocyte adhesion, chemotaxis, and phagocytosis ability, have been demonstrated with *in vitro* studies.[32,45] Hyperglycemia may also influence complement activity and suppress opsonization via competition with microorganisms for complement attachment. Lower C-reactive protein concentrations were also noted in response to intensive insulin treatment in critically ill subjects, suggesting decreased inflammation.[40] Additional evidence suggests alterations by blood glucose in inflammatory mediators and reactive oxygen species in other patient groups. Others have confirmed that the state of hyperglycemia is the actual determinant on clinical outcome and mortality, rather than the absolute amount of exogenous insulin provided.[46] These authors suggested the existence of a possible threshold level of less than or equal to 145 mg/dl for blood glucose control at which the protective advantages on mortality were derived. This suggests a more liberal goal for glucose levels than previous findings, which may help to reduce the associated risks for hypoglycemia.[46]

The possible advantages of blood glucose management on outcome in other clinical conditions have been extensively evaluated in the literature. Studies in burn patients have demonstrated lower incidences of bacteremia, fungemia, wound infection, and mortality in response to insulin-induced blood glucose control at levels less than 7.8 mmol/l (approximately 150 mg/dl).[9,25] Likewise, investigations of cardiac surgery patients, with or without diabetes, have determined correlations between preoperative hyperglycemia and a higher risk for infectious complications, increased length of stay, and higher hospital costs.[34,36,37]

Elevated blood glucose levels following acute myocardial infarction (AMI) have been associated with increased incidence of congestive heart failure, cardiogenic shock, hospital mortality, and poor clinical outcome, independent of prior diabetic status.[38] Research has shown admission glucose concentrations following AMI to be an independent predictor of cardiac injury and mortality.[34] Review of the literature demonstrated initial serum glucose levels after AMI of greater than 6.1 to 8.1 mmol/l to carry a 3.9-fold higher risk for mortality.[33,34] Evidence suggests a linear relationship between initial glucose readings and major complications in patients with acute coronary syndromes, without an identified glycemic threshold. The Diabetes and Insulin–Glucose Infusion in Acute Myocardial Infarction (DIGAMI) trial demonstrated blood glucose control at levels less than 12 mmol/l (approximately 240 mg/dl) in diabetic patients for up to three months following AMI to lead to significant improvements in long-term outcome.[47] Although the underlying mechanisms responsible have not been fully determined, impairment in endothelium-dependent coronary vascular relaxation, altered cardiac contraction, higher propensity for arrythmias, and prothrombotic status induced by impaired platelet function and alterations in plasminogen activator inhibitor-1 and thromboxane activity have been proposed.[34]

Similar relationships to that described previously have been identified following acute cerebral vascular events. Hyperglycemia upon hospital admission following cerebral vascular accident (CVA) has been found to correlate with decreased outcome at three months follow-up, regardless of other confounding variables, including age, the magnitude of the stroke, and diabetic status.[34] Likewise, initial serum glucose concentrations in cerebral ischemia have been associated with a two- to threefold higher mortality risk and poor functional recovery.[32,34] Possible underlying mechanisms for action include impaired endothelium-dependent relaxation, lactate-induced metabolic acidosis and free radical production, and the disruption of the blood–brain barrier secondary to fluid accumulation in the brain. Increased incidence of mortality from stress-induced hyperglycemia rather than diabetic status, despite similar blood glucose levels between groups has also been reported. Thus, the severity of the insult that gives rise to the hyperglycemic response may be a better risk predictor than the actual blood glucose level in this setting.[11]

37.6 NUTRITION SUPPORT IN CRITICAL ILLNESS

The provision of adequate nutrition support during critical illness is essential to promote healing, repletion, and recovery. It is important to avoid excessive administration of the total energy load to avoid complications associated with overfeeding, including hepatic dysfunction, hyperglycemia, azotemia, alterations in plasma lipid clearance, increased respiratory demands and impaired mechanical ventilator weaning, and augmented norepinephrine and urinary catecholamine secretion, to name some.[48] Excessive administration of total calories in parenterally fed acutely ill patients has been associated with hyperglycemia and a corresponding increased risk for infections.[32] Studies have demonstrated that energy expenditure in mechanically ventilated trauma patients does not correspond to the level of injury or stress. Thus, the use of the Harris–Benedict equation in this setting may lead to an overestimation of caloric requirements.[49] The efficacy of the use of hypocaloric feedings in mildly to moderately stressed obese patients in the promotion of wound healing, blood glucose control, and other indices of morbidity has been established.[50,51] Indirect calorimetry may be the most accurate means to estimate energy expenditure in this setting.[48] Specific restrictions on carbohydrate, protein, or lipid may be necessary, based on alterations with organ function, such as renal, hepatic, gastrointestinal, or other endocrinological disorders or stress manifestations. Micronutrients (vitamins, minerals, and electrolytes) should be supplemented to replete restore losses, correct for deficiencies, or compensate for various drug–nutrient interactions. The efficacy of supplementation with immune-enhancing agents (e.g., arginine, mRNA nucleotides, and omega-3-fatty acids) has also been investigated.[52,53] Immunonutrition has been shown to reduce the incidence of mortality and infection in critically ill septic patients. Also, the utility of supplementation with eicosapentaenoic acid (EPA), α-linolenic acid (GLA), and antioxidants in ARDS patients has been established. Administration of enteral feedings fortified with these nutrients was shown to reduce pulmonary neutrophil recruitment, improve oxygenation, decrease ventilator days and duration of ICU course, and reduce morbidity.[54] This effect has been demonstrated to be mediated by a reduction in IL-8 and leukotriene B4 levels in the bronchoalveolar lavage fluid. As discussed earlier, fish oil supplementation may also be important in attenuating the stress-induced suppression on IGF-1 concentrations.[12] Lastly, volume administration will need to be adjusted based upon the patient's specific requirements and clinical condition. The primary objective of nutrition support in the ICU setting is to aid with maintenance and repletion, thereby helping to reduce the incidence of morbidity and mortality. However, despite aggressive nutrition support interventions, the catabolic and hormonal processes outlined previously will likely persist until the underlying stress mechanism has resolved.[1]

37.7 CASE STUDY

E.C. is a 55-year-old obese male who is admitted to the surgical intensive care unit from an outside hospital, status post–Roux-en-Y gastric bypass completed five months earlier. He is currently septic and is experiencing complications from his recent surgery, including an enterocutaneous fistula at the gastrojejunal anastomatic site and an enteroenteric fistula originating from two loops of communicating proximal small bowel. He is chemically sedated, placed on mechanical ventilation for respiratory distress, and initiated on vasopressor support due to hemodynamic instability. The nutrition support team is consulted by the surgical service to initiate and manage the nutrition support regimen.

37.7.1 Subjective Information

The patient's family reports that he has only lost approximately 10 lbs. since his gastric bypass, despite the fact that his oral intake has been minimal since his surgical procedure. He has suffered from chronic diarrhea over the past several months and has experienced serous drainage from several areas on his wound site over the past three weeks. He has also been exhibiting progressively worsening shortness of breath and bilateral edema in his lower extremities.

37.7.2 Objective Data

- Past medical history:
  - COPD
  - Morbid obesity
  - Sleep apnea
  - Pulmonary hypertension
- Current pertinent medications:
  - Normal saline with KCL at 150 ml/h
  - Propofol at 15 ml/h
  - Octreotide 200 μg sq q8h
  - Piperacillin/tazobactam 4.5 g IV q8h
  - Famotidine 20 mg IV q12h
- Current laboratory values:
  - Blood glucose 154 mg/dl

- Potassium 3.4 mEq/dl (3.5–5.0)
- Phosphorous 4.6 mg/dl
- C-reactive protein 21 mg/dl
- Total protein 5.6 g/dl
- Albumin 1.4 g/dl
- Prealbumin 3.5 mg/dl
- BUN 23 mg/dl
- CO_2 39 mEq /dl
- Creatinine 0.5 mg/dl
- Magnesium 1.5 mEq/dl
- WBC 14
- Blood gas readings:
  - pH 7.52
  - PCO_2 34
- Vital signs:
  - CO 4.9
  - BP 100/50
  - MAP < 70

37.7.3 ASSESSMENT AND DISCUSSION

E.C. is likely profoundly nutritionally compromised at baseline, due to his history of poor oral intake and gastrointestinal losses resulting from malabsorption and chronic diarrhea and small bowel fistulas. He is also at high risk for further depletion based on his past surgical history, his current diagnosis and level of physiological stress, his inability to tolerate oral feedings due to mechanical ventilation, and his compromised gastrointestinal function. His current body weight is likely elevated due to fluid retention, thus masking true body mass weight loss.

There is likely a nutritional component to the low serum albumin and prealbumin concentrations. However, these levels are not reliable nutritional indicators in the acute care setting, because they may be influenced by many other confounding variables. These levels may be influenced by dilution, third spacing, and the current inflammatory process (identified by the elevated serum C-reactive protein concentration). Thus, visceral protein markers in the ICU setting provide little benefit in nutrition assessment and can be an unnecessary patient expenditure. Moreover, this patient's state of fluid overload may be significantly affected by nutritional variables. Hence, the low albumin and total protein levels observed may compromise oncotic pressure.

Based on the presence of multiple small bowel fistulas and chronic diarrhea and the requirement for vasopressor support (MAP < 70), the surgical service and nutrition support team agree to start parenteral nutrition support. This may be provided until the patient is hemodynamically stable and able to make the transition to enteral nutrition support below the site of the fistulas. Aggressive nutritional support for this patient may play a significant role in his ultimate outcome.

When determining the patient's current nutritional needs, the patient's energy goals are assessed at 14 kcal/kg/d of the patient's actual weight and 2 g/kg/d of protein based on ideal body weight, due to the patient's morbid obesity. An alternate method that may be used is using a 25% adjusted weight {[(Actual weight – IBW) × 25%] + IBW} in the Harris–Benedict equation and feeding at, or slightly below, the basal energy requirements. Weights obtained in the ICU setting are frequently influenced by volume overload and can therefore lead to an overestimation of energy and protein requirements. This patient would benefit from permissive underfeeding, based on his state of hemodynamic instability, baseline obesity, and acute sepsis. The low cardiac output with vasopressor support suggests that the patient is not hypermetabolic, but rather is hypercatabolic. Of note, the inclusion of the lipid-based calories derived by the propofol infusion needs to be considered when estimating caloric goals of nutrition support regimens.

As reviewed previously, aggressive blood glucose control to facilitate wound healing, nutritional repletion, and recovery is imperative. The serum blood glucose level is elevated at baseline, prior to the initiation of nutrition support and with the infusion of only saline-containing intravenous fluids. This patient is at further risk for hyperglycemia due to stress-induced excessive counterregulatory hormone and cytokine release, bedrest, and underlying obesity. The parenteral nutrition regimen may be modified accordingly in order to minimize the hyperglycemic response. The initial carbohydrate load may be restricted to 100 to 150 g the first day, and a higher percentage of fat calories may be provided. Insulin may be added via increments of 0.1 unit of insulin per gram of dextrose provided. Finger blood sugar readings may be monitored every 6 hours, and sliding-scale insulin supplementation to achieve blood sugar values 110 mg/dl in the ICU (with more liberalized blood glucose control in the less monitored setting of the general hospital ward). However, subcutaneous insulin is not likely to be as effective in this patient, because of his generalized edema and morbid obesity. Optimal glycemic control may require more aggressive therapy, such as a continuous intravenous insulin infusion. The parenteral nutrition dextrose composition may be advanced as tolerated toward the goal, as glycemic control permits. The fat concentration may then be adjusted accordingly, to an optimal level of ≤ 30% of the total calories provided.

This patient is at a moderate-to-high risk for a refeeding response (discussed in more detail in Chapter 2). He will need additional potassium, magnesium, phosphorous, and thiamin supplementation upon the initiation of nutrition support. The patient has multiple risk factors for hypophosphatemia, including refeeding syndrome, insulin administration, and respiratory and metabolic alkalosis (likely intracellular alkalosis). Because the patient is on a normal saline infusion and is not receiving a carbohydrate source prior to the initiation of nutrition support, the baseline serum level is not a reliable indicator of phosphorus needs. This patient's requirement for potassium may also be high because of refeeding syndrome (usually lasts ~72 hours), piperacillin/tazobactam (slight K$^+$ waster), and alkalosis. After the alkalosis has corrected and the patient has overcome the period of the refeeding response, potassium requirements will more than likely decrease. Octreotide also has a potential to decrease potassium requirements and growth hormone secretion, and to promote insulin resistance.

Some studies suggest that patient *may* benefit from androgen replacement therapy to promote tissue healing and anabolism. As described earlier, hypogonadism occurs early in critical illness, and replacement therapy has been associated with improved nitrogen retention and wound healing. Thus, supplementation with testosterone or testosterone derivatives (i.e., Oxandrolone, if enteral provision is an option) may be of benefit. The patient's prostate-specific antigen and liver function tests should be assessed prior to initiation of therapy.

This case presentation helps to illustrate the potential endocrine concerns that may influence nutrition requirements, metabolic function, and recovery in the critically ill patient. The provision of a nutrition support regimen that is individualized in accordance with the patient's clinical condition and particular requirements may help to shorten the length of stay in the ICU, decrease morbidity, improve survival, and decrease hospital cost.

REFERENCES

1. Vary TC: Regulation of skeletal muscle protein turnover during sepsis. *Curr. Opin. Clin. Nutr. Metabol. Care* 1998; 1: 217–224.
2. Ziegler, TR: Fuel metabolism and nutrient delivery in critical illness. In: Becker KL (Ed). *Principles and Practice of Endocrinology and Metabolism*. Philadelphia, J.B. Lippincott Co., 2001; pp 2102–2107.
3. Estívariz CF and Ziegler TR: Endocrinology of critical illness. In: Wass JAH, Shalet SM (Eds). *The Oxford Textbook of Endocrinology and Diabetes*. Oxford, Oxford University Press, 2002; pp 1457–1462.

4. Vrees MD and Albina JE: Metabolic response to illness and its mediators. In: Rombeau JL, Rolandelli RH (Eds). *Clinical Nutrition: Parenteral Nutrition* 3rd edition. Philadelphia, W.B. Saunders Co., 2001; pp 21–34.

5. Lavery G and Glover P: The metabolic and nutritional response to critical illness. *Curr. Opin. Crit. Care* 2000; 6: 233–238.

6. Van den Berghe, G: Neuroendocrine axis in critical illness. *Curr. Opin. Endocrinol. Diabet.* 2001; 8: 47–54.

7. Griffiths RD, Hinds CJ, Little RA: Manipulating the metabolic response to injury. *Br. Med. Bull. Intens. Care Med.* 1999; 55: 181–195.

8. Biolo G, Declan Fleming RY, Maggi SP, et al.: Inverse regulation of protein turnover and amino acid transport in skeletal muscle of hypercatabolic patients. *J. Clin. Endocrinol. Metabol.* 2002; 87: 3378–3384.

9. Hasselgren P: Glucocorticoids and muscle catabolism. *Curr. Opin. Clin. Nutr. Metabol. Care* 1999; 2: 201–205.

10. Webber J: Abnormalities in glucose metabolism and their relevance to nutrition support in the critically ill. *Curr. Opin. Clin. Nutr. Metabol. Care* 1998; 1: 191–194.

11. McCowen KC, Malhotra A, Bistrian BR: Endocrine and metabolic dysfunction syndromes in the critically ill. *Crit. Care Clin.* 2001; 17: 1–16.

12. Lang CH and Frost RA: Role of growth hormone, insulin-like growth factor-I, and insulin-like growth factor binding protein in the catabolic response to injury and infection. *Curr. Opin. Clin. Nutr. Metabol. Care* 2002; 5: 271–279.

13. Cooper MS and Stewart PM: Current concepts: corticosteroid insufficiency in acutely ill patients. *N. Engl. J. Med.* 2003; 348: 727–734.

14. Marik PE and Zaloga GP: Adrenal insufficiency in the critically ill: a new look at an old problem. *Chest* 2002; 122: 1784–1796.

15. Van den Berghe G: Dynamic neuroendocrine responses to critical illness. *Front. Neuroendocrinol.* 2002; 23: 370–391.

16. Van den Berghe, G and de Zegher, F: Anterior pituitary function during critical illness and dopamine treatment. *Crit. Care Med.* 1996; 24: 1580–1590.

17. Nierman DM and Mechanick JI: Hypotestosteronemia in chronically critically ill men. *Crit. Care Med.* 1999; 27: 2418–2421.

18. Van den Berghe G, Weekers F, Baxter RC, et al.: Five-day pulsatile gonadotropin-releasing hormone administration unveils combined hypothalamic-pituitary-gonadal defects underlying profound hypoandrogenism in men with prolonged critical illness. *J. Clin. Endocrinol. Metabol.* 2001: 86: 3217–3226.

19. Demling RH and DeSanti L: The rate of restoration of body weight after burn injury, using the anabolic agent oxandrolone, is not age dependent. *Burns* 2001; 17: 46–51.

20. Demling RH: Comparison of the anabolic effects and complications of human growth hormone and the testosterone analog, oxandrolone, after severe burn injury. *Burns* 1998; 25: 215–221.

21. Hart DW, Wolf SE, Ramzy PI, et al.: Anabolic effects of oxandrolone after severe burn. *Ann. Surg.* 2001; 233: 556–564.

22. Ramzy PI, Wolf SE, and Herndon DN: Current status of anabolic hormone administration in human burn injury. *JPEN* 1999; 23: S190–S194.

23. Wolf SE, Thomas SJ, Dasu MR, et al.: Improved net protein balance, lean mass, and gene expression changes with oxandrolone treatment in the severely burned. *Ann. Surg.* 2003; 237: 801–811.

24. Van den Berghe G: Endocrinology in intensive care medicine: new insights and therapeutic consequences. *Verhandelingen:* Koninklijke Academie voor Geneeskunde van Belgie 2002; 64: 167–187.

25. Mesotten D, Delhanty P, Vanderhoydonc F, et al.: Regulation of insulin-like growth factor binding protein-1 during protracted critical illness. *J. Clin. Endocrinol. Metabol.* 2002; 87: 5516–5523.

26. Van den Berghe G, Baxter RC, Weekers F, et al.: A paradoxical gender dissociation within the growth hormone/insulin-like growth factor I axis during protracted critical illness. *J. Clin. Endocrinol. Metabol.* 2000; 85: 183–192.

27. Pichard C, Kyle U, Chevrolet J, et al.: Lack of effects of recombinant growth hormone on muscle function in patients requiring prolonged mechanical ventilation: a prospective, randomized, controlled, study. *Crit. Care Med.* 1996; 24: 403–413.

28. Gamrin L, Essen P, Hultman E, et al.: Protein-sparing effect in skeletal muscle of growth hormone treatment in critically ill patients. *Ann. Surg.* 2000; 231: 577–586.

29. Jeevanandam M, Begay CK, Shahbazian L, et al.: Altered plasma cytokines and total glutathione levels in parenterally fed critically ill trauma patients with adjuvant recombinant human growth hormone (rhGH) therapy. *Crit. Care Med.* 2000; 28: 324–329.

30. Demling R: Growth hormone therapy in critically ill patients. *N. Engl. J. Med.* 1999; 341: 837–839.

31. Takala J, Ruokonen E, Webster NR, et al.: Increased mortality associated with growth hormone treatment in critically ill adults. *N. Engl. J. Med.* 1999; 341: 785–792.

32. Montori VM, Bistrian BR, McMahon MM: Hyperglycemia in acutely ill patients. *JAMA* 2002; 288: 2167–2169.

33. Van den Berghe G, Wouters P, Weekers F, et al.: Intensive insulin therapy in critically ill patients. *N. Engl. J. Med.* 2001; 345: 1359–1367.

34. Prieser J, Devos P, and Van den Berghe G: Tight control of glycemia in critically ill patients. *Curr. Opin. Clin. Nutr. Metabol. Care* 2002; 5: 533–537.

35. Van den Berghe G: Insulin therapy for the critically ill patient. *Clin. Cornerstone* 2003; 5: 56–63.

36. Guvener M, Pasaoglu I, Demircin, et al.: Perioperative hyperglycemia is a strong correlate of post-operative infection in type II diabetic patients after coronary artery bypass grafting. *Endocrine J.* 2002; 49: 531–537.

37. Estrada CA, Young JA, Nifong LW, et al.: Outcomes and perioperative hyperglycemia in patients with or without diabetes mellitus undergoing coronary artery bypass grafting. *Ann. Thorac. Surg.* 2003; 75: 1392–1399.

38. Wahab NN, Cowden EA, Pearce NJ, et al.: Is blood glucose an independent predictor of mortality in acute myocardial infarction in the thrombolytic era? *J. Am. Coll. Cardiol.* 2002; 40: 1748–1754.

39. Foo K, Deaner A, Knight C, et al.: A single serum glucose measurement predicts adverse outcomes across the whole range of acute coronary syndromes. *Heart* 2003; 89: 512–516.

40. Hansen TK, Thiel S, Wouters PJ, et al.: Intensive insulin therapy exerts anti-inflammatory effects in critically ill patients and counteracts the adverse effect of low mannose-binding lectin levels. *J. Clin. Endocrinol. Metab.* 2003; 88: 1082–1088.

41. Das UN: Insulin and the critically ill. *Crit. Care* 2002; 6: 262–263.

42. Gore DC, Chinkes D, Heggers J, et al.: Association of hyperglycemia with increased mortality after severe burn injury. *J. Trauma* 2001; 51: 540–544.

43. Van den Berghe G, Wouters PJ, Bouillon R, et al.: Outcome benefit of intensive insulin therapy in the critically ill: insulin dose versus glycemic control. *Crit. Care Med.* 2003; 31: 359–366.

44. McMahon MM and Rizza RA: Nutrition support in hospitalized patients with diabetes mellitus. *Mayo Clin. Proc.* 1996; 71: 587–597.

45. Finney SJ, Zekveld C, Elia A, et al.: Glucose control and mortality in critically ill patients. *JAMA* 2003; 290: 2041–2047.

46. Mesotten D and Van den Berghe G: Clinical potential of insulin therapy in critically ill patients. *Drugs* 2003; 63: 625–636.

47. McClave SA and Snider HL: Use of indirect calorimetry in clinical nutrition. *Nutr. Clin. Prac.* 1992; 7: 207–221.

48. Brandi LS, Santini L, Bertolini R, et al.: Energy expenditure and severity of injury and illness indices in multiple trauma patients. *Crit. Care Med.* 1999; 27: 2684–2689.

49. Dickerson RN, Rosato E, and Mullen JM: Net protein anabolism with hypocaloric parenteral nutrition in obese stressed patients. *Am. J. Clin. Nutr.* 1986; 44: 747–755.

50. Choban P, Burge J, and Flancbaum L: Hypoenergetic nutrition support in hospitalized obese patients: a simplified method for clinical application. *Am. J. Clin. Nutr.* 1997; 66: 546.

51. Braga M, Gianotti L, Radaelli G, et al.: Perioperative immunonutrition in patients undergoing cancer surgery. *Arch. Surg.* 1999; 134: 428–433.

52. Galban C, Montejo JC, Mesejo A, et al.: An immune-enhancing enteral diet reduces mortality rate and episodes of bacteremia in septic intensive care patients. *Crit. Care Med.* 2000; 28: 643–648.

53. Gadek JE, DeMichele SJ, Karlstad MD, et al.: Effect of enteral feeding with eicosapentaenoic acid, γ-linolenic acid, and antioxidants in patients with acute respiratory distress syndrome. *Crit. Care Med.* 1999; 27: 1409–1420.

54. Pracht ER, DeMichele SJ, Nelson JL, et al.: Enteral nutrition with eicosapentaenoic acid, γ-linolenic acid, and antioxidants reduces alveolar inflammatory mediators and protein influx in patients with acute respiratory distress syndrome. *Crit. Care Med.* 2003; 31: 491–500.

38 Feeding the Critically Ill Obese Patient

Joseph Lacy, Beverley Borjas, Rebecca Lee, and Jonathan P. Kushner
The University Hospital, Cincinnati

CONTENTS

38.1 INTRODUCTION

Obesity, body fat excess contributing to comorbidity, is a growing global menace that is beginning to rival protein-energy undernutrition as the most common form of malnutrition in the world [1,2]. Obesity is the most common chronic disease and may be the most significant public health problem in the U.S. today, affecting one-third of American adults [3]. Obesity's deleterious effects impinge on practically every organ system in the body and are responsible for ill health in millions. Overweight and obesity are associated with around 300,000 annual deaths [1]. Comorbidities associated with obesity are played out as decreased quality of life, increased work-lost days, hospital days, drug intervention, and physician visits secondary to organ dysfunction [4].

38.2 DEFINING OBESITY/OVERWEIGHT

The accepted standard for defining body weight is the body mass index (BMI), an estimate of body fat. Though not a technical measure of body fat, BMI correlates strongly with obesity, as well as with relative risk of death. Overweight is defined as individuals with a BMI > the 85th percentile

TABLE 38.1

The Third Report of the National Cholesterol Education Program Expert Panel on Detection, Evaluation, and Treatment of High Blood Cholesterol in Adults (ATP III)

Metabolic Syndrome — Defined by ATP III (> 3 of the following abnormalities) [8]:

Waist circumference greater than 102 cm in men and 88 cm in women

Serum triglyceride level of at least 150 mg/dl (1.69 mmol/l)

High-density lipoprotein cholesterol level of less than 40 mg/dl (1.04 mmol/l) in men and 50 mg/dl (1.29 mmol/l) in women

Blood pressure of at least 130/85 mm Hg or serum glucose level of at least 110 mg/dl (6.1 mmol/l)

(referencing weights of persons aged 20 to 29 years). Severely overweight constitutes persons 90th percentile or higher. A BMI > 27 kg/m² is commonly used to define obesity [5].

Adipose tissue distribution influences comorbid risk. Upper body or visceral adipose tissue (central or abdominal obesity) increases morbidity when compared to thigh, buttock, and lower extremity subcutaneous fat [5–7].

38.3 COMORBID CONDITIONS ASSOCIATED WITH OBESITY

Prevalent abnormalities, including visceral fat accumulation, insulin resistance, type 2 diabetes mellitus (DM), hypertriglyceridemia, and hypertension are referred to as the *metabolic syndrome* (Table 38.1 and Table 38.2).

Risk of disease has a curvilinear relationship with weight; with increased weight, prevalence of such illnesses increase proportionally [19–22]. In addition, wound infection, thromboembolic disease, myocardial infarction, respiratory failure requiring mechanical ventilatory support, sepsis, and sudden death are more frequent in this population [17]. Factors contributing to wound issues in trauma patients include the presence of a relatively avascular adiposity (reducing resistance to infection), increased local trauma related to abdominal wall retraction, and increased operative time secondary to large patient mass [11]. Despite the fact that obesity may increase the risk of wound dehiscence, the clinical incidence is < 1%, similar to that following standard abdominal operations [11]. Although obese persons may cope with increased morbidity, data suggest that obesity, even when severe, does not result in unacceptable operative risk [9].

Obesity may cause renal damage in otherwise healthy individuals. Elevated intra-abdominal pressure and altered intrarenal hemodynamics due to medullary compression by perirenal adiposity and increased intrarenal extracellular matrix may contribute to obesity-associated hypertension. Enhanced tubular sodium reabsorption — closely linked to activation of the sympathetic and renin–angiotensin system — may also be involved in obesity-induced hypertension [23].

Obese patients may be more accident-prone and suffer more skeletal fractures. Obese persons use seat belts less often and thus are predisposed to more severe accidental injuries [10].

38.3.1 EFFECT OF OBESITY ON IMMUNITY

The increase in obesity-associated comorbidity is due in part to an impaired immune response; severe obesity is characterized as a chronic inflammatory state associated with immune dysfunction [14,24]. Additionally, obesity may lead to increased autoimmune disorders [24]. Because immunity is impaired, septic event susceptibility may increase. Respiratory and cardiac dysfunction can manifest as prolonged ventilator dependence, recurrent pneumonia, myocardial infarction, congestive heart failure, or recurrent arrhythmias. Despite huge fat reserves and large body cell mass stores, the obese may develop protein-energy malnutrition (PEM) when stressed by critical illness and should be given prompt nutritional support [25]. Obesity increases nosocomial event risk in surgical patients, including wound infection, pneumonia, and *C. difficile* episodes. Following

TABLE 38.2
Organ/Tissue Sequelae of Massive Obesity [1,5,10,11,14–18]

Cardiovascular System
Accelerated atherosclerosis and angina pectoris
Cardiomegaly
Congestive heart failure
Coronary heart disease
Cor pulmonale
Hypertension
Pulmonary embolism
Varicose veins

Endocrine System
Dyslipidemia
Infertility
Metabolic syndrome
Polycystic ovary syndrome
Type 2 diabetes mellitus

Gastrointestinal System
Cholelithiasis
Colon cancer
Gastroesophageal reflux disease
Hernias
Nonalcoholic fatty liver disease
Reflux esophagitis

Genitourinary
Breast cancer
Endometrial hyperplasia and carcinoma of endometrium
Hypogonadism (M)
Prostate cancer
Infertility
Urinary stress incontinence

Immune System
Chronic inflammatory state (higher CRP, orosomucoid, and
  complement C3 and C4, irregularity in lymphocytes)
Depressed immune function:
Impaired cell mediated and
  humoral immunity
Reduced cutaneous delayed-type
  hypersensitivity (DTH) responses,
  mitogen-stimulated lymphocyte
  proliferation, and bactericidal
  capacity of polymorphonuclear
  leukocytes (PMN)
Higher incidence of infection and wound healing:
  C. difficile infection
  Donor site infection
  Nosocomial infection
  Respiratory infection
  Sternal dehiscence
Increased risk of certain forms of cancer:
  Breast — Colon
  Endometrium — Prostate
Increased prevalence of micronutrient deficiency remains
  controversial
Poor antibody response to immunization

Integument
Acanthosis nigricans
Cellulitis
Diminished hygiene
Intertrigo, carbuncles
Venous stasis of legs

Musculoskeletal System
Debilitating arthritis of back and weight-bearing joints
Immobility
Low back pain

Respiratory System
Asthma
Fatigue, dyspnea, diaphoresis
Hypoventilation (Pickwickian) syndrome
Obstructive sleep apnea

Neurological
Idiopathic intracranial hypertension
Meralgia paresthetica
Stroke

Specific to Females
Amenorrhea
Hirsutism
Infertility problems

Psychosocial
Depression
Social discrimination
Work disability

TABLE 38.3
Nutritional Modulation of Immune Response [66–76]

Possible Immuno-Enhancing Regimens	Possible Immunosuppressive Regimens
Meticulous glycemic control	Excessive omega-6 lipid
Key nutrients: arginine, glutamine, nucleotides, omega-3	Overfeeding
fatty acids, antioxidants	TPN
Pre- and postoperative therapy	

gastroplasty or gastric bypass, wound infection is the most common morbidity in obese persons [5]. Certain nutrients have been studied regarding their effects on the immune system (Table 38.3).

38.4 TRAUMA AND OBESITY

Once traumatized, obese patients appear to fare worse than nonobese counterparts. Specialized nutrition support is often required in such instances [9]. In a review of blunt trauma victims, the severely overweight had 42% mortality, compared with 5% for average weight and 8% for over-weight populations. Death was often attributed to fulminant respiratory failure [22].

Malnutrition and its consequences are difficult to avoid in the ICU and, once present, are difficult to treat. Patient selection for nutrition support is the same, irrespective of BMI. In obese patients with illnesses producing significant catabolism, nutrition support should be initiated [26]. In malnourished patients with ≥ 15% weight loss, parenteral nutrition is indicated when enteral therapy is not an option [27].

In patients who have undergone surgical procedures to reduce obesity, the risk of PEM, muscle wasting, reduced serum albumin, and total protein is greater the shorter malabsorptive segment (i.e., the common channel) [3]. Patients with a 75 cm common channel or less may exhibit increased parathyroid hormone (up to 18 months postoperatively) [29].

38.4.1 ENERGY NEEDS

Much obesity-specific nutritional therapy is inferred from general populations. Estimating energy expenditure is problematic in this population of patients [30]. Much of the body weight of severely obese patients is comparatively hypometabolic, and energy expenditure in critically ill persons is variable [28].

Most information regarding nutrient requirements of the obese pertains to energy needs in relation to weight loss, whether by a diet program or by surgical therapy. Debate smolders over the most useful weight measurement for calculating calories (kcal) for obese patients. Use of actual weight for predicting energy needs in overweight individuals may lead to overfeeding [31]. The adjusted body weight (ABW) formula accounts for altered body composition of the obese (addressing the fact that adipose tissue is less metabolically active) [13]. Predictive equations using IBW (based on normal populations) underestimate the resting energy expenditure (REE) of the obese and overestimate REE when actual body weight is employed [13]. More than 75% of obese subjects in Burge's study had initial measured energy consumption that differed from predicted rate (by Harris–Benedict equation) by > 10% [33]. The Ireton-Jones equation for estimating obese patients' energy needs more closely approximates measured indirect calorimetry results [32]. Indirect calorimetry, in most cases, maintains reliability in acute illness [34].

A high respiratory quotient in the fasting state (i.e., a tendency to oxidize more carbohydrate [CHO] than lipid) occurs in the obese [10]. Pulmonary function in the obese is characterized by decreased functional residual capacity, expiratory reserve volume, PaO_2, and an increase in the alveolar–arterial oxygen difference [11].

38.4.1.1 Hypocaloric Feeding

Energy-restricted protein-sparing nutrition support with outpatient weight-reduction dietary regimens is referred to as the *protein-sparing modified fast* (PSMF) [35]. Hypocaloric feeding benefit is attributed to creation of a semistarvation state. Total fasting achieves similar results, but protein-sparing differentiates it from the starvation state and decreases the negative nitrogen (N_2) balance seen in critical illness [36]. Obese persons have increased fat-free body mass and higher energy expenditure compared to normal-weight patients. The thermic effect of food appears to be normal or low in weight-stable obese patients, under usual dietary conditions accounting for 5 to 10% of daily energy expenditure. Intravenous glucose may impair thermic response [37].

The PSMF promotes endogenous fat combustion while maintaining N_2 homeostasis, providing effective weight loss in nonstressed obese patients. Relying on adequate protein delivery while intentionally underfeeding calories, the diet typically provides ≤ 50% of the REE and minimal or no CHO. Hypocalorically fed type 2 DM patients may trend toward decreased insulin requirements [38].

Semistarvation diets have successfully treated obesity in healthy individuals [13]. Hypocaloric feedings optimally should be used to achieve N_2 balance and glucose control rather than weight loss *per se*. Most studies suggest that weight loss in stressed obese patients receiving hypocaloric feeding is minimal. Results of these studies support hypocaloric feeding in patients greater than 130% of IBW and who have normal renal and hepatic function. The hypocaloric formula is administered at a rate providing 2 g of protein per kilogram IBW per day. Successful postoperative hypocaloric nutrition depends on adequate protein provision. Hypocaloric feedings supplying adequate protein to mild-to-moderately obese stressed patients appear capable of achieving N_2 balance (although study numbers are small). Elderly obese, trauma-stressed patients did not secure achievement of N_2 balance with this regimen [39]. Frankenfield et al. reported that, despite wide variation in energy intake among trauma patients receiving hypocaloric vs. eucaloric feedings, no N_2 loss attenuation was seen in either group [40]. Hypocaloric feeding benefit may include improved serum glucose, fluid balance, and ventilatory mechanics, along with decreased weight gain [13,41].

Shikora et al. used a PSMF (based on a diet reported by Baxter and Bistrian) providing protein at 1.5 g/kg of adjusted weight and a total of 60% required kcal. Nonprotein calories were given solely as dextrose. Despite exclusive use of dextrose, elevated blood glucose was rarely evidenced [25]. Administered glucose was within the maximal oxidation potential (5 to 7 mg kg −1 minute −1) [42]. Because less glucose is given with the PSMF, insulin secretion is decreased. Insulin is a potent antinatriuretic hormone and reduced serum levels favor diuresis. By encouraging diuresis and avoiding increased carbon dioxide production, the PSMF may improve respiration [25]. Additionally, weight loss alone in the severely obese can improve arterial blood oxygenation and reduce carbon dioxide retention.

Excessive glucose infusion is associated with lipogenesis. Glucose conversion into fat increases carbon dioxide production, resulting in increased respiratory demand. Importantly, hypocaloric feedings can be administered to mildly-to-moderately stressed hospitalized obese patients, achieving N_2 balance comparable to patients on conventional TPN formulas [33].

Obese persons' ability to use endogenous energy stores during stress is controversial. Any nutritional regimen must provide adequate calories to meet metabolic demands, or the body must mobilize endogenous energy stores for this purpose. Recommendations for nonprotein calorie intake vary widely. Pasulka and Kohl recommend a maximum of 25 kcal/kg. Baxter and Bistrain recommend feeding 300 to 500 kcal less than the measured or predicted energy expenditure in obese patients. Dickerson et al. fed an average of 880 nonprotein kcal to obese subjects, with approximately 14 kcal/kg IBW or 7 kcal/kg actual body weight (ABW). Patients in Burge's study received approximately 14 kcal/kg adjusted body weight (22 kcal/kg IBW) in the hypocaloric group and 25 kcal/kg ABW (42 kcal/kg IBW) in the control group. Burge's findings support that mildly-to-moderately stressed obese patients can liberate body fat for energy while receiving hypocaloric, high-protein nutrition support [33]. Many subjects in this study were postoperative, and some weight loss is attributable to normal postoperative diuresis of pre- and perioperative fluid. Moreover, hypocalorically fed patients may have manifested a decreased insulin response to glucose, resulting in decreased sodium retention and less weight gain. This indicates that mildly-to-moderately stressed patients receiving hypocaloric parenteral nutrition could achieve N_2 balance, compared to patients receiving normocaloric parenteral nutrition [33].

Das et al. saw a decrease in REE by 25% after massive weight loss in patients undergoing gastric bypass [43]. Yet drawing correlation from nonstressed clinical situations to stressed ones is done with trepidation.

Remaining to be demonstrated is comprehensive treatment resulting in improved fluid and electrolyte status, body composition changes, and length-of-stay differences [13].

38.4.2 Protein Needs

For severely stressed obese patients to reach optimal nutrient intake, macronutrients are prioritized: protein is given first, followed by CHO, and finally lipid. In addition to maintenance of normal needs, the stressed body requires increased N_2. During critical illness, caloric need in general increases marginally, but protein need can double or triple. Attenuating N_2 loss and improving retention of body protein should help to maintain or improve visceral function. Although this is likely true in the long term, it is difficult to establish in the short term [27].

Limited evidence suggests that the metabolic response to injury in obese patients differs from that in normal-weight individuals [44]. Traumatized obese patients mobilize more protein and less fat than nonobese subjects, perhaps because of a relative block in lipolysis and fat oxidation. Jeevanandam postulates that acutely injured obese patients have a reduced ability to mobilize fat stores and a limited capacity to oxidize fat. Although obese patients' energy needs may be comparable to their nonobese counterparts, nonobese patients exhibit an expected increase in net fat oxidation, but obese patients derive a significantly lower percentage of energy from fat. Additionally, plasma glycerol levels are reduced in the obese, whereas plasma free fatty acid levels are increased and whole-body lipolytic rate may be reduced [45]. Jeevanandam also observed increased energy production supplied from CHO and protein oxidation in obese subjects compared to nonobese. Urinary N_2 losses were significantly greater in obese patients (22.2 ± 3.2 g/d) than in nonobese controls (14.3 ± 1.7 g/d). These results underscore that posttrauma obese patients are not nutritionally protected because of their excess weight [45].

During stress, glucocorticoids alter homeostasis such that muscle protein is catabolized for energy. A 24-hour urine urea N_2 (UUN) helps to estimate protein need. Current practice for protein therapy in obese patients approximates 1.5 to 2 g of protein per kilogram IBW, depending on caloric content of the feeding [13].

Infusion of glucose-free amino acids as the sole nutritional source decreases net N_2 loss but does not prevent it [46]. Administering glucose nonprotein calories at only 50% of REE results in net protein anabolism, demonstrated by N_2 equilibrium or positive N_2 balance, an increase in serum proteins, and complete wound healing. Current literature on both obese and nonobese patients suggests that N_2 intake may be the more important factor in promoting positive N_2 balance [41]. Despite achieving positive N_2 balance, the efficiency of N_2 use appears low. This apparent efficiency is comparable to the findings of Greenberg, who provided protein without nonprotein calories to obese subjects and submitted that the efficiency of N_2 use is lower when energy is derived primarily from endogenous stores [46]. With increased energy intake, the effect on N_2 retention appears to attenuate. At constant protein intake, low energy intake improves N_2 balance by ~7.5 mg N_2/kcal supplied to unstressed depleted patients [46]. This anabolic effect decreases to 1 to 2 mg N_2 retained per additional calorie received when caloric intake exceeds 50 to 60% REE [42].

Protein intake was consistent within recommended levels: hypocaloric subjects received 2.0 g of protein per kilogram IBW. Pasulka and Kohl recommended an intake of 1.5 to 1.7 g of protein per kilogram IBW, as did Baxter [33]. Dickerson fed 2.13 g of protein per kilogram IBW to obese patients. These patients tended to be mildly-to-moderately stressed, with initial UUN values ranging from 1.6 to 15 g/d. Despite this, mean N_2 balance was positive in both groups and did not differ significantly [41].

When evaluated by group, the correlation with total body N_2 excretion, UUN, was maintained only in the control group (not in the hypocaloric group). This suggests that provision of adequate energy in the control group led to decreased protein catabolism, primarily in skeletal muscle. The hypothesis stands that mildly-to-moderately stressed obese patients can liberate body fat for energy while receiving hypocaloric, high-protein nutrition support [33].

38.4.3 FAT

Of concern in a population with an increased incidence of fatty liver is the hepatic dysfunction of critical illness. Such hepatic dysfunction may manifest as lipid intolerance, lipemic serum, hypercholesterolemia, and hypertriglyceridemia [26]. Additionally, altered distribution of lipophilic drugs may occur [10]. In theory, Kuppfer cells laden with fat may result in an impaired immune response [47]. During acute stress, the majority of energy requirements (up to 80%) are obtained from oxidation of free fatty acids liberated from adipocyte triglyceride stores [10].

Steatosis occurs in most obese patients; abnormal fatty infiltrate of hepatocytes is a linear function of body weight [48]. Excessive caloric or glucose infusion may contribute to fatty liver. The combination of excess glucose and hyperinsulinemia may promote hepatic triglyceride deposition.

Trauma can increase serum free fatty acid levels along with increasing serum triglycerides. It is noteworthy that a correlation exists between serum free fatty acid level and hypoxemia [22].

Lipid administration > 3 g/kg/d is associated with cholestasis (resolving after decreasing or discontinuing lipid infusion) [49]. Some proclaim that the rationale for providing parenteral lipid as a source of essential fatty acids does not appear justified, particularly if patients have a slightly negative energy balance. Around 10% of fat stores are composed of linoleic acid; the 2.0 to 3.5 g/d requirement for linoleic acid theoretically can be obtained from mobilization of 20 to 35 g/d (< 350 kcal/d) of endogenous fat. Plasma linoleic acid level is maintained after 10 to 14 days of an amino acid infusion (1.5 g/kg/d of protein) in nonobese postsurgical patients. Parnes et al. examined the effect of long-term (median: 20 days; range: 8 to 58 days) fat-free total parenteral nutrition in obese leukemic patients with negligible oral intake. Patients were fed an intravenous solution with 300 kcal/d less than estimated REE. No apparent signs of EFAD were seen, and the triene-to-tetraene ratio, an index of essential fatty acid deficiency, remained unchanged. Patients receiving maintenance energy did not have endogenous essential fatty acid release and, therefore, should be provided with a lipid source.

In patients exhibiting obesity-altered immunity, the potential negative impact of high linoleic acid intake on immune function must be considered. Excessive fat may affect immunocytes by direct mechanical effect or through altered prostaglandin and leukotriene synthesis [50–52]. The current recommendation for lipid administration in general patient populations is 1g/kg/d, or 25% to 30% of total calories [53].

It was initially presumed that stressed obese patients would be less able to mobilize endogenous fat for energy than stressed nonobese counterparts, but Dickerson et al. demonstrated N_2 balance in mild-to-moderately stressed obese patients receiving parenteral nutrition [18]. In fact, 68% of nonprotein energy expenditure may result from endogenous fat oxidation [41].

Patients with metabolic syndrome have higher circulating insulin, lower hepatic insulin extraction, greater insulin resistance, an elevated serum triglyceride, and a reduced high-density lipoprotein, which, in many respects, resembles the metabolic and hormonal profile of the physiologic response to injury.

Elevated serum triglycerides before or during parenteral lipid infusion may limit the use of exogenous lipid as a source of calories in some patients, including the obese. Additionally, obese patients may differ in metabolic response to severe trauma; some may have a comparative block in lipid mobilization and oxidation, resulting in preferential use of CHO calories fueled by increased breakdown of endogenous protein. Trials evaluating parenteral hypocaloric feedings in hospitalized obese patients (> 130% IBW) with various degrees of stress, showed that hypocaloric nutritional regimens providing 50% of nonprotein calories, compared with a control formula (while supplying adequate amounts of protein at 2 g/kg IBW per day), had equal efficacy in achieving positive N_2 balance. These data suggest that stressed obese patients are capable of using endogenous lipid stores for energy if provided adequate protein; thus it is prudent to note that at least hypocaloric nutrition support should be initiated early in stressed obese patients to preserve body cell mass and that such patients should not be expected to "live off their fat," as is commonly misconceived [9].

Whether the stressed obese patient on a hypocaloric feeding regimen can adequately mobilize and oxidize endogenous fat is controversial. In the nonstressed patient, decreased insulin secretion and insufficient caloric administration favor fat mobilization and oxidation. Nonetheless, critical illness may alter normal metabolic pathways. Critically ill obese patients not given nutrition support have demonstrated poor fat oxidation. In contrast, using indirect calorimetry Dickerson et al. estimated fat oxidation at 68% of nonprotein energy expenditure in a similar population of stressed obese patients receiving hypocaloric parenteral nutrition [41].

Indirect calorimetry reveals consistently low respiratory quotients, confirming endogenous fat oxidation during hypocaloric, high-protein feedings and use of endogenous caloric stores for energy needs [41].

Mobilization of stored lipid releases more than the 2 to 3.5 g of linoleic acid required daily. Even if lipolysis and fat oxidation are poor in stressed obese patients, most would only require intravenous nutrition for a limited period. For longer support, a lipid infusion can be given once weekly to prevent EFAD [25].

38.4.4 GLUCOSE AND INSULIN

Obesity results in myriad abnormal metabolic processes, the central of which involves insulin [44]. Abdominal obesity in particular is a marker for insulin resistance [12]. During stress, high insulin levels impede normal adaptive mechanisms. As a result, muscle protein is actively catabolized. Stressed obese patients may be less able to mobilize fat for energy than stressed nonobese patients, at least early post trauma [26].

A flourishing body of data links obesity to impaired immune function (see Table 38.2). Still, the exact effect of obesity on immunity remains obscure. Insulin resistance and glucose intolerance have been linked with hyperglycemia-related immune dysfunction. Excess administration of dextrose intensifies lipogenesis, which may lead to hepatic steatosis and resultant hepatic dysfunction. A glucose overabundance may increase CO_2 production, increasing respiratory work. If underlying respiratory dysfunction is present, then respiratory failure may ensue.

Baxter and Bistrian have recommended a minimum of 150 g/d dextrose to prevent ketosis and provide additional calories, with a maximum CHO intake of 300 g/d [54]. CHO stores are rapidly consumed following injury, and glucose-dependent organs are fueled by gluconeogenesis from glucogenic amino acids and glycerol, despite a loss of sensitivity to insulin as an initial metabolic defect in the obese [55]. The insulin resistance of obesity is both a cellular receptor and postreceptor phenomenon [56]. Because trauma elicits insulin resistance secondary to proinflammatory cytokine influence on the hormonal milieu, the injured obese are in particular likely to develop hyperglycemia during nutrition support, necessitating exogenous insulin coverage.

Adiposity, in tandem with often-accompanying anasarca in the critically ill, makes glucose control difficult by subcutaneous soluble insulin, thereby necessitating insulin infusion [10].

Eighty percent of people with type 2 DM are overweight. Weight loss not only decreases type 2 DM severity but also may result in euglycemia [13]. During injury, the body increases its nutrient substrate pool. Fat and protein oxidation rates are increased, plasma glycerol and free fatty acids rise, urinary urea excretion is increased, and N_2 balance is negative in the absence of nutrition support.

Yendamuri et al. studied trauma admission hyperglycemia as a prognostic indicator. Hyperglycemia independently predicted increased intensive care unit and hospital length of stay and mortality in the trauma population; hyperglycemia was associated with increased infectious morbidity. These associations held true for both mild and moderate hyperglycemia [57]. Van den Berghe et al. reported decreased mortality with vigilant insulin in critically ill surgical patients [58].

Excess parenteral glucose can enhance lipogenesis, causing hepatic steatosis and liver dysfunction. Hyperglycemia may adversely affect immunological function in patients, increasing untoward infectious risk, including sepsis [18,25].

The severely overweight are even more affected by operations because their heavy chest walls and increased intra-abdominal pressures augment respiratory work. Excess glucose administration can increase CO_2 production, which further increases respiratory work. For obese patients with underlying respiratory compromise, such a level of respiratory demand can lead to failure.

Addition of a nonprotein calorie source such as glucose may enhance protein sparing, at least in part due to attenuation of protein catabolism for gluconeogenesis. After rapid depletion of glycogen stores, the body relies on gluconeogenesis to provide glucose to glucose-dependent tissues, such as the immune system, the healing wound, and the peripheral nervous system.

The amount of glucose necessary to achieve maximal protein sparing is unknown. N_2 preservation increases with higher caloric administration, but the effect is blunted as energy delivery increases > 60% of REE [59]. It may be postulated that the total calories provided must exceed ~60% of the energy expenditure to be effective. A severely calorie-restricted diet (i.e., providing < 50% of energy expenditure) should be avoided [25]. One strategy provides ~60% of measured calories, along with adequate protein. When estimating energy expenditure, an adjusted body weight that assumes a larger-than-normal lean body mass may be employed. Again, only ~60% of required calories are provided. This achieves similar results suggested by Baxter, who based calorie provision on 8 to 12 kcal/lb actual weight minus 300 to 500 kcal at a maximum of 2000 kcal/d [25].

Gamble suggested 100 g of dextrose daily provides near-optimal protein sparing. Little further reduction in N_2 excretion was achieved by providing larger amounts (200 g) of dextrose. Less than 100 g will provoke unnecessary catabolism of tissue protein to provide energy and lead to excessive production of ketone bodies and the potential of inducing acidosis [27].

Hyperinsulinemia and exaggerated insulin response to glucose are among the hallmarks of obesity [60]. The central nervous system and other glucose-demanding tissue require about 125 g of glucose daily; this obligatory glucose need may be met via gluconeogenesis from protein catabolism (after depletion of glycogen stores) and glycerol. Dickerson demonstrated in obese patients (requiring parenteral nutrition for postoperative complications) that net protein anabolism could be achieved with hypocaloric, high-protein feeding. Patients received ~50% measured REE as nonprotein calories and 2.13 ± 0.59 g/kg IBW. With endogenous adipose stores supplying energy, patients lost weight while healing wounds and closing fistulae. Indirect calorimetry revealed low respiratory quotients, confirming endogenous fat oxidation for metabolic need during hypocaloric, high-protein parenteral nutrition. Although insulin can decrease proliferation of T-cells in diabetic persons [60], of significance, no changes were noted in the total lymphocyte count during the hypocaloric regimen [41].

38.4.5 MICRONUTRIENTS

Until more information is available on specific guidelines for obesity, it is recommended to saturate micronutrient stores. Daily nutrient guidelines were not formulated for a severely ill patient population; hence, adequacy of such should be viewed with suspicion. The American Medical Association guidelines for parenteral vitamin intake have been updated to include higher concentrations of vitamins.

An increase in reactive oxygen species-induced damage in lipid, protein, and amino acid occurs in the obese, as well as a decreased antioxidant status after glucose challenge [68,69]. Moreover, oxidant formation contributes to vascular disease and dysfunction. In contrast, exercise-dependent production of oxidants may stimulate adaptive responses that protect against development of such diseases [63]. Until proved otherwise, physical therapy should be a component of care in such patients.

Antioxidant therapy may be valuable in the regeneration of cytoprotective enzymes and the restoration of endothelial function in obesity [23]. A hypoenergetic diet rich in antioxidants (along with omega-3 fat) has shown benefit in obese patients with fatty liver [64].

38.4.6 FLUID

Abnormalities in cardiac function may predispose obese trauma patients to congestive heart failure during nutrition support. Appropriate fluid balance is imperative because a higher protein (or protein equivalent) regimen increases hydration need for optimum metabolism. In the ICU setting, pulmonary artery catheters are often placed to monitor hemodynamic status.

38.5 ROUTE OF FEEDING

38.5.1 PARENTERAL NUTRITION

The loss of anatomic landmarks secondary to subcutaneous fat in obese patients may make placing catheters for parenteral nutrition support difficult [9]. This may result in an increased risk of catheter-associated infection [10].

In patients requiring parenteral nutrition who are greater than 130% of IBW or have a BMI > 27 kg/m^2, the hypocaloric formula often provided includes 2 g protein/kg IBW/d in patients with normal renal and hepatic function [26]. This hypocaloric strategy may not be applicable to patients with significant renal or hepatic dysfunction, which generally mandates restriction of protein intake to avoid severe azotemia (BUN > 100 mg/dl) and hepatic encephalopathy. In such patients, protein is administered at a dose of 0.8 to 1.2 g/kg IBW/d and nonprotein calories provided at a quantity based on degree of stress [26].

38.5.2 ENTERAL NUTRITION

A large body of literature describes lowered complication rates and favorable effect on metabolic and immune function with enteral nutrition [65–75]. The infusion of intraluminal nutrients, important for maintaining gut mucosal integrity (and likely whole-body mucosal integrity), is a key factor for homeostasis and immunological competence. A growing number of studies demonstrate improved N$_2$ balance, lower infection rates, improved wound healing, and attenuation of the stress response with early enteral nutrition [36]. Patients receiving early enteral feeding, particularly following accidental injury, have fewer complications than comparable parenterally fed patients [27].

For obese patients relatively healthy prior to the onset of illness or for those undergoing elective surgery, common practice is to consider enteral or parenteral nutrition support after 5 to 7 days without oral intake [26]. Obese patients are more likely to face long periods of inadequate oral nutrition and to require nutrition support to avoid loss of body cell mass [54]. The window of opportunity for positive clinical outcome with enteral feeding probably varies for different disease states. Such parameters remain largely unknown in the obese population. In most cases, feeding is initiated shortly after achievement of hemodynamic stability (usually within 24 to 48 hours post admission).

Enteral nutrition support is not without caveat in the obese. The risk of aspiration pneumonia is greatly increased in the obese patient [10]. Obese patients have a higher gastric residual volume with lower intragastric pH than do the nonobese, placing obese persons at greater risk for pulmonary aspiration and pneumonitis, in part due to delayed gastric emptying and elevated acid secretory capacity [9]. For the seriously obese, the risks of feeding tube placement are not minimal. Increased adiposity of the soft tissues of the palate and pharynx may delay and even preclude simple blind placement. In addition, underlying conditions such as pulmonary insufficiency or severe degenerative joint disease may prevent the patient's remaining supine and cooperating for the procedure. Respiratory difficulties may further be compounded by the occlusion of a nostril with the tube (especially if a nasogastric drainage tube is already in place). Once placed, verification of tube position by auscultation may be unreliable because of muffled sound through a thickened abdominal wall. Patients weighing > 180 kg may be unable to undergo fluoroscopy because of their weight and size [36].

A hypocaloric enterally fed group had a shorter ICU stay, decreased duration of antibiotic days, and a trend toward decreased days of mechanical ventilation. No significant difference in N_2 balance or serum prealbumin was seen between groups [76].

Although hypocaloric protein-sparing was conceived for parenteral nutrition support, its attractive points lend to enteral therapy as well. The clinician can formulate a modular solution using protein and CHO or use a commercially prepared product [36].

38.6 CONCLUSION

Manipulating nutrients in the very sick with superimposed obesity proves a tenuous task. In supplying nutrition for the acutely ill obese, more questions than answers abound. Although much has been learned regarding the treatment of obesity, no clear-cut answer exists on how to best feed the critically ill obese patient. Much of nutrition support in the obese is inferred data; more studies may clarify the optimal recipe for nutrition support in the obese.

REFERENCES

1. Kushner, R.F., Medical management of obesity, *Sem. Gastr. Dis.*, 13, 123, 2002.
2. Deitel, M. and Shikora S.A., The development of the surgical treatment of morbid obesity, *J. Am. Coll. Nutr.*, 21, 365, 2002.
3. Choban, P.S. et al., Bariatric surgery for morbid obesity: why, who, when, how, where, and then what? *Cleveland Clinic J. Med.*, 69, 897, 2002.
4. Wolf, A.M. and Colditz, G.A., Current estimates of the economic cost of obesity in the United States, *Obes. Res.*, 6, 97, 1998.
5. Choban, P.S. et al., Increased incidence of nosocomial infections in obese surgical patients, *Am. Surg.*, 61, 1001, 1995.
6. Kissebah, A.H. et al., Relation of body fat distribution to metabolic complications of obesity, *J. Clin. Endocrinol. Metab.*, 54, 254, 1982.
7. Fujikora S. et al., Contribution of intra-abdominal fat accumulation to the impairment of glucose and lipid metabolism in human obesity, *Metab.*, 36, 54, 1987.
8. Ford E.S., Giles W.H., and Dietz W.H., Prevalence of the metabolic syndrome among U.S. adults, *JAMA*, 287, 356, 2002.
9. Choban, P.S. and Flancbaum, L., The impact of obesity on surgical outcomes: a review, *Am. Coll. Surg.*, 185, 593, 1997.
10. Varon, J. and Marik, P., Management of the obese critically ill patient, *Crit. Care Clin.* 17, 187, 2001.
11. Flancbaum L. and Choban, P.S., Surgical implications of obesity, *Annu. Rev. Med.*, 49, 215, 1998.

12. Little, P. and Byrne C.D., Abdominal obesity and the "hypertriglyceridaemic waist" phenotype, *BMJ*, 322, 687, 2001.

13. Burge, J.C., Obesity, in *Contemporary Nutrition Support Practice*, Matarese, L.E. and Gottschlich, M.M. Eds., Saunders, St. Louis, 2003, chap. 38.

14. Hanusch-Enserer, U. et al., Acute-phase response and immunological makers in morbid obese patients and patients following adjustable gastric banding, *Int. J. Obes.*, 27, 355, 2003.

15. Hulsewé, K.W. et al., Nutritional depletion and dietary manipulation: effects on the immune response, *World J. Surg.*, 23, 536, 1999.

16. Stallone, D.D., The influence of obesity and its treatment on the immune system, *Nutr. Rev.*, 52, 37, 1994.

17. Kim, J.J. et al., Surgical treatment for extreme obesity: evolution of a rapidly growing field, *Nutr. Clin. Pract.*, 18, 109, 2003.

18. Hostetter, M.K., Handicaps to host defense, *Diabetes*, 39, 271, 1990.

19. van Itallie, T.B., Health implications of overweight and obesity in the United States, *Ann. Intern. Med.*, 103, 983, 1985.

20. Kral, J.G., Morbid obesity and related health risks, *Ann. Intern. Med.*, 103, 1043, 1985.

21. Drenick, E.J., Sudden cardiac arrest in morbidly obese surgical patients unexplained after autopsy, *Am. J. Surg.*, 155, 720, 1988.

22. Choban, P.S., Weireter, L.J., and Maynes C., Obesity and increased mortality in blunt trauma, *J. Trauma*, 31, 1253, 1991.

23. Saxena, A.K, Renal repercussions of an emerging global "epidemic" of obesity, *BMJ*, 315, 997, 1997.

24. Cottam, D.R. et al., Effect of surgically-induced weight loss on leukocyte indicators of chronic inflammation in morbid obesity, *Obes. Surg.* 12, 335, 2002.

25. Shikora S.A. and Muskat, P.C., Protein-sparing modified-fast total parenteral nutrition formulation for a critically ill morbidly obese patient, *Nutr.*, 10, 155, 1994.

26. Choban, P.S. and Flancbaum, L., Nourishing the obese patient, *Clin. Nutr.*, 19, 305, 2000.

27. Wilmore, D.W., Postoperative protein sparing, *World J. Surg.*, 23, 545, 1999.

28. Shikora, S.A. and Jensen, G.L., Hypoenergetic nutrition support in hospitalized obese patients, *Am. J. Clin. Nutr.*, 66, 679, 1997.

29. Hamoui, N. et al., The significance of elevated levels of parathyroid hormone in patients with morbid obesity before and after bariatric surgery, *Arch. Surg.*, 138, 891, 2003.

30. Ireton-Jones, C.S. and Francis, C., Obesity: nutrition support practice and application to critical care, *Nutr. Clin. Pract.*, 10, 144, 1995.

31. Cutts, M.E. et al., Predicting energy needs in ventilator-dependent critically ill patients: effect of adjusting weight for edema or adiposity, *Am. J. Clin. Nutr.*, 66, 1250, 1997.

32. Ireton-Jones, C.S. et al., Equations for estimation of energy expenditure in patients with burns with special reference to ventilatory status, *J. Burn Care Rehabil.*, 13, 330, 1992.

33. Burge, J.C. et al., Efficacy of hypocaloric total parenteral nutrition in hospitalized obese patients: a prospective, double-blind randomized trial, *J. Parenter. Enteral Nutr.*, 18, 203, 1994.

34. Flancbaum, L. et al., Comparison of indirect calorimetry, the Fick method, and prediction equations in estimating the energy requirements of critically ill patients, *Am. J. Clin. Nutr.*, 69, 461, 1999.

35. Bistrian, B.R., Clinical use of a protein-sparing modified fast, *JAMA*, 240, 2299, 1972.

36. Shikora, S.A., Enteral feeding tube placement in obese patients: considerations for nutrition support, *Nutr. Clin. Pract.*, 12, 9S, 1997.

37. de Jonge, L. and Bray, G.A., The thermic effect of food and obesity: a critical review, *Obes. Res.*, 5, 622, 1997.

38. Choban, P.S. et al., Hypoenergenic nutrition support in hospitalized patients: a simplified method for clinical application, *Am. J. Clin. Nutr.*, 66, 546, 1997.

39. Liu, K. et al., Hypocaloric parenteral nutrition support in elderly obese patients, *Am. Surg.*, 66, 394, 2000.

40. Frankenfield, D.C., Smith, J.S., and Cooney, R.N., Accelerated nitrogen loss after traumatic injury is not attenuated by achievement of energy balance, *J. Parenter. Enteral Nutr.*, 21, 324, 1997.

41. Dickerson, R.N., Rosato, E.F., and Mullen, J.L., Net protein anabolism with hypocaloric parenteral nutrition in obese stressed patients, *Am. J. Clin. Nutr.*, 44, 55, 1986.

42. Wolfe, R.R. et al., Investigation of factors determining the optimal glucose infusion rate in total parenteral nutrition, *Metab.*, 29, 892, 1980.

43. Das, S.K. et al., Long-term changes in energy expenditure and body composition after massive weight loss induced by gastric bypass surgery, *Am. J. Clin. Nutr.*, 78, 22, 2003.

44. Jeevanandam, J., Ramias, L. and Schiller, W.R., Altered plasma free amino acid levels in obese traumatized man, *Metab.*, 40, 385, 1991.

45. Jeevanandam, M., Young, D.H. and Schiller, W.R., Obesity and the metabolic response to severe multiple trauma in man, *J. Clin. Invest.*, 87, 262, 1991.

46. Greenberg, G.R. et al., Protein sparing therapy in postoperative patients, *N. Engl. J. Med.*, 294, 1411, 1976.

47. Trahan, K.T. and Gore, D.C., Nutritional support, *Chest Surg. Clin. N. Am.*, 12, 227, 2002.

48. Buckwald, H., Lober, P.H., and Varco, R.L., Liver biopsy findings in seventy-seven consecutive patients undergoing jejunoileal bypass for morbid obesity, *Am. J. Surg.*, 127, 48, 1974.

49. Allardyce, D.B., Cholestasis caused by lipid emulsions, *Surg. Gynecol. Obstet.*, 112, 509, 1982.

50. Alexander, J.W., Immunonutrition: the role of ω-3 fatty acids, *Nutr.*, 14(7/8), 627, 1998.

51. Grimble, R.F., Nutrition modulation of cytokine biology. *Nutr.*, 14(7/8), 634, 1998.

52. Kinsella, J.E. and Lokesh B., Dietary lipids, eicosanoids and the immune system, *Crit. Care Med.* 18, S94, 1990.

53. Skipper, A., Parenteral nutrition, in *Contemporary Nutrition Support Practice*, Matarese, L.E. and Gottschlich, M.M. Eds., Saunders, St. Louis, 2003, chap. 18.

54. Baxter, J.K. and Bistrian, B.R., Moderate hypocaloric parenteral nutrition in the critically ill, obese patient, *Nutr. Clin. Pract.*, 4, 133, 1989.

55. Garrow, J., Importance of obesity, *BMJ*, 303, 704, 1991.

56. Grundy, S.M. and Barnett, J.P., Metabolic and health complications of obesity, *Dis. Mon.*, 36, 641, 1990.

57. Yendamuri, S., Fulda, J.G., and Tinkoff, G.H., Admission hyperglycemia as a prognostic indicator in trauma, *J. Trauma*, 55, 33, 2003.

58. Van den Berghe G. et al., Intensive insulin therapy in critically ill patients, *N. Engl. J. Med.*, 345, 1359, 2001.

59. Elwyn, D.H., Kinney, J.M. and Askanazi, J., Energy expenditure in surgical patients, *Surg. Clin. North Am.*, 61, 545, 1981.

60. Mito, N. et al., Effect of obesity and insulin on immunity in non-insulin-dependent diabetes mellitus, *Eur. J. Clin. Nutr.*, 45, 347, 2002.

61. Dandona, P. et al., The suppressive effect of dietary restriction and weight loss in the obese on the generation of reactive oxygen species by leukocytes, lipid peroxidation, and protein carbonylation, *J. Clin. Endocrinol. Metab.*, 86, 355, 2001.

62. Mohanty, P. et al., Glucose challenge stimulates reactive oxygen species (ROS) generation by leucocytes, *J. Clin. Endocrinol. Metab.*, 85, 2970, 2000.

63. Fenster, C.P. et al., Obesity, aerobic exercise, and vascular disease: the role of oxidant stress, *Obes. Res.*, 10, 964, 2002.

64. Okita, M. et al., Effect of a moderately energy-restricted diet on obese patients with fatty liver, *Nutr.*, 17, 542, 2001.

65. Alexander, J.W., Immunonutrition: the role of ω-3 fatty acids. *Nutr.* 14(7/8), 627, 1998.

66. Atkinson, S. et al., A prospective, randomized, double-blind, controlled clinical trial of enteral immunonutrition in the critically ill, *Crit. Care Med.*, 26(7), 1164, 1998.

67. Beale R.J. et al., Immunonutrition in the critically ill: a systematic review of clinical outcome. *Crit. Care Med.*, 27(12), 2799, 1999.

68. Braga M. et al., Preoperative oral arginine and n-3 fatty acid supplementation improves the immunometabolic host response and outcome after colorectal resection for cancer. *Surg.*, 132, 805, 2002.

69. Galbán C. et al., An immune-enhancing enteral diet reduces mortality and episodes of bacteremia in septic ICU patients, *J. Parenter. Enteral Nutr.* 22(1), 513, 1998.

70. Gianotti L. et al., A randomized controlled trial of preoperative oral supplementation with a specialized diet in patients with gastrointestinal cancer, *Gastroent.* 122, 1763, 2002.

71. Heys S. et al., Enteral nutritional supplementation with key nutrients in patients with critical illness and cancer: a meta-analysis of randomized controlled clinical trials, *Ann. Surg.* 229(4), 467, 1999.

72. Kudsk, K.A., Current aspects of mucosal immunology and its influence by nutrition, *Am. J. Surg.* 183, 390, 2002.

73. Marik P.E. et al., Early enteral nutrition in acutely ill patients: a systematic review, *Crit. Care Med.*,29, 2264, 2001.

74. Proceedings from Summit on Immune-Enhancing Enteral Therapy, supplement to *J. Parenter. Enteral Nutr.* 25(2) Mar–Apr, 2001.

75. Tepaske R. et al., Effect of preoperative oral immune-enhancing nutritional supplement on patients at high risk of infection after cardiac surgery: a randomised placebo-controlled trial, *Lancet* 358, 696, 2001.

76. Dickerson, R.N. et al., Hypocaloric enteral tube feeding in critically ill obese patients, *Nutr.*, 18, 241, 2002.

Section VIII

Professional Issues

39 Ethical Considerations

M. Patricia Fuhrman
Coram Healthcare

CONTENTS

39.1 INTRODUCTION

Ethical considerations in the intensive care setting revolve around the behaviors, expectations, and actions of the patient, the healthcare providers, and the legal system. The technological capabilities within the intensive care unit (ICU) to sustain life have increased the responsibilities of each of these entities to focus on what can be done vs. what should be done. Areas that appear to have the greatest challenges associated with them are effective communication among the patient, family members, and healthcare providers; surrogate decision making; provision of futile care; and termination of care. The turmoil stems in part from the replacement of the primary care physician with an intensivist and the absence of a long-standing relationship and familiarity with the patient and the family. The harsh reality is that 60% of deaths in the United States occur in acute care facilities; 75% of these deaths result after the decision to forgo life-sustaining medical therapy (1). Eighty-five percent of all cancer patients admitted to the ICU die while in the ICU (2). These statistics clearly demonstrate that difficult decisions concerning perpetuation and discontinuation of therapy occur daily in the ICU setting with critically patients, their families, and healthcare providers.

Difficult decisions abound in the ICU. Experience, training, and knowledge underscore the approach to treatment for most healthcare professionals. According to Valentin et al., critically ill men received an increased level of care with more invasive procedures than critically ill women who had a higher severity of illness (3). Interestingly, the higher level of care did not translate into improved outcomes over those of the female patients. It is unknown whether this bias in treatment was due to patient and family preferences or subjective decisions of healthcare clinicians (4).

The probability that a treatment will be successful based on population studies (evidence-based medicine) must be transcribed to the individual patient in the ICU. Technology can save lives, and

TABLE 39.1
Ethical Principles of Interacting with Patients

Beneficence
  Relieve suffering
  Enhance quality of life
  Provide peace of mind
Autonomy
  Communicate clearly and accurately in a timely manner
  Share information
  Obtain informed consent
Nonmaleficence
  Do no harm
Justice
  Provide care to which patient is entitled

Sources: From Herrmann, V.M., Nutrition support: ethical or expedient, and who will choose?, *J. Parenter. Enteral Nutr.*, 23, 195, 1999; Latimer, E.J., Ethical care at the end of life, *Can. Med. Assoc. J.*, 158, 1741, 1998.

it can increase pain and suffering for those who cannot be saved (5). Each of these potential outcomes must be measured equally in order to use the technology for the benefit and not to the detriment of the patient. An ethnographic study of three critical care units found that end-of-life care was determined by the administrative model (6). A surgeon-managed ICU was focused on "defeating death." An intensivist-managed ICU was focused on conserving resources and maximizing quality of life. Ideally a synergy between these two perspectives would champion life without increasing pain and suffering or squandering human and material resources. The four ethical principles for healthcare providers to follow when interacting with patients are listed and described in Table 39.1 (7,8).

39.2 COMMUNICATION

Communication, or the lack thereof, among healthcare providers, families, and patients has been a topic of concern among healthcare providers and patients (9–11). Hippocrates (460–370 BC) encouraged the physician to provide paternalistic care to the patient with "cheerfulness and sincerity" while "revealing nothing of the patient's future or present condition." The current healthcare environment encourages a patient-centered approach, with the patient an active participant in the decision-making process. Informed consent requires that the patient be told the whole truth, has the right to refuse treatment, has the right to read and copy the medical record, and has the right to privacy and human dignity (12). However, the timing and language used to communicate information can maintain an unequal distribution of information between the patient and the healthcare provider. It is important to remember that communication is not just revealing information to the patient and family but is also the art of listening and hearing what the patient and family comprehend and have to say. Healthcare providers should encourage patients to communicate their wishes for treatment when nearing the end of life.

Patients can communicate their wishes concerning medical care through advance directives. Healthcare professionals and family members can more readily follow the patient's wishes if the advance directive is specific and detailed as to the circumstances under which the patient does and does not want curative therapy or palliative care. Other topics often addressed in advance directives are preferences concerning withdrawing or withholding medical care (including nutrition), organ donation, and cardiopulmonary resuscitation and intubation. Do-not-resuscitate (DNR) provides specific guidelines for healthcare professionals in the event of cardiac arrest. Do-not-intubate (DNI) provides specific guidelines for healthcare professionals in the event of pulmonary failure. Durable power of attorney involves the legal appointment of someone to make decisions for the patient in the event the patient is unable to make decisions concerning his or her care.

The Joint Commission on Accreditation of Healthcare Organizations (JCAHO) standards include patient-focused functions related to patients' rights and organization ethics (13). The JCAHO standards address the patient's right to participate in decisions regarding his or her care, including the right to refuse treatment, including nutrition. The standards also state that the patient must be informed of the risks, benefits, and burdens of nutrition support. The patient should also have the opportunity to specify his or her preferences, goals, and values regarding medical care, including nutrition support, through advance directives. JCAHO reviewers look for a process within each facility that meets these standards.

Advance directives and do-not-resuscitate orders can be ineffectually communicated as a patient moves from one institution to another or from the care of one physician to another (14). Unwanted treatment can be avoided if the patient restates his or her wishes or if the surrogate decision maker is familiar with the patient's advance directives. The more comprehensive and specific the patient's advance directive, the more readily a surrogate can make decisions that are congruent with the patient's wishes. It is ironic that less than 1% of clinicians routinely offer end-of-life care plans to patients that provide terminal sedation in place of mechanical ventilation for patients with severe obstructive lung disease and that 98% of these clinicians, if faced with the same situation, would prefer terminal sedation for themselves (14).

Communication throughout the ICU stay is vital to making effective decisions concerning how best to provide care. A study by Lilly et al. examined the impact of intensive communication on mortality, morbidity, and length of ICU stay using counseling sessions during intensive care admission (9). The sessions were a noncoercive, patient- and family-centered, multidisciplinary process that kept the patient and family informed of the prognosis and progress of the patient in the ICU. The investigators discovered that intensive communication reduced mortality and ICU length of stay in the patients with the greatest probability of dying. Improved communication also prevented the inappropriate transition to comfort-care only in patients with APACHE scores in the third quartile who had a good probability for survival. The process also improved consensus among the healthcare providers, families, and patients.

However, communication can be stymied by the intensivist's usurpation of the primary care physician's role. The patient and family must now trust someone with whom they have no previously established relationship. This, combined with the focus on technology and the emotional and physical trauma in the ICU, can create mistrust and fear (15). Ideally, care is taken to be inclusive with the primary care physician when making decisions about continuation or discontinuation of care in the ICU. A prospective cohort multicenter study by Heyland et al. surveyed family members of patients who had been in the ICU on mechanical ventilation (11). The majority of family members were satisfied with the overall care and the overall decision making. Families were most satisfied with nursing skill and competency, as well as the level of compassion and respect given to the patient. The least level of satisfaction was with the atmosphere of the ICU waiting room and communication with the physician. The authors suggest that improvement in physician–patient communication may lead to greater satisfaction of family members and contribute to more effective utilization of resources in the ICU.

Another interesting aspect to communication involves the responsibility of the patient and family to ask questions and seek clarification of what is told to them and to specify preferences for approach to care, especially end-of-life care. Patients and family members report wanting to know the prognosis, but many patients do not ask for this information, and physicians often do not volunteer it without prompting from the patient and family (16). The patient and family should be prepared to address "how far to go" in the quest to sustain life. Discussions with family members and healthcare providers should begin when the patient's health begins to deteriorate and the patient's subjective assessment of the quality of life no longer meets desired goals (15). In the face of imminent death, the discussion can be impaired by medication, fear, unsubstantiated hope, and desperation. Advance directives enable the patient to appoint a surrogate decision maker in the event the patient is unable or incompetent to make decisions or to state clearly what treatments are acceptable and what treatments are unacceptable to the patient. The assumption is that this document will ensure that the wishes of the patient are carried out. However, it is important for the patient and family to realize that advance directives can change over time, as the patient's condition and response to therapy change (10).

Predicting death is a nonexact science. Patients with a terminal illness have a fairly precipitous trajectory of dying. Patients with chronic organ failure can experience a steady decline in function but may have intermittent periods of moderate to high levels of performance before a dramatic decrease immediately prior to death (17). Patients suffering from frailty have a lower level of function for a more prolonged period of time, with a steady decline over time. Death in all these cases often results after acute complications from the chronic condition (17).

Cultural and religious differences can affect the effectiveness of communication and decisions at the end of life. Family involvement in the decision-making process will depend on the background of the family (18). In North America, families are involved in making decisions, whereas in Europe, they are not routinely involved. In contrast, in the Far East, family wishes can override the patient's wishes. ICU deaths following the decision to withdraw or withhold therapy occurred in 34% of deaths in Spain (19) and in 50 to 53% of deaths in France (20,21). In Japan, decisions to withdraw or withhold treatment are rare (22,23). A study comparing four American ethnic groups (European Americans, African Americans, Korean Americans, and Mexican Americans) found that a positive attitude toward initiation of life support was highest with Korean Americans, followed by Mexican Americans, African Americans, and finally European Americans (24). Korean Americans expressed a strong commitment to keep a family member alive at all costs, despite a personal desire not to undergo aggressive life support measures. African Americans were more likely to want aggressive life support for themselves. Both groups expressed distrust of physicians. European Americans did not want aggressive life support for themselves or for others, expressing fear of losing autonomy following resuscitation. Groups less likely to want resuscitation were women, the less religious, the more educated, and those with a higher income or private health insurance.

Do not resuscitate (DNR) and do not intubate (DNI) are in essence requests "not to touch" in order to prevent clinicians from performing treatment that is expected to work (25). If the therapy were not anticipated to work, there would be no need to ask clinicians not to do it. Patients cannot refuse a saved life. Every patient should be asked specifically about their wishes concerning cardiopulmonary resuscitation (CPR) and pulmonary intubation. Patients and families need to understand that DNR and DNI do not mean that other therapies are also forgone. Conversations should expand past the DNR and DNI orders, because these focus only on what should *not* be done in the final moments of life. Patients and families must consider what palliative care should be done to improve the dying experience (25).

An institutional ethics committee is an invaluable resource for healthcare providers, patients, and families. The ethics committee should establish and implement the ethics guidelines by which the institution functions. The ethics committee not only provides support during a conflict or a difference of opinion between healthcare providers and patients but can also work with all parties involved to ease the process of making difficult decisions, particularly at the end of life. The ethics committee should be consulted early in the process in order to reduce the potential for conflict and disagreement. Members of an ethics committee will vary per facility but often include medical, surgical, and intensive care staff physicians; spiritual advisors; and an attorney. Other members or consultants can include nurses, social workers, administrators, and dietitians.

39.3 SURROGATE DECISION MAKING

Ideally, family members openly communicate their thoughts and feelings about medical management during end-of-life care. Clear directives should be recorded and shared, with little room for interpretation. However, this happens less than might be hoped with patients who are chronically ill and rarely with patients who were healthy prior to a traumatic event (26). When healthcare providers turn to the family for decisions when the patient is unable to provide direction, the family is often conflicted and indecisive. Communication is improved when the family speaks with one voice and has a consensus of what should and should not be done. Surrogate decision making should be according to the values and interests of the patient, based on intimate knowledge of the patient. However, surrogate decision making can be revocable if the decision is deemed to be contrary to what the patient would want or is outside the range of a societally acceptable decision (27). Surrogate decision making can be driven by compassion, fear, guilt, and religious and cultural influences.

Factors that influence decisions made by surrogates are (27):

- The patient's substituted judgment
- The patient's best interest
- The interests of the surrogate or family members
- Communication of healthcare providers
- The surrogate's relationship with the patient

Limits to surrogate decision making are based on general ethical principles (27):

- The surrogate must be capable of making the decision.
- The surrogate cannot make a decision that the patient could not make.
- The surrogate cannot choose to provide or continue futile interventions.

Surrogate consent is presumed when the patient is an infant or child. However, there is debate about when a child is old enough to participate more actively in informed consent. Children who have not reached the legal age of majority may have the capacity to make decisions based on their understanding of the problem and treatment risks, benefits, and alternatives (28). Adolescents have been shown to be capable of making intelligent medical decisions (29,30). Intensivists should include children in the discussion of medical treatment options, including life-prolonging treatments.

A survey of intensivists affiliated with American medical schools (respondents: 35% pediatric intensivists, 39% neonatologists, 26% medical intensivists) showed that the majority believed that family interests should be considered for the incompetent patient, even if the family's interests are not important interests of the patient (31). Physicians who treated children were more supportive of family-centered surrogate decision making than physicians who exclusively treated adults. Seventy-eight percent of survey respondents agreed that their duty was to protect their patients from the interests of others who had interests that competed with those of the patient. This protective, patient-centered surrogate decision-making philosophy was more predominant among physicians who were medical intensivists, more religious, and more opposed to healthcare rationing. The support for family-centered vs. patient-centered decision making from this study could be in part due to the fact that 76% of the survey respondents worked with infants and children who, by law, have decisions made by a family member or surrogate. Caveats of the study were the large pediatric response, limitation to academic ICUs, and the facts that the survey was not pilot tested (reliability) and there was only a 55% response rate (validity). However, the impact of decisions made at the end of life on family members and resources is likely to become more important not only for surrogate decision makers, but also for the competent patient (32).

39.4 ARTIFICIAL NUTRITION

Artificial nutrition includes enteral tube feeding and parenteral nutrition provided in an effort to maintain or improve nutritional status, to improve response to therapy, to improve outcomes such as survival, to correct metabolic abnormalities, and to provide comfort. Studies have failed to demonstrate that nutrition support provides a benefit or improved outcome at the end of life (33–35). Often, nutrition support is given for humane reasons rather than as medical treatment. The therapeutic effect of nutrition support can be independent of the effect of treatment on the disease process itself. It may improve quality of life for some patients. However, for other patients, the inherent complications of nutrition support (e.g., central access infection, hyperglycemia, aspiration pneumonia, and diarrhea) can increase discomfort, morbidity, and mortality (36). The goals of treatment with nutrition support must be weighed against the patient's or surrogate's wishes and the potential for benefit vs. burden for the patient.

Nutrition support is often legally categorized as medical treatment. It can be withheld or withdrawn, depending on the patient's and surrogate's wishes or the healthcare provider's recommendation or orders. However, many patients and families perceive nutrition support as food, with its connotation of love, nurturing, and comfort (36,37). Therefore, patients and families are reluctant to cease provision of nutrition support for fear that they will starve themselves or their loved one to death. Families and patients should be made aware that complete starvation has been reported to produce a sense of euphoria and well-being with no or only a mild sense of hunger (36).

Provision of nutrition support should only be done when there is an achievable goal and when it is in the best interest of the patient (37). When no physiological benefit is anticipated from nutrition support, healthcare providers are not obliged to provide it, even when requested. If nutrition support provides a physiological benefit but does not positively impact quality of life, such as during a permanent vegetative state, there is no obligation to recommend nutrition support. However, if the decision to withdraw nutrition support from the patient in a permanent vegetative state is not a consensus of family members or if it conflicts with state laws, the situation can result in a legal battle. Nutrition support should be recommended when it is anticipated that it will be beneficial for the patient. Nutrition support should contribute to the relief of pain and suffering. When the burden exceeds the benefit, the patient, surrogate, or healthcare provider can choose to withdraw nutrition support.

The voluntary cessation of eating and drinking by a competent patient who is physically capable of consuming nutrients is an expression of autonomy and must be respected. It can take one to three weeks or longer for the patient to die without food or beverage, depending on the underlying disease and the consumption of fluids. Controversy often occurs when the decision is being made by a surrogate for the incompetent patient, such as a patient in a permanent vegetative state. The withdrawal of nutrition is passive assistance in dying, because the patient is said to die from the underlying disease rather than the withdrawal of nutrition. However, it has been argued that anyone who stops eating and drinking will die; therefore, cessation of nutrient intake itself is an active means of dying (38). All competent patients have the right to refuse treatment, even if refusal will result in death. If the decision is made to withhold or withdraw nutrition, palliative measures must still be offered to control symptoms, particularly pain.

39.5 FUTILE CARE

Hippocrates wrote that the three major goals of medicine were cure, relief of suffering, and "refus[al] to treat those who are overmastered by their diseases" (39). The ability to support patients mechanically and chemically and, in fact, to be able to bring them back from the dead with cardiopulmonary resuscitation has challenged healthcare professionals to identify when a patient

TABLE 39.2
Resolving Futility Cases under the Texas Advance Directives Act, 1999

1. The patient/family must be given written information about hospital policy on the ethics consultation or medical committee review process.
2. The patient/family must be given 48 hours' notice of the meeting to discuss the patient's wishes/advance directives.
3. A written report must be provided to the patient/family following the meeting.
4. If the physician, patient, or patient's family/surrogate disagree with the decision, the physician must make a reasonable effort to transfer the care of the patient to another physician/facility.
5. If after 10 days, an alternate facility or physician cannot be found, the physician/hospital can withdraw or withhold futile care.
6. The patient/family or surrogate may ask a district or county court to delay the withdrawal of therapy. The court can grant an extension if there is evidence that a willing provider can be found if the time is extended.
7. If the patient/family does not request legal intervention or the court does not grant the extension, the physician/facility may withdraw futile care without fear of civil and criminal prosecution.

Source: http://www.tapm.org/vault/Texas%20Advance%20Directives%20Act.pdf

is indeed overmastered by disease. It has been argued that futile interventions can be unilaterally withdrawn or withheld by the physician. The support for this argument includes the following (27):

- Demanding futile care when the physician objects dismisses the integrity, autonomy, and expertise of the physician.
- Providing ineffective interventions wastes valuable healthcare resources that can be used more efficaciously and appropriately for others.

However, even when an ethics committee concurs that treatment is futile, physicians are often reluctant to stop life-sustaining treatments for fear of potential lawsuits from families who do not agree with the decision (40). In 1999, the Texas Advance Directives Act combined three laws dealing with end-of-life care to create a "legally sanctioned extrajudicial process for resolving disputes about end-of-life decisions" (40,41). The process for resolving futility cases, as outlined in this act, is in Table 39.2. This process enables the family to pursue treatment elsewhere, if available, and does not commit the physician or institution to providing futile care indefinitely when a family does not agree with withdrawing or withholding care.

39.6 WITHDRAWING AND WITHHOLDING CARE

Ethicists and lawyers view withholding and withdrawing treatment as equivalent actions with the same moral significance (42,43). However, families can view these two actions as very different ethically and morally. Any time a treatment is initiated in the ICU, there should be a clearly communicated timetable for reevaluation of appropriateness and effectiveness of care (14). Families need to also be reassured that withdrawing treatment does not mean withdrawing care. Symptom management is essential to provide comfort to the patient and support for family members.

A retrospective cohort analysis of Medicare patients who died of cancer in Massachusetts and Medicare cancer decedents in California found that chemotherapy was frequently given during the last three months of life (23% of cancer patients in Massachusetts and 20% of cancer patients in California) (44). There was no difference in the use of chemotherapy between patients with cancers responsive to chemotherapy and patients with cancers unresponsive to chemotherapy. This raises questions not only about futility of treatment but also appropriateness of treatment. The study did not address the reasons for treatment with chemotherapy during the last months of life. However, potential reasons include:

- Desperation of patients and families
- Quality-of-life improvement with palliation of symptoms
- Uncertain prognosis and response to treatment

Withdrawing or withholding care is not synonymous with physician-assisted suicide. Oregon is the only state in the U.S. to legalize assisted suicide, and 38 states outlaw its practice (45). Withdrawal of life support is done when treatment is futile and the disease takes its course and causes death. Physician-assisted suicide is the deliberate act of ending life when death may not be imminent. In Oregon, physician-assisted suicide is acceptable when it is anticipated that the patient has less than six months to live. The emphasis on better symptom management, particularly pain control, may decrease the desperation of patients who request physician-assisted suicide. Another issue that affects the patient's decision to seek physician-assisted suicide is the patient's perception that he or she is a physical, emotional, and financial burden for his or her family. The legality of physician-assisted suicide is currently being challenged on the grounds that prescribing lethal doses of drugs violates federal drug laws (45).

Terminal sedation is considered an "unintended" treatment effect of effective pain management at the end of life (38). The Supreme Court upheld that pain control in terminally ill patients should be managed, even when it requires increasing doses of medication that could result in unconsciousness and death (47,48). Ethically, terminal sedation is often thought a better solution to suffering than physician-assisted suicide and voluntary active euthanasia (49,50). This is in part due to the doctrine of double effect, which evaluates an action on the effect intended (pain control) vs. the effect foreseen but unintended (death) (51–54).

Important aspects of withdrawal and withholding of care, as well as terminal sedation, are that the patient and healthcare providers voluntarily participate; that the physician act in the patient's best interest, with the risk of causing harm weighed against the expected benefit; and that physicians provide intense palliative care within the legitimized options available (38).

39.7 ADDITIONAL ICU ISSUES

39.7.1 ORGAN DONATION

ICU staff are often the ones who must approach grieving family members about organ donation (55). The federal Conditions of Participation require that anyone involved in discussing organ donation with families undergo specific training (56). The law was designed to increase organ donation and ensure that every family is approached with the option of organ and tissue donation. Consent rate for donation is increased when the person making the request has special training in discussing the issue and when there is coordination and cooperation between the local organ procurement organization and the ICU staff (55). There are curricula developed for end-of-life care training, but there are few, if any, validated models specific for end-of-life care and organ donation. It is important to develop curricula with an interdisciplinary approach, including the physicians, nurses, hospital chaplains, and organ procurement organization transplant coordinators (55).

In the United States, the ethical framework for organ donation requires that the donor be dead before organs and tissues are harvested and that the patient's wishes concerning donation are respected. Ninety-nine percent of organs in the U.S. are from brain-dead donors; (57) 1% are from cardiac death donors. When approaching families with the request, it is important to decouple the discussion of brain death from the request for donation. Families need time to understand the implications of brain death before they can consider donation of organs and tissue (55).

TABLE 39.3
Issues Related to Performing Research on the Newly Dead (58)

Informed consent
  Consent can come premortem from subject or postmortem from surrogate.
Respectful treatment of the dead
  Clinicians must handle and treat the dead in a manner consistent with a living person.
Confidentiality
  Confidentiality of the individual as well as family members should be respected.
Scientific merit of the research
  Research should address an important question and methods/subjects/intervention should be appropriate to answer the
    question.
Conflicts of interest
  Investigators should not participate in determination of death or withdrawal of support or determine protocols needed to
    delineate how decisions are made.
Hospital resources
  Cadavers use ICU beds, resources, and nursing time
Financial burdens related to research activities
  Organ procurement for transplant takes precedence over research

39.7.2 RESEARCH ON THE NEWLY DEAD

Another issue that can arise in the ICU is research involving the newly dead. Although there are
scientific and ethical advantages to performing research on brain-dead subjects, some issues still
require oversight, as listed in Table 39.3 (58). Each facility should have policies and protocols in
place to clarify processes and areas of responsibility. Some institutions may choose to form a
standing committee on oversight for research on the newly dead (58,59). The creates a specific
committee to guide this area of practice, rather than using the ethics committee or institutional
review board, neither of which is routinely involved in oversight following the death of the patient.
It is important to treat the dead with respect and to communicate with the family.

39.7.3 GENETIC TESTING

Genetic testing and profiling could enable the healthcare provider to identify patients with a greater
genetic risk of mortality and morbidity. The identification of single-nucleotide polymorphisms
(SNPs) at key loci can be used to predict survival in septic patients presenting with similar illnesses
and injuries (60). SNP-determined regulation of the inflammatory response is a major determinant
of outcome with critical illness. High-risk patients could be triaged for closer monitoring and more
aggressive treatment. Issues revolve around who should be tested and who pays for testing. A
relatively safe and inexpensive method of screening could be with cord blood, which can be
collected and stored for analysis when needed. Alternative methods of obtaining access to DNA
include buccal scrapings, blood donations, and other minor tissue samples. The decision of who
pays becomes more complex when one considers the risk of having one's genetic profile available
to insurance companies and employers.

39.7.4 HEALTH INSURANCE PORTABILITY AND ACCOUNTABILITY ACT (HIPAA)

The Health Insurance Portability and Accountability Act (HIPAA) is administered by the Office of
Civil Rights within Health and Human Services (HHS) and was signed into law in 1996 (61). The
law encourages electronic transactions for healthcare businesses, which raises issues of security
and confidentiality of the patient information being transmitted. HHS published proposed regula-
tions to guarantee patients' rights under the new law in 1999. Following periods for comments,

the final rule was effective on April 14, 2001. Covered entities, such as healthcare plans, healthcare clearinghouses, and healthcare providers that conduct electronic billing and fund transfers, had two years (until April 14, 2003) to comply with the final rule's provisions (62). The final rule protects "all medical records and other individually identifiable health information used or disclosed by a covered entity in any form, whether electronically, on paper, or orally" (62). The patient must provide consent before a covered healthcare provider can use and disclose information about the patient. The goal of HIPAA is to maintain the privacy of the patient through institutional compliance with security measures. A detailed discussion of HIPAA is beyond the scope of this chapter. The reader is referred to the following Web sites for more details: http://www.hipaacomply.com and http://www.hhs.gov/news.

39.8 CASE STUDY

B.T., a 72-year-old obese African American female, presents to the emergency department in a tertiary university hospital with complaints of chest pain. She has not completed an advance directive and has not appointed a durable power of attorney. She tells the physician in the emergency department that she wants "everything done." Her daughter, who is accompanying her, agrees. [Case comment: at this juncture, the patient should have been encouraged to record her wishes and to record when she would no longer want aggressive treatment.]

B.T. is diagnosed with a myocardial infarction (MI) and is transferred to the cardiac ICU for observation. She remains stable in the ICU overnight and is transferred to the cardiology floor the next day. An angiogram indicates that she has three severely diseased vessels. Over the next couple of days, she is involved in discussions with her family and physician about the risks and benefits of a coronary artery bypass graft (CABG) surgery. B.T. consents to the surgery, despite her physician's warning concerning her substantial surgical risk due to her obesity, hypertension, mild renal insufficiency, and type 2 diabetes mellitus. [Case comment: in view of the risks associated with the surgery, it would have been prudent to have the patient complete advance directives and appoint someone with durable power of attorney. This would have been an excellent time to discuss the patient's ethnic and cultural perspectives, as well as her goals for therapy. This could also have been an opportunity to involve the ethics committee.]

B.T. survives the surgery and is transferred to the ICU on mechanical ventilation with inotrope support. Attempts to wean ventilator and inotrope support are not successful. Meanwhile, the patient's renal function rapidly deteriorates, and her serum glucose levels are poorly controlled. On day 4, enteral nutrition is initiated through a nasoenteric feeding tube. On day 5 post-CABG, B.T. develops a fever, leukocytosis, and purulent wound drainage, indicating a sternal wound infection. Several organisms are identified, and antibiotics are initiated. Three days later, the patient begins hemodialysis. Unfortunately, she cannot maintain her blood pressure with hemodialysis and is changed to continuous renal replacement therapy. On day 10 post-CABG, the patient aspirates her enteral feeding, and the decision is made to begin parenteral nutrition. In addition, the patient has poor vascular circulation to her extremities, raising concerns of potential ischemia of her toes and feet. [Case comment: the patient is deteriorating despite aggressive therapy.]

On post-CABG day 15, the physician consults with the family concerning how to proceed with medical treatment. The physician candidly discusses the patient's poor prognosis due to multiple organ failure, failure to wean off the ventilator, and severe vascular disease. The family insists on continued aggressive medical care — the preservation of life at all costs. [Case comment: families can have difficulty withdrawing care from a family member based on their cultural, ethnic, and religious beliefs.]

Concerned about the provision of futile care, the physician consults the institution ethics committee. The ethics committee works with the family and their spiritual advisor to identify what the patient would want based on the prognosis. The family will not consent to withdrawal of care but does agree to withhold additional treatments as more problems arise, and they agree to DNR in the event the patient suffers another MI. [Case comment: the physician agrees to continue treatments already in progress because the family has agreed not to institute any more therapies as the patient continues to deteriorate.] On day 22 post-CABG, the patient suffers another MI and expires.

39.9 CONCLUSION

Effective communication is the key to providing ethical and effective medical care in the ICU. Communication can be improved with routine meetings among the patient, family members, and healthcare providers to discuss the status of the patient and the options for care. Many patients and family members are overwhelmed by medical information and the ICU setting. Therefore, written explanations, audio or video tapes, and decision-making aids or algorithms may help to clarify the patient's condition and explain optimal patient management, depending on the patient's prognosis and desire for treatment. The greatest impediment to routine family meetings is the time limitation of the intensivist.

ICU clinicians require not only competent clinical skills but also compassion and understanding in order to deal with the ethical issues of end-of-life decision making by patients and their families. Dealing with withdrawing and withholding care, terminal sedation, futile care, organ donation, research on the newly dead, and genetic-based therapy require a well trained staff that understands the ethical issues involved. Clinicians not only deal with their own ethical and moral standards but must also be sensitive to the moral, ethical, and cultural standards of their patients and their families.

REFERENCES

1. Block, S., Psychological considerations, growth, and transcendence at the end of life: the art of the possible, *JAMA*, 285, 2892, 2001.
2. Pendergast, T.J. and Luce, J.M., Increasing incidence of withholding and withdrawal of life-support from the critically ill, *Am. J. Respir. Care Med.*,155, 15, 1997.
3. Valentin, A. et al., Gender-related differences in intensive care: a multiple-center cohort study of therapeutic interventions and outcome in critically ill patients, *Crit. Care Med.*, 31, 1901, 2003.
4. Tilford, J.M. and Parker, J.G., A gender bias in the allocation of intensive care unit resources? *Crit. Care Med.*, [editorial] 31, 2072, 2003.
5. Callahan, D., Living and dying with medical technology, *Crit. Care Med.*, 31(suppl.), S344, 2003.
6. Cassell, J. et al., Surgeons, intensivists, and the covenant of care: administrative models and values affecting care at the end of life — updated, *Crit. Care Med.*, 31, 1551, 2003.
7. Herrmann, V.M., Nutrition support: ethical or expedient, and who will choose?, *J. Parenter. Enteral Nutr.*, 23, 195, 1999.
8. Latimer, E.J., Ethical care at the end of life, *Can. Med. Assoc. J.*, 158, 1741, 1998.
9. Lilly, C.M. et al., Intensive communication: four-year follow-up from a clinical practice study, *Crit. Care Med.*, 31(suppl.), S394, 2003.
10. Mendelsohn, A.B. and Chelluri, L., Interviews with intensive care unit survivors: assessing post-intensive care quality of life and patient's preferences regarding intensive care and mechanical ventilation, *Crit. Care Med.*, 31(suppl.), S400, 2003.
11. Heyland, D.K. et al., Family satisfaction with care in the intensive care unit: results of a multiple center study, *Crit. Care Med.*, 30, 1413, 2002.
12. Annas, G.J., National bill of patient rights, *N. Engl. J. Med.*, 338, 695, 1998.
13. Joint Commission on Accreditation of Healthcare Organizations (JCAHO), *2002 Automated Accreditation Manual for Hospitals*, JCAHO, Oakbrook Terrace, IL, 2002. www.jcaho.org.
14. Lynn, J. and Goldstein, N.E., Advance care planning for fatal chronic illness: avoiding commonplace errors and unwarranted suffering, *Ann. Intern. Med.*, 138, 812, 2003.
15. Chaitin, E. et al., Physician–patient relationship in the intensive care unit: erosion of the sacred trust? *Crit. Care Med.*, 31(suppl.), S367, 2003.

16. Lamont, E.B. and Christakis, N.A., Prognostic disclosure to patients with cancer near the end of life, *Ann. Intern. Med.*, 134, 1096, 2001.

17. Lunney, J.R. et al., Patterns of functional decline at the end of life, *JAMA*, 289, 2387, 2003.

18. Levin, P.D. and Sprung, C.L., Cultural differences at the end of life, *Crit. Care Med.*, 31(suppl.), S354, 2003.

19. Esteban, A. et al., Withdrawing and withholding life support in the intensive care unit: a Spanish prospective multi-centre observational study, *Intens. Care Med.*, 27, 1744, 2001.

20. Pochard, F. et al., French intensivists do not apply American recommendations regarding decisions to forgo life-sustaining therapy, *Crit. Care Med.*, 29, 1887, 2001.

21. Ferrand, E. et al., Withholding and withdrawal of life support in intensive-care units in France: a prospective survey, *Lancet*, 357, 9, 2001.

22. Sirio, C.A. et al., A cross-cultural comparison of critical care delivery: Japan and the United States, *Chest*, 121, 539, 2002.

23. Nakata, U., Goto, T., and Morita, S., Serving the emperor without asking: critical care ethics in Japan, *J. Med. Philos.*, 23, 601, 1998.

24. Blackhall, L.J. et al., Ethnicity and attitudes towards life sustaining technology, *Soc. Sci. Med.*, 48, 1779, 1999.

25. Burns, J.P. et al., Do-not-resuscitate order after 25 years, *Crit. Care Med.*, 31, 1543, 2003.

26. Emanuel, E. and Emanuel, L., Proxy decision making for incompetent patients: an ethical and empirical analysis, *JAMA*, 267, 2067, 1992.

27. Arnold, R.M. and Kellum, J., More justification for surrogate decision making in the intensive care unit: implications and limitations, *Crit. Care Med.*, 31(suppl.), S347, 2003.

28. Zawistowski, C.A. and Frader, J.E., Ethical problems in pediatric critical care: consent, *Crit. Care Med.*, 31(suppl.), S407, 2003.

29. Hartman, R.G., Adolescent decisional autonomy for medical care, *Univ. Chicago Law School Roundtable*, 8, 87, 2001.

30. Ginsburg, K.R., Menapace, A.S., and Slap, G.B., Factors affecting the decision to seek health care: the voice of adolescents, *Pediatrics*, 100, 922, 1997.

31. Hardart, G.E. and Truog, R.D., Attitudes and preferences of intensivists regarding the role of family interests in medical decision making for incompetent patients, *Crit. Care Med.*, 31, 1895, 2003.

32. Nelson, J.L., Physicians and family interests, *Crit. Care Med.*, [editorial] 31, 2072, 2003.

33. Klein, S. and Koretz, R.L., Nutrition support in patients with cancer: what do the data really show? *Nutr. Clin. Prac.*, 9, 91, 1994.

34. Heys, S.D. et al., Enteral nutritional supplementation with key nutrients in patients with critical illness and cancer: a meta-analysis of randomized controlled clinical trials, *Ann. Surg.*, 229, 467, 1999.

35. Schols, A.M., Nutrition and outcome in chronic respiratory disease, *Nutrition*, 13, 161, 1997.

36. Winter, S.M., Terminal nutrition: framing the debate for the withdrawal of nutritional support in terminally ill patients, *Am. J. Med.*, 109, 723, 2000.

37. Planas, M. and Camilo, M.E., Artificial nutrition: dilemmas in decision-making, *Clin. Nutr.*, 21, 355, 2002.

38. Quill, T.E., Lo, B., Brock, D.W., Palliative options of last resort: a comparison of voluntarily stopping eating and drinking, terminal sedation, physician-assisted suicide, and voluntary active euthanasia, *JAMA*, 278, 2099, 1997.

39. Jecker, N.S., Knowing when to stop: the limits of medicine, *Hastings Cent. Rep.*, 21, 5, 1991.

40. Fine, R.L. and Mayo, T.W., Resolution of futility by due process: early experience with the Texas Advance Directives Act, *Am. Coll. Phys.*, 138, 743, 2003.

41. Texas Health and Safety Code 166.046(a) (Vernon Supp 2002). Accessed at http://www.capitol.state.tx.us/statutes/hs.toc.htm on July 6, 2003.

42. Meisel, A., Snyder, L., Quill, T., Seven legal barriers to end-of-life care myths, realities, and grains of truth, *JAMA*, 284, 2495, 2000.

43. Luce, J.M. and Alpers, A., Legal aspects of withholding and withdrawing life support from critically ill patients in the United States and providing palliative care to them, *Am. J. Respir. Crit. Care Med.*, 162, 2029, 2000.

44. Emanuel, E.J. et al., Chemotherapy use among Medicare beneficiaries at the end of life, *Ann. Intern. Med.*, 138, 639, 2003.

45. Foley, K. and Hendin, H., Conclusion: changing the culture, in *The Case Against Physician-Assisted Suicide: For a Right to End-of-Life Care*, Foley, K. and Hendin, H., Eds., John Hopkins University Press, Baltimore, 2002.

46. Letter from Attorney General John Ashcroft to Hugh C. Stelson, MD, President, Oregon Medical Association, November 6, 2001.

47. *Vacco v Quill*, 117 SCt 2293 (1997).

48. *Washington v Glucksberg*, 117 SCt 2258 (1997).

49. Trong, R.D. et al., Barbiturates in the care of the terminally ill, *N. Engl. J. Med.*, 327, 1678, 1991.

50. Byock, I.R., Consciously walking the fine line: thoughts on a hospice response to assisted suicide and euthanasia, *J. Palliat. Care*, 9, 25, 1993.

51. Council on Scientific Affairs, American Medical Association, Good care of the dying patient, *JAMA*, 275, 474, 1996.

52. American Board of Internal Medicine End of Life Patient Care Project Committee. *Caring for the Dying: Identification and Promotion of Physician Competency*, American Board of Internal Medicine, Philadelphia, 1996.

53. President's Commission for the Study of Ethical Problems in Medicine and Biomedical and Behavioral Research, *Deciding to Forego Life-Sustaining Treatment: Ethical, Medical and Legal Issues in Treatment Decisions*, U.S. Government Printing Office, Washington, DC, 1982.

54. The Hastings Center Report., *Guidelines on the Termination of Life-Sustaining Treatment and the Care of the Dying*, Hastings Center, Briarcliff Manor, NY, 1987.

55. Williams, M.A. et al., The physician's role in discussing organ donation with families, *Crit. Care Med.*, 31, 1568, 2003.

56. 42 CFR Part 482 [HCFA-3005-F] RIN: 0938-A195 Medicare and Medicaid programs; hospital conditions of participation; identification of potential organ, tissue, and eye donors and transplant hospitals' provision of transplant-related data: HCFA, Final rule, *Fed Regist.*, 6333856, 1998.

57. Department of Health and Human Services/Health Resources and Services Administration, Office of Special Programs/Division of Transplantation, and United Network for Organ Sharing: 2000 Annual Report of the United States Scientific Registry for Transplant Recipients and the Organ Procurement and Transplantation Network, Richmond, VA, 2000.

58. DeVita, M.A. et al., Research involving the newly dead: an institutional response, *Crit. Care Med.*, 31(suppl.), S385, 2003.

59. The Committee for the Oversight of Research Involving the Dead, Policy for research involving the dead, *Crit. Care Med.*, 31(suppl.), S391, 2003.

60. Pinsky, M.R., Genetic testing: costs and access to intensive care unit care, *Crit. Care Med.*, 31(suppl.), S411, 2003.

61. Health Insurance Portability and Accountability Act (HIPAA), Public Law 104-191, August 21, 1996.

62. U.S. Department of Health and Human Services, HHS Fact Sheet, http://aspe.hhs.gov/admn-simp/final/pvcfact2.htm, accessed October 17, 2003.

40 Quality and Performance Improvement

Mary Krystofiak Russell
Duke University Hospital

CONTENTS

40.1 INTRODUCTION

Quality in health care has been defined by the Institute of Medicine as the degree to which health services for individuals and populations increase the likelihood of achieving desirable outcomes and the degree to which they are consistent with current professional knowledge [1]. Graham defines quality as "the optimal achievable result for each patient, the avoidance of iatrogenic complications, and the attention to patient and family needs in a manner that is cost-effective and reasonably documented" [2].

The Joint Commission on Accreditation of Healthcare Organizations (JCAHO) defines performance improvement as "a continuous process ... [that] involves measuring the functioning of important processes and services, and, when indicated, identifying changes that enhance performance. These changes are incorporated into new or existing work processes, products, or services, and performance is monitored to ensure that the improvements are sustained" [3]. The 2004 JCAHO standards for performance improvement focus on the reduction of factors that contribute to unanticipated adverse events or outcomes, with the 2004 National Patient Safety Goals a prime component of this effort.

Two recent reviews describe in detail the history of quality assurance and continuous quality improvement in health care and the history of the JCAHO [4,5].

This chapter will:

- Describe the 2004 JCAHO standards and National Patient Safety Goals, as they relate to nutrition care teams
- Discuss the importance of performance improvement and several key performance and quality improvement initiatives that improve the work of nutrition support practitioners in both critical and intermediate care units

- Highlight the value of improving practice of implementation of clinical guidelines and standards
- Discuss the importance of a hazard analysis process for monitoring an enteral tube feeding program

Although hospital settings are used as examples, many of the tools and techniques can be applied to any healthcare setting.

40.2 2004 JCAHO STANDARDS

"Shared Visions — New Pathways" is the theme for the 2004 JCAHO standards. Safe, high-quality care has always been important to patients, healthcare organizations, and regulatory agencies, but the new standards place even more importance on the "shared vision" of the JCAHO and the organizations it surveys to provide such care all the time. "New pathways" refers to new and revised elements of the survey process, involving a new set of pathways to accreditation.

Adoption of the *tracer methodology* is a key component of the new pathways. The tracer is a new survey method in which patients are followed through the organization's processes and services from the patient's viewpoint; it is more focused on the execution and actual delivery of care and services than previous survey methods. Other important parts of the new survey process include [3]:

- Periodic performance reviews (PPRs) — These will be required after July 2005. The process (completed at 18 months following the organization's last survey) is accomplished via a tool by which the organization assesses and attests to compliance, and creates a corrective action plan with measures of success for any standards not fully met. These reviews are intended to help organizations gain a much clearer understanding of the relevancy of the standards, create more accountability for compliance, engage physicians more fully, and improve the consistency of the survey process. The reviews also help the organization to maintain itself in an "always ready" mode, continuously monitoring compliance and promptly identifying areas for improvement.
- Priority-focus process (PFP) — This process is an analysis to help the organization focus on areas, services, and issues of particular concern (such as those gathered via sentinel event reporting and core measure data). This process will help the survey to focus on those areas of most significance to the organization and will place emphasis on quality and patient safety concerns.
- PFP tool — An automated tool, supporting the process, that logically organizes the information provided by the healthcare organization and "shapes" the survey. Benefits of PFP include consistency and a more focused survey process, better preparation of surveyors, more on-site time for surveyors to educate organization members, and identification of tracers, which lead surveyors to appropriate clinical choices for analysis.
- Critical focus areas (CFAs) — Based on the assumption that systems that work well generate positive clinical outcomes, these areas are chosen based on the results of the PFP and will help surveyors to identify a hospital's most vulnerable situations. The 14 CFAs for 2004, which help shape and direct the tracer methodology used in the survey itself are:
  - Assessment and care/service
  - Communication
  - Credentialed and privileged practitioners
  - Equipment use
  - Infection control
  - Information management
  - Medication management

- Organization structure
- Orientation and training
- Rights and ethics
- Physical environment
- Quality improvement expertise and activity
- Patient safety
- Staffing
- Clinical/service groups (CSGs) — A method for categorizing patients into distinct, clinical populations on which JCAHO can gather data on the individual focus areas. They are part of the data that feed into the PFP.
- Elements of performance (EP) — Specific performance expectations and/or structures or processes that must be in place in order for a hospital to provide safe, high-quality care, treatment, and services. The scoring of EP determines a hospital's overall compliance with a standard.

The overarching goal of the new survey process is to "shift the paradigm from survey preparation to survey improvement," providing less focus on a specific score and more on using the standards to "achieve and maintain excellent operational systems."

The 2004 JCAHO standards are organized into 11 chapters (Table 40.1). Table 40.2 lists the significant highlights of the 2004 JCAHO standards that apply to nutrition services. Other standards are also relevant to providers of specialized nutrition support (SNS), specifically those in the Medication Management (MM) chapter. JCAHO notes that the term *medication* includes parenteral nutrition, but not "enteral nutrient solutions," which are defined by the Food and Drug Administration as medical foods. Providers of SNS, as well as all of their healthcare colleagues, must also be familiar with the JCAHO 2004 National Patient Safety Goals (Table 40.3).

40.3 PERFORMANCE IMPROVEMENT

Performance improvement (PI) must be an integral part of the management and direction of a healthcare organization. PI supports the mission, vision, values, and strategic plan and must be collaborative across disciplines. The JCAHO charges the leadership of the organization with setting the PI priorities, identifying how these priorities are adjusted in response to urgent or unusual

---

TABLE 40.1
Chapters Included in the 2004 JCAHO Hospital Standards

Chapter Title	Abbreviation
Ethics, Rights, and Responsibilities	RI
Provision of Care	PC
Medication Management	MM
Surveillance, Prevention, and Control of Infection	IC
Improving Organization Performance	PI
Leadership	LD
Management in the Environment of Care	EC
Management of Human Resources	HR
Management of Information	IM
Medical Staff	MS
Nursing	NR

Source: From JCAHO. Dept. Ed. Resources. With permission.

TABLE 40.2
Summary of 2004 JCAHO Nutrition-Related Standards for Hospitals

Nutrition care is primarily addressed in the chapter "Provision of Care, Treatment, and Services," known as PC. The following are excerpts; see www.jcaho.org for information about obtaining complete standards.

PC.2.20
The hospital delineates in writing the data and information gathered during assessment and reassessment.
Elements of performance for PC.2.20:
1. Scope, content, and criteria for assessment and reassessment.
2. Screening, assessment, and reassessment are within scope of practice, licensure laws, or certification of discipline doing them.
3. If applicable, separate specialized assessment and reassessment information is identified for the various populations served.
4. Information gathered during initial assessment includes the following as relevant to care, treatment, and services: each patient's nutrition and hydration status, as appropriate.
5. Hospital has defined criteria for when nutritional plans must be developed.

PC.2.120
The hospital defines in writing the time frame(s) for conducting the initial assessment(s).
Nutritional screening, when warranted by the patient's needs or condition, is completed within no more than 24 hours of inpatient admissions.

PC.4.10
Development of a plan for care, treatment, and services is individualized and appropriate to the patient's needs, strengths, limitations, and goals.
Elements of performance for PC.4.10:
1. Care, treatment, and services are planned to ensure that they are appropriate to the patient's needs.
2. Development of a plan for care, treatment, and services is based on the data from assessments.
3. Patient's evaluation is based on the patient's care goals and plan for care.
4. The goals of care, treatment, and services are revised when necessary.
5. Plans for care, treatment, and services are revised when necessary.

Note: Care plans must document goals, not simply interventions.

PC.5.50
Care, treatment, and services are provided in an interdisciplinary, collaborative manner.

Note: All staff members are expected to be able to articulate their understanding of the interdisciplinary plan of care as it is noted in the medical record.

PC.6.10
The patient receives education and training specific to the patient's needs and as appropriate to the care, treatment, and services provided.
Selected elements of performance for PC.6.10:
   As appropriate to the patient's condition and assessed needs and the hospital's scope of services, the patient is educated about nutrition interventions, modified diets, or oral health (many other things are cited here also).

PC.7.10
The hospital has a process for preparing and/or distributing food and nutrition products as appropriate to the care, treatment, and services provided.
Elements of performance for PC.7.10:

(continued)

TABLE 40.2 (CONTINUED)
Summary of 2004 JCAHO Nutrition-Related Standards for Hospitals

1. Food and nutrition products are provided for the patient as appropriate to care, treatment, and services.
2. Food and nutrition products are stored and prepared under proper conditions of sanitation, temperature, light, moisture, ventilation, and security.
3. Patient's cultural, religious, and ethnic food preferences are honored when possible, unless contraindicated.
4. Substitutes of equal nutritional value are offered when patients refuse the food served.
5. Responsibilities are assigned for all activities involved in safely and accurately providing food and nutrition products.
6. Foods brought in by patients are stored appropriately.
7. Special diets and altered diet schedules are accommodated.

Source: From JCAHO. Dept. Ed. Resources. With permission.

---

events, providing sufficient staff and resources, and tracking effectiveness of PI through measurement, assessment, monitoring, and analysis to identify opportunities for improvement. The PI standards themselves focus on collection of data, aggregation and analysis (including internal and external comparisons and identification of undesirable patterns and trends), identifying and managing sentinel events, use of analysis to drive change, and maintenance of an ongoing, proactive PI program to identify and reduce safety risks and adverse events. PI must look at "measures that matter" — those that focus on increasing staff efficiency and effectiveness, improve safety, or lower overall operating costs [7].

The following paragraphs and accompanying tables describe PI projects used by nutrition support practitioners at Duke University Hospital (DUH); the R. Adams Cowley Shock Trauma Center in Baltimore, Maryland; and University of Virginia Health System, Charlottesville (UVa).

At DUH, the FADE process (Figure 40.1) provides the structure for problem solving and PI. This process, developed by Organizational Dynamics Incorporated (ODI), consists of four steps:

*   *Focus* includes development of a problem statement, including the impact and desired outcome of the project.
*   *Analyze* involves collection of baseline data to determine how bad (or good) things actually are.
*   *Develop* includes asking what steps are needed to correct the problem.
*   *Execute* involves implementing the plan, monitoring results.

This is a circular process; if desired results are not achieved, the earlier stages of the process are revisited and studied further.

Before FADE can be applied, data collection helps to determine priorities for PI. In order to identify the current state and with the goal of justifying the services of a specialized nutrition support team, the DUH Nutrition Support Team retrospectively evaluated metabolic abnormalities found in total parenteral nutrition (TPN) patients managed by the team over a seven-year period (1992 to 1998). The purpose of this project was to identify the value added by a designated team approach to parenteral nutrition administration [8]. The metabolic abnormalities tracked included elevations in serum triglycerides, phosphorus, potassium, sodium, chloride, magnesium, ammonia, glucose, AST/ALT, alkaline phosphatase, bilirubin, and calcium; low levels of serum phosphorus, potassium, sodium, chloride, magnesium, glucose, albumin, calcium, copper, and zinc; acidosis, alkalosis, and volume overload. Although ~33% of the 2747 courses of TPN demonstrated metabolic abnormalities (primarily hyperphosphatemia, hyponatremia, hyperkalemia, and hyperglycemia), only 11 courses (0.4%) involved symptomatic events, 5 of which involved hyperkalemia. Identification of these symptomatic events (which are currently classified as adverse drug events and a

TABLE 40.3
JCAHO 2004 National Patient Safety Goals

Goal	Requirements	Scored as
Improve accuracy of patient identification	Use at least 2 patient identifiers (not the patient's room number) whenever taking blood samples or administering medications or blood products	PC 5.1.0, element of performance (EP) 4
	Prior to the start of any surgical or invasive procedure, conduct a verification "time out" to confirm the correct patient, procedure, and site	PC 13.20, EP 9
Improve the effectiveness of communication among caregivers	Implement a "read-back" process for taking verbal or telephone orders or critical test results	IM 6.50, EP 4
	Standardize abbreviations, acronyms, and symbols used throughout the organization, including a list of those *not* to be used	IM 3.10, EP 1
Improve the safety of using high-alert medications	Remove concentrated electrolytes (including KCl, KPO_4, NaCl > 0.9%) from patient care units	MM 2.20, EP 9
	Standardize and limit the number of drug concentrations available in the organization	MM 2.20, EP 8
Eliminate wrong-site, wrong-patient, wrong-procedure surgery	Use a preop verification process, such as a checklist, to confirm appropriate documents are available	N/A
	Implement a process to mark the surgical site and involve the patient in the process	
Improve the safety of using infusion pumps	Ensure free-flow protection on all general-use and PCA intravenous infusion pumps used in the organization	N/A
Improve the effectiveness of clinical alarm systems	Implement regular preventive maintenance and testing of alarm systems	N/A
	Ensure that alarms are activated with appropriate settings and are sufficiently audible with respect to distances and competing noises within the unit	
Reduce the risk of healthcare-acquired infections	Comply with the current CDC hand hygiene guidelines	N/A
	Manage as sentinel events all identified cases of unanticipated death or major permanent loss of function associated with a healthcare-acquired infection	

Note: For an explanation of EP, see Section 40.2.

Source: From JCAHO. Dept. Ed. Resources. With permission.

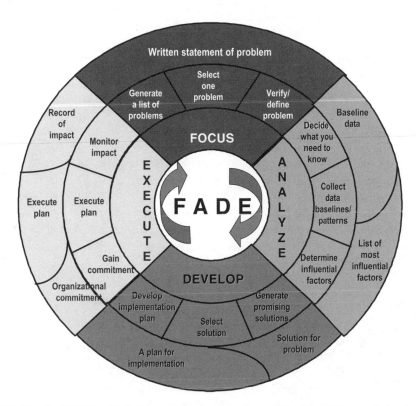

FIGURE 40.1 Detailed FADE wheel. (From Organizational Dynamics, Inc. With permission.)

part of the hospital balanced scorecard for quality evaluation) resulted in application of the complete PI process and changes to the TPN protocol.

The PI team of the Nutrition Services department at DUH applied the FADE process to an analysis of enteral tube feeding (ETF) documentation practices. The team began with the template developed by the Accreditation and Patient Safety Department that is based on the FADE methodology. They focused on the fact that important data, such as formula name, volume infused, intake and output records, stool, weight, and residual volume, were sometimes missing from the flow sheets of patients who received ETF. Missing data meant that clinical staff members were unable to make appropriate assessments of tolerance or the need for changes in formula composition or method of administration. The PI team created an audit tool and enlisted the Nutrition Services staff members as data collectors. The data confirmed the problems identified in the focus portion of the project and were presented to the Medical Nutrition Advisory Committee of the Pharmacy and Therapeutics Committee (Table 40.4). One of the problems identified in the analyze phase was that many nurses new to DUH were unfamiliar with the ETF policies and procedures. Therefore, the develop phase identified the need for an interdisciplinary committee to create an updated ETF protocol, and extensive education of all nursing staff once the new protocol was approved. Creation, revision, approval, and implementation of this protocol took more than two years. Follow-up data will compare the documentation practices with those initially demonstrated. If improvement is not noted, return to the analyze phase will be needed.

A different process, Goldratt's theory of constraints [9], was applied to the analysis of barriers to optimum nutrition care by Klein, Stanek, Wiles, and other interdisciplinary team members in a trauma center in Baltimore [10]. The goal of the process was to improve care systems in order to improve outcomes for trauma patients by providing them with nutrition support appropriate for their risk level and clinical conditions. The objectives were to identify the problem in the care

TABLE 40.4
Duke University Hospital, Results of Enteral Tube Feeding Performance Improvement Project Data Analysis

Parameter	% Yes	% No
Admission weight available?	88.1	11.9
If patient receiving ETF on admission, was this noted on universal admission assessment form?	16.6	83.4
Feeding tube flushes ordered?	78.3	21.7
Gastric residual volume checks ordered?	34.6	65.4
ETF order and ETF recorded match?	88.3	11.7
Tube flush order and tube flush recorded match?	79.9	21.1
Amount of ETF per hour or per bolus recorded?	87	13
Total ETF/24 hours recorded?	46.3	53.7
Gastric residual volumes recorded?	46.3	53.7
Last stool date, and/or stool volume in last 24 hours, recorded?	72.7	27.3
Presence/absence of bowel sounds recorded?	94.6	5.4
Feeding tube type noted?	73.1	26.9

Note: ETF = enteral tube feeding. N = 277 adult patients.

Source: From Duke University Hospital. With permission.

process that, if corrected, would yield the greatest positive change in outcomes, and to create and implement a realistic solution to the problem. Four steps defined this process:

- Identify symptoms of the problem
- Identify what to change
- Identify what to change to
- Define how to cause the change

At the end of a year-long process, monitoring and reassessment of nutritional status were identified as the "weakest links" in the nutrition care process, and a nutrition support care map was constructed [10]. Upon implementation, the care map was expected to improve compliance with JCAHO standards and reduce adverse outcomes related to nutrition care.

At the Digestive Health Center of Excellence at UVa, nutrition support specialists constantly question whether their protocols and procedures can be improved to enhance patient safety and the efficacy of the services provided. The team developed a protocol for intravenous insulin infusion (Table 40.5), a worksheet to monitor dose delivery of enteral tube feeding (Table 40.6), and a worksheet to monitor triglyceride concentration of patients receiving TPN (Table 40.7). Data collection is in progress; results of the analyze phase may suggest the need to develop new protocols, change existing ones, or create new educational programs for clinical staff.

40.4 CLINICAL GUIDELINES AND PRACTICE STANDARDS

Clinical practice guidelines exist for a variety of healthcare procedures and team members. JCAHO (2004 Hospital Standards, LD 5.1–5.4) encourages organizations to use guidelines (such as those from the Agency for Healthcare Research and Quality, the National Guideline Clearinghouse, and professional organizations) when designing or improving processes. Guidelines must be appropriate to the organization, with criteria consistent with its mission, vision, and values, and must be reviewed, revised, adapted, and approved by leadership before implementation. To benefit fully

TABLE 40.5
University of Virginia Health System
Adult Insulin Infusion Orders: Acute Care Units

MD Preparation for Insulin Infusion:

Discontinue previous insulin orders

Discontinue _____(oral diabetes agents)

Maintenance IV fluids (should contain glucose delivered via a dedicated IV line)

    D5NS _____ml/h

    D51/2 NS _____ml/h

    Other_____

Insulin Infusion Set-up:

Immediately prior to starting insulin infusion, obtain initial blood glucose (BG) test result per bedside meter.

Flush IV line with 25 ml of insulin solution before connecting infusion to patient. Piggyback insulin infusion into
  maintenance IV (use only pharmacy prepared insulin infusion).

Standard insulin solution prepared by pharmacy: 250 units of regular insulin in 250 ml NS.

  (1 unit :1 ml concentration)

Start Insulin Infusion Rate as follows:

0.5 units per hour for patients under 70 kg, or for patients previously diet controlled, taking oral diabetes agents, or taking
  30 units or less of insulin a day.

1 unit per hour for patients over 70 kg, or taking more than 30 units of insulin a day.

Other_____

MD Advice: Consider 3 to 5 units per hour initial dose with severe stress (e.g., sepsis, stroke), insulin resistance (e.g., use
  of greater than 75 units per day), high-dose steroids, etc. Adequate hydration, avoiding hypoglycemia, and measures to
  deal with underlying stress and infection are key to minimizing unstable glucose patterns.

MD Note: DKA is treated initially with 6 to 10 units per hour plus aggressive early hydration and cannot be managed
  alone with IV push insulin. Unlike simply poorly controlled DM, it is important to infuse glucose when BG < 200 mg/dl
  to avoid ketosis.

Decrease insulin infusion rate for patients with a **rapid decline in glucose:**

DOWNWARD TITRATION FOR RAPID DECLINE IN BLOOD GLUCOSE VALUES

Current Blood Glucose Value	Amount Blood Glucose Decreased within One Hour	Amount (%) to Decrease Insulin Infusion Rate
≥ 300 mg/dl	≥ 200 mg/dl	50
< 300 mg/dl	≥ 100 mg/dl	50
< 300 mg/dl	50–99 mg/dl	25

Test BG by bedside meter every hour until stable (range 100 to 150 mg/dl) for two consecutive readings, then every 2 hours.

Adjust Insulin Infusion rate as follows:

BG 80 mg/dl or less...................STOP infusion and follow Hypoglycemia Treatment Guidelines*

BG 81–100 mg/dl......................Decrease rate by 0.5 units per hour

BG 101–150 mg/dl.....................No change in the infusion rate

BG 151–200 mg/dl.....................Increase infusion by 0.5 units per hour

BG 201–250 mg/dl.....................Increase infusion by 1 unit per hour

BG above 250 mg/dl..................Increase infusion by 2 units per hour

Call physician if BG remains above 250 mg/dl for three consecutive hours.

If tube feeding is discontinued for any reason, reduce insulin infusion rate by 50%, and resume every 1 hour BG
  checks.

(continued)

TABLE 40.5 (CONTINUED)
University of Virginia Health System
Adult Insulin Infusion Orders: Acute Care Units

Nursing Practice Guidelines:

- A second licensed healthcare provider will **double-check** to verify the medication, the ordered dose and the dose programmed into the pump. The verification needs to be done at the following times:
  - **Initiation of therapy** for accuracy of the medication label, the ordered dose, and the dose programmed into the pump.
  - **All bag changes** for label accuracy compared to the physician's order, including concentration.
- Document the rate of insulin infusion and blood glucose results in a column on the CDFS with 2 initials for verification at appropriate times.
- Safety Recommendations:
  - In order to improve safety in the acute care settings, use of the Panel Lock 🔒 feature on the IVAC pump is recommended during any high-risk infusion. This feature will prevent unauthorized changes of pump settings. See IVAC owner's manual for further assistance.
  - If the patient receiving an insulin infusion has an order to travel off the unit for a procedure, the RN needs to assess the following factors:
    1. Can the procedure/test be done at the bedside? If so, consult with the MD about changing the order to "portable."
    2. The stability of the patient's condition and how the patient will tolerate being off the unit by considering estimated time off the unit, location of the procedure/test, stability of the patient's BG, and whether there is an RN at the procedure/test location to obtain BG and competently adjust insulin infusion.
    3. The RN needs to use his/her critical thinking skills/clinical judgment and collaborate with the MD.
  - Avoid flushing the line that would inadvertently **bolus** the patient with insulin. If the IV access needs to be flushed, attach the flush syringe at the most proximal point possible.

*Hypoglycemia Treatment Guidelines:

- Stop the infusion.
- If patient is conscious and able to eat or drink, give 15 g of carbohydrate (CHO), such as glucose tabs that equal 15 g CHO, 4 oz. juice or regular soda. Notify MD. Recheck BG in 15 min. Repeat 15 g CHO treatment and repeat BG check every 15 minutes until glucose is above 100 mg/dl.
- If patient is unconscious or unable to eat or drink, give 25 ml ($^1/_2$ amp) of Dextrose 50% slow IV push STAT/or 1 mg Glucagon IM STAT if no IV access. Notify MD. Recheck BG in 15 min, and repeat treatment if needed until BG is above100 mg/dl.
- **MD: Evaluate cause of hypoglycemic episode, determine appropriate monitoring schedule, and initiate order changes.**
- Restart infusion when patient's BG @_____.
- **Advice:** When restarting insulin infusion after hypoglycemia, begin at 50% of infusion rate prior to hypoglycemia.

MD Note: When converting to subcutaneous insulin injections, follow the **Adult Transition from IV Insulin Infusion to Subcutaneous Insulin Protocol** in MIS to be ordered by MD.

Approved by Pharmacy & Therapeutics Committee 04/25/2003.

---

from guideline use, organizations must evaluate the outcomes of patients treated and refine the guidelines as necessary. In 1996, Schwartz published the results of a performance improvement process applied to enteral and parenteral practice and outcomes that were enhanced using standards and guidelines available at that time. The article includes a nutrition support decision tree and patient outcome statements [11], citing guidelines and standards created by the American Society for Parenteral and Enteral Nutrition (ASPEN). Since publication of the article, ASPEN has created or revised guidelines for the use of SNS in adult and pediatric patients [12], standards for nutrition support of hospitalized adult patients [13], and standards for nutrition support dietitians [14], and developed standards for nutrition support of pediatric patients [15] and for nutrition support, nurses, pharmacists, and physicians [16–18]. Incorporation of the standards into clinical competency checklists for practitioners is important as a means of demonstrating staffing effectiveness.

TABLE 40.6
University of Virginia Health System

Aspect of Care: Periodic Assessment of the Effects of Nutrition Therapy　　　Data Gatherer _____　　　Area _____

Indicator: Tube-fed patients who are on dose delivery will receive at least 90% of the ordered volume of formula (5 days average).

Patient Name/Hx #	Day	Pt. Unit	Amt. cc's Received	Goal (cc)	% Goal Received	Compliant at ≥ 90% Y/N	Documentation Unclear Y/N	Comments (Reason TF held, etc.)
	(1)							
	(2)							
	(3)							
	(4)							
	(5)							
Avg:								

Source: From University of Virginia Health System. With permission.

TABLE 40.7
CQI-Triglycerides on TPN

Pt. name_____ Med Record #_____

Age_____ Male/Female/Other

Ht_____ Weight (please state whether this is actual or adjusted) _____

(Please give adjusted weight if you are using that for your calculations.)

Start of TPN_____

Triglyceride level_____ Date_____

Diagnosis _____

History _____

Hx. of hyperlipidemia? Yes/No

Hyperglycemia? _____

TPN order: _____

Changes made in TPN due to TG? _____

Source: From University of Virginia Health System. With permission.

40.5 HACCP STANDARDS

Although the Hazard Analysis Critical Control Point (HACCP) system for prevention-based food safety is not required by JCAHO [19], that organization does require that food and nutrition products be prepared, distributed, and administered safely and in a sanitary fashion. ETF must be included in evaluation of compliance with this standard. The interdisciplinary HACCP plan at New York– Presbyterian Hospital (Table 40.8) was created in 1996 and has been modified periodically. Table 40.9 illustrates the tool used to document compliance with the plan. Data collected with this tool are aggregated and reviewed to assess organizational compliance with HACCP; components of the tool may be used as a means to assess an individual's compliance with his or her duties in a pay-for-performance system.

40.6 CONCLUSION

High quality in health care has always been assumed. New reporting initiatives, highlighted in the media, and several high-profile sentinel events have significantly raised public awareness about healthcare quality. As a result, the demand for cost-effective and efficacious health care has never been greater. Regulatory agencies require the collection and analysis of data for performance improvement, the documentation of the competence of healthcare providers, and the use of appropriate standards and protocols to ensure patient safety and clinical quality. Consumers access data from these agencies and others when making decisions about where to seek health care. Nutrition support professionals in all practice settings must continuously evaluate and improve their practice in order to provide optimal nutrition care and ensure the best possible outcomes for patients.

TABLE 40.8
Hazard Analysis Critical Control Point (HACCP) Plan for Open System Enteral Feeding Preparation and Administration, New York–Presbyterian Hospital Department of Food and Nutrition

Flow Process	Hazard	Concern: CCP or CP	Control Criteria	Monitor Method: Procedure	Action Plan: Criteria Failure
Purchase	Contamination of enteral feeding products by chemical, microbiological, or particulate matter; breakdown in quality control at point of production.	CP (control point)	Purchase from approved, inspected and certified vendors, including Infant Formula Laboratory Service, Inc.	Monitor vendors for adherence to purchasing specifications. Inspect delivery upon receipt. Receive notification from vendors/FDA regarding quality control issues.	Reject delivery not adhering to specifications, without exception. Follow food recall procedures to address quality control issues.
Receiving	Contamination of enteral feeding products by chemical, microbiological, or particulate matter through improper receiving methods.	CP	Verify delivery based on receiving criteria. Immediately remove received enteral feeding products for appropriate storage.	Monitor receiving process and vendor adherence to specifications for delivery. Document vendor problems on Vendor Receiving Report.	Coach/counsel employees in proper receiving techniques. If necessary, revise receiving procedures according to HACCP guidelines.
Storage	Contamination of enteral feeding products by chemical, microbiological, or particulate matter due to improper storage and handling procedures.	CP	Liquid protein module: Verify adherence to temperature standards for freezer units prior to thawing and for refrigeration units during/after thawing. MCT module and all other products: Prevent from freezing and store at < 86°F. Verify the correct temperature for dry storage areas. Verify adherence to "first in first out" (FIFO) safety and sanitation standards in all storage areas. Remove dented cans from circulation.	Monitor temperatures in refrigeration/freezer units and dry storage areas. Monitor product expiration dates. Verify safety and sanitation process by conducting monthly safety and sanitation inspections.	Immediately remove enteral feeding products in affected refrigerator/freezer to a unit that is operating within standards; discard mixed or portioned product that has exceeded 2 hour limit of storage without temperature regulation. Shut down and repair refrigerators/freezers unable to maintain temperature standards. Remove products in affected dry storage areas to an area that meets temperature standard.

(continued)

TABLE 40.8 (CONTINUED)
Hazard Analysis Critical Control Point (HACCP) Plan for Open System Enteral Feeding Preparation and Administration, New York–Presbyterian Hospital Department of Food and Nutrition

Flow Process	Hazard	Concern: CCP or CP	Control Criteria	Monitor Method: Procedure	Action Plan: Criteria Failure
					Return to vendor/discard products that have exceeded expiration date as noted by the manufacturer. Return dented cans to vendor. Coach/counsel employees in monitoring and action procedures.
Thaw	Contamination of enteral feeding products due to inappropriate thawing and/or utilization of thawed item beyond specified time frame.	CCP (critical control point)	Thaw liquid protein module and unsweetened health shakes completely using approved method of thawing under refrigeration only. Do not thaw at room temperature. Label each unopened carton of liquid protein module with the date placed in the refrigerator for thawing. If unopened and unused after 5 days, the product is to be discarded. Unsweetened health shakes are labeled with an expiration date 12 days from transfer from freezer to thaw under refrigeration.	Monitor thawing temperature. Do not use until completely thawed. Verify thawing schedule to enteral formula production schedule.	Thaw fully if frozen and reject items of questionable quality. Discard thawed items that have exceeded expiration date. Coach/counsel employees in proper thawing methods. If necessary, revise thawing procedures according to HACCP guidelines.
Preparation	Introduction of microbes, chemicals, or particulates by process and/or equipment cross-contamination and/or employees.	CP	Train employees in proper enteral feeding product handling techniques and sanitation. Wash hands prior to preparing feedings or modular components. Prepare according to enteral formula recipe (attachment 1,2). Use tap water for reconstituting Pediatric Vivonex and Ceralyte. See Departmental HACCP Plan Section 4. Note: Sterile water is used for the preparation and dilution of enteral feedings for neonates. For adult and pediatric feedings, distilled or sterile water is used upon specific order only.	Verify cleaning and sanitizing process. Observe that separation of enteral feeding products and raw or processed food items and cleaning compounds is maintained. Verify adherence to enteral formula orders and recipes.	Discard questionable enteral formula ingredients. Reject ingredients not meeting acceptance criteria. Coach/counsel employees in proper enteral formula preparation methods. If necessary, revise enteral formula preparation procedures according to HACCP guidelines.

Step	Hazard	CCP	Control Measures	Monitoring	Corrective Action
			Food coloring/blue dye is not to be added to enteral feedings. Clean and sanitize equipment and utensils prior to use. Protect enteral feeding products from cross-contamination.		
Cold holding	Spores germinate and microorganisms multiply at temperatures above 40°F.	CCP	Seal, label, and date (date opened) opened cartons of liquid protein module used in EFPL. Store and hold under refrigeration at ≤ 40°F. Discard any open carton that has been unused after 48 hours of opening. Seal, label, and date (date opened) opened bottles of MCT oil used in EFPL. Store and hold in dry storage (do not refrigerate). Discard any open bottle that has been unused after 3 months of opening. Seal, label, and date (date opened) opened cans of Polycose and Promod. Discard any opened can that has been unused after 1 month of opening. Seal, label: formula, rate of administration, patient name, room #, and date (date prepared) all reconstituted mixed enteral formula and portioned protein, fat, or carbohydrate modules. With the exception of unopened cans of enteral formula, MCT oil and powdered CHO or powdered protein module (which are stored at room temperature), store any mixed, reconstituted, or portioned modules under refrigeration at ≤ 40°F until delivered to patient care units for administration. Verify temperature accuracy of refrigeration monitor. Inventory product to detect items at or near expiration.	Monitor refrigeration temperature and verify accuracy of temperature-monitoring device. Conduct daily inventory of prepared or open enteral feeding products to verify expiration and discard procedures.	Monitor refrigeration temperature for ≤ 40°F. If temperature standards are not being met, immediately remove prepared or open enteral feeding products to refrigerator that maintains the required temperature. Coach/counsel employees in enteral feeding product monitoring methods. Discard formulas that have exceeded shelf life criteria.

(continued)

TABLE 40.8 (CONTINUED)
Hazard Analysis Critical Control Point (HACCP) Plan for Open System Enteral Feeding Preparation and Administration, New York–Presbyterian Hospital Department of Food and Nutrition

Flow Process	Hazard	Concern: CCP or CP	Control Criteria	Monitor Method: Procedure	Action Plan: Criteria Failure
Delivery to nursing unit	Surviving microorganisms can grow in inadequately maintained mixed enteral feeding products. Spores that survive can begin to grow during the inadequate temperature delivery process. Chemical and particulates cannot be destroyed.	CP	After preparation, enteral feeding products, as required, will be stored under refrigeration until delivered to nursing units according to delivery schedule.	Monitor timeliness of delivery of enteral feeding products to nursing units.	Discard mixed or portioned product that has exceeded 2-hour limit of storage without temperature regulation. Coach/counsel employees in enteral feeding product delivery procedures. If necessary, revise delivery procedures according to HACCP guidelines.
Cold holding on nursing units	Surviving microorganisms can grow in inadequately maintained mixed or open enteral feeding products. Spores can survive and begin to grow during the inadequate refrigeration holding process. Chemical and particulates cannot be destroyed.	CCP	Verify that all mixed enteral formulas, modular components and open containers of enteral feeding products are sealed; labeled as to contents, patient name, room #; and dated. Store and hold mixed enteral feeding formulas and liquid protein module under refrigeration at ≤ 40°F in nourishment station refrigerators. Verify temperature accuracy of refrigeration monitor. Inventory product to detect items at or near expiration. All mixed enteral formulas, opened containers of formula, or containers of liquid protein module, MCT oil, CHO powder, or protein powder are discarded 24 hours after the production date by Food and Nutrition staff. Opened cans of enteral formula are to be discarded by Nursing staff and are not to be stored in the refrigerator.	Monitor refrigeration temperature and verify accuracy of temperature monitoring device. Conduct daily inventory of prepared or open enteral feeding products to verify expiration and discard procedures.	Monitor refrigeration temperature for ≤ 40°F. If temperature standards are not being met, immediately remove prepared or modular components to a refrigerator that maintains the required temperature. Coach/counsel employees in enteral feeding product monitoring methods. Discard formulas that have exceeded shelf life criteria.

Enteral feeding administration	All enteral feeding products, at room temperature, can support microbial growth. Formula manipulation or using procedures that increase handling of formulas or administration systems increases the potential for contamination.	CCP	Wash hands prior to handling feedings and administration systems.	Monitor staff for adherence to proper enteral feeding administration techniques.	Discard product that has exceeded limit for hang time. Coach/counsel staff on proper enteral formula administration procedures. If necessary, revise enteral formula administration procedures according to HACCP guidelines.
Enteral feeding administration (continued)			Avoid touching any part of the container or administration system that will come in contact with the feeding.		
			Inspect seals and reservoirs for damage prior to utilization.		
			Assemble feeding systems on a clean, dry, disinfected surface.		
			Avoid adding food coloring/blue dye to the feeding (use proper positioning and administration methods to avoid aspiration).		
			Avoid adding medications directly to the feeding. If necessary, flush tube after administration with tap water.		
			Follow approved guidelines for mixing and administration of modular enteral components (attachment 2).		
			Date/time each component of the system, also indicating patient name and formula (on feeding bag). Limit hang time of feeding to 4 hours for adults and pediatrics; for neonates, 8 hr for decanted formula and 4 h for mixed.		
			Empty feeding bags of product completely prior to pouring newly opened product into the bag.		
			Use administration sets with Y-ports and drip chambers and cap disconnected sets.		
			Position container to prevent reflux of feeding up the feeding set.		
			Irrigate feeding tube with tap water (or as specified).		
			Change adult and pediatric administration sets every 24 hours. For neonates, change syringe and connecting tube or feeding bag with each feeding.		

(continued)

TABLE 40.8 (CONTINUED)
Hazard Analysis Critical Control Point (HACCP) Plan for Open System Enteral Feeding Preparation and Administration, New York–Presbyterian Hospital Department of Food and Nutrition

Flow Process	Hazard	Concern: CCP or CP	Control Criteria	Monitor Method: Procedure	Action Plan: Criteria Failure
Sanitize (ongoing process through various stages of the system)	Destruction of microbes during the cleaning and sanitizing process. Introduction of microbes, chemicals, or particulates by cross-contamination and/or employees.	CP	Train employees in proper enteral feeding product handling techniques and sanitation. Clean and sanitize surfaces, equipment, and utensils prior to use. Protect products from contamination.	Verify cleaning and sanitizing process. Observe that separation of enteral feeding preparation and storage and sanitation processes is maintained.	Reclean and resanitize all preparation equipment. Coach/counsel employees in proper sanitation procedures. Discard enteral feeding products contaminated during sanitation process. If necessary, revise sanitation procedures according to HACCP guidelines.

Source: From New York–Presbyterian Hospital Department of Food and Nutrition. With permission.

TABLE 40.9
Quality Assessment and Improvement Program: HACCP Plan for Enteral Feeding Preparation and Administration, New York–Presbyterian Hospital Department of Food and Nutrition

Completed by/Title:_____ Date:_____ Unit/Room #: _____

Patient Name:_____ Patient History Number: _____

Current Enteral Feeding Order _____

Instructions: Review one patient on an enteral feeding. *For each "No" or "NA" explain in comments.

Direct Observation	Yes	No*	NA*	Comments
27. Enteral feeding product(s) received according to specification.				
28. Temperature standards for refrigeration and dry storage of enteral feeding product(s) met.				
29. Product usage according to FIFO; those exceeding expiration date returned/discarded.				
30. Liquid protein module and unsweetened health shakes thawed under refrigeration; products labeled with date placed in refrigerator for thawing.				
31. Unopened and unused thawed liquid protein module discarded after 5 days; open cartons discarded after 48 hours.				
32. Unopened and unused unsweetened health shakes discarded after 12 days.				
33. MCT oil, Polycose Powder, and Pro-Mod Powder stored at room temperature, labeled with date opened. Opened and unused bottles/cans discarded after 3/1 month(s).				
34. Employees wash hands prior to preparing enteral feedings or modular components.				
35. Cleaned and sanitized surface and equipment used to prepare enteral feedings or modular components.				
36. Enteral formula prepared according to recipe.				
37. Tap water used to reconstitute Pediatric Vivonex and Ceralyte; distilled or sterile water used in the preparation of enteral formulas upon specific order.				
38. Prepared enteral feedings kept separate from raw or processed food items and cleaning compounds.				

(continued)

TABLE 40.9 (CONTINUED)
Quality Assessment and Improvement Program: HACCP Plan for Enteral Feeding Preparation and Administration, New York–Presbyterian Hospital Department of Food and Nutrition

Direct Observation	Yes	No*	NA*	Comments
39. Reconstituted mixed enteral formulas and portioned protein, fat, and carbohydrate modules sealed and labeled (formula, rate of administration, patient name and room number, date prepared).				
40. Temperature standard for refrigerated storage of reconstituted, mixed enteral formulas and portioned protein, fat, and carbohydrate modules met.				
41. Inventory of reconstituted, mixed enteral formulas and portioned protein, fat, and carbohydrate modules reveals none is past expiration date.				
42. Nursing staff washes hands prior to handling feedings and administration systems.				
43. Nursing staff avoids touching any part of the container or administration system that will come in contact with the feeding.				
44. Nursing staff assembles feeding system on a disinfected surface and inspects seals/reservoirs for damage.				
45. Medications are not added to feeding unless necessary. If added, tube is flushed with tap water (or as specified) after administration.				
46. Date/time each component of feeding system also feeding bag is labeled with patient name and formula.				
47. Hang time of feeding limited to 4 hours.				
48. Feeding bags completely emptied of product prior to pouring newly opened product into the bag.				
49. Disconnected sets are capped.				
50. Container is positioned to prevent reflux of feeding up feeding set.				
51. Administration sets changed every 24 hours.				
52. Additional Comments:				

Source: From New York–Presbyterian Hospital Department of Food and Nutrition. With permission.

REFERENCES

1. Institute of Medicine. *Medicare: A Strategy for Quality Assurance*. Vol I. Lohr KN (ed). National Academy Press, Washington, DC, 1990.
2. Graham N.O. *Quality Assurance in Hospitals*. Aspen Publishers, Rockville, MD, 1990, 3–13.
3. Joint Commission Resources. *2004 Hospital Standards*, 2003 Education Program Workbook. Joint Commission Resources, Oakbrook Terrace, IL, 2003.
4. Marian M., Steiber M. Quality performance improvement, indicators, and standards, in *The Science and Practice of Nutrition Support: A Case-Based Core Curriculum*, Gottschlich M.M., Fuhrman M.P., Hammond K.A., Holcombe B.J., Seidner D.L., Eds, Kendall/Hunt, Dubuque, IA, 2001, chap. 36.
5. Winkler M.F., Hedberg A. Quality and performance improvement, in *Contemporary Nutrition Support Practice: A Clinical Guide*, Matarese L.A., Gottschlich M.M., Eds, W.B. Saunders, Philadelphia, 2003, chap. 43.
6. Joint Commission Resources. *2004 Advanced Hospital Standards and Survey Process Update*, 2003 Custom Education Program. Joint Commission Resources, Oakbrook Terrace, IL, 2003, chap. 1.
7. Joint Commission Perspectives on Patient Safety, December 2002.
8. Dodds ES, Murray JD, Trexler KT, Grant JP. Metabolic occurrences in total parenteral nutrition patients managed by a nutrition support team, *Nutr. Clin. Prac.*, 16, 78–84, 2001.
9. Dettmer HW. *Goldratt's Theory of Constraints: A Systems Approach to Continuous Improvement*. ASQC Quality Press, Milwaukee, 1997.
10. Klein CJ, Stanek GS, Wiles CE. Nutrition support care map targets monitoring and reassessment to improve outcomes in trauma patients, *Nutr. Clin. Prac.*, 16, 85–97, 2001.
11. Schwartz DB. Enhanced enteral and parenteral nutrition practice and outcomes in an intensive care unit with a hospital-wide performance improvement process, *J. Am. Diet. Assoc.*, 96, 484–489, 1996.
12. ASPEN Board of Directors and The Clinical Guidelines Task Force. Guidelines for the use of parenteral and enteral nutrition in adult and pediatric patients, *J. Parenter. Enteral Nutr.*, 22(supplement), 2002.
13. ASPEN Board of Directors. Standards for specialized nutrition support: adult hospitalized patients, *Nutr. Clin. Prac.* 17, 384–391, 2002.
14. ASPEN Board of Directors. Standards of practice for nutrition support dietitians, *Nutr. Clin. Prac.*, 15, 53–59, 2000.
15. ASPEN Board of Directors. Standards for hospitalized pediatric patients, *Nutr. Clin. Prac.*, 11, 217–228, 1996.
16. ASPEN Board of Directors. Standards of practice for nutrition support nurses, *Nutr. Clin. Prac.* 16, 56–62, 2001.
17. ASPEN Board of Directors. Standards of practice for nutrition support pharmacists, *Nutr. Clin. Prac.* 14, 275–281, 1999.
18. ASPEN Board of Directors. Standards of practice for nutrition support physicians, *Nutr. Clin. Prac.* 18, 270–275, 2003.
19. *The Complete HACCP Manual for Institutional Food Service Operations*, Food Services Associates, Dunkirk, NY, 1995.

41 Economic Considerations of Nutrition in the Critically Ill

Gail Cresci
Medical College of Georgia

Teresa R. Schmidt
AstraZeneca

CONTENTS

41.1 INTRODUCTION

As in other areas of health care, the validity of specialized nutrition support — total parenteral nutrition (TPN) and enteral nutrition (EN) — is questioned in terms of type, time, outcomes, and cost. Is it worth providing specialized nutrition support to hospitalized patients, and at what cost (1)? Today, this is a question that demands an answer from every clinician, in light of increasing healthcare costs and constraints of managed care.

Specialized nutrition support is a highly sophisticated therapy that carries significant expenses, including the price of its components, labor to compound the formula, expenses associated with gaining feeding access, assessment, and monitoring the patient's response to the therapy (2). Nutrition guidelines state that any patient unable to consume adequate nutrients orally (60% nutrition needs) for at least 5 days in the critically ill, or for 7 to 14 days in the general population, should be a candidate for specialized nutrition support (3).

Malnutrition negatively influences patient morbidity, mortality, and hospital length of stay. In a retrospective review, Kudsk et al. showed general surgery patients capable of receiving preoperative nutrition intake, but did not, had significantly increased postoperative complications, mortality rates, intensive care unit (ICU) and hospital lengths of stays, and requirement for TPN (4). Complications increased significantly as preoperative albumin levels dropped. Complications also were correlated with operative site, magnitude, and complexity of the procedures and preoperative albumin levels (Table 41.1). These increased complications equate to increased healthcare costs. Unfortunately, nutrition intervention is often not provided until malnutrition-related complications

---

TABLE 41.1
Surgical and Nutritional Risk Factors for Poor Surgical Outcomes (4)

High-Risk Procedures (Preoperative Serum Albumin < 3.25 g/dl)
Esophagectomy (total or partial)
Esophagogastrectomy
Intrathoracic anastomosis of the esophagus
Repair of esophageal stricture
Pancreatic duodenectomy
Distal pancreatectomy
Puestow procedure
Drainage pancreatic psuedocyst into stomach or small bowel

Lower-Risk Procedures (Preoperative Serum Albumin < 2.25 g/dl)
Partial gastrectomy (Bilroth I or II anastomosis)
Other partial gastrectomy
Total gastrectomy
Gastroenterostomy
Revision of gastric anastomosis
Closure of gastric fistula
Colorectal resection with anastomosis or abdominal perineal resection

---

arise and the patient has developed an advanced state of nutritional disrepair. This chapter will address the economic benefits of nutrition intervention for the critically ill patient.

41.2 ROUTE AND TIMING OF FEEDING

Presently, evidence and practice patterns support the use of enteral feedings over parenteral nutrient infusions in the critically ill patient. This is provided that the patient is hemodynamically stable and has a functional GI tract and enteral access. When compared to TPN, enteral feeding is associated with decreased infectious complications, length of stay, and costs (5–10). (See Chapter 12 for details.) It is ideal, but often impractical or impossible, to provide full nutrient delivery to the critically ill patient by the enteral route. Provision of as little as one-third (25 to 40%) of the nutrient requirements delivered enterally has shown benefits over TPN (11). Some patients cannot tolerate enteral feedings, and in them TPN is essential because it is more advantageous in reducing complications than not feeding at all. Buzby et al. provided perioperative TPN after major abdominal or thoracic surgical procedures in the severely malnourished patient (12). They found that malnourished patients who received TPN had fewer noninfectious complications than the control group who did not receive TPN (p = 0.03, relative risk 0.12, 95% confidence interval, 0.02 to 0.91), with no concomitant increase in infectious complications.

Moore et al. found TPN associated with a significantly greater number of total postoperative infections and septic complications than EN, 39.3% vs. 18.6%, respectively (7). Pneumonia, the most frequently occurring infection in the meta-analysis, was higher in those fed via TPN than EN (14.3% vs. 5.8%). Kudsk et al. found enteral patients experienced significantly less septic morbidity than patients receiving TPN (5). Enteral patients developed significantly fewer pneumonias (11.8% vs. 31%), abscesses (1.9% vs. 13.3%), or line sepsis (1.9% vs. 13.3%) when compared to parenteral patients.

The time to initiation of enteral feeding is also associated with patient outcomes, including incidences of infectious complications. Enteral feeding started within 12 to 48 hours following injury or ICU admission in fluid resuscitated patients resulted in decreased infectious complications

TABLE 41.2
Guidelines for TPN Use in the Critically Ill (3)

Indications	Contraindications
Ischemic bowel or hypotension	Functioning GI tract and hemodynamically stable
Bowel obstruction distal to GI access, prolonged ileus	Inability to obtain central venous access
Severe GI hemorrhage	Treatment anticipated less than 5 days in a patient without severe malnutrition
Severe complicated acute pancreatitis	Prognosis does not warrant aggressive nutrition support
Severe colitis or diarrhea	
High output fistula or ostomy (> 1 l/d)	
Short bowel syndrome	
Inability to gain enteral access	

TABLE 41.3
Reasons for Inappropriate TPN Use

Arguments against early enteral feeding
    Fear of visceral ischemia/necrosis
Perceived intolerance issues
    Dysmotility
    Diarrhea
    Reflux
    Aspiration
"Most" patients do not need
Expensive with questionable benefit
Unable to obtain enteral access

(7,9,13), as well as improved digestion and absorption (14–18), nitrogen balance (14,19), glycemic control (7,20), gut immune function (15–18), and reduced hospital costs (7,10,21–25).

41.3 SELECTION OF CANDIDATES FOR SPECIALIZED NUTRITION SUPPORT

The early identification and immediate nutritional intervention in patients at nutritional risk is the best way to minimize the costly and harmful effects of protein-calorie malnutrition (26–28). In hospitalized patients in the U.S., it was found that the additional costs arising as a result of malnutrition were $5575 for a surgical patient and $2477 for a clinical patient (1,29). Because the route of feeding can make a difference in patient complication rate, morbidity, and cost, it is very important to select only the most appropriate patients for TPN based on established guidelines (Table 41.2). Despite guidelines to aid the decision making of candidates for TPN and EN, inappropriate use of TPN continues for various reasons (Table 41.3).

41.3.1 INAPPROPRIATE TPN

The inappropriate use of TPN has been reported to occur in medical and surgical patients (22,24,30,31). Fessler et al. reported that, based on clinical guidelines for appropriate TPN usage, 27% of TPN and 32% of peripheral parenteral nutrition orders were inappropriate during a 6-month review period (22). Multidisciplinary nutrition support team work can be responsible for a reduction in treatment costs when certain procedures are adopted, with a goal of improved clinical outcomes and consequently reduced costs (32–35). Inappropriate use of PN is less likely when patients are followed up formally by a team with expertise in nutrition and metabolic support (23,24). Trujillo et al. reported that 82% of TPN initiations after metabolic support team consultation were appropriate, compared with only 56% of TPN initiations without consultation (24).

Often the reason for inappropriate TPN use is the absence of optimal enteral access. Although gastric feeding access is quick and easy to obtain, many critically ill patients do not tolerate gastric feedings and clinicians prefer to feed into the small intestine. Ability to gain small bowel enteral access in critically ill patients relies on the clinical skill at the institution. There are numerous techniques for gaining enteral access for ICU patients (see Chapter 15 for details). For ICU patients requiring short-term access or as a bridge until longer-term access is obtained, small bowel enteral access can be successfully obtained at the bedside (36). Placement of these tubes requires trained personnel; dietitians and nurses make ideal candidates for placement. Cresci et al. found a reduced use of inappropriate use of TPN in critically ill trauma patients once an enteral access protocol (36) and ASPEN guidelines (3) for TPN were implemented (37). Inappropriate TPN use decreased from 35% without an enteral access protocol to 12% when a protocol including guidelines for nutrition support was strictly enforced.

41.4   ECONOMIC IMPACT OF SPECIALIZED NUTRITION SUPPORT

41.4.1   FEEDING PROTOCOLS

Implementation of enteral feeding protocols (Table 41.4) not only benefit the patient because they are more likely to be fed in the GI tract vs. intravenously, but they also benefit the institution by reducing costs. Schwartz projected a cost savings of nearly $700,000 annually occurring because enhanced enteral and parenteral nutrition practice resulted in reduced overall hospital and intensive care unit lengths of stay (38). Projected cost savings involving enteral and parenteral solutions were identified at $55,000 annually. Charges for TPN can range from $200 to 1,000/d, compared with enteral feeding, which is usually less than or equal to $50/day (39). Szeluga et al. reported an average 28-day enteral feeding program cost $1,169 for bone marrow transplantation vs. $2,575 for TPN (40). Another study concluded enteral feeding costs of $170 per day vs. $308 per day for PN for patients with severe head injury (41). Fessler projected costs savings of $23,000 annually by eliminating the use of inappropriate TPN (22).

41.4.2   INFECTIOUS AND NONINFECTIOUS COMPLICATIONS

Parenteral feeding and delayed enteral feeding are associated with increased infectious and noninfectious complications. Infectious complications are associated with high morbidity, mortality, and costs. Reduction of complications, both infectious and noninfectious, is now becoming a prime focus in critical care medicine. The added cost of a single ICU infection can be estimated at $21,000 (42). These infectious complications become even more important with the rise of bacterial flora resistant to one or multiple antibiotics. The increased microbial resistance has made many antibiotics relatively ineffective in the ICU setting; therefore, the push for prevention of infections is becoming a subject of growing interest and attention (43). In addition to infectious complications, the adverse impacts and cost associated with noninfectious complications are often marked. For example, Waitzberg et al. have recently demonstrated that anastomotic leaks, though frequently noninfectious, are the most costly postoperative complication in the surgical patient population (44). The epidemiology of postoperative nosocomial infections is changing. In the 1960s, postop wound infections were responsible for 46% of infections. During the 1970s and 1980s, urinary tract infections (UTIs) were the most common (43). Currently, 43% of postop nosocomial infections are from pneumonia,

TABLE 41.4
Sample Enteral Feeding Protocol for ICU Patients

Purpose: Enteral nutrition is the optimal route of feeding in hospitalized patients because it has been shown to:

1. Provide better maintenance of gut integrity and reduce infection
2. Attenuate the hypermetabolic response to stress
3. Decrease hospital length of stay
4. Reduce hospital costs

Goal: Initiate enteral tube feedings within 48 hours of hospital admission

Indications: Candidates are all patients who are not anticipated to consume adequate nutrients (at least 60% of nutrition needs) within 5 days of admission. Enteral access should be obtained within 48 hours of admission after adequate resuscitation.

1. Mechanical ventilation
2. Neurologic dysfunction
3. Gastric atony from surgery or other cause
4. Unable to consume adequate nutrients orally

Contraindications

1. Bowel obstruction distal to site of enteral access
2. Hemodynamic instability
3. Splanchnic hypoperfusion
4. Major upper GI hemorrhage caused by varices or ulcer disease with vessel visible with endoscopy
5. Prolonged ileus
6. High output ostomy, fistula, diarrhea (> 1.5 l/d)

Permission: Nurse or dietitian will obtain physician order ASAP for use of protocol within 48 hours of admission.

Feeding Route

1. If preexisting enteral access available, use it (surgical G/J tube, PEG).
2. Bedside placement of small bowel feeding tube is preferred if not contraindicated. Trained and certified dietitians and nurses should initiate feeding tube placement. Physicians may also place feeding tubes.
3. Gastric feeding may be utilized if patient has < 2 aspiration risk factors. Risk factors for aspiration:
   a. Documented aspiration
   b. Decreased level of consciousness
   c. Mechanical ventilation
   d. Emesis
   e. Absent gag reflex
   f. Inability to elevate head of bed > 30 degrees
   g. Persistent high gastric output or residuals (> 1 l per 24 hours)
   h. Neuromuscular disease and/or structural abnormalities of the digestive tract
   i. History of gastroparesis, poor GI motility

Guidelines for Enteral Feeding Protocol Use

1. ICU patients meeting the indications for early enteral feeding will be enrolled in enteral feeding protocol.
2. Use an appropriate enteral formula recommended by the registered dietitian.
3. Enteral feedings should begin at full strength at 20 ml/h and advanced every 6 to 8 hours if tolerated. Consult the dietitian for nutrition assessment and goal tube feeding rate.

(continued)

TABLE 41.4 (CONTINUED)
Sample Enteral Feeding Protocol for ICU Patients

4. Elevate the patient's head of bed at least 30 degrees at all times. Enteral feedings do not need to be halted for routine nursing care (wound dressing changes, bed change, bathing, PT, OT), as long as head of bed can remain elevated properly for gastric feedings.
5. Flush feeding tubes with 60 ml warm water every 4 hours and after each medication to maintain tube patency. Avoid delivering medications via feeding tube if possible.
6. Monitor closely for signs of feeding intolerance:
   a. Increasing abdominal distention
   b. Emesis
   c. Nausea
   d. Excessive diarrhea (> 1 l/d)
   e. Formula reflux into gastric tube or increased gastric residuals (> 400 ml in 4 h)
7. Check laboratory values to monitor metabolic and nutritional status
   a. Prealbumin every Monday, Thursday
   b. BMP, Mg, PO4 every morning
   c. CMP, triglyceride every Monday
8. Adjust IVF for desired total volume input in 24 hours. Note enteral formulas are not 100% free water and should not be counted as such (on average, 80% volume is free water).

Enteral Feeding Orders
- Insert feeding tube per protocol.
- Once feeding tube placement confirmed via KUB, initiate feedings as indicated below.
- Consult dietitian for nutrition assessment.

Route of Feeding (Select One)

☐ Naso/oro enteric feeding tube   ☐ PEG/gastrostomy   ☐ Also NGT as
☐ Naso/oro gastric feeding tube   ☐ Jejunostomy   ☐ LIWS or clamped

Select the Desired Formula

Product	Kcal/ml	g pro/l	% Free Water	Product	Kcal/ml	g pro/l	% Free Water
Isosource VHN	1.0	62	85	Peptinex DT	1.0	50	83
Nutren 1.0	1.0	40	85	Vivonex Plus	1.0	45	85
Fibersource HN	1.2	53	81	Impact with Glutamine[a]	1.3	78	81
Comply	1.5	60	77	Oxepa[a]	1.5	62.7	78
				Nepro[a]	2.0	70	70

Feeding Schedule:

☐ Initiate feedings at full strength at _____ ml/h (suggested 20 ml)
☐ Advance feeding rate by _____ml per hour every _____ hours, to goal of _____ml/h
   (suggested 20 ml/h every 6 hours advancement)
☐ Or, bolus feeding (for gastric feedings only)
   Bolus _____ ml every _____ hours for a total of _____ ml/24 hours
☐ Adjust IVF by _____ ml/h
   IV MVI, trace element packet, and 40 μg selenium to 1st bag IVF until goal tube feeding tolerated

(continued)

TABLE 41.4 (CONTINUED)
Sample Enteral Feeding Protocol for ICU Patients

Orders for Tube-Feeding Protocol (Using a Single Line Strike through Any Orders Not to Be Used)

☐ Strict daily input and output; record daily weights on flow chart.

☐ Keep head of bed elevated at least 30 to 45 degrees.

☐ Give formula at room temperature. Hang formula for a maximum of 8 hours and change enteral administration set every 24 hours.

☐ Check residuals every 4 hours if feeding gastrically.

☐ Hold gastric feedings if residuals are greater than _____ ml. Return residual to patient if less than ____ 400 ml (suggested 400 ml). Recheck residuals in 4 hours; if residual greater than ____, call physician.

☐ Flush feeding tube with _____ ml water every _____ hours and before and after medications (suggested 60 ml q 4 h for patency)

☐ If feeding tube is clogged/dislodged and attempts to unclog are unsuccessful, replace ASAP and confirm with KUB.

☐ Record persistent nausea, vomiting, and/or diarrhea on flow sheet; notify physician if continues > 4 h.

☐ DO NOT stop tube feeding for routine nursing care, wound dressings, bathing, etc.

☐ Implement mouth care protocol.

☐ If feedings are held, call MD for maintenance IVF orders until feeds are resumed.

☐ Obtain serum basic metabolic panel, Mg, PO4 level q am.

☐ Obtain serum prealbumin level every Monday and Thursday.

☐ Obtain serum comprehensive metabolic panel and serum triglyceride level every Monday.

MD Signature_____ Date_____ Time_____

[a] Formulas must be approved by dietitian, attending physician.

with wound infections accounting for approximately 15% (45). This trend dramatically changes the potential morbidity of a postop nosocomial infection, because pneumonia carries a much higher mortality than does UTI or wound infection. The economic impact of caring for patients with an infection, specifically, has been shown to be $42,651, compared with $18,064 for patients without an infection (46). Infections were shown to add $12,542 to mean hospital costs due to longer postoperative length of hospital stay (46).

Patients suffering trauma, sepsis, or major surgery exhibit depressed immune function and are at high risk of developing nosocomial infections and other major morbidities. Enteral nutrition, specifically with the use of formulas with added nutrients such as glutamine, arginine, dietary nucleotides, and omega-3 fatty acids, has been shown to improve immune functioning, (47,48) which ultimately decreases mortality, morbidity, and resource utilization. Several immune-modulating formulas are commercially available worldwide (see Chapter 16). Demonstrated benefits of using these formulas in the appropriate patient populations include decreasing the incidence of complications (both infectious and noninfectious), ventilator days, ICU length of stay, and overall length of stay, when compared with those patients receiving an isocaloric control diet (49–52). There are no data to support similar outcomes with the use of PN. Recently, it has been shown that immune-modulating formulas are a cost-effective way for hospitals to improve clinical outcomes while reducing resource consumption and total cost (53). For the medical patient population, based on a 51% decrease in risk of infectious complications and a decreased length of hospital stay of 9.7 days, net cost savings (after accounting for the increased costs of administering immune-modulating formula) are $2066. The same calculations were done for surgical and trauma patients, with $688 and $308 net cost savings per patient, respectively. These figures assume a base infection rate of 5%. Expected cost savings vary markedly for deviations in base infection rate and slightly for differences in facility type or region of the country.

41.5 SUMMARY

When properly indicated and managed, specialized nutrition support significantly contributes to reductions in patient morbidity and hospital costs. Applying the principles of economic science to manage health care resources does not necessarily mean that one should spend less, but that the resources should be used in a more efficient manner (1). Nutritionists need to take an active role in not only acting as the patient advocate for nutritional care, but also doing so by practicing optimal health economics.

REFERENCES

1. Waitzberg DL, Baxter YC. Costs of patients under nutritional therapy: from prescription to discharge. *Curr. Opin. Clin. Nutr. Metab. Care* 7: 189–198, 2004.
2. Chiolero R, Kudsk K. Current concepts in nutrition delivery in critically ill patients: route, insulin and economics. *Curr. Opin. Clin. Nutr. Metab. Care* 7: 157–159, 2004.
3. ASPEN Board of Directors. Guidelines for the use of parenteral and enteral nutrition in adult and pediatric patients. *JPEN* 26 (Suppl): 18SA, 19SA, 92SA, 2002.
4. Kudsk K, Tolley E, DeWitt C, et al. Preoperative albumin and surgical site identify surgical risk for major postoperative complications. *JPEN* 27: 1–9, 2003.
5. Kudsk KA, Croce MA, Fabian TC, et al. Enteral versus parenteral feeding: effects on septic morbidity after blunt and penetrating abdominal trauma. *Ann. Surg.* 215: 503–511, 1992.
6. Christensen ML, Hancock ML, Gattuso J, et al. Parenteral nutrition associated with increased infection rate in children with cancer. *Cancer* 72: 2732–2738, 1993.
7. Moore FA, Feliciano DV, Andrassy RJ, et al. Early enteral feeding, compared with parenteral, reduces postoperatie septic complications: the results of a meta-analysis. *Ann. Surg.* 216: 172–183, 1992.
8. Heyland DK, MacDonald S, Keefe L, et al. Total parenteral nutrition in the critically ill patient: a metaanalysis. *JAMA* 280: 2013–2019, 1998.
9. Marik PE, Zaloga GP. Early enteral nutrition in acutely ill patients: a systemic review. *Crit. Care Med.* 29: 2264–2270, 2001.
10. Braga M, Gianotti L, Gentilini O, et al. Early postoperative enteral nutrition improves gut oxygenation and reduces costs compared to total parenteral nutrition. *Crit. Care Med.* 29: 242–248, 2001.
11. Border JR, Hassett J, LaDuca J, et al. The gut origin septic state in blunt multiple trauma (ISS = 40) in the ICU. *Ann. Surg.* 206: 427–448, 1987.
12. Buzby, GP, et al. Perioperative total parenteral nutrition in surgical patients, *NEJM* 325: 525, 1991.
13. Lewis SJ, Egger M, Sylvester PA, et al. Early enteral feeding versus "nil per os" after gastrointestinal surgery: systemic review and meta-analysis of controlled trials. *Br. Med. J.* 323: 773–776, 2001.
14. Berger M, Gryllaki M, Weisel PH, et al. Intestinal absorption in patients after cardiac surgery. *Crit. Care Med.* 28: 2217–2223, 2000.
15. Li J, Kudsk K , Gocinski B, et al. Effects of parenteral and enteral nutrition on gut-associated lymphoid tissue. *J. Trauma* 39: 44–52, 1995.
16. Faries PL, Simon RJ, Martella AT, et al. Intestinal permeability correlates with severity of injury in trauma patients. *J. Trauma* 44: 1031, 1998.
17. Houdjuk APJ, Rijnsburger ER, Jansen J, et al. Glutamine-enriched enteral diet increases splanchnic blood flow in the rat. *Am. J. Physiol.* 267: G1035–G1040, 1994.
18. Buchman AL, Moukarzel AA, Bhuta S, et al. Parenteral nutrition is associated with intestinal morphologic and functional changes in humans. *JPEN* 19: 453–460, 1995.
19. Rombeau JL, Takala J. Summary of round table conference: gut dysfunction in critical illness. *Intens. Care Med.* 23: 476–479, 1997.
20. Brundin T, Branstrom R, Wahren J. Effects of oral vs IV glucose administration on splanchnic and extra splanchnic O_2 uptake and blood flow. *Am. J. Physiol.* 271: E496–E504, 1996.

21. Lipman TO. Grains vs veins: is enteral nutrition really better than parenteral nutrition? A look at the evidence. *JPEN* 22: 167–182, 1998.

22. Fessler TA. Appropriateness of adult parenteral nutrition use in a large hospital. *Nutr. Clin. Pract.* 16: 153–157, 2001.

23. Roberts MF, Levine GM. Nutrition support team recommendations can reduce hospital costs. *Nutr. Clin. Pract.* 7: 227–230, 1992.

24. Trujillo, EB, et al. Metabolic and monetary costs of avoidable parenteral nutrition use, *JPEN* 23: 109, 1999.

25. Trice S, Melnik G, Page C. Complications and costs of early postoperative parenteral versus enteral nutrition in trauma patients. *Nutr. Clin. Pract.* 12: 114–119, 1997.

26. Braga M, Gianotti L, Vignali A, et al. Artificial nutrition after major abdominal surgery: impact of route of administration and composition of the diet. *Crit. Care Med.* 26: 24–30, 1998.

27. Braunschweig C, Gomez S, Sheenn PM. Impact of declines in nutritional status on adult patients hospitalized for more than 7 days. *J. Am. Diet. Assoc.* 100: 1316–1322, 2000.

28. Gianotti L, Braga M, Frei A, et al. Health care resources consumed to treat postoperative infections: cost saving by perioperative immunonutrition. *Shock* 3: 325–330, 2000.

29. Laramee SH. Position of the American Dietetic Association: nutrition services in managed care. *J. Am. Diet. Assoc.* 96: 391–395, 1996.

30. Anderson CF, MacBurney MM. Application of ASPEN clinical guidelines: parenteral nutrition use at a university hospital and development of a practice guideline algorithm. *Nutr. Clin. Pract.* 11: 53–58, 1996.

31. Maurer J, Weinbaum F, Turner J, et al. Reducing the inappropriate use of parenteral nutrition in an acute care teaching hospital. *JPEN* 20: 272–274, 1996.

32. Faubion WC, Wesley JR, Khalidi N. TPN catheter sepsis: impact of the team approach. *JPEN* 10: 642–645, 1986.

33. Hassel JT, Games AD, Shaffer B, Harkins LE. Nutrition support team management of enterally fed patients in a community hospital is cost-beneficial. *J. Am. Diet. Assoc.* 94: 993–998, 1994.

34. Hedberg A, Lairson D, Aday L, et al. Economic implications of an early postoperative enteral feeding protocol. *J. Am. Diet. Assoc.* 99: 802–807, 1999.

35. McQuiggan M, Marvin R, McKinley B, Moore F. Enteral feeding following major torso trauma: from theory to practice. *New Horizons* 7: 131–146, 1999.

36. Cresci GA. Bedside placement of small bowel feeding tubes in hospitalized patients: a new role for the dietitian. *Nutrition* 19: 843–846, 2003.

37. Cresci GA. Enteral feeding protocol use decreases inappropriate TPN usage. *Nutrition* (submitted for publication) .

38. Schwartz D. Enhanced enteral and parenteral nutrition practice and outcomes in an intensive care unit with a hospital-wide performance improvement process. *J. Am. Diet. Assoc.* 96: 484–489, 1996.

39. Kirby DF. Decisions for enteral access in the intensive care unit. *Nutrition* 17: 776, 2001.

40. Szeluga DJ, Stuart RK, Brookmeyer R, et al. Nutritional support of bone marrow transplant recipients: a prospective, randomized clinical trial comparing total parenteral nutrition to an enteral feeding program. *Cancer Res.* 47: 3309, 1987.

41. Ott L. et al. Postpyloric enteral feeding costs for patients with severe head injury: blind placement, endoscopy, and PEG/J versus TPN. *J. Neurotrauma* 16: 233, 1999.

42. Graves N. Economic and preventing hospital acquired infection. *Emerging Infectious Dis.* 10: 561–568, 2004.

43. Martindale R., Cresci G. Preventing infectious complications with nutritional intervention. *JPEN* 29(1), 2005.

44. Waitzberg DL, Saito H, Plank LD, et al. Clinical effects of immunonutrition in elective surgery: a systematic review and meta-analysis of randomized controlled trials. Working paper, Department of Gastroenterology, University of Sao Paulo Medical School, Sao Paulo, Brazil, 2003.

45. Wallace W, Cinot M, Nastanski F, Gornick W, Wilson S. New epidemiology for postoperatic nosocomial infections. *Am. Surgeon* 66: 874–878, 2000.

46. Heyes SD, Walker LG, Smith I, et al. Enteral nutrition supplementation with key nutrients in patients with critical illness and cancer. *Ann. Surg.* 229, 467, 1999.

47. Mora RJF. Malnutrition: organ and functional consequences. *World. J. Surg.* 23: 530–535, 1999.

48. Hall JC, Heel K, McCauley R. Glutamine. *Br. J. Surg.* 83: 305–312, 1996.
49. Cresci G. Targeting the use of specialized nutritional formulas in surgery and critical care. *JPEN* 29(1), 2005.
50. Beale RJ, Bryg DJ, Bihari DJ. Immunonutrition in the critically ill: a systematic review of clinical outcomes. *Crit. Care Med.* 27(12): 2799–2805, 1999.
51. Gianotti L, Braga M, Nespoli L, et al. A randomized controlled trial of preoperative oral supplementation with a specialized diet in patients with gastrointestinal cancer. *Gastroenterology* 122: 1763–1770, 2002.
52. Braga M, Gianotti L, Nespoli L, et al. Nutritional approach in malnourished surgical patients. *Arch. Surg.* 137: 174–180, 2002.
53. Strickland A, Brogan A, Krauss J, Martindale R, Cresci G. Is the use of specialized nutritional formulations a cost effective strategy? A national database evaluation. *JPEN* 29(1), 2005.

Index

A

Very low-density lipoprotein (VLDL), 54, 59
VIP, *see* Vasoactive intestinal peptide
Vitamin(s), 109
    drug–nutrient interactions involving, 348
    fat-soluble, 293
        absorption of, 110
        toxicity of, 111
    FDA requirements for parenteral, 315
    inflammatory response and, 111
    parenteral, 292
    requirements
        pediatric, 395
        transplant recipients, 465
    shortages, 292
    water-soluble, 293
        absorption of, 110
        toxicity from, 111
Vitamin C deficiency, 110
Vitamin E
    absorption, reduced, 121
    excess, 110
    oxidized, 118
VLDL, *see* Very low-density lipoprotein
VOD, *see* Veno-occlusive disease

W

Warfarin resistance, 351
Wasting
    AIDS, 173, 597
    cancer and, 173
    diseases, essential amino acids and, 35
    geriatric, 408
    rapid, 32

Water-soluble vitamins, 293
    absorption of, 110
    toxicity from, 111
Weight history, 73
Weir Equation, 556
Wernicke–Korsakoff syndrome, 315
Whey-to-casein ratio, 375, 384
Whole-body nitrogen balance, 35
Withdrawing of care, 627
Wound(s)
    classification, 436
    closure, gradual, 436
    healing, *see also* Burns and wound healing
        arginine and, 438
        delayed, 438
        effects of pharmacologic agents on, 448
        enteral feeding and, 214
        poor, 155, 389
    infection, 663
    sources of, 435

Y

Yeast RNA, 182
Y-port, 237

Z

Zinc
    deficiency
        infant, 378
        prolonged labor and, 362
    requirements, 293